Eat for
EXTRAORDINARY
Health
&HEALING

Eat *for* EXTRAORDINARY Health &HEALING

THE EDITORS OF
RODALE BOOKS

RODALE

© 2016 by Rodale Inc.

Printed in the United States of America

Rodale Inc. makes every effort to use acid-free ♾, recycled paper ♻.

Book design by Joanna Williams

Library of Congress Cataloging-in-Publication Data is on file with the publisher.

ISBN 978-1-62336-719-0 direct mail hardcover

4 6 8 10 9 7 5   direct mail hardcover

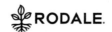

We inspire health, healing, happiness, and love in the world.
Starting with you.

contents

Foods

Beans and Legumes 2

Black Beans 2
Lentils 3
Mung Beans 4
Red Beans 4
Split Peas 6
White Beans 6

Beverages 8

Coffee 8
Kefir 9
Milk (Plant-Based) 12
Tea 13
Water 16
Wine 17

Dairy Products 20

Eggs 20
Milk (Dairy) 21
Yogurt 23

Fruits 25

Apples 25
Aronia Berries (Chokeberries) 27
Avocados 28
Blueberries 30
Cherries 32
Citrus Fruits 34
Cranberries 36
Cucumbers 38

Gac Fruit 38
Grapes 39
Papayas 42
Pineapples 43
Pomegranates 44
Raspberries 46
Strawberries 47
Tomatoes 48
Watermelon 49

Herbs and Spices 51

Basil, Holy Basil 51
Black Pepper 52
Capers 53
Cilantro/Coriander 54
Fenugreek 55
Garlic 56
Ginger 58
Ginseng 60
Licorice 62
Oregano 63
Parsley 65
Rosemary 66
Sage 67
Thyme 68
Turmeric 69

Nuts 72

Almonds 72
Brazil Nuts 73
Peanuts 73

Pecans 74
Pistachios 75
Walnuts 76

Oils **78**

Extra-Virgin Olive Oil (EVOO) 78
Flaxseed Oil 81
Red Palm Oil 81
Virgin Coconut Oil (VCO) 84

Seafood and Fish **86**

Oysters 86
Salmon 87
Sardines 89
Tuna 90

Seeds **92**

Chia Seeds 92
Flaxseeds 93
Pumpkin Seeds 94
Sesame Seeds 95
Sunflower Seeds 96

Sweets **98**

Chocolate 98
Honey 100

Vegetables **103**

Artichokes 103
Asparagus 105
Beets/Beetroot Juice 108
Broccoli 110
Brussels Sprouts 112
Cabbage 112
Carrots 115
Cauliflower 116
Fennel 118
Greens 119
Mushrooms 123
Onions 125
Peppers, Bell 127
Peppers, Chile (Hot Peppers) 128
Sauerkraut 130
Sea Vegetables and Seaweeds 131
Soy Products 133
Sweet Potatoes 136

Whole Grains **139**

Barley 139
Buckwheat 140
Oats 142
Quinoa 144
Sorghum 145

Conditions

Acid Reflux **148**

Acne **151**

Adrenal Exhaustion/Adrenal Fatigue **153**

Allergic Rhinitis (Hay Fever) **156**

Alzheimer's Disease **160**

Anxiety **165**

Arthritis and Joint Pain **171**

Asthma **174**

Attention Deficit Hyperactivity Disorder
   (ADHD) **176**

Back Pain **180**

Bladder Infections/Urinary Tract Infections
   183

Bronchitis **186**

Bruises **188**

Burns **189**

Bursitis **192**

Cancer 196

Cold Sores 212

Colds 214

Constipation 218

Coughs 220

Dandruff 222

Decreased Libido 224

Dementia 226

Depression 232

Diabetes 238

Diarrhea 245

Diverticulitis 248

Dry Eyes 250

Dry Mouth 252

Dry Skin 254

Earache 257

Eczema 259

Erection Problems, Erectile Dysfunction 263

Fatigue 266

Fibrocystic Breasts 270

Fibromyalgia 272

Flatulence 276

Food Allergies 278

Fungal Infections (General, Yeast Infections, Candidiasis) 281

Fungal Infections (Nails) 284

Gallstones 287

Gastritis 290

Gingivitis 293

Glaucoma 297

Gout 300

Hair Loss 304

Halitosis 307

Headaches/Migraines 309

Heart Disease (Cardiovascular Disease) 313

Heartburn 322

Hemorrhoids 325

High Blood Pressure (Hypertension) 327

High Cholesterol 334

Hives 339

Hyperhidrosis (Excessive Sweating) 341

Hypoglycemia 343

Indigestion 345

Infertility 348

Influenza 352

Insect/Spider Bites and Stings 354

Insomnia 357

Irritable Bowel Syndrome 360

Kidney Stones 364

Lightheadedness 368

Lupus 370

Macular Degeneration 374

Memory Loss (Short Term) 377

Menopause 381

Menstrual Cramps (Dysmenorrhea) 384

Motion Sickness 386

Muscle Cramps 388

Nausea 390

Osteoporosis **392**

Overweight and Obesity **396**

PMS (Premenstrual Syndrome) **404**

Pneumonia **407**

Psoriasis **410**

Shingles **413**

Sinusitis **415**

Sore Throat **417**

Stress **419**

Stroke **423**

Sunburn **427**

Thyroid Disease **429**

Tinnitus **432**

Tooth Decay **435**

Ulcers (Peptic) **439**

Vaginitis **442**

Varicose Veins **444**

Vertigo **446**

Warts (Common) **448**

Wounds **450**

Wrinkles **454**

Extraordinary People, Extraordinary Healing   **458**

Endnotes   **463**

Index   **504**

foods

Let food be thy medicine and medicine be thy food.
—Hippocrates

Since ancient times, the healing powers of whole, nutritious foods have been regarded as the most powerful medicine. Here you'll find 90 of the best foods for ultimate health and healing, complete with lists of the nutrients, vitamins, and benefits they provide, all backed by the latest research. Read on to learn more about these timeless remedies.

beans and legumes

black beans

Black beans are rich in protein, folate, fiber, and iron, and they're a good source of magnesium, phosphorus, manganese, and thiamin. Black beans contain higher amounts of bioactive components, such as saponins and flavonoids, than most other types of beans. Saponins have been shown to induce cell death in several types of cancer and to inhibit cancer cell proliferation, especially when combined with flavonoids. Flavonoid-rich black bean extracts have been shown to inhibit the growth of colon, breast, liver, and prostate cancer cells via apoptosis (cell death), while leaving normal cells intact.[1] And despite their reputation as a top cause of flatulence, beans play a key role in supporting gastrointestinal health because of their high fiber content. Eating a high-fiber diet prevents constipation, and it has been shown to decrease your risk of colorectal cancer. Further, as fiber leaves you feeling full, beans can play a valuable role in weight management and overall health.

In one study, 12 subjects with metabolic syndrome consumed one of three meals on three different occasions: a meal with black beans, a meal with no beans but matched fiber content (FM), or a meal with no beans but matched antioxidant capacity (AM). The mean 5-hour insulin response after the black bean meal was 10 percent lower than after the FM meal and a whopping 34 percent lower than after the AM meal.[2]

As black bean extracts have previously been shown to reduce glycemia and food intake in both human and animal studies, researchers compared the effect of 100 milligrams of black bean extract to a placebo on several metabolic markers in 12 volunteers. Three hours after meal consumption, black bean extract reduced postprandial glucose, insulin, and C-peptide excursions; suppressed ghrelin secretion; and enhanced satiety, curbing the desire to eat.[3]

Legumes of all types—beans, chickpeas, lentils, and peas—have been found to lower LDL ("bad") cholesterol.[4] Black beans are low in sodium (though be cautious of added sodium in canned beans), low in fat, sugar free, cholesterol free, high in fiber, and high in flavonoids. They also have good levels of magnesium, which controls blood pressure, so they provide excellent cardioprotective benefits.

lentils

Yellow, black, red, orange, green, brown, spotted . . . the array of lentils can be overwhelming. But you really can't miss when it comes to the nutritive value of these tiny disc-shaped powerhouses. The pulses—the dried seeds of legume plants—we know as lentils grow all over the world and have been eaten for thousands of years, and for good reason. Lentils are high in protein, fiber, manganese, and folate, and they're good sources of iron, potassium, phosphorous, copper, and thiamin, as well. With their high protein content—not to mention the added benefits of having zero fat, cholesterol, or sodium—lentils make an excellent meat substitute, and they're an important part of the heart-healthy Mediterranean diet. Unlike dried beans, lentils do not require soaking before cooking, so prep time is minimal. Here's a look at what some of the

latest research studies have found out about this versatile, time-honored culinary classic.

The phenolic compounds in lentils have been shown to have an antioxidant effect and to inhibit alpha-glucosidase and pancreatic lipase, two enzymes associated with glucose and lipid digestion, suggesting that lentils have the potential to help control weight and blood glucose levels.[5]

A recent randomized, crossover trial of overweight diabetic patients found that replacing two servings of red meat 3 days a week with non-soy legumes such as lentils, chickpeas, beans, and peas resulted in a reduction in high-sensitivity C-reactive protein, interleukin-6, and tumor necrosis factor alpha—all markers of inflammation. The study period lasted 8 weeks, and the decrease in inflammation occurred regardless of weight loss.[6]

A similar study conducted by many

power pairs
lentils and lemon

Let's iron out the facts: If you're at risk for iron deficiency, like most premenopausal women are, consider adding some lemon juice to your lentils or beans. Eating these iron-rich foods with foods high in ascorbic acid and carotenoids, like lemon, considerably increases the amount of iron absorbed.[7]

of the same researchers found that replacing two servings of red meat 3 days a week with non-soy legumes such as lentils, chickpeas, beans, and peas also resulted in improved lipid profiles and glycemic control among diabetes patients. More specifically, the legume-based diet significantly decreased fasting blood glucose, fasting insulin, triglyceride concentrations, and LDL cholesterol.[8]

mung beans

These small, green legumes are related to peas and lentils. Like many beans, mung beans are rich in fiber, folate, and protein, and they're also a good source of vitamin K, magnesium, manganese, and phosphorous. They're also easily digestible, have a low glycemic index, and cook more quickly than most other beans. Mung beans are an extremely versatile food, used in both sweet and savory dishes. They can be eaten whole, added to stews and soups, ground into mung bean paste or a hummuslike dip, or used as an ingredient in dishes as diverse as beverages, pancakes, noodles, and pastries. Mung bean extract is used in cosmetic and health products, and mung beans are germinated to make sprouts—a use that's becoming increasingly popular in the United States. One cup of raw, sprouted mung beans contains about 30 calories and nearly 8 grams (g) of protein.[9] A cup of cooked mung beans contains 212 calories and more than 49 g of protein.[10]

Mung bean extract has shown potent antiviral capabilities. One study compared the effect of mung bean extract to two common antiviral medications, ribavirin and acyclovir, on the respiratory syncytial virus (RSV) and the herpes simplex virus 1 (HSV-1). Mung bean extract showed significant direct antiviral action against both viruses and provided some measure of prophylactic protection, as well. These findings point the way toward safe, inexpensive alternatives to conventional antiviral drugs.[11]

Mung bean sprouts have been shown to have high antioxidant activity and excellent anti-oxygenic properties, making them effective ingredients in anti-aging products.[12]

Mung bean extract has demonstrated cytotoxic (cell-killing) effects against hepatocellular carcinoma, a common liver cancer, and cervical cancer, the second-most-frequent cancer occurring in women worldwide.[13]

red beans

There are actually several types of red beans: the common red kidney bean (which comes in light, dark, and speckled varieties); the smaller, rounder red bean that resembles the pinto bean; and the adzuki (or azuki) bean, which is native to Asia and is famously used in sweet red bean paste and red bean ice cream. All of these beans are legumes, and they're all high in fiber, contain no cholesterol, and provide an excellent vegetarian source of protein. In addition to a high total antioxidant capacity, they exhibit further surprising health benefits.[14]

Red bean extract has been shown to exert strong antioxidant and anti-inflammatory effects.[15]

A hemagglutinin (a compound that causes red blood cells to aggregate) made from northern red beans was found to exert immunostimulatory effects and antiproliferative activity against breast, liver, and nasopharyngeal (upper throat behind the nose) cancer cells.[16]

High-fiber, low-GI (glycemic index)

beans by the book

GO FOR THE FIBER. While virtually all dried beans are good sources of fiber, some varieties stand out from the pack. Black beans, for example, contain 6 grams of fiber in a half-cup serving. Chickpeas, kidney beans, and lima beans all weigh in at about 7 grams of fiber, and black-eyed peas are among the best, with about 8 grams of fiber.

ENJOY THEM CANNED. In general, the dry beans that you cook for yourself have a slight edge over canned beans in terms of retaining nutrients, says Joe Hughes, PhD, assistant professor in the nutrition and food sciences program at California State University in San Bernardino, whose research is centered on beans. However, the average American these days just doesn't have the time needed to cook dry beans. If you only have time for canned beans, then by all means eat canned beans, he says. However, canned beans may be higher in sodium, so if that's a concern, drain and rinse canned beans before using them.

USE GAS-DEFLATING SPICES. Has the fear of uncomfortable and embarrassing gas kept you from reaping beans' nutritional benefits? Try spicing them with a pinch of summer savory or a teaspoon of ground ginger. According to some university studies, these spices may help reduce beans' gas-producing effects.

READ THE LABEL. Some canned refried beans contain a lot of fat, and some contain little to none, says Dr. Hughes. Be sure to pick a kind that's low in fat—it will still taste great.

GO DARK. Buy darker beans for more disease protection. In general, the darker the beans, the more powerful the antioxidants they contain, says Dr. Hughes.

foods such as red beans have been shown to reduce LDL cholesterol, control the postprandial glucose response, and decrease oxidative stress—thus positively influencing some of the top cardiovascular risk factors. Dietary patterns that include low-GI and low glycemic-load foods such as beans are associated with a lower risk of cardiovascular disease (CVD), even after adjusting for other CVD risk factors.[17]

split peas

Split peas are green or yellow, they cook more quickly than whole peas, and, unlike many other legumes, they don't require soaking. Split peas are high in protein, folate, and fiber, and they're a good source of potassium, manganese, and thiamin. One cup of cooked split peas contains 16 g of protein and a whopping 65 percent of your recommended daily value of fiber.[18] With their high fiber content, low fat content, and low glycemic index score, split peas are an ideal weight-loss food that will keep you feeling full longer. Their health benefits should not be overlooked.

The protein in yellow peas has been shown to suppress appetite—thus decreasing further food intake—and regulate glycemic response.[19]

A 28-day study that compared the effects of flours made from whole yellow peas, fractionated yellow peas, and whole wheat found that consuming whole or fractionated flour equivalent to ½ cup of peas a day reduced insulin resistance in overweight subjects. Further, whole pea flour reduced central adiposity (belly fat) in women.[20]

There is some evidence that, when exposed to water, yellow and green pea protein yields bioactive peptides including angiotensin I–converting enzyme inhibitors, which help relax blood vessels and control blood pressure.[21]

Split peas contain a variety of polyphenolic compounds that have antioxidant and anticarcinogenic activity, saponins that may exhibit cholesterol-lowering effects, and galacto-oligosaccharides, which may exert beneficial prebiotic effects in your large intestine.[22] Prebiotics are indigestible fiber compounds that stimulate the growth of healthy bacteria.

white beans

"White beans" can refer to any type of bean that's white or creamy in color; examples include cannellini (sometimes referred to as white kidney beans), navy, and great northern beans. Cannellini beans, native to Italy, are the largest of the three and retain their shape when cooked, so they're a great choice for salads or other dishes in which beans are

**super-
charge
your
meals**

More and more research is showing just how important beans are for your diet. To start getting more of these small fiber-filled nuggets into your meals, add them to dishes that can use some extra creaminess. For example, to make your berry smoothie a little creamier throw some cannellini beans into the blender.

kept whole. Navy beans break down easily, so they're great choices for soups and stews; they're also typically used in baked bean recipes. Great northern beans, like cannellini beans, hold their shape well, and they have a slightly nuttier flavor than the rest. In a pinch, you can safely use any of these types in recipes that call for white beans, and they all have a high level of fiber, protein, manganese, and folate. White beans are also a good source of thiamin, iron, magnesium, phosphorus, and copper. They're an excellent vegetarian source of iron, as they provide more bioavailable iron than red or other colored beans.[23] Here are some other interesting reasons to eat white beans.

Many foods tend to lose some of their nutrient content during the cooking process, but a recent study found that heat actually increases the antioxidant activity of white beans. Gallic acid and chlorogenic acid in particular, both of which have powerful antioxidant effects, were present in high quantities.[24]

White beans produce an alpha-amylase inhibitor, which slows the absorption of carbohydrates and starches by inhibiting enzymes responsible for their digestion, thus reducing the glycemic index of foods and prolonging your sense of satiety.[25] Low-glycemic diets are effective at preventing type 2 diabetes and obesity, and one study observed that a 10 percent drop in the GI of a diet results in a 30 percent increase in insulin sensitivity.[26]

beverages

coffee

The news for coffee lovers could hardly be any better: A large observational study in the journal *Circulation* found that drinking coffee was associated with a lower risk of death. Researchers examined the associations between consumption of total, caffeinated, and decaffeinated coffee with risk of total and cause-specific mortality among 74,890 women in the Nurses' Health Study (NHS), 93,054 women in the Nurses' Health Study 2, and 40,557 men in the Health Professionals Follow-Up Study. They found that, compared to nondrinkers, drinking 1 to 5 cups a day was associated with a lower risk of mortality generally. Significant inverse associations were also observed between coffee consumption and deaths due to cardiovascular disease, neurological diseases, and suicide. The protective effects were more pronounced among people who'd never smoked. (And if you're wondering, researchers found no association between risk of mortality and drinking more than 5 cups a day.)[1] One word of caution: All the research you'll read here concerns coffee and coffee alone. In other words, you won't be doing yourself any favors by adding heaps of sugar and cream to your daily joe.

If protection against death by any cause isn't enough for you, take a look at the surprising array of health benefits provided by America's favorite pick-me-up, which is brimming with free-radical-scavenging antioxidants and polyphenols.

Coffee is amazingly protective against liver cancer. A recent study found that women who drank 2.5 or more cups of coffee per day and men who drank 3.5 or more were 72 percent less likely to develop liver cancer than those who drank less than ⅓ cup a day.[2]

Several studies have shown that coffee has a protective effect against type 2 diabetes (T2D). In one of the largest studies, researchers examined data from more than 1.1 million people and found that coffee consumption was inversely related to the risk of T2D in a dose-dependent manner: The more coffee consumed, the less likely you are to develop T2D. At 6 cups a day, the risk of T2D was 33 percent lower. The effect was present for both caffeinated and decaf coffee.[3]

Researchers have discovered an

inverse relationship between caffeinated coffee and suicide. Based on data from more than 208,000 people, researchers found that compared with those who don't drink coffee, the risk of suicide was 45 percent lower for those who drank 2 to 3 cups of coffee a day and 53 percent lower for those who drank 4 or more cups a day.[4]

A 10-year study of 50,000 women found that those who drank 2 to 3 cups of caffeinated coffee a day were 15 percent less likely to have depression than women who drank little coffee. Women who drank 4 or more cups a day had a 20 percent lower risk of depression.[5]

Caffeinated coffee has been associated with a decreased risk of melanoma, breast cancer, uterine cancer, and colon cancer.[6] Decaf and regular coffee appear to have a protective effect against lethal prostate cancer.[7]

A metastudy based on data from nearly 1,280,000 participants found that moderate coffee consumption was inversely significantly associated with the risk of cardiovascular disease (CVD). Three to five cups per day was the optimal "dose" for the lowest CVD risk, though heavy coffee consumption did not cause increased CVD risk.[8]

There's even evidence that coffee protects against age spots caused by sun damage.[9]

It also seems to decrease oxidative DNA damage, which helps prevent cancer.[10]

kefir

Kefir is a fermented, probiotic-rich beverage that has been steadily gaining popularity in the United States because of its potent health benefits. The word *kefir* is Russian in origin, meaning "pleasure drink" because of its ability to promote health and good mood.[11] Kefir is usually made with milk, though there is also a water version. Because the milk version is far more popular and easy to

(continued on page 12)

Q. What's the number one nutrient you feel people are lacking, and what are the best ways for them to include it in their diets?

A. Omega-3 fats. Data show it's one of the most important components of diets in those who live the longest, healthiest lives. Further, a recent Harvard study showed that low omega-3s may be responsible for up to 96,000 deaths per year!

Q. What food combinations do you recommend for overall health?

A. I'd say aim to eat protein, fiber, and/or fat with every single meal and snack. That may mean an apple and nut butter, Greek yogurt and berries, nuts, or salmon and veggies. There are a lot of mix-and-match options, but combining these nutrients provides your body with what it needs throughout the day and slows absorption so that you have long-lasting energy.

Q. Have you had a client heal him- or herself with food?

A. My mother has genetically high triglycerides. Normal levels should be under 150, and when she was pregnant with me, hers peaked at 5,000. For most of her adult life they were around the 600 to 800 mark, until she added one thing to her diet—more omega-3 fats. She's always been otherwise healthy, but since she began to include omega-3 fats, she has lowered her levels to just over 200.

Q. Do you recommend sneaking healthy foods into diets? If so, how?

A. Yes! Make foods fun. With two little kids, I'm always looking for (and finding) lots of ways I can add unique foods to their diet. The other day, I built up breakfast as "super-exciting" and with "magic energy." I made black wild rice with coconut cream, toasted pecans, mango, and banana. With that excitement, our 4- and 6-year-olds came running down the stairs and gobbled up all that healthy fiber, good-for-you-fat, and protein.

Q. What are your food recommendations for weight loss?

A. At every meal, at least half of your plate should be vegetables.

Q. What are the top 5 to 10 foods everyone should be eating?

A. I recommend wild salmon; nuts; berries; dark, leafy greens; wild sardines; oatmeal; beans; beef; mushrooms; and cruciferous veggies, like Brussels sprouts and cauliflower.

Q. If we were to go to the grocery store with you, what would we always find in your shopping cart?

A. That's easy—veggies, fruit, cottage cheese, almond milk, cow's milk, cheese, eggs, coffee, crackers, pasta, bread flour (to make our pizza dough), and San Marzano tomatoes for our sauce.

Q. What's your favorite indulgence?

A. Friday night at the Mohr house is pizza Friday. We start making the dough the night before, or sometimes after the girls get home from school we open a bottle of wine (not for the girls) and go to town. The pizza might just be cheese or it could have any variety of toppings we think sound appealing.

Q. What do you select when you eat out at different restaurants or eateries?

A. At Italian restaurants, I choose either lasagna, Zuppa de Pesce (a thick fish soup), or pasta and sausage. If I'm eating at a Mexican eatery, you'll find guacamole and chips with steak fajitas on my plate. And I choose coconut bowls or pad Thai with chicken at Thai restaurants.

Q. Are there any natural home remedies you use?

A. I mince a clove of raw garlic, let it sit for a bit, and mix it with applesauce to mask that lovely flavor. I'll eat this a couple of times each day if I feel like I'm getting a cold. Either it makes me healthier or no one comes around.

Q. What's your favorite grab-and-go snack?

A. Nuts. They're portable, they taste great, and they're great for you.

find commercially, we'll be discussing the milk kefir here. Cow, goat, or sheep milk can be used to make kefir. It's now readily available in most grocery stores and comes in a variety of flavors, though it's quite easy (and economical) to make at home with a starter kit or with certified live kefir grains. On its own, kefir has a slightly sour taste, but you can add flavor to it if you wish or use it in smoothies, shakes, or ice cream. Some people have even substituted kefir when a recipe calls for regular dairy or coconut milk; just keep in mind that heating kefir will kill off most, if not all, of its healthy bacteria. Many people who are lactose intolerant are able to tolerate kefir, as there is very little lactose left over after the fermentation process. Though the vitamin content of kefir is influenced by the type of milk that's used, as well as by the particular probiotic strains it contains, it generally contains calcium, magnesium, phosphorous, vitamin A, vitamin D, and, in lesser amounts, vitamins C, K, B_1, B_2, and B_5. Kefir has been used in a variety of therapeutic roles, including as an antimicrobial, an anti-inflammatory, for the treatment of peptic ulcers, as an anticarcinogen, to support and enhance the immune system, and to lower cholesterol.[12]

A preliminary study on the effect of kefir on performance and recovery during endurance training found that athletes who consumed kefir improved their times in a 1.5-mile run and had lower C-reactive protein levels (a marker of inflammation).[13]

A study of kefir consumption in 40 patients with osteoporosis found significant improvement in a number of markers of bone health after 6 months. Parathyroid hormone, which promotes bone remodeling, increased significantly in the kefir group but declined in the control group, and the kefir group experienced significant improvement in hip bone mineral density.[14]

In vitro studies have shown that kefir has chemopreventive (cancer-preventing) effects against breast cancer, colorectal cancer, gastric cancer, leukemia, and melanoma. Preliminary animal studies have shown that kefir can inhibit tumor growth and actually diminish tumor size in sarcomas and breast cancer.[15]

milk (dairy)

See: Dairy Products (page 20)

milk (plant-based)

Those who are lactose intolerant, have a milk allergy, follow a vegan lifestyle, or simply don't like the taste of dairy milk have plenty of delicious and nutritious options with the variety of plant-based milks that are now available, including almond, hemp, oat, flax, spelt, soy, rice, coconut, cashew, and hazelnut milk. Plant milks are low in sodium, don't have the saturated fat that dairy milk does, and are cholesterol-free (or contain only trace amounts). Soy milk is perhaps the most popular variety of plant-based milk and is certainly the most well researched, due in part to its abundance of isoflavones, which have known anticancer and antiestrogenic properties. Soy milk is typically also the closest to dairy milk in terms of macronutrient content, with comparable protein and sometimes even more calcium than dairy milk. When choosing a plant-based milk, look for milks that have been fortified with calcium, vitamin D, and vitamin A; some plant milks are also fortified with iron or vitamin B_{12}, two nutrients that can be difficult to obtain from nonanimal sources. Many dieticians also particularly recommend soy milks that are organic and made with non-GMO ingredients so as to avoid exposure to toxic herbicides that are commonly used with conventionally raised soy. Consider these additional benefits.

In a study of patients with type 2 diabetes and kidney disease, those who consumed soy milk for 4 weeks experienced a significant reduction in systolic blood pressure compared to those who drank cow's milk.[16]

Soy foods, including soy milk, with their high levels of isoflavones, are associated with a reduced risk of ovarian cancer.[17]

Soy protein lowers LDL ("bad") cholesterol, and soy isoflavones improve endothelial function and may slow the progression of subclinical atherosclerosis.[18]

In a study of 9,514 breast cancer survivors over an average follow-up time of 7.4 years, researchers found that soy isoflavone consumption was inversely related with tumor recurrence.[19]

tea

We'll just come right out and say it: Tea is one of the healthiest beverages on the planet. In fact, after you take a look at the research, you may come to the conclusion that it's *the* healthiest beverage. A zero-calorie drink that's been consumed for millennia, there are hundreds of varieties of tea to choose from, and if you're new to tea it can be overwhelming. So before we get to the science, here are a few basics.

Every true (meaning nonherbal) tea is brewed from the dried leaves of the *Camellia sinensis* bush—it's how the leaves are processed that determines what type of tea is made. Green tea, for instance, is made from the unoxidized leaves of *C. sinensis*. White tea is the least processed: It's made from the hand-plucked, unopened buds of *C. sinensis*. Oolong tea is partially oxidized and goes through a complex production process. Black tea is fully oxidized and has the strongest flavor. Pu-erh tea is a black tea that's fermented and then aged. Newcomer purple tea, exclusive to Kenya, was specifically developed as a medicinal tea and has very high levels of antioxidants. Herbal teas are distinguished from "true" teas in that they are made from roots, flowers, seeds, or leaves, and they do not contain caffeine. All of these production processes result in teas with an extraordinary range of flavors and polyphenolic contents. Among the polyphenols in tea are catechins, theaflavins, tannins, and flavonoids. The most potent catechin is a compound known as epigallocatechin gallate, or EGCG, and it's found in abundance in green tea.

Tea is so rich with health benefits and so much research has been conducted on it that entire books have been written on its healing potential. It's been credited with antioxidative, anti-inflammatory, antimicrobial, anti-carcinogenic, antihypertensive, neuro-protective, antiaging, antibacterial, antifungal, cholesterol-lowering, triglyceride-lowering, and metabolism-stimulating properties. Studies have found that tea's polyphenols play a preventive role against a staggering range of conditions, including cancer, diabetes, arthritis, cardiovascular disease (particularly atherosclerosis and coronary heart disease), stroke, obesity, neurodegenerative disorders, psychiatric disorders, and even genital warts.[20] The following is but a taste of the remarkable benefits of what many have called "the world's healthiest drink."

A meta-analysis of 10 trials with a total of 834 participants found that both green and black tea consumption can reduce systolic and diastolic blood pressure in hypertensive and prehypertensive individuals.[21]

A metastudy involving nearly 23,000 people found an inverse relationship between tea consumption and depression. For every 3 cups of tea consumed per day the risk of depression fell by 37 percent.[22]

A meta-analysis of 37,445 cases of diabetes among 545,517 people found that an increase of 2 cups of tea a day was associated with a 4.6 percent lower risk of type 2 diabetes.[23]

A study of the association between tea and physical function in adults over 55 found that tea consumption was positively associated with better balance, better gait, and improved scores in an assessment of instrumental and basic activities of daily living.[24]

A meta-analysis of nearly 195,000 people, 4,378 of whom had suffered a stroke, found that those who drank 3 or more cups of green or black tea per day had a 21 percent lower risk of stroke than those who drank less than 1 cup per day.[25]

A longitudinal study of 490 people over the age of 60 with normal cognitive function tracked subjects' consumption of green tea, black tea, and/or coffee over a period of almost 5 years. Researchers found that there was a lower incidence of mild cognitive impairment (MCI) and dementia among those who drank green tea. Compared to those who drank no green tea, those who drank green tea daily had a 68 percent decreased risk of MCI or dementia, and those who drank green tea one to six times per week had a 53 percent decreased risk. There was no association found between cognitive function and drinking black tea or coffee.[26]

Research suggests that catechins in both green and black tea can help prevent neurodegenerative disorders such as Alzheimer's disease, Parkinson's disease, and dementia in part by neutralizing free radicals and inflammation.[27] More recent research has found that, in addition to their antioxidant and anti-inflammatory effects, tea polyphenols can also directly interfere with aggregation of the alpha-synuclein protein involved in Parkinson's and modulate intracellular signaling pathways.[28] Epigallocatechin gallate (EGCG), a major component of green tea, can inhibit the production of amyloid beta fibrils (the main components of the amyloid plaques in those with Alzheimer's disease) and can even remodel already-existing amyloid beta fibrils into smaller aggregates that are nontoxic.[29]

Green tea extract provides effective protection against ultraviolet (UV) radiation, and in vitro studies have shown that EGCG can inhibit melanoma cell growth, migration, and invasion.[30]

--- power pairs ---

green tea and toast

Eating a starchy breakfast can lead to a midmorning energy crash. Start sipping 12 ounces of green tea as you munch on your morning toast—it's been shown to blunt the before-lunch blood-sugar dip we all know so well. And adding a squirt of lemon to your green tea increases your body's ability to absorb the tea's antioxidants.[31]

Tea polyphenols (including EGCG) and polysaccharides have been linked to the prevention of many other cancers, including lung, colon, esophagus, oral-digestive tract, bladder, stomach, small intestine, kidney, pancreas, skin, prostate, and breast.[32]

Green tea powder is an effective natural means to combat halitosis, as tea polyphenols have been shown to have antimicrobial and deodorant effects. In one study, green tea was as effective as toothpaste in reducing halitosis. Green tea has been associated with improved periodontal health, and because of its antimicrobial power, it has an anticavity effect.[33]

water

Water accounts for up to 75 percent of an adult's weight. We all know that staying sufficiently hydrated is essential for every system of your body, so it's easy to overlook water's healing effects or take them for granted. But water's influence on your health and wellness really can't be overestimated. Drinking water can help prevent kidney stones, kidney infections, urinary tract infections, dry mouth, dry eyes, dizziness and lightheadedness, fatigue, headaches, and constipation. It can also flush toxins from your body; lubricate your joints; keep your skin clear and

moisturized; maintain collagen; regulate body temperature; boost your mood; enhance physical performance; improve your focus; aid in weight loss by keeping you feeling full; and, obviously, prevent and treat dehydration. There is no firm consensus on how much water is recommended per day, in part because it varies by person. Factors such as weight, age, environmental conditions, exercise, and work demands, as well as pregnancy and lactation, all affect how much water you need. As a general reference point, adults under normal conditions should aim for between 2.5 and 3 liters of water per day. Pregnant and lactating women need more, as do athletes, those with physically demanding jobs, and those in hot climates or conditions. Remember that thirst is a reliable guide, and urine that is pale yellow indicates that you're sufficiently hydrated. In the case of water, more, not less, is better. Here's why.

Even mild dehydration—a body water loss of 1 to 2 percent—has been shown to impair cognitive abilities. Cognitive impairments stemming from dehydration include poor concentration, delayed reaction time, short-term memory problems, moodiness, and anxiety.[34]

Young men underwent voluntary exercise-induced mild dehydration (body water loss of 1 percent) and then completed a cognitive test and a mood states questionnaire. Researchers found that, compared to those who were sufficiently hydrated, the dehydrated volunteers made more errors and their working memory was adversely affected. Further, their tension or anxiety and fatigue increased while at rest, and fatigue was greater during exercise.[35]

Volunteers who were deprived of water for 24 hours experienced decreased alertness and increased sleepiness, fatigue, and confusion. When volunteers resumed drinking water, confusion subsided and alertness increased immediately.[36]

A study of 120 healthy young women who recorded all fluid and food intake for 5 consecutive days found that higher habitual water intake was associated with better moods. More specifically, those with the lowest water intake (about 1.5 liters a day) reported the highest Total Mood Disturbance scores and a higher incidence of depression. Those with the highest water intake (about 3.1 liters a day) had the lowest Total Mood Disturbance scores and also reported the least depression, tension, and confusion.[37]

Water plays a vital role in wound healing by hydrating epithelial cells so they can migrate and close a wound; acting as a solvent for minerals, vitamins, amino acids, glucose, and other molecules and enabling them to diffuse in and out of cells; and removing toxins from cells. Further, increased water intake may increase tissue oxygenation.[38]

Studies have shown that a urine output of at least 2.5 liters a day is protective against kidney stones. A recent meta-analysis confirmed that water is the best beverage to consume to prevent kidney stones. Increasing water intake can dilute urine concentration, decrease uric acid, remove salt, and reduce calcium oxide supersaturation.[39]

wine

Wine—and red wine in particular—has gained a lot of attention as a healing beverage because it's a staple of the heart-healthy Mediterranean diet and because it's rich in resveratrol, that polyphenolic compound that's made headlines for protecting cardiovascular health and (possibly) turning back the clock on aging. But though red wine has a higher total phenolic content, there's still an abundance of phenolic compounds in both red and white wine, many of which exert an antioxidant effect. Examples include catechins, flavonols, tannins, anthocyanins (red wine only), hydroxycinnamates, stilbenes (including resveratrol), and gallic acid and caffeic acid, which have shown strong free-radical-scavenging ability, just to name a few.

Though there are plenty of healthy compounds in wines of all types, there's also plenty of reason to use caution when partaking of this healing beverage. Regular consumption that surpasses a moderate level leads to myriad health problems, including cirrhosis, alcohol dependence, increased risk of certain cancers (such as breast, liver, colon, mouth, and esophagus), hypertension, increased susceptibility to infection, greater risk of mental health problems, and eventually, premature death. The World Health Organization has observed that the harmful use of alcohol is a causal factor in more than 200 diseases and injuries.[40] Moreover, as alcohol is a well-known intoxicant, over-consumption can lead to a range of negative behavioral and social consequences, some of them very serious or even lethal, such as accidents or injuries.

With such potential negative consequences, the obvious question is: What's a *healthy* amount to drink? Though alcohol can affect people differently, mostly because of differences in weight and gender, the most widely accepted definition of moderate, health-promoting alcohol consumption is up to one drink a day for women and up to two drinks a day for men. One standard drink equals 14 grams of pure alcohol, which is the amount found in a 5-ounce glass of wine (12 percent alcohol content).[41] Exceeding these recommendations can have negative health consequences. But there's plenty of reason to raise an occasional glass, as the latest research can attest.

A study of more than 5,500 adults found that drinking two to seven glasses of wine per week led to less depression. The researchers caution that drinking more than this may have the opposite effect and contribute to depression.[42]

Epidemiological studies have demonstrated a 20 to 40 percent lower cardiovascular disease incidence among drinkers of alcoholic beverages compared with nondrinkers. Drinking one to two drinks per day is a negative risk factor for atherosclerosis, myocardial infarction, and ischemic stroke.[43]

A study of 26,662 people ages 25 to 97 who were followed for an average of 12.5 years found that those who drank three or more units of liquor each week had a 53 percent higher risk of venous thromboembolism (VTE) compared to nondrinkers. On the other hand, those who drank three or more units of wine per week had a 22 percent reduced risk of VTE.[44] Why does wine provide more health benefits than liquor? Because it's chock-full of polyphenols that exert an antioxidant effect.[45]

A study of 2,900 women with an average age of 46 found that moderate wine consumers (one glass a day) had significantly lower levels of C-reactive protein (a marker of inflammation), fibrinogen, factor VII, and plasminogen activator inhibitor type 1 (all involved in clotting) than women who drank little or no wine. Researchers concluded that moderate wine consumption may protect against cardiovascular disease that occurs through inflammatory and clotting pathways.[46]

In a small (24 subjects) but fascinating study, researchers set out to determine the oxidative and inflammatory effects of red wine when paired with different types of meals. They had subjects consume two meals on opposite ends of the health spectrum: a McDonald's meal or a Mediterranean meal, with and without red wine. They found that values for oxidized LDL cholesterol significantly decreased after the Mediterranean meal, and adding red wine supersized, if you will, the protective effect. On the other hand, the consumption of the McDonald's meal increased the values of oxidized LDL, while pairing red wine with the McDonald's meal actually brought the values back toward baseline levels. Researchers also found that expression of oxidative stress genes and inflammation genes was positively altered after the Mediterranean meal, as well as with either meal paired with red wine, probably due to the additional antioxidant compounds.[47] While this study doesn't give you license to eat a Big Mac every day as long as you pair it with a nice Merlot, it *does* show the health-boosting power of red wine's antioxidants—even against a supersize serving of fat and calories.

A metareview revealed that regular and moderate wine consumption (one to two glasses per day) is associated with decreased incidence of cardiovascular disease, hypertension, diabetes, and certain cancers, such as colon, breast, lung, and prostate. Wine polyphenols are able to control cell apoptosis (cell death) in these cancers through the increase of reactive oxygen species (oxygen-containing cells) and the decrease of cell growth.[48]

dairy products

eggs

Once maligned for their high cholesterol content, eggs are making a comeback as a healthy food. Though technically not a dairy product (but sold in the dairy section), eggs are a great source of protein, riboflavin, selenium, choline, B vitamins, and vitamin D, a nutrient that can be challenging to get in sufficient quantities through your diet. And more recent research has indicated that the cholesterol obtained through food sources only accounts for about 20 percent of our blood cholesterol levels. The Scientific Report of the 2015 Dietary Guidelines Advisory Committee plainly states, "Cholesterol is not considered a nutrient of concern for overconsumption."[1] And it turns out that the cholesterol you do get from egg yolks may be far outweighed by the health benefits eggs provide. Consider.

A study that was just released found that eating whole cooked eggs along with carotenoid-rich foods enhances carotenoid absorption. In this study, volunteers ate a raw mixed salad of tomatoes, carrots, baby spinach, romaine lettuce, and goji berries with no eggs, one and one-half eggs, or three eggs. Those who ate the salad that was high in eggs had the highest absorption of carotenoids. Compared to the no-egg salad, the salad that was high in eggs resulted in a four- to fivefold increase in lutein and zeaxanthin and a three- to eightfold increase in alpha-carotene, beta-carotene, and lycopene.[2]

---

power pairs

eggs and salad

Your favorite breakfast food is also an "eggcellent" salad topper. Adding eggs to your greens enhances your absorption of carotenoids, including lutein, lycopene, and beta-carotene, which protect your eyes and can decrease your cancer risk and sharpen your memory. Make sure your egg includes the yolk, as that's where most of the benefits are to be found.[3]

- A study based on data from 2,332 middle-aged men found that eggs may actually help prevent type 2 diabetes (T2D). Over an average follow-up period of 19.3 years, researchers found that the men with the highest consumption of eggs had a 38 percent lower risk of T2D compared to men with the lowest egg consumption.[4]
- In an observational study of 382 adult patients undergoing coronary angiography, researchers found a significant association between eating more than one egg per week and a lower coronary atherosclerotic burden (less advanced coronary artery disease).[5]
- In a 12-week study that compared the effect of whole egg consumption (three per day) to a zero-fat, zero-cholesterol egg substitute in those with metabolic syndrome, all of the participants experienced improvements in dyslipidemia (cholesterol levels), waist circumference, weight, and body fat percentage. But the egg group also experienced reductions in the inflammatory markers tumor necrosis factor alpha and serum amyloid A.[6]

milk (dairy)

Dairy milk is any milk that comes from a mammal, but most often it refers to cow's milk, which is the convention we'll follow here. Cow's milk is not universally recommended, as many people are lactose intolerant or have a milk allergy—and beyond that, dairy products are known to be inflammatory. The other serious words of caution involve the high saturated fat content in whole-fat dairy products and dairy's hormone content: Increasing evidence indicates that some of the naturally occurring steroid hormones (such as estrogens and insulin-like growth factor 1) in dairy milk play a role in the development of breast, prostate, and endometrial cancer.[7] The latest version of the Harvard T. H. Chan School of Public Health's Healthy Eating Plate actually recommends limiting milk and dairy to one to two servings a day, as a high intake of dairy is associated with an increased risk of prostate cancer and possibly of ovarian cancer.[8]

Taking all of this into consideration, as dairy milk is a nutrient-dense food with demonstrable health benefits, we're including it in our list of healing foods. (If you'd rather eschew dairy entirely, there are plenty of health benefits to be gained from plant-based milks; see Beverages on page 8.) Milk is an excellent source of protein, phosphorous, calcium, riboflavin, and vitamin D (most commercial milks are fortified with vitamin D) and a good source of potassium, selenium, and vitamin B_{12}. Whole-fat milk contains 5 grams (g) of saturated fat per

sardines and cheddar cheese

Chowing down on a yummy, cheesy fish sandwich could just melt the fat right off your tummy. Studies show that when foods high in calcium and vitamin D are eaten together, your fat metabolism is stimulated,[9] especially around your abdomen. Sardines are ridiculously high in vitamin D, while Cheddar cheese is one of the best sources of calcium on the market—making this a powerhouse sandwich just waiting to be eaten.

---

cup (that's 23 percent of your recommended daily value) and 146 calories, so many people opt for low-fat or skim milk, which contains 0 g of saturated fat and 86 calories. And though per capita dairy milk consumption has been falling over the past 2 decades, milk continues to be an extremely popular beverage in the United States,[10] so let's look at some of the latest research on its health benefits.

- A study that followed 477,122 adults over 11 years found that milk consumption was inversely related to colorectal cancer risk. Both high-fat and low-fat dairy provided this protective benefit.[11]

- The abundant nutrients in milk—calcium, phosphorous, vitamin D, and protein—are known to support bone health. In addition, whey protein and milk basic protein promote bone formation, suppress bone resorption, and increase bone mineral density, making milk an effective dietary means with which to delay or prevent osteoporosis.[12]

- A metastudy based on 22 trials found an inverse association between dairy consumption and overall risk of cardiovascular disease and stroke. Low-fat dairy and cheese significantly reduced the risk of stroke and coronary heart disease.[13]

- Interestingly, a recent study of more than 15,000 adults found that full-fat dairy products and total dairy consumption were protective against metabolic syndrome—but no protective effect was found for low-fat dairy. Researchers concluded that the beneficial effects were mediated by the saturated fatty acids in dairy.[14]

See also: Kefir (page 9), Milk (Plant-Based) (page 12)

yogurt

Yogurt may be one of the most popular superfoods, in part because of the wide variety of products commercially available. With dozens of flavors and textures, there's a yogurt to suit everyone. Though yogurt experienced a surge in popularity in the United States beginning in the 1970s and another peak more recently, as Americans took to thick, Greek-style yogurt, some form of yogurt has been eaten for centuries. It's made from the bacterial fermentation of milk; at a minimum, yogurt will contain the bacterial cultures *Lactobacillus bulgaricus* and *Streptococcus thermophilus,* though some companies include additional strains. Most often it's made from cow's milk, but milk from goats, yaks, buffalo, camels, and other mammals is used around the world. Yogurt made from plant-milk sources (such as soy milk, rice milk, or almond milk) is now available, but because the fermentation process converts lactose to lactic acid, even those who are lactose intolerant can often consume yogurt without a problem. Yogurt is an excellent source of calcium, phosphorous, and riboflavin and a good source of protein, vitamin B_6, vitamin B_{12}, and potassium. But its main claim to fame as a superfood is based upon its probiotic content—those millions of "beneficial bacteria" that bring a plethora of health benefits.

There are hundreds of yogurt products available on store shelves, and some types certainly are healthier than others. To get the most health benefit, avoid any yogurt with artificial sweeteners or other artificial ingredients, and be wary of yogurts with added sugars, even if the product advertises itself as "all natural." Even those that have been sweetened with fruits and fruit juices can be packed with unwanted calories and sugar. To ensure that you're getting the full probiotic benefit, look for the National Yogurt Association's "Live & Active Cultures" seal, which indicates that the product contains at least 100 million live cultures per gram at the time of manufacture and that it has not undergone heat-treating, which kills off the probiotics you want.[15] (Companies

super-charge your meals

Chicken and tuna salads are healthy lunch options until we mix in heaping tablespoons of mayonnaise. To get the same amount of creaminess plus an extra helping of calcium, swap the same amount of plain Greek yogurt for mayonnaise. The added protein in the Greek yogurt will keep you fuller longer, also.

are required to say on the label if their yogurt has been heat-treated.)

- An assessment of long-term weight gain in nearly 121,000 volunteers over a period of 12 to 20 years found that there was an inverse association between higher yogurt consumption and weight gain: Those who ate more daily servings of yogurt gained nearly a pound less on average over a 4-year period.[16]

- Cross-sectional studies reveal that yogurt consumers tend to have a better body mass index (BMI), waist circumference, systolic blood pressure, fasting glucose level, triglyceride level, and HDL cholesterol level.[17] Similarly, a meta-analysis of the effect of probiotics on cardiovascular risk factors found that probiotics reduced total cholesterol, LDL ("bad") cholesterol, BMI, waist circumference, and inflammatory markers. The effect was strongest when the medium was yogurt or fermented milk, when consumption lasted for at least 8 weeks, and when there were multiple strains of probiotics present in the probiotic food.[18]

- Because it contains zinc, vitamin B_6, protein, and healthy probiotics, yogurt helps to enhance your immune system. Studies have shown that probiotics alone enhance innate immunity, the severity and duration of respiratory infections, and gut-associated immunity.[19]

- The results of two multiyear, large European studies conducted with nearly 366,000 subjects found that fermented dairy products, including yogurt, provide some protection against type 2 diabetes. When researchers examined dairy intake according to fat content, they found that people who consumed low-fat fermented dairy products had a lower risk of new-onset diabetes over 11 years compared to people who didn't consume these foods. Yogurt accounted for 87 percent of those low-fat fermented foods.[20]

- Recent research has established a clear connection between the gut microbiota and a variety of health conditions, including obesity, diabetes, schizophrenia, autism, anxiety, and depression. Though more research in human volunteers is needed, there is promising evidence that probiotics confer antidepressant and anti-anxiety effects.[21] In response to chronic stress, probiotics have been shown to decrease hypothalamic–pituitary–adrenal axis and autonomic nervous system activity.[22]

fruits

apples

Ranging from tart to sweet, pale yellow to bright green to rich burgundy, there are more than 7,500 varieties of apples. Full of fiber, vitamins C and E, polyphenols, and flavonoids, apples are a true superfood of health and healing. Research has indicated that consumption of apples and apple products is associated with a reduced risk of asthma, Alzheimer's disease, cardiovascular disease, colorectal cancer, lung cancer, prostate cancer, and type 2 diabetes. Apples have also been shown to positively affect lipid metabolism, weight management, vascular function, and inflammation, and to lower total cholesterol.[1] Along with capers, onions, tea, and wine, apples are one of the best dietary sources of the powerful dietary flavonoid quercetin, which boasts an incredible array of health benefits. Quercetin from apple consumption seems to be particularly protective against the development of lung cancer and colon cancer,[2] and it's been shown to induce cell death in colon cancer cells in vitro and to reduce tumor volume.[3] Apple oligosaccharides have likewise been shown to induce apoptosis (cell death) and cell cycle arrest in colon cancer cells.[4]

Though it's generally best to eat the whole form of a food, juices can be a convenient way to get fruit polyphenols into your diet when certain fruits are out of season. Evidence suggests that apple juice provides the most health benefits when it's 100 percent apple juice of the "nonclarified" variety—in other words, apple cider. Cloudy apple juice or apple cider is unfiltered and has a higher content of pectin and procyanidin, showing more antioxidant activity than the clear juice found in most store bottles. Apple juice has shown protective effects against colon cancer in in vitro studies,[5] but its more valuable role is in cancer *prevention,* as many chemotherapeutic agents lose their efficacy once cancer has progressed to an invasive stage.[6] The apple polysaccharides in cloudy apple juice have been shown to be effective in inducing colorectal cancer cell death.[7] Here are other benefits to keep in mind.

An Italian study of more than 6,000 people found that consuming one or more fresh, medium-size apples a day was associated with a reduced risk of cancer compared to eating less than one apple a day. More specifically, a reduced risk of the following cancers was observed (percent reduction in parentheses): oral cavity and pharynx (18 percent), esophagus (22 percent), colorectal (30 percent), larynx (41 percent), breast (24 percent), ovary (24 percent), and prostate (7 percent).[8]

Small studies have consistently shown that apples play a role in reducing oxidative stress,[9] and a large, multiyear study released in 2015 shines new light on the antioxidant effect of apples. Researchers examined the diets of 792 people with an average age of 69.5 to determine the relationship between diet and individual foods and biomarkers of systemic inflammation (C-reactive protein [CRP] and fibrinogen). They found that a lower CRP score was associated with a higher overall healthy dietary pattern score; a higher intake of fresh fruit, including flavonoid-rich apples and citrus fruits; as well as a combination of fruits and vegetables, dietary vitamin C, and flavanones. Fibrinogen levels were inversely associated with the Mediterranean diet, fruit intake, and combined fruit and vegetable intake.[10]

Apples and other flavonoid-rich foods have been associated with reduced asthma prevalence and severity, and drinking apple juice once a day

clean your fruit

Since the peel of fruits and vegetables is rich in fiber, it makes sense to eat this part of the produce rather than peeling it off and throwing it away. However, the peel may also harbor unhealthy dirt, bacteria, and other contaminants.

So before you sink your teeth into any fruit or veggie (even if you are going to peel it), you should clean it first. If the vegetable has outer leaves, such as lettuce, discard them. Wash firm fruits and vegetables under warm, clean running water. Rinse veggies that will go into salads with cool water, to preserve crispness. Don't bother with soap, detergent, or washes commercially marketed for produce, says the FDA. If the piece of produce is sturdy enough to handle a little scrubbing, clean it with a sanitary produce brush as well.

If you're eating more delicate fruit, like berries, pour them into a colander and hose them off with a kitchen sink sprayer. Jostle the colander from time to time to turn the berries so you can wash them all over.

has been shown to reduce wheezing in asthmatic children.[11]

Researchers found that a compound in apple skins and green tomatoes can prevent muscle atrophy and weakness. It works by turning off a protein called ATF4, which acts upon genes to trigger the normal muscle wasting associated with aging. What gives these fruits such power? Ursolic acid in apple peels and tomatidine compounds in green tomatoes. In the study, researchers found that mice who ate a diet containing both of these compounds for 2 months saw a 10 percent increase in muscle mass and a 30 percent increase in muscle strength. In effect, mice without the ATF4 protein were resistant to aging.[12]

aronia berries (chokeberries)

Aronia berries, also known as chokeberries, are known for their tart taste and their incredibly high antioxidant content. The main types are red and black; a third, lesser-known variety of purple chokeberries is a hybrid of the red and black varieties. Raw berries can be eaten directly off the bush, but they're also used in juices, wines, teas, jams, syrups, and many other products. Traditionally, black aronia berries were used by the Potawatomi Native Americans to treat colds,[13] and with their

many polyphenols—anthocyanins, proanthocyanidins, quercetin, chlorogenic acid, flavonoids, and hydroxycinnamic acids among them[14]—it's easy to see why. Their total polyphenolic content is among the highest measured for any plant, and their many health benefits stem in large part from their strong antioxidant activity. Research is still ongoing, but aronia berries have already been shown to exert antioxidative, anti-inflammatory, antimutagenic, anticancer, cardioprotective, hepatoprotective (protective against liver damage), gastroprotective, antidiabetic, antibacterial, antiviral, radioprotective (protective against radiation), immunomodulatory, vasorelaxant, and antithrombotic (protective against blood clots) properties.[15] Let's look at the results of a few studies on aronia berries.

Postmenopausal women with abdominal obesity consumed 100 milliliters (ml) of an aronia juice supplement along with their regular diets every day for 4 weeks. By the end of the study, volunteers had a significant decrease in body mass index (BMI), waist circumference, and systolic blood pressure; a higher level of omega-3s; and a better ratio of omega-6 to omega-3 fatty acids.[16]

In a study of 29 women ages 25 to 48 who drank 100 ml of aronia berry juice daily for 90 days, all subjects experienced a visible difference in subcutaneous skin tissue thickness, with an average reduction of nearly 2 millimeters. Translation? A reduction in cellulite! Furthermore, after 45 days approximately half of the women had a reduction in dermal edemas (swelling), and by the end of the study, *none* of the subjects had any signs of edema.[17]

Aronia has also been shown to lower blood pressure. Researchers studied the effect of aronia berry juice on 24-hour ambulatory blood pressure in hypertensive subjects. Twenty-three subjects ages 33 to 67 enrolled in the study, and they drank 200 ml of the juice daily for 4 weeks. At the end of the study, the average 24-hour and awake systolic and diastolic blood pressure were significantly decreased, and subjects experienced a reduction in triglyceride levels, total cholesterol, and LDL ("bad") cholesterol, as well.[18]

In an in vitro study, aronia berry extract exhibited an anti-inflammatory effect on human aortic endothelial cells by inhibiting cell adhesion molecules, a proinflammatory signaling pathway (NF-κB), and the production of reactive oxygen species.[19]

In volunteers with metabolic syndrome, 1 month of aronia berry extract supplementation significantly inhibited ADP-induced platelet aggregation, reduced the potential for clot formation and lysis (breakdown of cell membranes), and had a positive effect on lipid profiles.[20]

avocados

Avocados once got a bad rap because of their relatively high fat content, but approximately 70 percent of that fat is comprised of monounsaturated fats (MUFAs). Unlike saturated fats, which are found in foods like red meat, fried food, butter, and cheese, MUFAs can actually reduce LDL cholesterol and decrease inflammation. And despite their high fat content, studies have shown that people do *not* tend to gain weight after adding avocados to their diet. In fact, avocados are often recommended as an effective food for weight management, in part because of their

super-charge your meals

Avocados can supercharge any meal of the day, even dessert. Search recipes for brownies, cakes, and even puddings that slip avocado into the mix to get your dose of monounsaturated fats and chocolate all in one sitting.

avocados 101

For the avocado newbie, here are a couple of important buying and preparation tips.

HELP THEM RIPEN. Like bananas, avocados ripen better off the tree, so they are picked and sold unripe. Once you get them home, leave them on the counter for several days or until the fruit is slightly soft. Or, if you're in a hurry to use them, place them in a paper bag with an apple or banana to soften. Never place hard avocados in the refrigerator, or they will ripen too slowly.

MAKE A PIT STOP. To open an avocado, cut it lengthwise, rotating the knife all the way around the seed. Then twist the halves in opposite directions to separate them. To remove the pit, slip the tip of a spoon underneath, and pry it free. Or poke the tip of a knife into it and twist.

very low sugar content and their high fiber content, which promotes satiety. One California avocado contains less than half a gram (g) of sugar and 9.2 g of total dietary fiber.[21] The benefits are plentiful.

A study of overweight individuals found that adding half a Hass avocado to a normal lunch increased satisfaction by 23 percent and decreased the desire to eat by 28 percent compared to a lunch without avocado. Though the avocado added about 112 calories, the effect of feeling full lasted for up to 5 hours, discouraging between-meal snacking.[22]

A large study based on data from 17,567 participants found that, compared to those who don't eat avocados, avocado consumers had a lower body weight, BMI, and waist circumference, and their HDL ("good") cholesterol was higher. What's more, they had an overall better diet quality and nutrient intake, and their odds for metabolic syndrome were 50 percent lower.[23]

Preliminary in vitro evidence indicates that some of the compounds in avocados, especially glutathione, exhibit anticancer activity. A large population-based case-controlled study showed a significant correlation between increased glutathione intake and decreased risk of oral and pharyngeal cancer. With 19 milligrams (mg) of glutathione per one-half fruit, avocados are one of the best sources of this powerful antioxidant.[24]

A study recently published in *Cancer Research* found promising results for a brand new way to fight leukemia:

Avocatin B, a lipid derived from avocados, was effective in killing acute myeloid leukemia stem cells, while leaving normal stem cells untouched.[25]

Avocados are packed with the carotenoids lutein and zeaxanthin, which have been linked to a decreased risk of the cartilage defects that indicate osteoarthritis as well as a decreased risk of age-related eye diseases. Now consider that the Women's Health Initiative observational study found that MUFA-rich diets protect against age-related eye dysfunction; avocados offer up a double dose of protection for eye health. There's also evidence that lutein and zeaxanthin provide some protection against skin damage from UV radiation—and a study of 716 women found that a diet high in dietary fat was associated with greater skin elasticity.[26] Less osteoarthritis, better protection against age-related eye conditions, and fewer wrinkles? Sounds like an antiaging superfood!

blueberries

Blueberries are a rich source of flavonoids, notably anthocyanins, caffeic acid, flavanols, and hydroxycinnamates. They're also a great source of manganese, vitamin C, vitamin K, copper, and fiber. One cup of blueberries contains 24 percent of the recommended daily value of vitamin C and 14 percent of the recommended daily value of fiber, all for just 84 calories. Blueberries are consistently on top 10 lists of "superfoods," and with good reason.

Researchers examined data from 93,600 women ages 25 to 42 over 18 years of follow-up and found that eating ½ cup of blueberries or strawberries at least three times a week was associated with a decreased risk of heart attack. Those who ate the most berries were 32 percent less likely to have suffered a heart attack than the women who ate the least.[27]

Postmenopausal women with prehypertension and stage 1 hypertension

power pairs
spinach and blueberries

Whip up a smoothie with spinach and blueberries and drink it before and after you exercise. The nitrate present in spinach helps muscles work more efficiently during exercise, while blueberries are known to decrease muscle soreness after exercise.[28]

who ate 22 g of freeze-dried blueberry powder daily for 8 weeks experienced significant decreases in systolic and diastolic blood pressure and pulse wave velocity (a measure of arterial stiffness). Nitric oxide, a powerful vasodilator, was greater in the blueberry group, as well. A control group experienced none of these positive changes.[29] Blueberry powder is commercially available and can be used in smoothies, added to granola or granola bars, stirred into yogurt, sprinkled onto oatmeal or any other hot cereal, or used in baked goods.

Blueberry fruits and extracts have been shown to inhibit the growth of tumor cells, inhibit cancer cell proliferation, and induce cancer cell death. Breast cancer, esophageal cancer, melanoma, ovarian cancer, colon cancer, liver carcinoma, and prostate cancer are among the types of cancer that have been studied in connection with blueberries and shown to respond positively.[30]

Remarkably, a single serving of blueberries (300 g) was shown to protect against DNA damage from oxidative stress. Compared to controls, healthy male volunteers saw an 18 percent reduction in peroxide-induced cell damage just 1 hour after consumption.[31] Oxidative stress has been linked to a number of degenerative conditions, including Alzheimer's disease, atherosclerosis, cancer, and premature aging.

A study compared 6 weeks of blueberry consumption (2 cups per day) to carrot juice consumption in adults 60 years old and older. Compared to the carrot juice group, the blueberry group demonstrated significant improvements in their performance of a challenging mobility test. They also performed better in three additional measures of the test: gait speed, number of step errors during a single-task adaptive gait test, and gait speed during a dual-task adaptive gait test. These results suggest that blueberries can improve age-related declines in functional mobility.[32]

cherries

There are hundreds of varieties of cherry trees worldwide, but not all produce edible fruit. Of those that do, cherries are generally divided into two main categories: sweet and tart (or sour). In the United States, Bing and Rainier cherries are among the most well-known sweet cherries, and Montmorency are the most popular type of tart cherry. Like any fruit with a red, blue, or purple hue, cherries are rich in anthocyanins, flavonoids that boast an abundance of health benefits. Cherries also contain vitamin C, fiber, and potassium, and tart cherries are good sources of vitamin A. Acerola cherries, also known as West Indian cherries, deserve special mention for their exceptionally high levels of vitamin C: 1 cup of acerola cherries contains 1,644 mg of vitamin C, or 2,740 percent of the recommended daily value.[33]

Cherries have gained a well-deserved reputation as a healing food for the treatment and prevention of certain types of arthritis,[34] especially gout, a type of inflammatory arthritis that occurs when an excess of uric acid accumulates in certain joints.[35] They're also a natural treatment for insomnia because they boost melatonin levels.[36] But cherries provide other health benefits, some of them surprising.

Most studies on cherries and arthritis have focused on oral consumption of tart cherries. But a new study shows that a topically applied cream made with sour cherry extract is an effective, low-cost treatment for osteoarthritis (OA). Study participants with OA of the knee applied 2.5 ml of sour cherry extract cream to each knee twice a day for 2 months. The topical cream was shown to reduce joint pain, inhibit the expression of inflammatory cytokines, decrease the amount of C-reactive protein, and increase leukocyte heme oxygenase-1.[37]

With its high content of anthocyanins and other flavonoids that act as antioxidants and anti-inflammatories, tart cherry juice has been shown to reduce inflammation, reduce oxidative stress, alleviate muscle soreness, and even prevent muscle damage for those engaged in rigorous exercise.[38]

Tart cherry juice has been shown

to promote postexercise muscle recovery in a number of studies, but recent research also demonstrates its efficacy at reducing upper respiratory tract symptoms associated with rigorous exercise. In this study, runners consumed Montmorency cherry juice or a placebo before and after a marathon. Inflammation scores were lower in the cherry juice group, and these runners reported *no* upper respiratory tract symptoms after the marathon, whereas 50 percent of the runners who drank a placebo reported symptoms 24 and 48 hours after the race.[39]

Researchers in China isolated three new compounds (tetranorditerpenes) from the acerola cherry. In vitro tests found that all three compounds demonstrate cytotoxic activity against breast cancer, hepatocellular carcinoma,

cherries 101

Fresh cherries are their ever-loving, mouthwatering best from May through July. To get the sweetest taste from the harvest, here are some tips you may want to try.

- **CHECK THE STEMS.** When buying cherries, make sure that the stems are green. Dark-colored stems are a tip-off that cherries have been sitting in the bin too long.
- **BUY IN SMALL QUANTITIES.** Cherries are highly perishable. Even when properly stored in the refrigerator, they'll only keep for a few days. So plan on buying only what you're going to eat right away.
- **STORE THEM DRY.** Washing cherries ahead of time can cause them to spoil in the refrigerator. So it's best to store them dry, and then wash them as needed. It's important, however, to wash them thoroughly. Cherries are often coated with a mixture of insecticides, antifungal oils, and moisture seals that producers use to keep them fresh.
- **USE UP THE EXTRAS.** When you're tired of munching cherries, you may want to try a little juice. Simply pit and crush the cherries. Heat them in a saucepan, then press the mixture through a strainer. Refrigerate several hours, then pour the clear juice into glasses to serve, adding sugar to taste.

myeloid leukemia, lung cancer, and colon cancer cells.[40]

citrus fruits

Citrus fruits are well-known superstars of health and healing, mainly due to their high vitamin C content, but it's the flavonoids that deserve much of the credit. These polyphenolic molecules include subclasses such as flavanones, flavonols, flavones, flavan-3-ols, isoflavones, and anthocyanins. Many research studies have demonstrated an association between a flavonoid-rich diet and a reduced incidence of diseases such as cancer, type 2 diabetes, neurodegenerative disorders, and osteoporosis. Citrus flavonoids have also been shown to lower LDL cholesterol and reduce inflammation. In patients with peripheral artery disease, 500 ml of orange juice a day for 28 days reduced circulating high-sensitivity C-reactive protein (hsCRP) by 11 percent, and another study showed that drinking blood orange juice for just 7 days improved endothelial function and reduced circulating cytokines such as CRP, interleukin-6 (IL-6), and tumor necrosis factor alpha (TNFα).[41]

Oranges are usually the first citrus fruit that comes to mind, but dozens of citrus fruits grow all over the world, from the amanatsu of Japan to the yuzu that's native to China and used in many types of Asian cuisine. In addition to oranges, the most common citrus sources in the United States include grapefruit, clementines, mandarin oranges, tangerines, tangelos, lemons, and limes. All of these fruits are rich in vitamin C, and any of the fruits that we eat whole (as opposed to using in small quantities for flavoring) are good sources of fiber, as well. If you want to expand your citrus fruit palate, choices such as pomelos, ugli fruit, kumquats, and blood oranges are usually easy to find in supermarkets. Here are some highlights from research studies on common citrus fruits.

A study of 48 healthy postmenopausal women demonstrated that drinking 340 ml of grapefruit juice daily had a beneficial effect on arterial stiffness. The study was conducted for 6 months, and researchers observed lower pulse wave velocity (a measure of arterial stiffness) in the women who drank grapefruit juice but not in the women who consumed a placebo drink. The positive effect is likely due to grapefruit flavanones.[42]

Based on data from more than 69,600 women collected over 14 years of follow-up, researchers observed that a high flavanone intake was associated with a 19 percent lower risk of ischemic stroke in women. In this study, flavanones came primarily from oranges, grapefruits, and their juices.[43]

In a study of adults with an average age of 67, researchers observed a significant improvement in global cognitive function after 8 weeks of drinking 500 ml of high-flavanone, 100 percent orange juice on a daily basis.[44]

There is also evidence linking orange juice consumption to bone health. In a study that examined data from nearly 14,000 people age 4 and up, researchers found that orange juice consumers had higher serum levels of a variety of nutrients, including magnesium, potassium, carotenoids, and vitamin C, compared to those who did not consume orange juice. Adult OJ drinkers also had a higher level of calcium, and OJ consumption was positively associated with femur bone mineral density in children and femur bone mineral content in both children and adults. In this study, a little more than half of the OJ consumed was fortified with calcium and vitamin D. Though nonfortified OJ provides a host of health benefits, OJ fortified with calcium and vitamin D is recommended for bone health, especially as adequate levels of vitamin D can be difficult to obtain through diet.[45]

Based upon an average of 11.9 years of research on 2,915 subjects who were free of diabetes at the outset of the study, researchers found that each two-and-a-half–fold increase in flavonol intake was associated with a 26 percent lower incidence of type 2 diabetes, and each two-and-a-half–fold increase in

zest for life

Whether you're making a lemon meringue pie or simply adding flavor to salads or store-bought lemon yogurt, be sure to add plenty of zest. The healing compound limonene makes up about 65 percent of oils in the zest, says Michael Gould, PhD, professor of oncology and medical physics at the University of Wisconsin Medical School in Madison.

Zest can be added to just about anything, including sautéed vegetables like onions and mushrooms or as a topping for tabbouleh or rice pilaf. Zest can even be added to dry ingredients when baking, especially zucchini and banana bread.

flavan-3-ol intake was marginally associated with an 11 percent lower incidence of type 2 diabetes. In this population, the main sources of flavonols were tea, apples, and pears; flavones came from orange juice, oranges, and red wine; flavanones came from oranges and orange juice; and flavan-3-ols came from tea, apples, pears, and bananas.[46]

The Kaffir lime, also known as the makrut lime, possesses a variety of beneficial health effects. Kaffir lime peel, used in an essential oil or as a crude extract, has shown an inhibitory effect against common microbial pathogens such as *Salmonella*, *Escherichia coli* (commonly known as *E. coli*), *Staphylococcus,* and *Candida albicans.* It's also been shown to be effective against *Propionibacterium acnes* and to reduce inflammation, which leads to fewer blemishes and less post-acne scarring. The juice of Kaffir limes has been shown to have a high antioxidant content, and in an in vitro model, it has exhibited an anticancer effect.[47]

A study of 101 middle-aged women examined the effect of walking and lemon consumption on blood pressure and found, not surprisingly, that both had a positive effect on blood pressure. But those with higher lemon consumption had a higher serum concentration of citric acid, and citric acid has been shown to promote the absorption of calcium and magnesium, which also played a role in the lower blood pressure observed.[48]

Juice from blood oranges, which is higher in lycopene than regular orange juice is, has been shown to improve risk factors for metabolic syndrome. Studies followed subjects who consumed red orange juice daily for 8 weeks and experienced a decrease in LDL cholesterol and C-reactive protein and an increase in antioxidant activity. Normal-weight volunteers experienced a reduction in insulin resistance and systolic blood pressure, while overweight volunteers experienced a reduction in diastolic blood pressure.[49]

cranberries

Cranberries are a good source of vitamin C, manganese, and fiber, but it's their phytonutrient content that makes them a super healing food. They're a particularly good source of anthocyanins, which give cranberries their vibrant red color and help fight off inflammation. If you opt for cranberry juice, the unsweetened variety saves you from loading your diet with unwanted sugar and calories, but if its notorious tartness is too much, you can combine it with another juice, such as orange or blueberry. Cranberry supple-

how to prepare cranberries

Buying and preparing cranberries is the ultimate no-brainer. If it were any easier, they'd be called fast food.

Whole cranberries usually come in 1-pound bags. The berries are long keepers; they'll last a month or more when kept in the refrigerator and over a year when stored in the freezer. You don't even have to wash them because washing cranberries prior to storage will cause them to spoil.

When preparing fresh cranberry sauce, here's all you need to do.

1. Put a pound of cranberries (4 cups) in a medium saucepan, and cover with 2 cups of boiling water. Return to a boil, cover the pan, and continue cooking for about 4 minutes, or until the skins burst.
2. Stir in sugar to taste. Because the berries are so tart, you'll probably use about 2 cups of sugar.
3. Return the pan to the heat, and bring to a boil. Immediately remove from the heat. Allow to cool before serving.

ments can deliver an even higher dosage of active polyphenols, as can dried cranberries. Their additional health benefits are worth considering.

In research studies, cranberries have been shown to play a role in preventing recurrent UTIs (urinary tract infections)[50] and in inhibiting certain types of cancer, including esophageal, prostate, ovarian, neuroblastoma, breast, colon, lung, and liver.[51]

The same mechanism that makes cranberries effective at preventing recurrent UTIs—their ability to prevent bacteria from adhering to surfaces and from colonizing—makes them gum-disease fighters because they prevent plaque from adhering to teeth and gums.[52]

There's now evidence that cranberries can enhance immune system function, as well. In a recent study, those who drank 450 ml of a cranberry beverage daily for 10 weeks experienced a fivefold increase in gamma delta T cells, which are part of your immune system's first line of defense. In volunteers who developed a cold or flu over the study period, those who drank the cranberry beverage experienced significantly fewer symptoms than those who drank a placebo.[53]

cucumbers

Cucumbers, an important part of the traditional Mediterranean diet, are about 95 percent water and are extremely low in calories: Half a sliced cucumber, including the peel, contains a mere 8 calories. Thus they're a great option for keeping yourself hydrated and feeling full, making them an effective weight-loss snack to eat any time of day. Their high water and fiber contents also make them a great healing food to prevent or treat constipation and to keep your kidneys flushed. Nutrient-wise, 100 g of cucumber contains 16 percent of your daily recommended value of vitamin K, which plays a key role in blood clotting and building strong, healthy bones. Research shows that cucumbers are great at fighting cancer and treating skin.

Along with squash, pumpkins, and melons, cucumbers (*Cucumis sativus*) are members of the plant family Cucurbitaceae, and cucurbitacins—biochemical compounds produced by Cucurbitaceae plants as part of their natural defense system—have shown powerful cytotoxic and antitumor-growth activity.[54]

Cucumbers have a high concentration of lactic acid, an alpha hydroxy acid proven effective at maintaining skin health, which is one of the reasons it's often used in skin-care treatments.[55]

Cucumber has exhibited potential as an antiwrinkle agent because of its antioxidant properties, its ability to inhibit melanin production, and its ability to prevent the breakdown of elastin. At high concentrations it also exhibits some protection from sun damage.[56]

gac fruit

Gac fruit may be unfamiliar to Western palates, but this brilliant red fruit, native to Vietnam and grown throughout South Asia, is emerging as a true superfood. Gac fruit contains 70 times the lycopene of tomatoes; it has the highest concentration of beta-carotene of any fruit or vegetable; and it's also a rich source of zeaxanthin, a carotenoid that is beneficial for eye health. Gac fruit also contains lutein, phenolic acids, and the flavonoids myricetin, rutin, luteolin, and apigenin.[57] The edible fruit (known as arils) and the seeds contain oleic and linoleic fatty acids, suggesting gac fruit's potential to reduce LDL ("bad") cholesterol and inhibit the formation of arterial plaques. The fruit, the seeds, and the leaves have been used in traditional medicine for thousands of years to protect eye health; strengthen the immune system; reduce inflammation; and treat dry eyes, cancer, boils, mastitis, and skin infections.[58]

Gac fruit is still somewhat hard to find in the United States. You're more likely to see it as an ingredient in a supplement than in its whole form at your local health food store, but gac fruit and its products are available as gac oil, gac oil capsules, gac powder, frozen fruit (arils), or as a juice or juice ingredient. Gac fruit and gac fruit products can be ordered online and can be found in some specialty stores and Asian markets. Some enterprising health enthusiasts are growing gac fruit for themselves, cultivating it from seeds, branches, or roots. Research on gac fruit is still in the early stages, but existing studies already confirm its health benefits.

Gac extract has been shown to exhibit nearly three times the antioxidant power of vitamin C and up to 11.8 times the antioxidant power of vitamin E. Gac fruit extract is also far more effective at inhibiting tyrosinase, an enzyme involved in melanin synthesis, than vitamins C and E, highlighting its potential as an antiaging remedy. Used in an antiwrinkle cream, gac fruit extract was shown to reduce roughness and increase skin hydration.[59]

One of the most exciting areas of research into the health benefits of gac fruit is its potential as a cancer fighter due to its high content of carotenoids and phenolic compounds. In vitro and animal studies have shown that gac fruit extract inhibited the growth of colon and liver cancer cells, and extract from gac fruit seeds has been shown to inhibit the growth of and induce apoptosis in breast cancer cells.[60]

Recent in vitro studies confirmed gac fruit seed extract's efficacy in inhibiting the proliferation of lung cancer cells and in inducing apoptosis in gastric cancer cells.[61] Gac fruit seed extract has also exhibited in vitro anticancer activity against lung carcinoma, breast carcinoma, esophageal carcinoma, and melanoma cells by inhibiting proliferation.[62]

grapes

Grapes contain more than 1,600 health-promoting polyphenolic compounds, including anthocyanins, catechins, ellagic acid, flavanols, flavonols, lutein, lycopene, melatonin, proanthocyanidins, quercetin, stilbenes (including resveratrol), and phenolic acids. Black grapes are particularly high in resveratrol,[63] and red grapes have a higher phenolic content than yellow-green grapes because of their anthocyanin content. Grapes are one of our most powerful

(continued on page 42)

Q. What's the number one nutrient you feel people are lacking, and what are the best ways for them to include it in their diets?

A. Americans lack quality fiber. A great way to increase soluable and insoluable fiber intake is to eat whole grains, legumes, fruits, vegetables, and cocoa nibs.

Q. What food combinations do you recommend for overall health?

A. Eat salads with a source of fat, like avocado or olive oil. The fat-soluble vitamins and phytonutrients (such as lycopene) are better absorbed. Also, according to one study in Italy, drinking either red or white wine with fish helps you to absorb more omega-3 fatty acids.

Q. Have you had a client heal him- or herself with food?

A. I recently had a patient who went to China for a yearlong business trip. He rarely exercised, endured significant stress, and ate lots of fast food. When he returned, he'd gained 17 pounds and had chest pain when he exercised. I put him on a plant-based Mediterranean-style diet. Approximately 6 months later he had lost more than 20 pounds and was working out and performing daily stress-reduction exercises pain-free.

Q. Do you recommend sneaking healthy foods into diets? If so, how?

A. I recommend combining certain foods, such as making organic almond and pis-tachio cookies, adding lemon to drinking water, and adding legumes to salads.

Q. What are your food recommendations for weight loss?

A. I recommend high-protein foods, which are nutritious and make you feel full, like eggs; fish; organic, grass-fed beef; and organic, free-range poultry. Also, nutrient-dense foods such as green, leafy vegetables and sweet potatoes, which are naturally low in calories. These foods deliver real nutrients as opposed to the empty calories of highly processed foods.

Q. What are the top 5 to 10 foods everyone should be eating?

A. Everyone should be getting more legumes, olive oil, whole wheat grains, pecorino cheese, garlic, cocoa nibs, wine, turmeric, green tea, tomatoes, and almonds.

Q. What are the top 5 foods everyone should be avoiding?

A. We should avoid predator fish, like tuna and swordfish, due to high mercury levels. Nonorganic soy, soda (I recommend sparkling water and natural juice or lemon for flavor), and creamy sauces or salad dressings should all be avoided. Finally, don't eat pizza with too many toppings.

Q. What are the top foods men should be eating? What are the top foods for women?

A. Men should eat organic, grass-fed lean beef; shellfish (a source of zinc, which is helpful for testosterone levels); and milk and whey. (They are good sources of leucine, which is needed for muscle health.)

Women should eat cruciferous vegetables (for their anticancer properties), sardines (for omega-3s, vitamin D, and calcium), and kale (for calcium, vitamin C, and carotenoids).

Q. What are the top foods for people in their thirties?

A. They should eat lots of fish, legumes, and nuts.

Q. What are the top foods for people in their forties?

A. Consume more sweet potatoes (for beta-carotene), Brazil nuts (for selenium), and red wine, which is good for your heart.

Q. What are the top foods for people in their fifties?

A. They should eat more fruits and vegetables and have less animal fat and salt intake.

Q. What are the top foods for people in their sixties?

A. Once you hit your sixties, increase your intake of high-fiber foods and legumes, which are a good source of iron. Eat more sardines; they're a good source of vitamin D and calcium.

Q. What are the top foods for people in their seventies?

A. People in their seventies should increase their intake of whole grains, fish, and lean meats. If you notice a reduction in appetite, snack on organic peanut butter; it's a useful source of good fats.

Q. If we were to go to the grocery store with you, what would we always find in your shopping cart?

A. I never leave the grocery store without buying a wide variety of vegetables, fruits, lemons, extra-virgin olive oil, avocados, red wine, artichokes, wakame, cocoa nibs, turmeric, natto, kombucha, and kefir.

Q. What's your favorite indulgence?

A. I love poached pear with vanilla bean, cinnamon, and anise in a wine sauce.

Q. What do you order in a restaurant?

A. At my favorite Italian restaurants, I order handmade, organic ancient grain pasta with organic San Marzano tomato sauce. If I'm eating Mexican, I'll order a pinto bean salsa salad, and I'll have a curried red lentil stew with vegetables if I'm at an Indian restaurant.

Q. Are there any home remedies you use?

A. If I'm getting sick, I eat 52 cloves of garlic and ginger soup, which works as a natural "flu shot." Garlic-infused olive oil drops are a great cure for otitis (inflammation of the ear). Taken orally, they can prevent upper respiratory infections in children and adults.

dietary antioxidants. With their high concentration of flavonoids, they play a role in suppressing oxidative stress and reducing oxidative damage. Grape polyphenols have also been shown to decrease chronic inflammation by reducing reactive oxygen species and modulating inflammatory pathways, and the proanthocyanidins in grape seeds scavenge free radicals, prevent lipid peroxidation, and inhibit formation of proinflammatory cytokines.[64] With their ability to reduce chronic inflammation and insulin resistance, grapes can play a role in preventing obesity-related metabolic diseases.[65]

Older adults with mild cognitive impairment drank Concord grape juice or a placebo daily for 16 weeks. The volunteers who drank grape juice performed better on tests of memory function, and fMRI scans revealed greater activation in the anterior and posterior regions of their right hemispheres.[66]

Grapes and grape products, such as red wine and grape juices, exert a cardioprotective effect by enhancing endothelial function, decreasing LDL oxidation, improving vascular function, altering blood lipids, and modulating inflammatory processes.[67]

A long-term study of nearly 290,000 people, 12,198 of whom developed type 2 diabetes (T2D), found that greater consumption of whole fruits—grapes, apples, and blueberries, in particular—

was associated with a significantly lower risk of type 2 diabetes. All of these fruits contain high levels of anthocyanins, which are associated with a lower risk of T2D, and grapes provide the extra benefit of resveratrol, which has been shown to increase insulin sensitivity. This study also offers a word of caution: The consumption of fruit juice was associated with a higher risk of developing T2D, most likely because of juice's higher glycemic load and the loss of nutrients during the juicing process.[68]

In vitro and in vivo studies have demonstrated the effectiveness of resveratrol in exerting antiproliferative effects in several types of cancer, including breast, prostate, liver, colorectal, intestinal, skin, lung, blood, and thyroid.[69]

Many studies have shown that grape phenolic compounds inhibit platelet aggregation. This is true of phenolics found in the fruit, skin, and seeds of grapes, but some studies have suggested that the effect is greater when components from grape skin and seeds are present in combination, as they are in red wine or grape juice.[70]

See also: Wine (page 17)

papayas

Papaya, sometimes referred to as pawpaw, originated in Mexico and now grows in many tropical climates. Papaya is one of the best dietary sources of vitamin C. One cup of papaya chunks contains more than 88 mg of vitamin C, which surpasses the 75 mg per day recommended for women and nearly satisfies the 90 mg per day recommended for men.[71] Papaya is also rich in vitamin A and is a good source of fiber and folate. Red-fleshed papaya is a great source of lycopene, a carotenoid antioxidant that has anticancer and cardioprotective effects.[72] Besides being a great vitamin source, papaya demonstrates strong healing properties.

In a study that assessed the post-prandial bioavailability of carotenoids from raw, red-fleshed papaya, tomato, and carrots, beta-carotene was found to be about three times more bioavailable from papaya than from tomatoes or carrots, and the bioavailability of lycopene was found to be about 2.6 times higher in papaya than in tomatoes. Higher concentrations of vitamin A were also observed after the papaya meal.[73]

Extracts from papaya seeds and leaves have been shown to demonstrate an antimycotic (antifungal) effect against fluconazole-resistant *C. albicans*,[74] the fungus responsible for most yeast infections.

Papaya seed extract has been shown to accelerate wound healing, decrease inflammation and oxidative damage to tissues, and inhibit microbial activity in wounds.[75]

Though clinical trials in humans are limited, in vitro studies have shown promising anticancer effects from papaya flesh extract (breast cancer), papaya seed extract (leukemia), papaya juice (breast and liver cancer), and papaya leaf extract (breast, colon, stomach, pancreatic, ovarian, uterine, blood, cervical, lung, and lymph cancers).[76]

See also: Tomatoes (page 48), Watermelon (page 49)

pineapples

Pineapple is part of the Bromeliaceae family, which gives you a clue as to one of its roles as a healing food. Pineapple is one of the richest food sources of the enzyme bromelain, which has anti-inflammatory effects. There is also emerging evidence of bromelain's anti-cancer capabilities and its use in treating coagulation-related diseases, asthma, and allergies.[77] Pineapple stem has the highest levels of bromelain, but it's present in the fruit and juice, as well. Bromelain is available in concentrated form as a supplement. Pineapple is also a good source of vitamin C, manganese, and fiber.

Bromelain has been used in health care to treat a number of inflammatory conditions, including arthritis, ulcers, wounds, bronchitis, sinusitis, hematomas, and oral inflammation. It was shown to alleviate pain and swelling and to decrease healing time in all of these conditions.[78]

Pineapple contains melatonin, the hormone that regulates sleep cycles and helps to prompt sleep. A study found that drinking pineapple juice raised serum melatonin concentrations as well as antioxidant capacity in healthy volunteers. The highest melatonin concentration was observed 120 minutes after drinking the juice.[79]

A recent study showed that fruit juices can attenuate some of the metabolic stress response and inflammation associated with eating high-fat meals. In a study of 14 overweight volunteers who drank an antioxidant-rich fruit juice including pineapple along with a high-fat meal, both uric acid and thiol (an organosulfur compound) production decreased compared to those who drank a placebo juice.[80]

pomegranates

Although the white pith of pomegranates is edible, most people forgo that for

sweet on the inside

With its tough skin and sharp edges, the pineapple doesn't give up its sweetness easily. To choose the best fruit and get to the "heart of gold" inside, here's what you need to do.

- ◼ BUY IT FIRM. Find a fruit that's plump and firm. Avoid pineapples that are bruised or have soft spots. Surprisingly, shell color is not always a reliable indicator of ripeness. The stem end should have a sweet, aromatic fragrance and not smell fermented.
- ◼ LOOK FOR FRESHNESS. The leaves on pineapples should be crisp and deep green, without yellowed or browned tips. Don't bother testing the fruit by pulling a leaf from the crown. Contrary to popular wisdom, a leaf that comes off easily doesn't indicate that the fruit is ripe.
- ◼ REVEAL THE FRUIT. When you get the pineapple home, cut off the top and bottom ends, then place the pineapple in a shallow dish to catch the juices as you slice off the spiny skin vertically. You can then cut it into rounds and remove the tough center core.

the delicious and nutrition-packed seeds. Technically, what you're eating is the pomegranate's seeds *and* arils: It's the deep red, jewel-like arils that surround the slightly tart seeds. But whatever you call them and however you remove these jewels, pomegranates and pomegranate juice are well worth the effort: Research confirms their superfood status. Pomegranate seeds are a great source of fiber, vitamin C, and vitamin K, but it's the polyphenolic compounds that confer an abundance of healing effects. Pomegranate juice has been found to have three times the antioxidant activity of red wine and green tea.[81] Pomegranates are a rich source of anthocyanins, potent antioxidants that give pomegranate arils their brilliant red color, and hydrolyzable tannins, which account for 92 percent of the antioxidant activity of the whole fruit. Pomegranate fruit, juice, bark, leaves, flowers, and roots have been used to treat everything from AIDS to cancer, from allergies to cardiovascular conditions.[82] Pomegranate extracts have been found to have strong anti-inflammatory, antioxidant, and antitumor properties in vivo and in vitro, and extracts and juice have been shown to exert an antibacterial effect.[83]

A study of 28 overweight or obese volunteers ages 40 to 65 who drank 500 ml of pomegranate juice a day for 4 weeks demonstrated an impressive range of improved cardiovascular and metabolic factors compared to those who consumed a placebo. In the pomegranate juice group, both systolic and diastolic blood pressure dropped anywhere from 0.5 to 22 mmHg for systolic and up to 12 mmHg for diastolic pressure. Subjects also experienced improved insulin resistance, reduced fasting plasma insulin, and decreased pulse wave velocity (a measure of arterial stiffness). A trend toward lower free cortisol levels was also observed, indicating a lower overall stress level.[84]

An in vitro study showed that pomegranate polyphenols decreased secretion of the proinflammatory cytokines tumor necrosis factor alpha and interleukin-6 by up to 37 and 94 percent, respectively. These results demonstrate that pomegranate consumption can counteract progressive intravascular inflammation and the development of atherosclerosis.[85]

In vitro studies have demonstrated pomegranate's effectiveness in fighting prostate cancer, breast cancer, lung cancer, colon cancer, skin cancer, liver cancer, bladder cancer, brain cancer, and leukemia.[86] Its anticancer activity is thought to be due to its high polyphenolic content, including ellagitannins (including punicalagin, a powerful bioactive compound unique to pomegranate), ellagic acid, and other flavonoids, such as quercetin.[87]

Pomegranate can help prevent and treat type 2 diabetes by reducing oxidative stress and lipid peroxidation and decreasing fasting blood glucose levels. Compounds in pomegranate, including punicalagin and ellagic, gallic, oleanolic, and ursolic acids, have been shown to exert antidiabetic actions.[88]

raspberries

The most well-known type of raspberry is the popular red variety, but raspberries range in color from yellow to golden, purple, and black. All of the varieties are delicious, but the darker the berry, the higher the level of anthocyanins, powerful flavonoids that exert antioxidant effects. Raspberries are also rich in fiber and manganese and provide a good source of vitamin K. Red raspberries are the best dietary source of ellagic acid, a phenol antioxidant known for its anticancer effects. Due to their high flavonoid and phenolic content, raspberries and their seeds have demonstrated potent anti-inflammatory and antioxidant effects.

A study that followed 2,332 men for more than 19 years and examined the association between their intake of fruits, berries, and vegetables and their risk of type 2 diabetes found that berries were the most protective, reducing the risk of developing T2D by as much as 35 percent.[89]

Patients with metabolic syndrome who ate 750 mg of black raspberries per day for 12 weeks experienced significantly decreased total serum cholesterol and inflammatory cytokines (tumor necrosis factor alpha and interleukin-6) and improved vascular endothelial function.[90]

Fatty, calorie-rich meals are known to induce metabolic stress and trigger an inflammatory response. Researchers designed a study to see if freeze-dried

power pairs

raspberries and grapes

Satisfying your sweet tooth could help you beat cancer. Raspberries and grapes are both high in antioxidants, and science shows that when it comes to antioxidants, two is better than one. Raspberries contain ellagic acid, which is known to enhance the effect of quercetin, found in grapes. When combined, these antioxidants are cancer-fighting machines.[91]

black raspberries could attenuate this response. Overweight or obese men in group 1 ate 45 g per day of freeze-dried black raspberries for 4 consecutive days. Group 2 did not eat berries. After a 14-hour postprandial visit, men in group 1 ate a high-fat, high-calorie breakfast with black raspberries while group 2 ate only the high-fat, high-calorie breakfast. After a 2-day washout period, the groups switched to the opposite protocol. In all subjects, black raspberries were found to positively modulate interleukin-6, reducing postprandial inflammation resulting from a high-fat, high-calorie meal.[92]

strawberries

Strawberries boast a high antioxidant and flavonoid content, including caffeic acid, ellagic acid, anthocyanins, tannins, catechin, quercetin, kaempferol, gallic acid derivatives, vitamins C and E, and carotenoids.[93] They're also a good source of fiber, folate, potassium, and manganese. As a healing food, strawberries are best known for their antioxidant and anti-inflammatory effects, due in part to their very high vitamin C content. They're especially effective at inhibiting cyclooxygenase-2 (COX-2), the main promoter of inflammatory prostaglandins and an enzyme that plays a role in neurodegenerative diseases such as Alzheimer's and Parkinson's.[94] In the short term, eating strawberries increases plasma antioxidant capacity, improves circulating inflammatory markers, and improves your postprandial glycemic response. Longer-term consumption of strawberries is associated with an improved lipid profile, a reduction in chronic inflammation, and an improvement in cognitive performance.[95] And there's even more good news.

Greater intakes of strawberries and blueberries are associated with slower rates of cognitive decline. Frequent berry consumption has been shown to delay cognitive aging by as much as 2.5 years.[96]

An in vitro study demonstrated the photoprotective properties of strawberry extract in human dermal fibroblasts. The extract also increased cellular viability and decreased DNA damage.[97]

In a study of 500 volunteers who ate 500 g of strawberries per day for 30 days, strawberry consumption lowered total cholesterol, LDL cholesterol, and triglycerides; decreased markers of oxidative stress, oxidative hemolysis (rupture of red blood cells), and number of activated platelets; and increased antioxidant capacity.[98]

In a study of patients with type 2 diabetes, those who consumed 2 cups a day of a freeze-dried strawberry beverage for 6 weeks (equivalent to 500 g of fresh strawberries per day) experienced improved glycemic control and antioxidant status and reduced lipid peroxidation and inflammatory response.[99]

tomatoes

When it comes to superfoods, it's hard to argue with the health-promoting benefits of tomatoes. Packed with vitamin A, vitamin C, and the cancer-fighting and cardioprotective antioxidant lycopene—and a good source of vitamin K, potassium, and fiber—they make everyone's list of healthiest foods. And they're extremely versatile—delicious consumed raw, cooked, or as a juice, there's a tomato-based recipe that appeals to everyone. One word of caution: Watch out for the high sodium content in many commercially prepared tomato juices. Low-sodium and no-salt-added options are available and preferable. The overall health benefits are numerous.

Researchers asked a group of 35 women, ages 18 to 20, to eat a raw, ripe tomato every day before lunch for 4 weeks. At the conclusion of the study, participants had lost an average of more than 2 pounds, and their body fat had decreased by an average of 1.54 percent. What's more, their fasting blood glucose, triglycerides, total cholesterol, and uric acid levels all decreased.[100]

Research has also shown that eating tomato products with a meal can lower lipemia-induced oxidative stress and its associated inflammatory response. On two separate occasions, 25 people consumed high-fat meals containing either a tomato product or a tomato-free alternative; their postprandial responses were then monitored at several points through blood samples. Researchers found that tomato significantly reduced high-fat meal-induced LDL oxidation and a rise in interleukin-6, a proinflammatory cytokine and marker of inflammation.[101]

Lycopene is found in higher concentrations in tomato juice than in fresh tomatoes. A recent study focusing on the health benefits of tomato juice found that 93 middle-aged women who drank 200 ml of unsalted tomato juice twice a day for 8 weeks experienced significant positive changes in the following areas: (1) decreased menopausal symptoms, (2) an improved score on the Hospital Anxiety and Depression Scale (HADS), (3) a slight increase in heart rate, which went hand in hand with (4) an increase in resting energy expenditure (REE), and (5) a decrease in serum triglyceride levels in the women who had high triglycerides at the outset of the study.[102]

In a study conducted at the China Medical University in Taiwan, researchers found that a daily glass of tomato juice had a direct positive effect on waist circumference, cholesterol, and inflammation. Women ages 20 to

30 consumed 280 ml of tomato juice daily for 8 weeks. On average, their waists shrank by 1.6 cm, and they lost more than a pound of fat. They also experienced lower cholesterol, a reduction in BMI, and a decrease in MCP-1 levels (a marker of inflammation). And all of this happened in spite of no other changes to their overall diets.[103]

See also: Papayas (page 42), Watermelon

watermelon

Watermelon, that quintessential summer fruit, is one of our very best sources of naturally occurring lycopene, the cancer-fighting and cardioprotective antioxidant that gives fruits their red color. The other health-promoting compound in watermelon that's been the subject of much research is citrulline, an amino acid that's converted into

sun-dried DIY

Come February, the juiciest, vine-ripened tomatoes are but a wistful summer memory. Cheer up. Even when fresh tomatoes are out of season, sun-dried tomatoes are a great way to get the delicious taste all year and are a nice change of pace from the Roma, grape, and cherry tomatoes you can find just about year-round in the supermarket.

Unfortunately, sun-dried tomatoes can be expensive. To enjoy their rich taste without paying an exorbitant price at the supermarket, you may want to take advantage of the abundance of vine-ripened tomatoes available in summer at a low price, and dry some yourself. Here's how.

1. Choose ripe, unbruised tomatoes. Wash them thoroughly and cut off the stems and butt ends.
2. Place each tomato on its side, and cut into ¼-inch slices.
3. Put the slices on a baking sheet and place in a 120° to 140°F oven for about 24 hours. The tomatoes are done when they're leathery, yet still pliable.
4. Pack the dried tomatoes into small jars, plastic freezer bags, or plastic containers, and refrigerate or freeze until you're ready to use them. If you're using glass jars, make sure they're at room temperature before putting them in the freezer to prevent them from breaking.

Be sure to discard any tomatoes that develop black, yellow, or white spots, which could be mold that sometimes develops during the drying process.

arginine. Citrulline has been found to prevent muscle soreness, and because its by-product, arginine, relaxes blood vessels and boosts nitric oxide, some researchers have postulated a "Viagra-like effect" from eating watermelon.[104] Though studies with human subjects are limited, one study did find that citrulline supplementation (1.5 g a day) improved erection hardness in men with mild erectile dysfunction.[105] Citrulline is found in watermelon flesh and seeds, but its highest concentrations can be found in watermelon rind. Watermelon is also rich in vitamin C and is a good source of vitamin A and fiber. At 92 percent water, watermelon will keep you hydrated and prevent constipation, and it contains fewer than 50 calories per cup. The health findings will keep you eating it year-round.

A recent metastudy based on 17,517 cases of prostate cancer among 563,299 subjects found that higher lycopene consumption and higher circulating levels of lycopene significantly reduced the risk of prostate cancer.[106]

A study had athletes drink half a liter of watermelon juice an hour before engaging in exercise. Researchers gave one test group natural watermelon juice, a second group pasteurized watermelon juice enhanced with 6 mg of citrulline, and the final group a placebo. The groups that ingested the watermelon drinks reported no muscle soreness 24 hours after exercising, while the placebo group did experience muscle soreness. What's more, the group that drank unpasteurized watermelon juice absorbed 19 percent of the citrulline, while the group with the citrulline-enhanced watermelon juice only absorbed 13 percent, suggesting that it's better to treat yourself to the naturally occurring citrulline in fresh watermelon.[107]

A 12-week study on obese, hypertensive adults found that citrulline-rich watermelon extract reduced brachial and aortic systolic blood pressure and myocardial oxygen demand during the cold pressor test, during which subjects' hands were immersed in cold water for about a minute.[108]

A 6-week study on menopausal women found that watermelon supplementation (6 g per day of L-citrulline and L-arginine) resulted in decreased arterial stiffness and aortic blood pressure.[109]

See also: Papayas (page 42), Tomatoes (page 48)

herbs and spices

basil, holy basil

There are well over 100 varieties of basil, all of them part of the *Ocimum* genus and part of the Lamiaceae or mint family of plants. The basil that's most familiar to Americans is called sweet basil, though plenty of people now cook with Thai basil, lemon basil, or spicy cinnamon basil. Holy basil (*Ocimum sanctum or O. tenuiflorum*), is also known as tulsi; it's native to India and has long been used for religious and medicinal purposes. It's used as a culinary herb in Thai cooking, too. Basil is extremely easy to grow and complements a wide range of dishes. It's eaten fresh or dried, raw or cooked, and is cultivated for its essential oil as well as for making tea. Basil is an excellent source of vitamin A and vitamin K and a good source of manganese, copper, and iron. But many of its healing effects stem from its polyphenolic compounds—basil essential oil has shown some of the highest total antioxidant activity and thus highest antibacterial activity among more than a dozen common essential oils.[1] There is some evidence that organic cultivation methods using biofertilizers result in higher levels of phenolics and total flavonoids in basil than inorganic methods do.[2] The additional research is encouraging.

- Both common basil and holy basil essential oil have demonstrated antifungal, antibacterial, antiparasitical, insect-repelling, and in vitro anticancer activity.[3]

- Preclinical studies have also shown that holy basil and some of its phytochemicals prevented chemical-induced skin, liver, oral, and lung cancers and mediated these anticancer effects by increasing antioxidant activity, altering gene expressions, inducing cancer cell death, and inhibiting angiogenesis (the growth of new blood vessels) and metastasis. Its phytochemicals were also shown to prevent radiation-induced DNA damage.[4]

- Studies have confirmed sweet basil and holy basil's anti-inflammatory effects. Holy basil extract and essential oil demonstrated antiulcer and antisecretory effects that could heal gastric ulcers, and they were found to be effective at preventing hepatic steatosis (the buildup of fat in your liver).[5]

■ Volunteers who consumed a holy basil extract daily (1,200 milligrams [mg]) for 6 weeks experienced improvement in a number of stress-related symptoms, such as forgetfulness, sleeping difficulties, frequent exhaustion, and sexual problems of recent origin. With this last symptom, holy basil produced remarkable results: Compared to those who took a placebo, holy basil reduced sexual problem scores by 87.5 percent. Overall, holy basil extract was found to be 39 percent more effective at managing the symptoms of stress than a placebo.[6]

■ Holy basil leaf extract also appears to have cognition-enhancing properties. Compared to those who took a placebo, volunteers who took 300 mg of holy basil extract per day for 30 days showed significant improvement in tests of cognitive function and anxiety.[7]

black pepper

Perhaps you wouldn't think of humble black pepper as a healing food, but a closer look reveals that *Piper nigrum* is a good source of manganese, which plays a

basil basics

Your friend with the green thumb hands you a bouquet of fresh basil, still warm from the sun. It smells heavenly—but how do you use it? Here are a few suggestions.

■ TEAR IT GENTLY. Basil is delicate. Rough handling will cause the leaves to blacken around the edges, says Mildred Mattfeldt-Berman, PhD, RD, LD, of St. Louis University. She recommends handling it gently—and as little as possible—before you put it into your recipe.

■ KEEP IT HAPPY IN THE FRIDGE. To store fresh basil for the short term, wrap the lower stems with a damp paper towel, place it in an unsealed

plastic bag, and store in your vegetable drawer.

■ FREEZE IT FOR LATER. For long-term storage, fill an ice cube tray with basil leaves, top off the little compartments with water, and put the tray in a sealed freezer container. When you need basil, you'll have premeasured chunks that you can drop into a soup or sauce, says Dr. Mattfeldt-Berman.

key role in healthy metabolism. Piperine, an alkaloid that gives pepper its kick, has demonstrated anti-inflammatory, antioxidant, immunomodulatory, antiasthmatic, antiulcer, antiamoebic (parasite-fighting), and chemopreventive (cancer-fighting) effects.[8]

■ Several studies have found that piperine has strong potential as a natural antidepressant. It works by acting as an MAOI, or monoamine oxidase inhibitor, elevating brain serotonin and brain-derived neurotrophic factor (BDNF) levels and positively modulating the hypothalamus-pituitary-adrenal axis.[9]

■ Black pepper's anticancer effects were demonstrated in an in vitro study. Black pepper extract of 200 mcg/ml and its active ingredients at 25 mcg/ml inhibited lipid peroxidation by 45 to 85 percent, COX enzymes (involved in inflammation) by 31 to 80 percent, and cancer cell proliferation by 3.5 to 86.8 percent. Researchers concluded that overall, these results suggested that black pepper and its constituents exhibit anti-inflammatory, antioxidant, and anticancer activities.[10]

See also: Turmeric (page 69)

capers

Capers may be most familiar to American palates as the small, pealike, pickled accompaniment to salmon dishes. Capers are actually the unopened flower buds of the *Capparis spinosa,* or caper bush. We originally included capers in our list of healing foods because of their chart-topping amounts of the powerful antioxidant quercetin—these tiny little buds contain more quercetin by weight than any other plant. But it turns out there's a lot more to capers than their quercetin content. Their other phenolic compounds include rutin, which has anti-inflammatory effects and is used to treat varicose veins, and the flavonol kaempferol, which has demonstrated a range of anticancer effects. Capers are usually sold in a vinegar brine and are high in sodium, but you can rinse them to remove some of the excess salt. In addition to their use as a garnish, capers can be sprinkled whole onto salads, or you can add ground capers to sauces to lend a tangy, slightly spicy flavor. This little-used superfood will make its way onto tables everywhere based on this research.

■ Quercetin has been shown to exert a range of health benefits, including lowering blood pressure, acting in cancer prevention and treatment, reducing inflammation, supporting the immune system, and acting as an antiallergy treatment.[11] Capers, at 180 mg of quercetin per 100 g (and only about 20 calories for that amount) are a low-calorie, low-cost, and delicious means of boosting your quercetin intake.

- Capers have been used traditionally in Iran to treat diabetes. A randomized controlled trial was established to test their antidiabetic effects. Type 2 diabetes patients on standard diabetic therapy were divided into two groups: One received 400 mg of caper fruit extract three times a day for 2 months while the other received a placebo. Those in the caper group experienced significant decreases in fasting blood glucose levels, glycosylated hemoglobin, and triglyceride levels.[12]

- A protein isolated from caper seeds was shown to inhibit the proliferation of liver, colon, and breast cancer cells in vitro. It also inhibited HIV-1 reverse transcriptase (an enzyme involved in replicating human immunodeficiency virus).[13]

cilantro/coriander

Cilantro and coriander are the same plant, *Coriandrum sativum*, but cilantro refers to the leaves and coriander refers to the seeds. Many people use the two terms interchangeably, but if you're referring to the whole plant, most experts agree that the correct term is coriander. (If a recipe calls for fresh coriander, use the cilantro leaves!) Cilantro (the leaves) is eaten fresh or dried, and dried coriander (the seeds) can be bought whole or ground. The leaves and seeds are both used to make essential oil and can be found as an extract, as well. Traditionally, coriander was used as a digestive to settle the stomach and treat indigestion. Coriander is a good source of vitamin K and a rich source of folates, making it an all-natural means of alleviating vitamin B_9 deficiency, and both the leaves and seeds exhibit strong antioxidant activity.[14] It also contains an impressive range of phytochemicals, including alkaloids, flavonoids, terpenoids, sterols, saponins, and phenolic compounds, and it displays potent antimicrobial activity.[15] Coriander seeds are a good source of fiber, copper, iron, manganese, and magnesium.

- In one study, researchers investigated the antioxidant, anti-inflammatory, and antiproliferation properties of raw and roasted coriander seeds. Both raw and roasted seeds showed comparable antioxidant and anti-inflammatory activities, and both inhibited the growth of gastric, prostate, colon, breast, and lung carcinoma cells in vitro.[16]

- Coriander essential oil has exhibited antifungal activity against *Candida* species responsible for oral candidiasis[17] and vaginal yeast infections and antibacterial activity against a range of bacteria responsible for vaginal infections, including *Escherichia coli* (commonly known as *E. coli*) and *Staphylococcus aureus*.[18]

- In a study using an animal model as well as an in vitro test of human dermal cells, coriander leaf extract was shown to exert protection against ultraviolet radiation and to help to prevent skin from photoaging. Human cells that were treated with coriander leaf extract exhibited higher procollagen (a precursor to collagen) production and lower levels of matrix metalloproteinase-1 (which breaks down interstitial collagen) than untreated cells.[19]

- Antidiabetic effects have been observed from ingesting coriander essential oil. It appears to stimulate insulin secretion and enhance glucose uptake and metabolism by muscles.[20]

fenugreek

The leaves and seeds of fenugreek are edible, and both can be eaten fresh or dried. It has a bitter, rather unusual taste, and toasting the seeds brings out its pungent flavor. The use of fenugreek is known in both ancient medicine and contemporary complementary medicine as a way to stimulate lactation, induce labor, and treat various digestive complaints. In clinical trials it has been widely studied for its antidiabetic benefits.

- In a study on the effect of fenugreek on dysmenorrhea (painful menstrual cramps), 51 women took 900 mg of fenugreek seed powder three times a day for two consecutive menstrual cycles, while 50 women took a placebo. Those in the fenugreek group experienced significantly greater reductions in pain, and the duration of pain decreased between the two cycles. Other common dysmenorrhea symptoms, such as headache, fatigue, and nausea, decreased as well.[21]

- Fenugreek was shown to increase sexual desire and arousal in healthy menstruating women. In this study, women ages 20 to 49 took a 600 mg fenugreek seed extract once a day over two menstrual cycles, while another group took a placebo. Those in the fenugreek group experienced a significant increase in free testosterone and estradiol and reported increased sexual desire and arousal compared with the placebo group.[22]

- Fenugreek seed extract was shown to be effective against fluconazole-resistant *C. albicans*, the most common cause of candidiasis.[23]
- A number of studies have shown that fenugreek seeds, which are high in soluble fiber, and fenugreek extracts decrease blood glucose levels in diabetic patients.[24]

garlic

Garlic has so many health-promoting benefits that you'd nearly swear it's supernatural. But while no clinical trial has proven its ability to repel vampires or protect against evil spirits, research has proven that garlic is a true superfood. It's difficult to know where to begin when describing garlic's healing powers, but just to whet your appetite for this pungent *Allium*, take a look at this list of scientifically proven effects. Garlic has antibacterial, antiviral, antiprotozoal, antiparasitic, and antifungal effects; reduces inflammation; lowers blood pressure; lowers serum cholesterol; lowers triglycerides; helps to prevent atherosclerosis; inhibits platelet aggregation and acts as an antithrombotic; increases fibrinolytic activity (breaking down of blood clots); scavenges free radicals; displays some of the most potent cancer-preventing effects of any food; reduces blood glucose levels; protects your liver from various toxins; strengthens your immune system; potentially reduces the frequency of the common cold and cuts its duration; and, believe it or not, improves the aroma of sweat.[25] Yes, this was proven by a study in which 42 male "odor donors" were given a low or high amount of raw garlic (study 1 and 2) or garlic capsules containing 1,200 mg of garlic extract (study 3) to consume and then wore underarm pads for 12 hours to collect body odor. Researchers then recruited 82 brave women who judged the samples for "pleasantness, attrac-

power pairs
garlic and onions

Garlic and onions may give you stinky breath, but they're a great addition to grains. When added to whole grains like brown rice and wheat pasta, these pungent veggies more than tripled the body's absorption of zinc and iron. We'd say the bad breath is worth it.[26]

tiveness, masculinity, and intensity." Contrary to what you may expect, the women found the samples from men who'd had a higher raw garlic dosage—12 g, or the equivalent of four fresh cloves—to be more pleasant, more attractive, and less intense; they found the samples from garlic capsules (study 3) to be more attractive and less intense. The low-dose garlic from study 1 (6 g of fresh garlic) produced no significant differences in ratings.[27] Has science just turned up a new cologne ingredient with aphrodisiac properties? We'll let you be the judge.

Garlic's infamously pungent smell is released when the cloves are cut or crushed—and so is the sulfur compound allicin, which is responsible for so many of garlic's health-promoting effects. Raw, crushed garlic and fresh, raw garlic extract are more effective than cooked garlic or heated garlic extract, as cooking decreases the allicin levels.[28] Adding garlic toward the end of the cooking process retains more of the

garlic—the good way

Unless you have taste buds of steel, it's difficult to eat a lot of raw garlic at one sitting. Not to mention the havoc that loads of garlic can wreak on some people's digestive systems. But you can substantially boost your garlic intake without hurting your tongue or stomach in the process by roasting it.

Unlike eating raw garlic cloves, roasting gives the bulb a sweet, caramelized taste—garlic at its most polite, in other words. It delivers just a hint of the sulfuric odor and taste rather than the full blast.

To roast garlic, cut the top from the garlic bulb to expose just the tips of the cloves. Rub the bulb lightly with a little olive oil, and wrap in a piece of aluminum foil. Leave some air space around the bulb, but seal the edges tightly. Roast in a 350°F oven for about 45 minutes, or until very tender. (You can also "roast" garlic in the microwave; use the high power setting and cook, uncovered, and without oil, for about 10 minutes, turning twice during the cooking process.)

To eat roasted garlic, simply squeeze the root end firmly to push the cloves out of their skins. You can spread the garlic on bread or toss it with cooked pasta or vegetables. If you're not eating it right away, you can refrigerate roasted garlic in a tightly covered container for up to 1 week.

allicin. Garlic contains a higher concentration of sulfur compounds, noted for their anticancer effect, than any other *Allium,* as well as enzymes, amino acids, and minerals such as selenium and manganese.[29]

■ A 5-week study of garlic's effect on cognition and memory was conducted on healthy volunteers. One group received a 400 mg capsule of garlic powder twice a day for 5 weeks; the other group received a placebo. Garlic supplementation was found to improve visual memory and increase attention.[30]

■ A meta-analysis of seven randomized, controlled trials revealed that garlic has a significant blood-pressure-lowering effect on both systolic and diastolic blood pressure.[31]

■ A meta-analysis of 8,621 cases of gastric cancer and 14,889 controls found that any amount of garlic intake was associated with a reduced risk of gastric cancer; a high intake was correlated with the most significant risk reduction.[32]

■ A meta-analysis based on data from 513 subjects found that garlic intake (whole garlic or extract) results in a significant reduction in fasting blood glucose concentrations.[33]

■ A meta-analysis based on 13 trials found that if garlic is consumed for 2 months or more, it's effective in reducing total cholesterol by up to 23 points and LDL cholesterol by up to 15 points in those with elevated cholesterol (200 or more). An 8 percent reduction in total serum cholesterol is associated with a 38 percent reduction in risk of coronary events at 50 years of age.[34]

■ A meta-analysis of nine epidemiological studies found that *Allium* vegetables, garlic especially, decreased the risk of prostate cancer.[35]

ginger

Ginger root (*Zingiber officinale*) has been used for thousands of years, as both a food and a medicine. It has a warm, spicy, and slightly sweet taste and is a principal ingredient in curries. Ginger can be used in several forms, including fresh, dried, powdered, pickled, candied, crystallized, or preserved, and it is used to make tea, beer, sauces, essential oils—and, of course, gingerbread cookies and other baked goods. The brightly colored accompaniment to sushi is sliced ginger that's been pickled in sweet vinegar. Ginger's most famous medicinal use is as a natural, safe, and quite effective means of treating nausea and vomiting associated with morning sickness, postoperative recovery, and medication therapy, including chemotherapy and antiretrovirals.[36]

Many of ginger's health-giving benefits come from its two major classes of bioactive compounds, gingerols and shogaols. Gingerols are more abundant in fresh ginger and give it its spicy, aromatic flavor, and shogaols are more abundant in dried ginger. When ginger is cooked, gingerols convert to a component called zingerone. A recent review on zingerone alone observed that it acts as an anti-inflammatory, antidiabetic, antilipolytic (counters fat cell process), antidiarrheal, antiaxiolytic (lessens anxiety), antispasmodic, antithrombotic, and antimicrobial. It also stimulates appetite, protects against radiation, and inhibits reactive nitrogen species, which play a key role in causing Alzheimer's disease and many other inflammatory disorders.[37] Ginger in any form exerts strong antioxidant and anti-inflammatory properties and has been used as a natural analgesic. It holds much promise as a healing food.

■ A meta-analysis of Zingiberaceae (the plant family of ginger, turmeric, and cardamom) extracts' effects on chronic pain found that they are clinically effective pain relievers and are safer to use than nonsteroidal anti-inflammatory drugs (NSAIDS). In this study, "chronic pain" was defined as pain that lasts for 24 hours or longer. Researchers observed a relationship between Zingiberaceae extracts and

ginger goodness

Ginger comes in a variety of forms, including fresh, dried, crystallized, and powdered. It's best to use it fresh, advises Charles Lo, MD, a doctor of Chinese medicine in private practice in Chicago. "Fresh ginger is more active than dried," he says. To find the freshest ginger and get the most healing compounds, shop for ginger that looks healthy. "Avoid ginger with soft spots, mold, or dry, wrinkled skin," Dr. Lo advises.

Make a ginger marinade for meats. Mix fresh ginger, minced garlic, olive oil, and light soy sauce for a marinade for chicken, beef, or fish, says Janet Maccaro, PhD, ND, a holistic nutritionist in Ormond Beach, Florida. "They use ginger for a marinade in Japan, and it's a wonderful way to get the health benefits," she says.

pain relief: Higher doses gave better pain relief.[38]

- A metareview of oral ginger as a treatment for osteoarthritis found that ginger consumption produced a significant reduction in pain and disability. And compared to a placebo, patients given ginger were more than twice as likely to discontinue treatment for osteoarthritis.[39]

- In vitro studies have shown ginger's anticancer power against colorectal, prostate, skin, cervical, gastrointestinal, pancreatic, breast, and non-small cell lung cancers, among others.[40]

- Type 2 diabetes patients who received 2 g a day of ginger powder for 12 weeks experienced significantly improved fasting blood sugar and other positive effects on various indicators of glycemic status and oxidative stress, further highlighting ginger's role in alleviating some of the risk of chronic complications in diabetes.[41]

- Another study found that type 2 diabetics who consumed three 1 g capsules of ginger powder daily for 8 weeks experienced a 10.5 percent decrease in fasting blood sugar and improved insulin resistance.[42]

- Ginger has shown beneficial effects on ameliorating heavy menstrual bleeding (HMB). Ninety-two women experiencing HMB were assigned to either a ginger intervention group that took 250 mg capsules three times a day or a placebo over three menstrual cycles. Those in the ginger group experienced a significant reduction in menstrual blood loss.[43]

See also: Turmeric (page 69)

ginseng

There are eleven species of ginseng, and three among them—Korean ginseng, American ginseng, and Chinese ginseng—are most commonly used. The active compounds in ginseng largely responsible for its health benefits are called ginsenosides, and a great deal of recent research focuses on their potential role in treating central nervous system disorders. Ginseng has been used for thousands of years for a variety of health conditions, and it is perhaps best known as a natural means of fighting fatigue, boosting your immune system, and promoting longevity. Ginseng root can be eaten raw or steamed, but it's most often used in its dried form and can be used in a tea or other drinks, eaten in cooked dishes, or taken as a supplement or an extract. It's no surprise that it's been the subject of much research.

In vitro studies have shown that ginsenosides provide direct neuroprotective effects against glutamate and amyloid beta stimulation. In animal models, ginsenosides were observed to reduce the accumulation of amyloid beta. (Glutamate, a nerve cell messenger, can become toxic to neurons at elevated levels, and amyloid beta is implicated in the development of Alzheimer's disease.) Ginseng has also been shown to attenuate chronic neuroinflammation.[44]

A study of 61 patients with Alzheimer's disease found that Korean red ginseng improved cognitive function. The patients were divided into three groups: One took a low dose of ginseng (4.5 g a day), one took a high dose (9 g a day), and one served as a control group. The group taking the low dose of ginseng showed no difference at 12 or 24 weeks compared

herbal essence

To preserve the healing powers of herbs, you have to dry and store them properly. Here's how.

- When drying leaves or flowers, tie small bunches of herbs together, and hang them upside down in a dry, well-ventilated area such as an attic or large pantry. To prevent herbs from getting dusty, hang them inside paper bags with holes punched in the sides to allow air to circulate. Be careful not to crush the herbs, which will cause the precious oils to dissipate.

- When drying roots, cut them into thin pieces, thread them on a length of string, and hang them to dry.

- To dry seeds, hang the entire plant upside down in a hole-punched paper bag, and allow it to dry; as the plant dries, the seeds will fall to the bottom of the bag.

- To keep dried herbs fresh, store them in tightly sealed jars in a cool, dark place. When they are properly stored, dried herbs will retain their potency for a year or more.

to the control group, but the high-dose ginseng group showed a significant improvement in Alzheimer's disease assessment scores and mini mental state examination scores. Maximum improvements were obtained by week 24 and remained steady for 2 years.[45]

- A study of 90 adults with idiopathic chronic fatigue found that a ginseng extract—specifically 1 to 2 g per day of a 20 percent ethanol extract of *Panax ginseng* taken for 4 weeks—improved mental and physical fatigue. Ginseng also significantly lowered serum total reactive oxygen species and malondialdehyde levels (both associated with oxidative stress) and significantly increased the total glutathione (a powerful antioxidant) content and glutathione reductase (the related enzyme) activity compared with the placebo.[46]

- A study found that ginseng can have a positive effect on fatigue associated with multiple sclerosis (MS). MS patients received 250 mg of ginseng or placebo capsules twice a day for 3 months. Those in the ginseng group experienced reduced fatigue and reported better scores on an assessment of quality of life.[47]

licorice

When it comes to licorice, many people think of the black, supersweet candy—it's 50 times as sweet as sugar—but what we're talking about here is the root of the *Glycyrrhiza glabra* plant. Licorice root is indeed used as a sweetener, but its true power lies in the medicinal effects of a compound called glycyrrhizic acid, or just glycyrrhizin. In fact, we'll begin our discussion of licorice with a few contraindications that illustrate the potency of glycyrrhizin: Experts agree that women who are pregnant or breastfeeding should avoid licorice, as should those with heart, liver, or kidney disease; hormone-sensitive cancers; erectile dysfunction; or diabetes. Licorice has the potential to raise blood pressure, decrease potassium levels, and cause salt and water retention. Licorice can interfere with many medications, including blood pressure medications, MAO inhibitors (a common type of antidepressant), ACE inhibitors and diuretics, insulin, oral contraceptives, warfarin (Coumadin), digoxin, and corticosteroids.[48] But don't let these warnings scare you away from occasional use of licorice. The unwanted side effects are more likely to occur with long-term use and/or at very high dosages. There is also a form of licorice from which the glycyrrhizin has been removed, called deglycyrrhizinated licorice (or DGL), that's available as an herbal supplement and has far fewer potential contraindications than the whole food.

Licorice can be consumed in its whole form; many people simply chew the root in order to gain its healing benefits. But it's also available in dried or powdered forms, as an extract, and as a tea. More than 20 triterpenoids and more than 300 flavonoids have been identified in licorice.[49] Let's look at the impressive array of healing effects that licorice confers.

- Licorice has long been used as an herbal remedy for gastrointestinal complaints, and research has shown that it stimulates the production of gastric mucus, lending a protective coating to your esophagus, stomach lining, and any existing ulcers, making your digestive tract more resistant to irritating stomach acid.[50] Licorice is also recommended to relieve the symptoms of GERD (gastroesophageal reflux disease).[51]
- Fifty people experiencing a range of dyspeptic symptoms were divided into two groups, one who took a commercially available extract of *G. glabra* (75 mg) and one who took a placebo twice a day for 30 days.

When assessed at days 15 and 30, those in the *G. glabra* group experienced a significant reduction in symptoms including abdominal pain, belching, bloating, early satiety, nausea, vomiting, regurgitation, heartburn, and loss of appetite.[52]
- Glycyrrhizin exhibits strong liver-protecting effects. It has anti-inflammatory, antiviral, and chemopreventive (cancer-fighting) effects and can inhibit liver cell death and necrosis.[53]
- Licorice displays potent antibacterial, antiviral, and immunoregulatory properties, highlighting its role in treating infectious diseases.[54]

oregano

Oregano is one of the most frequently used herbs in Mediterranean cuisine, and it contains a high concentration of antioxidants.[55] The predominant compounds in oregano are carvacrol and thymol, which have antimicrobial properties and antioxidant effects.[56] Oregano can be consumed fresh or dried, and oregano essential oil is a popular complementary medicine remedy to prevent and treat respiratory infections, treat skin conditions, and fight fungal and bacterial infections.

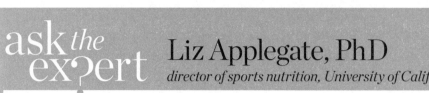

Liz Applegate, PhD

director of sports nutrition, University of California, Davis

Q. What's the number one nutrient you feel people are lacking, and what are the best ways for them to include it in their diets?

A. We don't get enough live bacteria and probiotics. And as far as traditional nutrients, people are not eating enough vitamin D. With some kefirs, which are loaded with probiotics, you get more probiotics for your buck. Most dairy products are also fortified with vitamin D.

Q. What food combinations do you recommend for overall health?

A. The most notable combination is iron and vitamin C. If I see someone has breakfast cereal, I make sure they eat a piece of fruit with that. Iron is better absorbed when it has been exposed to vitamin C.

Q. Have you had a client heal him- or herself with food?

A. I had a patient whose blood cholesterol was creeping up. He was a regular exerciser and he ate fairly well, but he was bothered by his high blood cholesterol. He didn't eat a lot of soluble fiber, which can essentially create a sinkhole for your body's cholesterol. When he finally started eating a serving of beans and oats every other day, his blood cholesterol went down. He's no longer on medication and his blood cholesterol is currently in the healthy range.

Q. Do you recommend sneaking healthy foods into diets? If so, what are some tips?

A. When people frequently eat canned soup, I tell them to add a baggie's worth of chopped spinach or kale in the bowl and microwave it so they also get a serving of greens.

Q. What are your food recommendations for weight loss?

A. The biggest recommendation I can give is to eat foods that are high in fiber and low in calories and to make vegetables fill half your plate. Also, eat on a small plate, and use small utensils so your serving sizes will appear more satisfying.

Q. If we were to go to the grocery store with you, what would we always find in your shopping cart?

A. You'll always find coffee. Two to four cups a day can lower your risk for diabetes, as well as Parkinson's disease. And there are always probiotics and organic, plain kefir. I always have a variety of nuts, and if I didn't have a garden I'd always be buying greens like kale, as well as any seasonal fruit.

Q. Are there any natural home remedies you use?

A. I usually look to ginger tea as a stomach soother, whether I need it because I've had too much garlic at a meal or because I'm stressed at my job.

- In an in vitro study, oregano essential oil was shown to be highly toxic to human colon adenocarcinoma,[57] the most common type of colon cancer.

- Another in vitro study demonstrated oregano oil extract's ability to destroy leukemia cells.[58]

- Yet another in vitro study showed that oregano extract was particularly effective against cervical, lung, and again, leukemia cells.[59]

- Both in vitro and in vivo research have shown that oregano oil is effective at combating many types of fungi, including *Candida albicans*, which is the cause of around 90 percent of yeast infections. The topical application of oregano oil is effective against stubborn nail fungus.[60]

- Greek oregano extract exhibited strong in vitro antibacterial activity against *Staphylococci* bacteria, including the MRSA (methicillin-resistant *Staphylococcus aureus*) strain. Its essential oil exhibited strong antibacterial activity against *Escherichia coli* (*E. coli*), *Salmonella*, and *Klebsiella pneumoniae*.[61]

parsley

Both flat-leaf and curly parsley are among the most popular herbs in the world. Dried and fresh parsley are used in a wide variety of dishes, and it's incredibly easy to grow, especially the flat-leaf variety. Parsley is an excellent source of vitamin K, and it's a good source of vitamins A and C and iron, as well. It has an impressive antioxidant content and is an excellent source of the flavones apigenin and luteolin, which fight inflammation and have been identified as chemopreventive (cancer-fighting) agents. A review of the pharmacological benefits of parsley identified antioxidant, hepatoprotective (liver-protecting), brain protective, antidiabetic, analgesic, spasmolytic (providing smooth muscle spasm relief), immunosuppressant, antiplatelet, gastroprotective, cytoprotective, laxative, estrogenic, diuretic, hypotensive, antibacterial, and antifungal activities caused by this delicious common herb.[62] Clearly, parsley has much going for it on a cellular level.

- Apigenin was shown in an in vitro study to inhibit DNA synthesis and promote cell cycle arrest in breast cancer. Even at a low dose, it demonstrated the potential to prevent and slow breast cancer.[63] In a different study that compared different phytoestrogens, apigenin was found to be the most effective at inhibiting the growth of breast cancer cells, including HER2-positive (active cancer) ones.[64]

■ Parsley essential oil was shown to be highly effective at eradicating *Vibrio* bacteria, which is responsible for many types of foodborne infections.[65]

■ Genins isolated from parsley have been shown to exert potent anti-platelet activity, demonstrating parsley's role in preventing thrombosis (blood clots) and other cardiovascular disease.[66]

rosemary

Rosemary is a woody, evergreen herb with a strong pinelike aroma and taste. Its needle-shaped leaves are used fresh or dried, and though it is very low in traditional vitamins and nutrients, it's packed with powerful phenolic compounds that give it an impressive array of healing effects. The diterpenes in rosemary—in particular carnosic acid, carnosol, and rosmanol—have demonstrated promising anticancer activity.[67] Rosemary has one of the highest antioxidant contents of any herb, and its cognitive-promoting effects have been studied extensively. (In fact, it's long been known as the "herb of remembrance" and has been used as a memory enhancer for centuries.) Research has shown that rosemary can improve circulation, relieve pain, and control blood lipid and antilipid peroxidation, or the creation of damaging free radicals.[68] Its primary phenolic acid is rosmarinic acid, which research has credited with anti-inflammatory, antiviral, antibacterial, antidepressant, anticarcinogenic, and chemopreventive (cancer-fighting) properties.[69]

■ Twenty-eight adults with an average age of 75 took four different

─────── power pairs ───────
rosemary and grilled meats

If you like your meat well-done, you're at higher risk for ingesting cancer-causing compounds. But if you add rosemary to your burgers before you throw them on the grill, the herb can help break up the potent carcinogens that form during the cooking process.[70]

doses of powdered rosemary or a placebo, with a 7-day washout between each course. Interestingly, the lowest dose of rosemary (750 mg) had a positive effect on measures of cognitive performance, while the highest dose (6,000 mg) had a significantly impairing effect. The 750 mg dose is actually closest to the level used in cooking.[71]

- In a study of a number of different herbal extracts, rosemary was found to have the highest antioxidant content and free radical scavenging ability, highlighting its potential as a chemopreventive (cancer-fighting) healing food. When tested in vitro, rosemary extract strongly inhibited the proliferation of cervical cancer cells.[72]

- A metareview found that rosemary is able to suppress the development of tumors in several organs, including the colon, breast, liver, and stomach, as well as melanoma and leukemia cells. Its anticancer effects are thought to be due to its phenolic compounds carnosol, carnosic acid, ursolic acid, and rosmarinic acid.[73] Rosemary extract has also been found to enhance the effects of the conventional breast cancer chemotherapy drugs tamoxifen, trastuzumab, and paclitaxel.[74]

sage

Sage, like basil, is a member of the Lamiaceae family and has been valued since antiquity for its culinary and medicinal uses. Its fresh leaves have a fuzzy texture, and dried sage is more common in cooking; dried sage also has a more potent flavor. In addition to its use as a savory herb, sage is available as a tea, an essential oil, and in supplement form. Both sage and clary sage are common essential oils; they're from the same plant family, but clary sage is a bit milder than common sage. Sage is a good source of vitamin K, and its primary phenolic acid is rosmarinic acid, which has demonstrated a range of powerful health benefits, including anti-inflammatory, antiviral, antibacterial, antidepressant, anticarcinogenic, and chemopreventive (cancer-fighting) properties.[75]

- A study of 22 menopausal women found that inhaling clary sage essential oil lowered cortisol levels and increased serotonin concentrations, resulting in an overall antidepressant-like effect.[76]

- Healthy female volunteers ages 40 to 50 drank 300 ml of sage tea twice a day for 4 weeks.

Researchers found that the sage tea lowered volunteers' LDL and total cholesterol levels, increased HDL cholesterol, and increased antioxidant activity.[77]

■ In another study, 40 patients with type 2 diabetes took a 500 mg capsule of sage leaf extract twice a day for 3 months, while 40 more took a placebo. At the end of the study, those in the sage group experienced reduced fasting glucose, HbA1c, total cholesterol, triglycerides, and LDL cholesterol, as well as increased HDL cholesterol compared to baseline, with no adverse effects.[78]

■ A metareview showed that both common sage and Spanish sage exert beneficial effects on cognitive performance in healthy subjects as well as in patients with dementia or cognitive impairment. The authors of this study acknowledge that its weakness is that it lacks specific detail on the herbal products used— results from studies on whole sage, essential oil, and sage extracts are included in the review—but it still highlights sage's potential role in enhancing memory and other cognitive functions and in treating neurodegenerative illnesses.[79]

thyme

Thyme is a member of the mint family, and like basil and rosemary, its primary phenolic acid is cancer-fighting rosmarinic acid. It exhibits very high antioxidant activity all around, due to the presence of polyphenols such as rosmarinic acid, gallic acid, caffeic acid, luteolin, and chlorogenic acid. Rich in vitamin K and vitamin C, thyme is used fresh or dried in cooking, as an effective ingredient in cough syrups, and as an herbal tea ingredient. It's also highly valued as an essential oil with antioxidant and antimicrobial properties.

■ In a recent in vitro study, thyme extract was shown to inhibit the proliferation, adhesion, migration, and invasion of human colorectal cancer cells.[80]

■ Thyme extract is a powerful anti-inflammatory. It's able to work on a cellular level to inhibit nuclear factor-kappa beta, interleukin-6 release, nitric oxide release, COX-1 activity, and COX-2 activity—all of which play a role in inflammation and pain.[81]

■ Thyme essential oil (topically applied) is arguably the best essential oil for treating stubborn nail fungus (onychomycosis) due to its high concentrations of thymol and carvacrol, which work synergistically to exert potent antifungal effects.[82]

turmeric

Turmeric (*Curcuma longa*), the mildly spicy root that's common in South Asian cuisine, has demonstrated so many healing effects that we highly recommend you add this superfood to your diet this very day. Turmeric is available fresh, dried, and as a supplement, and it's used to make herbal tea. A famous drink called "golden milk" is actually a tealike beverage traditionally made with turmeric and coconut milk and/or coconut oil and sometimes other spices, such as cinnamon or ginger. One extremely helpful tip when using turmeric is to combine it with black pepper to increase its healing effects: Black pepper increases the bioavailability of curcumin, its active compound, by up to 2,000 percent.[83]

Turmeric, a member of the ginger family (Zingiberaceae), has been used for thousands of years to treat conditions including but not limited to: bacterial, viral, fungal, and parasitic infections; inflammation of any type;

menstrual problems; cancer; overweight and obesity; depression; acute or chronic pain; diabetes; arthritis; indigestion; high cholesterol; inflammatory bowel disease; blood clots; diarrhea; liver problems; flatulence; fibromyalgia; neurological disorders; pancreatitis; asthma; bronchitis; cardiovascular disease; chronic kidney disease; swelling and water retention; psoriasis; and even leprosy.[84] The active component in turmeric that gets the lion's share of the credit for its healing effects (and that supplies its bright yellow pigment) is curcumin. Many thousands of clinical trials have been conducted on curcumin and have confirmed its astonishing healing powers. The following is but a brief survey of the latest research on turmeric, one of our most powerful superfoods.

- Both in vitro and in vivo studies have demonstrated curcumin's clinical therapeutic potential as an anticancer agent. Among the cancers that responded positively to curcumin are colorectal, liver, oral, pancreatic, lung, breast, uterine, cervical, thymic, ovarian, prostate, bladder, kidney, renal, brain, gastric, head and neck, non-Hodgkin's lymphoma, and leukemia.[85]

- In an 8-week study of 117 patients with metabolic syndrome, 59 were assigned a daily dose of curcuminoids (1 g) combined with 10 mg of piperine (black pepper) to enhance bioavailability, while 58 were assigned a placebo. Those in the experimental group experienced significantly improved superoxide dismutase (SOD) activities and significantly reduced concentrations of malondialdehyde (MDA) and C-reactive protein, indicating significantly improved oxidative and inflammatory status.[86]

- Both in vitro and in vivo studies have demonstrated curcumin's efficacy at preventing the development of cataracts; with its strong antioxidant properties, it's able to scavenge the free radicals responsible for cataractogenesis.[87]

- A study of patients with type 2 diabetes found that curcumin significantly reduced pulse wave velocity, increased levels of serum adiponectin, and decreased levels of leptin, thus lowering their overall atherogenic risk. Participants took three 250 mg capsules of curcumin per day (or a placebo) for 6 months.[88]

- Patients with rheumatoid arthritis were divided into three groups: one received 500 mg of curcumin, one received 50 mg of diclofenac sodium (an NSAID), and one received a combination of the two. While all patients showed changes in their Disease Activity Scores (DAS), the curcumin-only group showed the highest percentage of improvement in the DAS as well as in an assessment that evaluated tenderness and swelling of joints—and with zero adverse effects.[89]

- Though more research is needed, in vitro studies have shown that amyloid beta metabolism, which plays a role in the development of Alzheimer's disease (AD), is positively altered by curcumin, and animal studies have shown that curcumin may influence brain function and the development of dementia because of its antioxidant and anti-inflammatory properties, as well as its ability to influence amyloid beta metabolism. Researchers are hopeful that if curcumin interventions are begun early—in those with early AD or even in those with no cognitive impairment—they can be a powerful therapy for preventing Alzheimer's.[90]

- The topical application of turmeric paste is a traditional way to treat wounds. Curcumin has been shown to speed wound healing by enhancing granulation tissue formation, collagen deposition, tissue remodeling, and wound contraction. Further, its antimicrobial effects ward off infection.[91]

■ A meta-analysis of curcumin's effect on patients with major depressive disorder found that curcumin therapy was able to produce a significant reduction in depressive symptoms. Subgroup analyses revealed that curcumin was most effective in middle-aged patients, when given at higher doses, and when given for longer durations.[90]

See also: Black Pepper (page 52), Ginger (page 58)

almonds

Almonds are a great source of monounsaturated fats (MUFAs), fiber, protein, phosphorous, vitamin E, magnesium, copper, and manganese. An ounce and a half of almonds provides nearly 75 percent of the daily value of vitamin E recommended for adults.[1] They've been shown to reduce cardiovascular disease risk by lowering LDL ("bad") and total cholesterol, reducing inflammation, regulating glucose, and exerting an antioxidant effect. The benefits don't stop there.

- Eating almonds increases oleic acid and MUFA levels, both of which are known to reduce coronary heart disease (CHD) lipid risk factors. In a study of hyperlipidemic subjects, almond intake was found to reduce CHD risk scores, increase HDL ("good") cholesterol, and decrease the overall estimated 10-year CHD risk.[2]

- MUFA- and antioxidant-rich almonds have been shown to improve oxidative status, both in the short term and after long-term consumption.[3] Reducing the effects of oxidative stress on cells helps decrease your risk of inflammatory-related conditions, some types of cancers, and premature aging.

- Previous studies have shown that almonds decrease LDL cholesterol, so researchers designed a study to determine the effect of almonds on the total lipid profile in adults on statin therapy. One group ate 100 grams (g) of almonds a day, while a control group ate no almonds. At the end of

---

power pairs

almonds and kefir

Kefir is the new yogurt, according to scientists. Like yogurt, this dairy product provides your gut with tons of beneficial bacteria and probiotics. To give the friendly bacteria a boost, add some chopped almonds to a bowl of kefir. Research shows that the fiber in almond skin acts as a prebiotic, which feeds the probiotics found in kefir, helping them keep your gut happy and healthy.[4]

4 weeks, though the almond group ate significantly more calories, they experienced a 4.9 percent reduction in non-HDL cholesterol, while the control group experienced a 3.5 percent increase in non-HDL cholesterol. The almond group also experienced improvements in LDL cholesterol and triglyceride levels, though the improvements were not statistically significant.[5]

brazil nuts

Brazil nuts are our richest food source of selenium. Selenium is a trace element that works like an antioxidant, and it plays an important role in cognition and the healthy functioning of your thyroid, immune system, and reproductive system. One ounce of Brazil nuts, which is equivalent to six to eight nuts, provides 777 percent of your daily recommended value of selenium.[6] Brazil nuts are also rich in copper, magnesium, manganese, and phosphorous, and they're a good source of fiber and thiamin. Here's further reason to add them to your diet.

- In dialysis patients, supplementing the diet with just one Brazil nut a day for 3 months was shown to reduce oxidative stress and inflammation. When researchers followed up with the subjects after 12 months, they found that some, but not all, of the benefits were attenuated—and that resuming consumption of just one Brazil nut a day could easily improve their antioxidant status.[7]

- Another study showed that Brazil nuts can quickly improve your lipid profile. Each subject was tested four times, in response to 0, 5, 20, or 50 g of Brazil nuts and at different times after consumption. Volunteers experienced an increase in selenium levels 6 hours after consumption and lower LDL cholesterol and higher HDL cholesterol levels 9 hours after consuming 20 or 50 g of Brazil nuts.[8]

peanuts

Peanuts may well take the prize for America's most popular nut . . . even though they're actually legumes. Yes, this protein-packed food is eaten, prepared, and marketed much like tree nuts are, though it grows in the ground and is closely related to other legumes, such as peas and beans. Here, we're taking the most common usage—not to mention a cue from their name—and grouping peanuts with true nuts.

Regardless of how you categorize them, peanuts are eaten in their whole form, ground as the source of our most popular nut butter, and pressed for their oil, which research has shown to have cardioprotective and anti-inflammatory properties.[9] Peanut flour can be used as a gluten-free alternative, and peanuts make a nice lactose-free nut milk. And while true tree nuts such as almonds and walnuts tend to be pricey, peanuts are a more affordable alternative. This is great news because it turns out peanuts boast an array of health benefits. Peanuts are high in calories and fat but contain little saturated fat and no cholesterol. They're also high in protein, niacin, and manganese and are one of our best sources of biotin, which is necessary for cell growth and metabolism. Additionally, peanuts are a good source of folate, magnesium, phosphorous, arginine, and copper. They also contain two important phytonutrients, resveratrol and phytosterols. Resveratrol (found in even larger amounts in red wine and grapes), is an anti-inflammatory, anti-cancer, and heart-healthy antioxidant, and phytosterols have a cholesterol-lowering effect. And there's more good news.

- A recent cohort study and meta-analysis found that tree nut and peanut consumption was linked to lower mortality. This conclusion was based upon 120,852 men and women ages 55 to 69 who were followed for 10 years. Researchers found that total tree nut and peanut consumption was related to lower overall and cause-specific (cancer, diabetes, cardiovascular, respiratory, neurodegenerative diseases, etc.) mortality. Interestingly, peanut butter did not exhibit this protective effect.[10]

- Another study that examined the relationship between nuts and mortality—this one based on just over 206,000 subjects—also found that nut consumption was associated with lower overall mortality and cardiovascular disease mortality. Peanuts figured heavily in this study, and the researchers pointed out that with their affordability, eating peanuts can be considered a cost-effective measure to improve cardiovascular health.[11]

- Peanut skins have proven to be a rich source of cardiovascular-protective proanthocyanidins, consisting mostly of a subtype called procyanidins. Peanut procyanidins have a natural hypolipidemic, or lipid-lowering, effect.[12]

pecans

Pecans are rich in manganese and are a good source of protein, fiber, copper, vitamin E, and thiamin. They're also rich in both polyunsaturated and mono-unsaturated fats,[13] both of which have been shown to reduce cholesterol and decrease your risk of heart disease and type 2 diabetes. The fruit, leaves, and shells of pecans are used for medicinal purposes; pecans are known for their antihyperglycemic and antihyperlipid-emic effects[14] and certainly warrant further research.

■ Pecan consumption has been shown to increase antioxidant biomarkers and to decrease oxidized LDL and the ratio of malondialdehyde (a bio-marker of oxidative stress) to tri-glycerides.[15]

■ Pecan shell extracts are used as antimicrobials[16] and to treat various toxicological diseases. An analysis of the aqueous extract of pecan shells revealed a high content of total poly-phenols, condensed tannins, and antioxidant capacity, as well as the ability to inhibit iron-induced lipid peroxidation in vitro, highlighting pecan shells' efficacy in protecting your liver.[17]

pistachios

Pistachios are members of the cashew family and are distinctive among nuts because they have a grassy green color due to the presence of chlorophyll. But that's not all that distinguishes them: Compared to other nuts, pistachios have a lower fat and calorie count and the highest levels of vitamin E, vitamin K, vitamin B_6, phytosterols, xanthophyll carotenoids, potassium, copper, iron, magnesium, and thiamin.[18] Pistachios are also a good source of protein, fiber, phosphorus, and manganese. Research shows that pistachios exert anti-inflammatory activity and improve endothelial function. Adding pistachios to a high-glycemic meal can lower the overall postprandial glycemic response.[19] As the research shows, there are additional blood sugar (and blood pressure) management advantages.

■ In a 24-week study of 60 adults with metabolic syndrome, the half who ate daily unsalted pistachios equiva-lent to 20 percent of improvements in waist circumference, fasting blood glucose levels, total cholesterol, LDL cholesterol, high sensitivity C-reactive protein and tumor necro-sis factor alpha (both markers of inflammation), free fatty acids, thio-barbituric acid reactive substances (by-products of lipid peroxidation), and adiponectin levels.[20]

■ In a study on the effect of pistachios in diabetic patients, those who

super-charge your meals

If you're a big pistachio fan but are tired of eating them the same way every day, we have a delicious solution for you. Swap them in for the pine nuts when you are making homemade pesto. In addition to adding a burst of green color, you'll be getting an extra dose of vitamins as well.

consumed 25 g of pistachios twice a day as a snack experienced a significant decrease in HbA1c and fasting blood glucose concentrations. Pistachio consumption also decreased systolic blood pressure, BMI, and C-reactive protein levels.[21]

- A large metastudy on the effects of tree nuts, soy nuts, and peanuts on blood pressure found that nut consumption leads to a significant decrease in blood pressure in those with diabetes. Pistachios had the strongest effect, and they were found to lower both systolic and diastolic blood pressure.[22]

- Pistachios may also help to keep those with prediabetes from developing type 2 diabetes. In a crossover trial, 54 prediabetic subjects consumed two diets, each for 4 months: a pistachio-supplemented diet (57 g per day) or a control diet. After the pistachio diet, the subjects' metabolic profiles improved on a variety of parameters: Fasting glucose, insulin, insulin resistance, fibrinogen (a protein that

helps form blood clots), oxidized LDL cholesterol, and platelet factor 4 (a cytokine involved in blood coagulation) all significantly decreased.[23]

walnuts

Walnuts have been extensively researched for their health-promoting benefits, and studies have confirmed their ability to fight cancer, support cardiovascular health, prevent overweight and obesity, prevent metabolic-related illnesses (especially diabetes), support brain health, and decrease inflammation. Walnuts and walnut oil are also two of the best vegetarian sources of heart-healthy omega-3 fatty acids, and they're also good sources of copper, protein, fiber, melatonin, and manganese. And among a variety of other nuts, walnuts are the best in class when it comes to polyphenol antioxidant content.[24] Adding walnuts to your diet, research shows, can potentially turn back the clock.

- Walnuts have been shown to decrease LDL cholesterol by as much as 16 percent, lower diastolic blood pressure by as much as 3 mmHg, lower triglycerides, improve endothelial function, decrease oxidative stress and some markers of inflammation, and increase the excretion of cholesterol,[25] making them a super-food for cardiovascular health.

- The antioxidant-rich Mediterranean diet was shown to enhance cognitive function in the elderly, and walnuts in particular were associated with better working memory.[26]

- A study of 46 overweight adults with visceral adiposity (abdominal fat) and one or more signs of metabolic syndrome found that daily consumption of 56 g of walnuts improved endothelial function, reduced blood pressure, and did not lead to weight gain over the 8-week study period.[27]

- A study of 40 healthy subjects found that 8 weeks of a walnut-enriched diet (43 g per day) resulted in decreased non-HDL cholesterol and apolipoprotein B, the main protein constituent in LDL cholesterol.[28]

- Alpha-linolenic acid, an anti-inflammatory omega-3 fatty acid found in abundance in walnuts, has been shown to inhibit cell proliferation in breast, colon, bladder, and prostate cancer cells.[29]

extra-virgin olive oil (evoo)

Extra-virgin olive oil is an unrefined oil and is of the highest quality of any type of olive oil. The "extra-virgin" refers to the processing, or in this case, the *lack* of processing, as extra-virgin olive oil is produced simply by pressing the olives. An integral part of the heart-healthy Mediterranean diet and rich in beneficial monounsaturated fats, EVOO is used for cooking, as a salad dressing, for drizzling atop dishes, and as a dip. Olive oil polyphenols have a powerful antioxidant effect, and olive oil's inflammation-fighting power is well documented. As a healing food, EVOO is at the top of its class, with proven benefits for cardiovascular health, neurological health, bone health, metabolic health, and skin health. It has demonstrated an anticancer effect and may even play a role in protecting against depression. EVOO has been the subject of tens of thousands of clinical trials and research studies; the following is but a representative list of some of the latest research on this delicious superfood.

- A 22-year study of more than 145,000 women found that EVOO helped protect against type 2 diabetes (T2D). Substituting olive oil (8 g per day) for margarine, butter, or mayonnaise was associated with a 5, 8, and 15 percent lower risk of T2D, respectively.[1]

- Oleocanthal, a phenolic compound found in EVOO, was shown in an in vitro study to induce cell death in cancer cells as rapidly as half an hour after administration—and

power pairs

leafy greens and olive oil

Who says fat is the enemy? Research has found that pairing vegetables with a source of healthy fat enhances absorption of nutrients and antioxidants,[2] meaning you get more bang for your buck. Drizzle olive oil over your salad to ensure that no nutrient gets left behind.

A long list of health benefits is associated with apple cider vinegar, but how to incorporate it into your healthy diet? Start small by swapping balsamic for apple cider vinegar when making homemade oil and vinegar salad dressing.

without being toxic to noncancerous cells. In this particular study, the types of cancer studied were pancreatic, prostate, and breast.[3]

- A small (18 participants) but fascinating study that compared a diet rich in butter to a diet rich in EVOO revealed that the butter-rich diet increased cardiovascular risk while the EVOO diet decreased the risk of metabolic syndrome and coronary heart disease. Study participants followed each of the diets for 28 days. The butter-rich diet increased cardiovascular disease risk in 77.8 percent of the patients, but in 61.1 percent of the patients, the risk decreased after switching to the EVOO diet. This study demonstrates how harmful even *1* month of a diet high in saturated fat can be.[4]

- A study of 7,216 people ages 55 to 80 at high risk of cardiovascular disease assessed the association between intake of olive oil and cardiovascular disease and mortality. Participants were randomized to one of three diets—the Mediterranean

plus additional olive oil, the Mediterranean plus nuts, or a low-fat diet—and were followed for an average of 4.8 years. The results were striking: (1) Participants who consumed the highest amounts of regular olive oil and extra-virgin olive oil experienced a 35 percent and 39 percent cardiovascular disease risk reduction, respectively. (2) Higher baseline total olive oil consumption was associated with a 48 percent reduced risk of cardiovascular mortality. (3) For each 10 gram-a-day increase in EVOO consumption, cardiovascular disease risk decreased by 10 percent, and cardiovascular mortality risk decreased by 7 percent. (4) There were no significant associations observed between cardiovascular events and the low-fat diet group. Extra-virgin olive oil intake had the strongest protective effect of any of the interventions against cardiovascular disease risk and mortality.[5]

- A 1-year study of women with moderate hypertension found that the Mediterranean diet supplemented with

olive oil by the grade

Some olive oils are quite rare and exquisitely flavored—and exquisitely priced. Others are much more affordable and, of course, the flavors reflect that. Many cooks keep two (or more) kinds of olive oil in the kitchen—a gourmet oil for drizzling on salads or pastas and a heartier oil to use for cooking.

- **EXTRA-VIRGIN** is the Cadillac of olive oils. It's usually used as flavoring oil and not for cooking. When buying extra-virgin olive oil, look at the color. The deeper the color, the more intense the olive flavor is.

- **PURE (ALSO CALLED VIRGIN) OLIVE OIL** is paler than extra-virgin and has a milder flavor. It's usually used for low- to medium-heat frying.

- **LIGHT OLIVE OIL** is often used by people who want the heart-healthy benefits of monounsaturated fats but don't want the strong olive taste. It stands up to heat well, so you can use it for light frying.

EVOO resulted in lower systolic and diastolic blood pressure and improved endothelial function.[6]

- Adhering to the Mediterranean diet, which relies on EVOO as its main source of fat, has long been known to protect against cognitive decline associated with aging. Now new research is revealing the power of EVOO's phenolic compounds to prevent the progression of Alzheimer's disease by counteracting amyloid aggregation and toxicity.[7]

- Numerous studies have noted that rates of osteoporosis are significantly lower in regions where olive oil is regularly consumed. New research helps explain why: Olive oil is very high in oleoyl serine, a lipid that stimulates bone formation and prevents bone resorption.[8]

- Pairing olive oil with tomatoes appears to increase the bioavailability of the lycopene in tomatoes. Volunteers drank either tomato juice with 10 percent olive oil or plain tomato juice. Lycopene isomers increased significantly in subjects consuming tomato juice with oil. Subjects' LDL and total cholesterol decreased significantly within 6 hours.[9] This synergistic effect of two major ingredients of the Mediterranean diet provides another angle on why this diet is so beneficial to your health.

flaxseed oil

Flaxseed oil (also known as linseed oil), is an ancient oil that was once virtually unheard of in American kitchens, but it has become a popular ingredient in salad dressings and smoothies these days. Some people stir flaxseed oil into yogurt, and though it's probably the least-tasty option, some eat a tablespoon of flaxseed oil straight up, especially to treat constipation. Flaxseed oil is better used as an ingredient rather than as a cooking oil, as it's easily oxidized by heat, and it should be refrigerated after opening, as heat, light, and air can cause it to spoil quickly. Cold-pressed flaxseed oil sold in an opaque container is recommended because it has been exposed to minimal heat during the extraction process and its packaging has protected it from light damage.

Besides having a delightful nutty flavor, flaxseed oil has a high concentration of alpha-linolenic acid (ALA), an omega-3 acid that has demonstrated a wide range of health benefits.

- Many studies have shown that ALA is associated with a decreased risk of cardiovascular disease. It's thought to exert its cardioprotective effects by reducing plaque calcification; lowering lipids; maintaining endothelial function; and exhibiting anti-thrombotic, antiarrhythmic, and anti-inflammatory effects.[10]

- Flaxseed oil consumption has been shown to lower LDL ("bad") cholesterol, particularly in those with high triglyceride levels.[11] It has also been shown to increase HDL ("good") cholesterol and to lower total cholesterol, suggesting that flaxseed oil has a positive effect on your lipid profile generally.[12]

- Flaxseed oil consumption has also been shown to improve the condition of your skin. In a study of healthy volunteers, daily supplementation with flaxseed oil led to decreased skin sensitivity, transepidermal water loss, roughness, and scaling and increased skin hydration and smoothness.[13]

See also: Flaxseeds (page 93)

red palm oil

Red palm oil has been used for thousands of years, but it's really just beginning to gain wide acclaim in the United States. Derived from the fruit of the oil

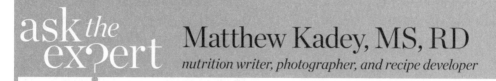
Q. What's the number one nutrient you feel people are lacking, and what are the best ways for them to include it in their diets?

A. A big one is vitamin D. Some great sources are fatty fish like salmon, sardines, mackerel, and herring. But people rarely eat enough of these fish. I personally love stinky swimmers and always seem to have some smoked mackerel or pickled herring on hand.

Q. What food combinations do you recommend for overall health?

A. I am a big proponent of eating your vegetables with some healthy fat, such as olive oil, avocado, or nuts. The fat will increase your absorption of fat-soluble antioxidants like beta-carotene and lycopene, which are present in colorful veggies.

Q. Do you recommend sneaking healthy foods into diets? If so, how?

A. Smoothies are a great way to sneak in all sorts of body-friendly items such as leafy greens, avocado, spices, and flaxseed. And I also look for ways to work vegetables into more than salads. For example, grated carrot can be a standout addition to a pot of simmering steel-cut oats, and you can work pureed beets into chocolate baked goods. I'll also swap out half of the ground beef in recipes like pasta sauce and tacos for meaty mushrooms, as studies show that this is a great way to improve nutrition and even flavor.

Q. What are your food recommendations for weight loss?

A. For me, it mostly comes down to eating predominately uncompromised whole foods like fruits, vegetables, whole grains, nuts, and fish—foods that contain just one ingredient. I believe these are the most conducive to achieving and maintaining weight loss.

Q. What are the top 5 to 10 foods everyone should be eating?

A. First, dark, leafy greens. Also, fatty, omega-3-rich and sustainable fish—wild

palm tree, it gets its reddish hue from its high levels of carotenoids, including alpha-carotene, beta-carotene, and lycopene. Red palm oil has been used as a supplement to boost blood levels of vitamin A and beta-carotene.[14] You should use only the unrefined form of red palm oil, as the refining process strips away many of its health-promoting compounds. Despite having a high saturated fat content (50 percent), red palm oil has not been found to promote cardiovascu-

salmon, sardines, and sablefish. Fermented foods such as yogurt, kefir, and sauerkraut are also essential, as are berries (such as blueberries and raspberries), avocados, nuts, and whole grains (such as teff, quinoa, steel-cut oats, and spelt).

Q. What are the top 5 to 10 foods everyone should be avoiding?

A. That's easy: sweetened drinks, highly processed meats, sugary boxed cereals, refined grains (such as white bread and white pasta), and store-bought baked goods. It's okay to make your own.

Q. What are the top foods for people in their thirties?

A. Sorry, I don't really believe foods should differ that much based on what decade you were born in. Whole, unprocessed foods are the way to go regardless of your age. Of course, a woman in her thirties will need to worry more about consuming iron (from beef, teff, or legumes) than a woman in her seventies. It's best if people meet with a nutrition professional to determine their individual needs.

Q. If we were to go to the grocery store with you, what would we always find in your shopping cart?

A. Well, being a professional recipe developer, that all depends on what recipe feature I am working on. So if it is a feature on plant protein, you'll see my cart loaded with items like beans and hemp seeds.

Truth be told, I try to do most of my personal shopping at farmers' markets, where I can get better prices and higher quality fruits, veggies, and meats.

Q. What's your favorite indulgence?

A. Nut butter and dark chocolate— separate or served together.

Q. What's your favorite grab-and-go snack?

A. I've become a big fan of roasted chickpeas—great crunch and plenty of satiating fiber.

lar disease, probably because of its high concentration of antioxidants, including the above-mentioned carotenoids, as well as tocotrienols, tocopherols, and vitamin E, and its ratio of saturated to unsaturated fat.[15] All of these wonderful nutrients and vitamins translate into wonderful health benefits.

- Palmitic acid, the main saturated fat in palm oil, has cardioprotective and antihypertensive effects. Palm oil's vitamin E tocotrienols are powerful antioxidants that inhibit cholesterol synthesis, as well.[16]

- Red palm oil has been shown to lower cholesterol, reduce your risk of arterial thrombosis and/or atherosclerosis, inhibit platelet aggregation, reduce oxidative stress, and lower blood pressure.[17]
- Red palm oil phenolics have been shown to exert anticarcinogenic activities in various cancer types, including breast, colon, lung, pancreatic, prostate, and skin cancers.[18]

virgin coconut oil (vco)

A growing body of evidence suggests that virgin coconut oil (VCO) can play a role in reducing your risk of cardiovascular disease. As opposed to conventional coconut oil, virgin coconut oil is obtained from the fresh, mature kernel of coconut and is not subjected to a chemical refining process; this preserves the vitamins, minerals, and antioxidants that would otherwise be stripped away. VCO is a rich source of medium-chain fatty acids (MCFAs), which are rapidly absorbed in your intestine and thus do not negatively impact cholesterol levels, but which do provide an easily metabolized source of energy. VCO's phenolic content is higher than that of regular coconut oil, and with its abundance of antioxidant and anti-inflammatory effects, it helps to prevent the progression of atherosclerosis. There is also evidence that virgin coconut oil helps prevent platelet aggregation.[19] But there are even more reasons to add virgin coconut oil to your diet.

- A recent study examined the effects of extra-virgin coconut oil in 116 adults with coronary artery disease. For the first 3 months of the trial, subjects received the same nutritional treatment. During the next 3-month span, subjects were divided into two groups: a diet group and a diet plus 13 milliliters (ml) of extra-virgin coconut oil a day group. While all of the subjects experienced a reduction in BMI, waist circumference, body weight, and glycemic profile after the first 3 months of the study, the people who consumed extra-virgin coconut oil maintained their improvements and exhibited a greater reduction in waist circumference, as well as improved HDL cholesterol levels.[20]
- Virgin coconut oil has also been used to enhance the quality of life of and to relieve chemotherapy side effects in women with breast cancer. In a study of women with stage

III or IV breast cancer, 30 women were given 10 ml of virgin coconut oil twice a day after 1 week of each chemotherapy cycle from the third until the sixth cycle. A control group of 30 women did not receive coconut oil throughout their chemotherapy. At the end of the study, the coconut oil group had less fatigue, fewer breathing difficulties, fewer sleep difficulties, and less loss of appetite compared to the control group. They also exhibited improvements in breast functioning and symptom scores for body image, sexual function, future perspective, breast symptoms, and systemic chemotherapy side effects, resulting in higher scores in assessments of overall functioning and quality of life.[21]

■ A study that was just released demonstrates coconut oil's efficacy in combating the most common fungal pathogen, *Candida albicans*. Researchers fed mice who'd been colonized by *C. albicans* beef tallow, soybean oil, or coconut oil. Not only did coconut oil reduce colonization, it also altered the metabolic programming of *C. albicans* cells, and the effect was present even when the diet also contained beef tallow. Researchers believe their findings could pave the way for coconut oil to become the first dietary intervention to reduce *C. albicans* colonization in humans. This is good news indeed, considering that this is a fungal pathogen whose mortality rate can reach 40 percent when infection becomes systemic.[22]

seafood and fish

oysters

One of the main health benefits of oysters is their high zinc content: They contain more zinc per serving than any other food.[1] Zinc is crucial for healthy immune system function, and it plays a key role in wound healing. But oysters are also a high-potency source of copper and vitamin B_{12}, rich in iron, and a good source of protein, omega-3s, vitamin C, calcium, and manganese. Even with this high nutritional profile, they're a low-calorie, low-cholesterol, low-fat food.

Both farmed and wild oysters are approved by the Monterey Bay Aquarium Seafood Watch, which monitors seafood supply and recommends sustainable seafood and fish sources, though farmed oysters are in more abundant supply.[2] Oysters can be eaten raw or cooked; interestingly, cooking oysters appears to reduce their allergenicity.[3] Here are a few more reasons to eat oysters.

freshness check

Shellfish are extremely perishable. Even when properly stored, they stay fresh for only a day or two. In addition, they cook very quickly. The difference between "just right" and "yuck" is often measured in minutes—or less. Here are a few tips to have the freshest catch every time.

- BUY THEM LIVE. Since shellfish go bad so quickly, it's best to buy them alive and cook them the same day. To keep them fresh after bringing them home from the store, be sure to store them in the refrigerator until you're ready to start cooking.
- CHECK FOR DONENESS. Few foods are less appetizing than undercooked shellfish. Lobsters and crabs turn bright red when they're done, usually in about 15 to 20 minutes. Clams, mussels, and oysters are nearly done when the shells open. Letting them cook for another 5 minutes will finish the job.

- The recommended daily value of zinc for adult males is 11 milligrams (mg) and 8 mg for adult females. Pregnant and lactating women should consume 11 and 12 mg of zinc per day, respectively.[4] A 3-ounce serving of canned oysters contains more than 77 mg of zinc, 3 ounces of wild oysters cooked with moist heat contain nearly 67 mg, and six medium raw oysters (about the same weight) contain 33 mg of zinc.[5]

- A meta-analysis of studies on zinc intake based on approximately 400,000 participants found that higher zinc intake was associated with a reduced risk of colorectal cancer.[6]

- A natural phenolic antioxidant called 3,5-dihydroxy-4-methoxybenzyl alcohol (DHMBA), sourced from Pacific oysters, was found to protect liver cells from cell death caused by oxidative stress.[7]

salmon

Salmon is the perennial spotlight stealer when it comes to a fish source of healthy omega-3 fatty acids. Salmon is a favorite in American diets, and it boasts very high levels of protein, selenium, riboflavin, niacin, vitamin D, vitamin B_3, and vitamin B_{12}, and it is a good source of vitamin B_6, pantothenic acid, iodine, phosphorous, potassium, and thiamin, as well. And yes, it's chock-full of those omega-3s: Along with wild herring and wild mackerel, wild-caught salmon contains more than 1,500 mg of omega-3s per 3-ounce serving. (By comparison, oysters, mussels, and canned tuna and sardines contain anywhere from 500 to 1,000 mg per 3-ounce serving, while the same serving size of shrimp, lobster, or tilapia contains fewer than 200 mg of omega-3s.)[8] Alaskan salmon is approved by the Monterey Bay Aquarium Seafood Watch, which monitors seafood supply and recommends sustainable seafood and fish sources.[9] The health benefits of omega-3 polyunsaturated fatty acids (PUFAs) are legion, and they include—but aren't limited to—cardiovascular protection, protection of joints and cartilage, improved mood, improved cognition, attenuated age-related neurodegeneration, less inflammation, decreased risk of macular degeneration and dry eye, lower risk of cancer, lower blood triglycerides, attenuation of ADHD symptoms, and benefits to skin health. To gain cardiovascular and other benefits of seafood-derived omega-3s, the American Heart Association (AHA) recommends eating at least two 3.5-ounce servings of fish per week, preferably oily/fatty fish such as salmon, herring, and mackerel.[10] Further, the AHA

salmon and tomatoes

Whoever said eating protein-rich foods was the key to strong muscles clearly hasn't put tomato sauce on their salmon. The phytochemicals in tomatoes and the omega-3 fatty acids in salmon are a strength-inducing dynamic duo. When ingested together, they work to stimulate muscle proteins, increasing your lean muscle mass and giving you arms to envy.[11]

recommends one serving of fish per day for those with coronary heart disease.[12] This research would motivate anyone to eat the recommended amount.

- Dietary omega-3 PUFAs have been shown to decrease neuroinflammation, reduce the oxidative stress responses that occur with age and neurodegenerative diseases, and improve cognitive performance.[13] A recent meta-analysis found that a greater consumption of fish was associated with a 35 percent lower risk of Alzheimer's disease. Every 100 g increase in fish consumption per week was associated with an 11 percent lower risk of Alzheimer's.[14]

- Vitamin B$_{12}$ and fish oil—both in abundant supply in salmon—have been shown to work synergistically to lower blood homocysteine concentrations.[15] Elevated homocysteine levels are associated with an increased risk of cardiovascular disease.

- Omega-3 fatty acids have been shown to significantly reduce the risk of sudden death caused by cardiac arrhythmias and all-cause mortality in patients with coronary heart disease. Omega-3 fatty acids are also used to treat hyperlipidemia and hypertension, two major risk factors in cardiovascular disease.[16]

- Omega-3s and the carotenoids lutein and zeaxanthin, which are all found in salmon, have been linked with a reduced risk of age-related macular degeneration.[17]

- Proteoglycans (a type of protein) sourced from salmon cartilage were shown to speed wound healing by stimulating cell proliferation and cell migration.[18]

- Omega-3 fatty acids have been shown to be an effective nutritional therapy for nonalcoholic fatty liver disease, and oily fish such as salmon are among the best exclusive sources of omega-3s (i.e., salmon does not contain omega-6s).[19]

sardines

Sardines are very rich in vitamin B_{12}—a 3-ounce serving contains more than 300 percent of the recommended daily value! They're also a good source of protein, phosphorous, selenium, vitamin D, and omega-3 fatty acids. According to the Monterey Bay Aquarium Seafood Watch, wild-caught Pacific sardines caught off the coast of the United States or Canada are the most sustainable.[20] Little fish have big benefits.

■ Vitamin B_{12} deficiency is associated with Alzheimer's disease, dementia, Parkinson's disease, and overall cognitive impairment.[21] Sardines, with their high levels of vitamin B_{12}

the freshness test

While fresh fish delivers some of the most delicate flavors imaginable, it goes bad in a hurry. One day may be all it takes to turn a beautiful, flavorful fish into a dish you'd rather forget. To get the best taste from fish every time, here's what you can do.

■ FOLLOW YOUR NOSE. Fresh fish should smell just slightly briny. Off odors develop in the gut cavity first. When buying fish, always take a sniff in the belly area to make sure the fish is clean and fresh. Incidentally, beware of fish that has been pre-wrapped in plastic. Unless the fish has been frozen, it can go bad very quickly.

■ LOOK AT THE EYES. When buying whole fish, look at the eyes; if the fish is fresh, they will be clear, bright, and bulging. Eyes that are slightly milky or sunken are an indication of the condition of the fish—that freshness is waning.

■ CHECK THE GILLS. The gills should be moist and bright red, almost burgundy. If they are gray or brown, the fish is old, and you should pass it by.

■ PRESS THE FLESH. The flesh on fresh fish should be firm and springy. If you press it with your finger, and the indentation remains, the fish is old and won't deliver the best flavor.

garlic and fish

Sure, eating fish offers more heart protection than eating red meat does. But what about the fishy cholesterol-raising side effects? Sprinkle garlic on your whitefish next time you enjoy a seafood dinner—in one study where people took fish oil supplements, added garlic prevented the increase in LDL or "bad" cholesterol that sometimes occurs.[22]

as well as their omega-3 fatty acids, which have been shown to decrease neuroinflammation and improve cognitive performance,[23] may provide twice the neurocognitive protection.

■ Sardines are highly recommended for people with epilepsy, not only because they contain an abundance of heart-healthy long-chain fatty acids (these fatty acids have the potential to reduce seizures), but also because of their strong potential role in preventing SUDEP, or sudden unexpected death in epilepsy. Evidence suggests that omega-3 fatty acids improve a number of cardiovascular risk factors and decrease the overall risk of cardiac death, and as SUDEP results from cardiac arrhythmias and/or abnormalities, omega-3s can play a powerful protective role in preventing SUDEP.

Sardines are an easily obtained, low-cost way to add healthful omega-3s to your diet.[24]

tuna

Tuna is rich in vitamin B_{12}, protein, and selenium, and it's a good source of vitamin B_6, vitamin D, phosphorous, and omega-3s. Albacore and skipjack tuna are approved by the Monterey Bay Aquarium Seafood Watch, which monitors seafood supply and recommends sustainable seafood and fish sources; yellowfin and bigeye are good alternatives if the others aren't available.[25] No matter the type, do exercise caution when consuming tuna, because of its mercury levels—though one bit of good news is that albacore tuna caught off the coast of the western United States and Canada has some of the lowest levels of mercury, as these fish are caught earlier in their life cycles than tuna caught elsewhere. If you're unsure of your tuna's source or you can't find this type of tuna, limit consumption to no more than once per week or no more than once per month, if you're pregnant or lactating.[26] Further findings are compelling.

- Tuna-derived triacylglycerol, a dietary lipid, has shown anticarcinogenic activity in in vitro studies.[27]
- Long-term consumption of omega-3 fatty acids can improve arterial stiffness, a known marker of cardiovascular disease.[28]
- The marine-derived omega-3 fatty acids eicosapentaenoic acid (EPA) and docosahexaenoic acid (DHA) are known to exert anti-inflammatory effects,[29] highlighting their potential for treating a range of inflammatory-related illnesses, including inflammatory bowel disease, irritable bowel syndrome, arthritis, and rheumatoid arthritis, as well as neurodegenerative diseases such as Alzheimer's disease.[30]

chia seeds

At only about 1 millimeter in diameter, chia seeds are the smallest seeds on our list, but they pack a powerful punch. The chia plant is a member of the mint family, and it's cultivated commercially for its highly nutritious seeds. Rich in fiber, protein, omega-3 fatty acids, magnesium, phosphorous, manganese, and selenium, as well as a good source of calcium, riboflavin, folate, iron, copper, thiamin, and niacin, there's far more to chia seeds than meets the eye. What's more, a recent analysis revealed that chia's phenolic content and antioxidant activity are higher than previously thought; its major phenolic compound is rosmarinic acid, but chia also contains protocatechuic ethyl ester acid, caffeic acid, gallic acid, and the isoflavone daidzein.[1] Once found only in specialty stores, chia seeds are now readily available at most any supermarket. Chia seeds are often eaten whole, but they can be purchased in ground form, as well. They're used to make flour, and their oil is extracted for cooking. Chia seeds can be sprinkled on yogurt, cold cereal, oatmeal and other hot cereals, or salads; stirred into smoothies; or used in baking. Just remember that chia seeds swell dramatically when they come into contact with a liquid. The good news about chia goes beyond its superfood qualities.

- Hypertensive individuals who were not on blood pressure medication were randomly divided into one of three groups: chia flour plus blood pressure medication, chia flour only, or a placebo. The subjects in the chia groups ate 35 grams (g) a day of chia flour for 12 weeks. Both chia groups experienced a reduction in mean clinical blood pressure and lipid peroxidation, and the group who had chia

super-charge your meals
Chia seeds can be a challenge in smoothies or puddings if you're not a huge fan of the texture. To still get all the healing benefits of these tiny seeds, add them to your favorite blueberry muffins or zucchini bread recipe. Another way to hide chia seeds is to sprinkle them on top of a salad.

flour only experienced a reduction in ambulatory blood pressure, as well.[2]

■ Chia oil contains 83 percent polyunsaturated fatty acids (PUFAs), particularly alpha-linolenic acid (an omega-3 fatty acid). This is the highest value among edible oils. Chia oil also has the lowest amount of saturated fatty acids of any edible oil.[3] PUFAs are known to have a number of health benefits, including protection against cardiovascular disease, depression, inflammation, arthritis, certain cancers, high blood pressure, and metabolic disorders.[4] Chia seeds provide an excellent vegetarian source of healthy PUFAs.

flaxseeds

Flaxseeds lend a nutty flavor and an extra dose of fiber to baked goods, and they can be sprinkled on top of yogurt, oatmeal, or other hot cereals or stirred into cold cereal. Ground flaxseeds can also be combined with water to make a substitute for eggs in baking. Naturally gluten-free, ground flaxseeds can replace some of the conventional flour called for in baked goods. Flaxseeds may be best known for their high concentration of alpha-linolenic acid, an omega-3 fatty acid, but they're also a good source of fiber, magnesium, manganese, and dietary lignans, which have a high antioxidant level and a phytoestrogenic effect. It's no wonder interest in their health benefits has spawned much research.

- A study of 6,369 women found that the consumption of flaxseeds or flax bread was significantly associated with a reduced risk of breast cancer. The protective effect is thought to be due to lignan phytoestrogens.[5]
- Flaxseed lignan phytoestrogens have also been shown to have a protective effect on urinary incontinence in postmenopausal women. Researchers studied 1,789 women age 50 and older and analyzed the flax-derived lignan phytoestrogens and soy-derived isoflavones in their urine. Women with higher concentrations of flax-derived lignans had a decreased likelihood of urinary incontinence, while no association was observed between soy-derived isoflavones and incontinence.[6]
- Lignans have also been associated with a lower risk of depression in women ages 45 to 55.[7]

- Lignans appear to reduce chronic inflammation, as well. In a study of 4,656 adults, lignans were shown to be inversely related to concentrations of C-reactive protein and white blood cell count, two markers of inflammation.[8]
- A metastudy of 14 trials on the effect of flaxseed (whole, oil, lignans, or fiber) on blood pressure found that consumption of flaxseed does decrease both systolic and diastolic blood pressure; the effect appears to be greatest when flaxseeds are consumed whole for 12 weeks or more.[9]

See also: Flaxseed Oil (page 81)

pumpkin seeds

Tossed with a little sea salt and extra-virgin olive oil, roasted pumpkin seeds make a delicious all-natural snack. Pumpkin seeds are loaded with heart-healthy polyunsaturated fats (PUFAs) and monounsaturated fats (MUFAs), and they're one of the best vegetarian sources of zinc. They're also rich in fiber, protein, and iron and are a good source of manganese, magnesium, and phosphorous. Did you know:

- Pumpkin seed oil was shown to have a beneficial effect on overactive

super-charge your meals

In addition to pumpkin seeds, canned pumpkin has some hidden benefits, too. Substituting canned pumpkin for half of the butter in a brownie recipe, for example, can slash the fat, and add wonderful moisture to your mix. You don't even notice the change (unless it's for the better perhaps!)

bladder? Forty-five volunteers with overactive bladder consumed 10 g of pumpkin seed oil extract a day for 12 weeks. At both 6 and 12 weeks after intervention, scores on all parts of an overactive bladder symptom questionnaire—namely daytime frequency, nighttime frequency, urgency, and urgency incontinence—were significantly improved.[10]

- Men with androgenetic alopecia (hair loss) were given 400 milligrams per day of pumpkin seed oil or a placebo for 24 weeks. Those who took the pumpkin seed oil experienced mean hair increases of up to 40 percent.[11]

- Pumpkin seeds have been shown to contain globulins (a type of protein) that possess significant antidiabetic and hypoglycemic properties.[12]

sesame seeds

Sesame seeds are rich in manganese and fiber and are a good source of calcium,

iron, magnesium, and phosphorous. They may be best known to the American palate as a topping on hamburger buns or rolls, but these seeds, which come in shades of ivory, yellow, red, brown, and black, have many other uses. Sesame is one of the principal ingredients in tahini, which is used in hummus and can be used in salad dressings. Whole sesame seeds can be sprinkled onto salads or stirred into hot cereals, cold cereals, and yogurt, and whole or ground sesame seeds can be used in baking— sesame seeds are naturally gluten-free. Cooking with sesame oil brings a warm, nutty flavor to dishes, and sesame seeds can be used to make a plant-based milk. Besides adding delicious flavor to your meals, sesame seeds have great health-boosting qualities.

- Sesame seeds have been shown to reduce inflammation. In a study of 50 patients with osteoarthritis of the knee, 25 received 40 g per day of a placebo powder and 25 received 40 g per day of sesame seeds for

2 months. Those in the sesame group experienced a significant decrease in malondialdehyde and C-reactive protein—markers of oxidative stress and inflammation.[13]

■ A study of prehypertensive individuals examined the effects of black sesame meal. One group ingested capsules containing 2.5 g of black sesame meal each day for 4 weeks, while the other group ingested a placebo. Black sesame meal significantly decreased systolic blood pressure and malondialdehyde levels, and it increased vitamin E levels.[14]

■ Sesame seeds are high in the antioxidant lignans sesamin, sesamolin, sesaminol, and sesamol, which have exhibited antihypertensive, anticancerous, and cholesterol-lowering effects.[15]

sunflower seeds

Sunflower seeds are rich in antioxidant vitamin E and are a good source of magnesium, phosphorous, copper, manganese, selenium, thiamin, vitamin B_6, and folate. They can be purchased unshelled or shelled, and many people enjoy a few handfuls of shelled sunflower seeds as a heart-healthy, low-carb, gluten-free, zero-cholesterol snack. Sunflower seeds are also a popular addition to salads, baked goods, and hot and cold cereals, or try adding them to vegetable side dishes. Ground sunflower seeds can be added to smoothies and protein drinks and used in baking. Sunflower seed oil, with its high vitamin E content, is also used in skin-care products, and on its own it can be used as an all-natural treatment for dry skin. The benefits don't stop there.

■ A study that compared the effects of olive oil and sunflower seed oil on skin found that sunflower seed oil was far superior. One group of adults applied six drops of olive oil to their forearms twice a day for 5 weeks; a second group did the same, but with olive oil on one arm and sunflower seed oil on the other. Olive oil caused a reduction in stratum corneum (the outer layer of skin) integrity and mild erythema (redness). But sunflower seed oil preserved stratum corneum integrity, did not cause erythema, and improved hydration in the same volunteers.[16]

■ Postmenopausal women with type 2 diabetes added 30 g a day of either almonds or sunflower kernels to their regular diets for 3 weeks, and then after a 4-week washout period switched to the other intervention for 3 weeks. Total cholesterol and LDL ("bad") cholesterol decreased significantly with both interventions, but the sunflower intervention also produced a significant drop in systolic blood pressure and greater reductions in apolipoprotein B100 concentration (a protein associated with LDL cholesterol). However, the sunflower seed intervention also reduced apolipoprotein A1 (a protein associated with "good" HDL cholesterol) and HDL cholesterol itself. But given the host of positive effects, researchers concluded that adding almonds *and* sunflower seeds to your diet is beneficial to cardiovascular health.[17]

sweets

chocolate

Yes, it's true, chocolate is a healing food. It's also true that the darker the chocolate, the better it is for you. That's because dark chocolate contains a higher cocoa content, which means more heart-healthy cocoa flavonols and more phenolic compounds. Technically, this means that unsweetened, 100 percent cocoa baking chocolate is the healthiest chocolate, but if that's too much pucker for your palate, look for chocolate that contains at least 70 percent cocoa solids. And don't worry about *occasionally* indulging in milk chocolate: All chocolate contains serotonin-like monoamines and tryptophan, which is the precursor to serotonin, the famous mood-boosting neurotransmitter.[1]

Research has credited chocolate with such health benefits as reducing oxidative stress, lowering blood pressure, increasing vasodilatation, increasing platelet activity, exerting antidiabetic effects, relieving stress, reducing inflammation, improving exercise recovery, and even exerting antiobesity effects.[2] Chocolate boasts large concentrations of flavonoids, epicatechin, catechin, and procyanidins; dark chocolate even contains higher amounts of flavonoids than tea or wine.[3] In terms of nutritional profile, dark chocolate—we're talking at least 70 percent cocoa solids—is a rich source of copper and manganese and a good source of fiber, iron, potassium, zinc, phosphorous, and magnesium. One ounce of dark chocolate contains about 170 calories and 12 grams (g) of fat, so it's an energy-dense food, but it's much more than that, too. Take a look at the healing power of chocolate.

- Cocoa polyphenols may actually counteract obesity-related metabolic conditions (cardiovascular disease, hypertension, and type 2 diabetes) by reducing inflammation and regulating lipid and energy metabolism.[4]

- Based on data from more than 7,800 people, researchers found that compared to people who ate chocolate once per month or less, people who ate chocolate one to four times a month, two to six times a week, or more than once a day had a lower risk of diabetes by 13 percent, 34 percent, and 18 percent, respectively. They concluded that the risk of diabetes decreased as the frequency of chocolate intake increased, up to two to six 1-ounce servings of chocolate per week.[5]

■ Nearly 21,000 people were followed for an average of 11.9 years, during which time 14 percent experienced a stroke or coronary heart disease. Researchers found that those who ate more chocolate typically had a lower weight, lower waist-to-hip ratio, lower blood pressure, lower markers of inflammation, and less prevalence of diabetes, and they were also more physically active. Compared to those who ate no chocolate, the people who ate more chocolate—some of them up to 100 g a day!—had an 11 percent lower risk of cardiovascular disease and a 23 percent lower risk of stroke. Interestingly, these results included both milk and dark chocolates. Researchers speculate that the health benefits of chocolate come from its flavonoids, calcium, and fatty acids.[6]

■ A study on overweight men shed light on how dark chocolate can protect against atherosclerosis. Over 4 weeks, the men, ages 45 to 70, ate 70 g of dark chocolate per day. One group ate a chocolate with elevated flavanols, while the other ate regular chocolate; both contained the same amount of cocoa. In the end, both

types of flavanols produced the same cardiovascular benefits: an increase in flow-mediated dilation (more responsive bloodflow), a decrease in augmentation index (a measure of arterial stiffness and thus a good predictor of disease), a reduced white blood cell count, and reduced adhesion of white blood cells to arterial walls.[7] Chocolate has also been shown to decrease platelet aggregation and reduce platelet adhesion, highlighting its potential role in preventing and treating atherosclerosis.[8]

■ A study on 90 elderly individuals without cognitive dysfunction compared the effects of consuming cocoa drinks containing varying levels of flavanols for 8 weeks. Those in the high-flavanol (993 mg) and in the intermediate-flavanol (520 mg) groups experienced improvements in lipid peroxidation, insulin resistance, and blood pressure, and they scored better on tests of cognitive function than those in the low-flavanol (48 mg) group. Researchers concluded that regular cocoa flavanol consumption can reduce some measures of age-related cognitive dysfunction, possibly through an improvement in insulin sensitivity.[9]

■ Clinical and epidemiological studies have found that dark chocolate has a positive effect on blood pressure, lipids, mitochondrial structure and function, and inflammation due to enhanced nitric oxide bioavailability (which improves endothelial function). According to the latest research, much of the health benefit comes from the flavanol epicatechin, which is found in high concentrations in dark, but not milk, chocolate.[10]

honey

Honey is a true healing superfood. Used medicinally for millennia, honey boasts an astonishing array of health benefits, including anti-inflammatory, antioxidant, antitumor, antifungal, antiviral, antibacterial, antiwrinkle, antitussive, anti-insomnia, antiulcer, anticaries, antigingivitis, immune-supporting, and wound-healing properties.[11] [12] Before we get to the research, one of the first questions many people ask is which type of honey is best for health. What you may not know is that there are thousands of distinct types of honey worldwide—their differences depend on what type of flower the nectar came from, where those plants were grown, and what the climatic conditions were for a particular year. All of these factors influence the taste, appearance, and even the nutritional content of honey, and thus far, we're just talking

about raw honey. Heat processing and filtration can reduce some of honey's healing benefits, such as antioxidant capacity or antibacterial power.[13] Many health-care professionals recommend raw honey because it hasn't been filtered or processed, and many recommend local honey because of its antiallergenic effect, though evidence on this is mixed. One honey consistently recommended is manuka honey from New Zealand, which has such strong antimicrobial properties that it's considered a medical grade honey. (To avoid an adulterated product whose healing power will be compromised, look for certified 100 percent raw manuka honey, and prepare to pay quite a bit more than for processed, conventional honey.) Another honey that has gained a great deal of attention in the medical community is tualang honey, a multifloral rain forest honey from Malaysia that is actually higher in phenolics and flavonoids than monofloral manuka honey.[14]

"Nature's sweetener" is composed mainly of fructose and glucose, but natural honey also contains amino acids; vitamins C, B_1, B_2, and B_6; pantothenic acid; potassium; calcium; magnesium; phosphorous; sodium; sulfur; enzymes; flavonoids; fructooligosaccharides (which serve as prebiotic agents); phenolic acids (such as ellagic acid and gallic acid); tocopherols; catalase; and superoxide dismutase—among many more. These compounds work synergistically to confer a powerful antioxidant effect.[15] There are very few contraindications for honey, but children under 12 months should not consume it. And though they are rare, allergic reactions to bee pollen or bee proteins are possible.

■ The topical application of honey has been shown to speed the healing of wounds, ward off infection, reduce inflammation, exert a wound debriding action (making wounds easier to clean), and discourage swelling and wound exudation (overleakage).[16]

■ Honey has been shown to inhibit more than 80 species of bacteria. Its antibacterial effect is thought to be due in part to its hydrogen peroxide content and the presence of methylglyoxal, an organic compound that acts against a number of pathogenic microorganisms.[17] The concentration of methylglyoxal is up to 100 times higher in manuka honey than in conventional honey.[18]

■ Emerging research indicates that the polyphenols in raw honey exert a neuroprotective effect by protecting neurons against oxidative injury and inflammation, stimulating adult

sweet swap

Even though honey and sugar can be used interchangeably in most recipes, you may have to make some adjustments. For example:

■ Honey is sweeter than sugar, so you can substitute 1 cup honey for 1¼ cups of sugar if you reduce the liquid in the recipe by ¼ cup.

■ When using honey for baking, add a pinch of baking soda. This will neutralize honey's acidity and help the food to rise. (If the recipe contains sour cream or sour milk, however, you can forgo the baking soda.)

■ When using honey instead of sugar in jams, jellies, or candies, increase the cooking temperature just a bit to allow the extra liquid to evaporate.

There are many different flavors of honey, and it's important to match the type to the recipe. Orange blossom honey, for example, has a light, delicate flavor and is best used for foods with mild tastes, like a honey nut cake. Honey produced from buckwheat flowers, however, has a considerably stronger flavor. It's a good choice for spreading on bread or when making whole grain desserts.

neurogenesis, helping to improve memory, improving hippocampal synaptic plasticity, and attenuating oxidative stress involved in neuro-degeneration and age-related memory deficits. Ellagic acid, which is known to have chemopreventive (cancer-fighting) effects, has also been shown to restore lipid perox-ides, nitric oxide, and the total anti-oxidant status of your brain to normal levels. Two other honey polyphenols, gallic acid and chrysin, have been shown to exert antianxiety effects, which help prevent anxiety-related memory disturbances.[19]

Honey can even provide some mea-sure of pain control. In a study of tonsillectomy patients, those who received honey in addition to acet-aminophen experienced less pain, required less acetaminophen, experi-enced less waking at night, and were able to return to their normal diets sooner than the control group who received only acetaminophen.[20]

Honey is a time-honored and highly effective natural means to remedy coughs associated with upper respi-ratory infections.[21]

Honey has been shown to be effective at treating ringworm, athlete's foot, and conditions arising from *Malasse-zia* yeasts, such as seborrheic derma-titis and dandruff.[22]

Though it is rich in sugars, honey appears to be an effective comple-mentary treatment for diabetes. In a 12-week study of people with type 1 diabetes, those who ate honey daily (0.5 milliliter per kilogram of body weight) experienced significant decreases in subscapular skinfold thickness, fasting serum glucose, total cholesterol, serum tri-glycerides, and low-density lipopro-tein, as well as significant increases in fasting C-peptide and 2-hour post-prandial C-peptide.[23] Honey in mod-eration is recommended as a sugar substitute for diabetics.[24]

Both honey and a combination of honey and bee pollen (1 tablespoon per day for 14 days) were found to be effective at treating hot flashes as well as a range of postmenopausal symptoms in breast cancer patients receiving antihormone treatments.[25]

In vitro studies have shown that tualang honey has antiproliferative effects against breast cancer, osteo-sarcoma, cervical cancer, and both acute and chronic myeloid leukemia cells.[26]

vegetables

artichokes

Artichokes have been used as a source of medicine as far back as 4 BCE,[1] and modern research confirms that this prickly plant boasts a plethora of health benefits. Few other vegetables contain as many phytonutrients as artichokes. They're an excellent source of fiber, folate, vitamin C, and vitamin K and a good source of the essential minerals magnesium, phosphorous, and potassium and the flavonoids quercetin, gallic acid, cynarin, silymarin, and rutin.

how to cook an artichoke

At first glance, the artichoke is kind of like *The New York Times* crossword puzzle—it looks inviting and intriguing, but you may not be sure if you're up to the challenge. Appearances can be deceptive. If you follow a few easy tips, preparing and eating artichokes is simple.

- When shopping for artichokes, look for those that are bright green—not brown—to ensure freshness and lots of nutrients.
- Dirt is easily lodged beneath their scaly leaves, so it's important to rinse artichokes thoroughly before cooking them.
- Pull off tough, outer, lower petals. With a sharp knife, slice off the stems so that they're level with the bottoms of the artichokes. You can also trim off the spiny tips of the leaves using scissors if you like.
- Stand the artichokes in a large saucepan. Cover them halfway with water and simmer, covered, for 30 to 40 minutes. Or place them on a steaming rack, and steam for the same amount of time.
- To test for doneness, pull on a center petal. If it comes out easily, the artichoke is done.
- To eat the leaves, hold them by the tip, curved side down, and draw them between your teeth to remove the tender flesh.
- When the leaves are gone, use a fork or spoon to scoop out the hairy layer, called the choke. Discard the hairy choke, then dig into the best part—the tender heart.

Ancient physicians used artichoke to treat jaundice and prevent and treat diseases of the liver, and to this day medicines made from artichoke leaf extract are used to improve liver function, enhance the flow of bile, lower cholesterol, and treat gastrointestinal conditions such as indigestion and irritable bowel syndrome (IBS).[2]

And that's just the beginning for this powerful healing food. Artichoke has also been shown to lower blood glucose, exert antioxidant and anti-inflammatory effects, stimulate the growth of the helpful probiotic strain *Bifidobacterium bifidum,* induce apoptosis (cell death) of leukemia cells in vitro, and prevent atherosclerotic plaque deposits by lowering cholesterol.[3] Take a look at some of the clinical evidence for this superfood.

- Overweight subjects who consumed 250 milligrams (mg) of artichoke leaf extract twice a day for 8 weeks experienced significantly lower total cholesterol, lower LDL ("bad") cholesterol, and higher HDL ("good") cholesterol.[4]

- Two hundred and eight adults with irritable bowel syndrome consumed either 320 or 640 mg of artichoke leaf extract daily for 2 months. By the end of the trial, IBS incidence for both dosage groups had fallen by 26 percent, and participants reported a significant shift from a bowel habit pattern of "alternating constipation/diarrhea" toward "normal." Further, their dyspepsia score fell by 41 percent, and they reported a 20 percent improvement in overall quality of life.[5]

- Artichoke leaf extract exhibits strong anticancer properties against pleural mesothelioma, a type of lung cancer with a very poor survival rate. Researchers found that it exerts an in vitro and in vivo antitumor effect by strongly affecting mesothelioma growth, migration, and invasion.[6]

- The compounds chlorogenic acid, inulin, and caffeoylquinic acid found in artichoke have demonstrated blood-sugar-lowering effects. But artichoke consumed as a whole food may increase the effect, due to its high quantities of nourishing fiber.[7]

- Artichoke has long been known to increase the secretion of bile, which aids in digestion and helps rid your body of toxins. In one small, placebo-controlled trial, bile flow was increased by 127 percent in volunteers half an hour after they consumed a 1,920 mg artichoke extract supplement; after 1 hour, bile flow increased by 152 percent.[8]

- A recent in vitro study found that artichoke polyphenols were effective in suppressing the growth of MDA-MB-231 cancer cells, a type of highly aggressive breast cancer. Previous in vitro studies have also shown artichoke polyphenols' anticancer effect on certain types of colon, gastric, ovarian, prostate, lung, skin (melanoma), brain (glioblastoma), bone, and bone marrow (leukemia) cancers.[9]

asparagus

Fans of this stalky perennial vegetable eagerly anticipate the arrival of spring, when asparagus spears emerge. From that point, asparagus season will last anywhere from 4 to 12 weeks, depending on geographical location. While we most often think of pale green shoots when it comes to asparagus, this delicate-flavored veggie can range from white (this occurs when asparagus is raised without light and thus cannot produce chlorophyll) to a dark purple. Asparagus can be eaten raw, but most people find it tastier grilled, roasted, or steamed, and it's a popular ingredient in quiches, soups, stir-fries, and stews. Because of its high antioxidant content, especially the powerful antioxidant glutathione, some people use asparagus juice as an ingredient in detox juice preparations.

Asparagus is a good source of folate, fiber, vitamin A, vitamin C, and vitamin K, and it's very low in calories, sodium, and sugar. But it has other surprising health benefits, too.

■ Asparagus has been shown to exert a phytoestrogenic effect. A phytoestrogen is any plant compound similar to ovarian or placental

how to cook asparagus

Since most of asparagus's nutrients are in the tip, if you're going to cook it on the stovetop, it's better to cook it upright in a tall container, says Gertrude Armbruster, PhD, RD, of Cornell University. Add a few inches of water to the pot, cover with a lid, and bring to a simmer. Keeping the tips out of the water will not only preserve nutrients but will also help the stalks cook evenly and more quickly.

Pamela Nisevich Bede, MS,

co-owner of Swim, Bike, Run, Eat! LLC

Q. What food combinations do you recommend for overall health?

A. Eat calcium with vitamin D because the two work together for best absorption. Similarly, you'll want to consume your iron with vitamin C, as these two nutrients also have a synergistic relationship.

Q. Have you had a client heal him- or herself with food?

A. When I worked in pediatrics, I had a young patient who suffered seizures that were so severe that it limited her development. She came to be [developmentally] delayed for her age and unable to communicate well. She was listless and didn't play like other kids. We changed her diet to include limited carbohydrates and just enough protein to meet her daily needs. Her seizures were greatly reduced and eventually stopped. Within a year, she was able to communicate, walk, and play.

Q. What are your food recommendations for weight loss?

A. I've never met anyone who couldn't shed pounds because their intake of fruits and vegetables was too great. Certainly some choices are better than others—no juices, no sugar-laced items, limited starchy veggies, and limited dried fruit, please—but when it comes to produce, just about everything gets the green light!

Q. What are the top 5 to 10 foods everyone should be eating?

A. Spinach, tart cherries, beets, carrots, and popcorn all top my list.

Q. What are the top 5 to 10 foods everyone should be avoiding?

A. We should be avoiding pop (soda), French fries, and white bread.

Q. What are the top foods men should be eating? And the top foods for women?

A. Most women ages 19 to 50 need to work on their iron intake, and foods like lean red meat and legumes can be great sources of this critical nutrient. If you're relying on foods like spinach to boost iron intake, be sure to combine them with a vitamin C–rich food (like citrus) for best absorption.

estrogens and their active metabolites, and studies have shown a lower incidence of breast cancer in populations with higher exposure to phytoestrogens.[10]

Asparagus extract has also been used to stimulate lactation. In a study of 60 mothers with deficient lactation, those who consumed an asparagus root extract for 30 days saw a three-

Both genders need to work on boosting their intake of potassium. Once again, the new Dietary Guidelines consider the potassium intake of Americans to be subpar. Find potassium in dairy products and produce, such as strawberries and watermelon.

Q. If we were to go to the grocery store with you, what would we always find in your shopping cart?

A. Spinach, bananas, 1% milk (I find it to be a good compromise between watery skim and indulgent whole milk), and chicken breasts.

Q. What's your favorite indulgence?

A. Craft beer and peanut butter–filled pretzels.

Q. What do you select when you eat out at different restaurants or eateries?

A. I love steamed vegetables and marinara sauce with meat at Italian restaurants. I usually hold the pasta because I'd rather have more colorful, filling, and low-calorie veggies. When eating at a Mexican restau-rant, I choose a taco salad containing lots of lettuce, black beans, grilled lean protein, guacamole, and plenty of grilled vegetables. And if I know I'm going to the movies, I'll be sure to plan a long run or hard workout in the hours before movie night so I don't feel as guilty ordering my absolute favorite: popcorn (hold the butter).

Q. Are there any natural home remedies you use?

A. I believe in a daily multivitamin, a nutrient-dense diet, and plenty of exercise to keep my immune system strong and to fend off bugs.

Q. What's your favorite grab-and-go snack?

A. A serving of fruit and a handful of graham crackers.

fold increase in the hormone prolactin and a subsequent increase in milk production. Accordingly, the babies of the mothers in the asparagus group gained more weight than the babies whose mothers were in the control group: There was a mean percentage weight increase of 16.13 in the asparagus group compared to 5.68 in the control group.[11]

Asparagus root extract has demonstrated effective antimicrobial activity against a variety of pathogens, including *Escherichia coli*, commonly known as *E. coli*, which causes a wide array of illnesses; *Salmonella typhimurium*, which is responsible for food poisoning; *Candida albicans*, the most common cause of fungal infections; *Staphylococcus aureus*, the leading cause of skin infections; and the *Malassezia* fungus, responsible for dandruff and dermatitis.[12]

beets/beetroot juice

Though it's the taproot portion of this versatile vegetable that most people mean when they refer to beets, both the leaves (which can be eaten raw in salads or prepared the way you'd cook any other green) and the richly colored root are edible. Red beets (or beetroots) are the most common variety, but there are also albino or white beets, jewel-toned golden beets, yellow beets, and a range of specialty beets that have been cultivated for a variety of different tastes, colors, and purposes. Beets are rich in manganese, pantothenic acid, and folate, and they're a good source of phosphorous, vitamin C, potassium, and fiber, as well. Beets and beetroot juice are also known for their high concentrations of nitrates, which are vasodilators; numerous studies have demonstrated that nitrates lower blood pressure and enhance exercise performance.[13] Beetroot juice has become increasingly popular as a healing food because unlike cooked beets, which lose some of their phytonutrients during the cooking process, beetroot juice maintains its phytonutrient content.

Beetroot juice has been shown to lower blood pressure, increase plasma nitrate concentration, and help your body respond better to exercise. On six separate occasions, 10 healthy men engaged in moderate- or severe-intensity exercise 2.5 hours after consuming 70, 140, or 280 milliliters (ml) of either beetroot juice or a placebo. The placebo and the 70 ml of beetroot juice did not alter the response to exercise, but 140 ml of beetroot juice reduced oxygen consumption by 1.7 percent during moderate-intensity exercise, and 280 ml reduced it by 3.0 percent. Additionally, time to task failure—the point at which a muscle becomes fatigued—was extended by 14 and

Wondering whether to eat beets raw or cooked? Studies have shown that the antitumor power of beets is diminished by heat. So peel and grate beets, and toss them into salads, or cook them lightly to get the most nutrients.

Another discovery is that beets are nearly as nutritious out of the can as they are fresh from the ground. So you can enjoy their health benefits in and out of season.

12 percent, respectively, for 140 ml and 280 ml of beetroot juice.[14]

- In a similar study, healthy subjects consumed 140 ml of beetroot juice daily for 6 days. After moderate- to severe-intensity exercise performed on days 4, 5, and 6, subjects experienced an increased rate of VO_2 kinetics (the time it takes for oxygen delivery to respond to exercise) and an increase in time to task failure.[15]

- Similar positive effects can be seen in those who aren't healthy. In a study of patients with heart failure who drank beetroot juice or a placebo, those who drank the beetroot juice experienced enhanced nitric oxide bioavailability and an accompanying increase in muscle power. Though this was a small study, it confirms that the ingestion of the inorganic nitrate found in beetroot juice increases nitric oxide production, even in those whose cardiovascular systems are compromised.[16]

- But all the credit doesn't go to beetroot juice alone: A study of whole beet consumption found that eating

super-charge your meals

Beets are an awesome source of vitamin C, manganese, and fiber. But many people can't seem to get these nutritious root vegetables onto their plate. Start small by shredding a raw beet, similar to a carrot, and sprinkling it on your salad. You'll get a nice hint of the beet flavor that's not too overwhelming.

whole beets improves running performance. In this study, runners ate 200 g of beets or a calorie-matched placebo 75 minutes before running 5 kilometers (km). Runners who ate beets ran faster, and their running velocity during the last 1.1 km was 5 percent faster than that of the runners who ate the placebo.[17]

See also: Greens (page 119)

broccoli

Broccoli is frequently cited as one of the world's healthiest foods, and if you look at its nutrient profile, you can see why. At just 81 calories per cup and only a trace amount of fat, this member of the Brassica family beats out its cruciferous cousins for highest concentration of the antioxidant vitamin C. It's also an excellent source of vitamin K, folate, and chromium, and it's a good source of vitamin A and fiber.

Like all cruciferous veggies, broccoli is known for its high content of glucosinolates, which are sulfur-containing compounds. When glucosinolates break down (such as from chewing or cutting) they form biologically active compounds called isothiocyanates, and of all the cruciferous vegetables, broccoli contains the highest amount of the isothiocyanate compound sulforaphane. If you only remember one word from this list of compounds, let it be sulforaphane, as it's been shown to be effective at preventing and/or treating a variety of health conditions, from bacterial infections (including *Helicobacter pylori* infection) to cardiovascular disease, and in reducing oxidative stress and hyperglycemic damage in diabetics.[19] Sulforaphane has also been

power pairs

broccoli and eggs

If your menstrual cycle is wreaking serious emotional havoc, whip up an omelet with broccoli. Consuming calcium (found in the broccoli) and vitamin D (found in the eggs) together is known to ease premenstrual syndrome (PMS) symptoms. And there's an added bonus: Calcium and vitamin D help reduce your risk of osteoporosis.[18]

just right broccoli

One of the problems with cooking broccoli is consistency—or, more specifically, a lack thereof. Broccoli consists of both tough stalk and tender florets, the result being that it ends up with parts either overdone or underdone.

To help ensure even cooking it's helpful to cut broccoli into little spears. First, cut off and discard the thick, woody part of the stalk, generally from the bottom up to where the broccoli florets begin to branch. Then cut any large florets and stems in half lengthwise.

If you find that the stems are still too tough for eating, either trim them farther up from the bottom or peel them with a vegetable peeler before cooking.

shown to exert anti-inflammatory effects by inhibiting the production of cytokines, cell-signaling molecules involved in the inflammatory response.[20] But sulforaphane's main claim to fame is its proven effectiveness at every stage of carcinogenesis, from inhibiting cancer cell proliferation and differentiation to causing cancer cell death to reducing the risk of mutations that give rise to malignancies in the first place. It also exerts anti-inflammatory and antibacterial effects that are relevant to cancer prevention.[21] Here's more good news about broccoli.

- A wide range of studies—in animals, in humans, and in vitro—have demonstrated an inverse relationship between broccoli intake and various cancers. Studies have proven the inhibitory effects of sulforaphane on colon cancer, pancreatic cancer, leukemia, and prostate cancer, and eating broccoli sprouts has been shown to reduce the incidence of breast cancer and prostate cancer, as well as reduce tumor growth.[22]

- There is also an indication that broccoli sprouts can play a preventive role in cardiovascular disease. In a small clinical trial, 12 subjects consumed 100 g of broccoli sprouts daily for 1 week and experienced lower LDL and total cholesterol and lower markers of oxidative stress.[23]

- Broccoli sprouts have been shown to reduce nasal allergic inflammation in response to pollution,[24] and sulforaphane derived from broccoli was shown to lower the incidence of airway inflammation in some asthmatics.[25] In a study that examined the effect of broccoli sprouts on smokers with influenza, researchers found that ingesting a shake made with broccoli sprouts significantly reduced virus-induced markers of inflammation and even reduced virus quantity. All of these results demonstrate the antioxidant and anti-inflammatory powers of broccoli-derived sulforaphane.

brussels sprouts

Brussels sprouts look like miniature cabbages, and their taste is quite similar to green cabbage. These two veggies are actually close cousins: Both are cruciferous vegetables from the *Brassica* genus, and Brussels sprouts are actually a type of cabbage from the Gemmifera group of *Brassica oleracea*. Brussels sprouts are a high-potency source of vitamin C and vitamin K and a good source of vitamin A, manganese, folate, and fiber. Like all of the *Bras-*

sica vegetables, Brussels sprouts are high in sulforaphane, a phytochemical that has demonstrated powerful anti-carcinogenic properties. What's more . . .

- Cruciferous vegetables such as Brussels sprouts contain sulforaphane and indole-3-carbinol, which have been shown to work on a cellular level to prohibit the proliferation and viability of various kinds of cancer.[26]
- Sulforaphane also exerts a cardio-protective role by acting as an antioxidant and anti-inflammatory. Clinical trials have shown sulforaphane-mediated protection against hypertension, atherosclerosis, tissue damage after a heart attack, diabetes, and diabetes-related complications such as neuropathy, cardiomyopathy, and angiopathy.[27]

See also: Broccoli (page 110), Cabbage

cabbage

If your idea of cabbage is the over-boiled stuff leached of color and texture (not to mention nutrients) or the leafy green that is only palatable served with ham hock, you're in for a

For such tiny vegetables, Brussels sprouts sure cause some large culinary conundrums. Not only is it challenging to cook them just so, but it's also likely that you'll smell up the house while you do it.

It doesn't have to be this way. If you follow these tips, you'll get the health benefits of Brussels sprouts without the hassles.

■ MARK THE SPOT. To allow the tough stems to cook as quickly as the leaves, make an "X" on the bottom of each stem, using a sharp knife. Then steam them for 7 to 14 minutes, until they're just tender enough to poke with a fork.

■ QUELL THE SMELL. The big sulfur smell thrown off by these little cabbages discourages some people from taking advantage of their healing power. Try tossing a rib of celery in the cooking water. It will help neutralize the smell.

■ USE THEM FAST. Although Brussels sprouts will keep for a week or more in the refrigerator, they start getting bitter after about 3 days, which may discourage you and your family from eating them and reaping their benefits. Buy only as many as you'll use in the next few days.

treat. There are actually many varieties of cabbage—from napa to savoy, from pale green to brilliant purple—and many ways to prepare this versatile vegetable. Cabbage can be eaten raw; used in salads, stews, soups, or noodle dishes; and braised, boiled, sautéed, steamed, stir-fried, and even pickled, such as in sauerkraut or kimchi. Cabbage is part of the Brassicaceae family of vegetables, which also includes common cruciferous vegetables such as cauliflower, broccoli, kale, turnips, kohlrabi, and mustard greens. Brussels sprouts and bok choy are also in this family, and, while they are specific veggies in their own right, they are also actually types of cabbage. Cabbage is rich in vitamin C, vitamin K, and fiber; has zero fat and cholesterol; and is very low in calories, sugar, and sodium.

■ Cabbage, like other cruciferous vegetables such as broccoli and

As produce goes, cabbage is a cook's best friend. It's versatile, inexpensive, readily available, and easy to prepare. Sure, there's that cabbagy smell, but that's easily remedied.

The next time you're cooking cabbage, add a celery rib or whole English walnut (in the shell) to the pot. This will help neutralize the powerful odor. Or simply cook the cabbage quicker, stir-frying it in a skillet or wok rather than boiling it for a long time. Long cooking times release more of the strong-smelling sulfur compounds.

Brussels sprouts, contains a phytochemical called sulforaphane, a type of organosulfur compound. As you've no doubt gathered from its name, it's this compound that's responsible for cabbage's sulfurous smell. But any aroma is well worth it: Sulforaphane has been shown to inhibit the growth of cancer cells.[28] Savoy cabbage and red cabbage are particularly high in glucosinolates, the precursor to sulforaphane.

■ Cabbage and other cruciferous vegetables have been shown to reduce systemic inflammation. A study of more than 1,000 middle-aged women assessed the association between cruciferous vegetable consumption and markers of inflammation and oxidative stress. The vegetables identified in this study included bok choy, green cabbage, napa cabbage, cauliflower, and radish. Researchers found that a higher intake of cruciferous vegetables was associated with significantly lower concentrations of the pro-inflammatory biomarkers tumor necrosis factor alpha, interleukin-1 beta, and interleukin-6. These results held even after adjusting for a wide range of variables, including socioeconomic status, dietary and nondietary lifestyle factors, BMI, health conditions, and medication use.[29]

■ Kimchi, the traditional Korean fermented cabbage dish, has been shown to improve fasting blood glucose and to lower cholesterol. In this particular study, the effects were more profound in those who had high LDL and total cholesterol at baseline, and results were dose-dependent: The more kimchi subjects ate, the greater the improvement to their lipid profiles.[30]

See also: Broccoli (page 110), Brussels Sprouts (page 112), Sauerkraut (page 130)

carrots

When it comes to health benefits, this popular root vegetable is perhaps most often associated with eye health. And while carrots can't improve visual acuity, as part of an overall antioxidant-rich diet they can play a role in reducing your risk of age-related macular degeneration and its associated vision loss.[31] Carrots are rich in alpha-carotene and beta-carotene, which your body converts to vitamin A during digestion. One cup of chopped raw carrots contains 428 percent of the recommended daily value of vitamin A,[32] and carrots are a good source of vitamin C, vitamin K, and folate, as well. Naturally sweet, carrots make for a delicious juice that's popular on its own and as an ingredient in smoothies and cleansing juices.

Clinical trials on carrots have revealed a variety of healing effects.

- A metastudy of carrot consumption and the risk of prostate cancer concluded that a high consumption of carrots was inversely associated with prostate cancer risk. An increase of one serving per week, or 10 g of carrots per day, resulted in a 4 to 5 percent decrease in the risk of prostate cancer in the study population.[33]

better beta-carotene

Roasting carrots brings out their flavors. Toss 1¼-inch pieces of a carrot with salt, pepper, and a little extra-virgin olive oil. Bake, covered, for 20 minutes at 400°F. Uncover and bake for 30 minutes longer.

Adding olive oil is important. Beta-carotene needs a small amount of fat to make the trip through your intestinal wall and into your body, says John Erdman, PhD, of the University of Illinois in Urbana. So the next time you're serving carrot sticks, you may want to accompany them with a small amount of a dip, such as ranch dressing. (As if you needed an excuse!)

In vitro studies of wild carrot extract demonstrated a significant antiproliferative effect against human breast and colon cancer cells and a cytotoxic effect against acute myeloid leukemia cells.[34] (By the way, wild carrots are quite different from the cultivated carrots we've been discussing. The roots of wild carrots are edible only when they're very young, and in the United States, wild carrots are better known as Queen Anne's lace, a noxious weed.)

Carotenoids provide some measure of natural sunscreen protection. In clinical tests, a sunscreen made with purple carrot exhibited good ultraviolet (UV) blocking, underscoring its potential as a natural ingredient in sunscreen and cosmetics products.[35]

cauliflower

Cauliflower, though most widely known and eaten as a white vegetable, also boasts beautiful orange, green, and purple varieties. Orange cauliflower contains more vitamin A than other varieties, and purple cauliflower contains anthocyanins, the same pigments with antioxidant properties found in red wine, red cabbage, red grapes, and berries. All types of cauliflower are rich in vitamin C and vitamin K and are good sources of folate, fiber, and potassium. Like other members of the Brassicaceae family, cauliflower plays a role in preventing cancer and it exhibits antioxidant and anti-inflammatory effects. Much of the credit goes to its naturally occurring phytochemicals, called isothiocyanates, which have been shown to induce cell death and inhibit cell proliferation in various types of cancer. Consuming cruciferous vegetables at least once per week has been shown to significantly decrease the risk of cancers of the oral cavity and pharynx, esophagus, colon and rectum, breast, and kidney.[36]

Though cruciferous vegetable intake is associated with a lower risk of cancer generally, cruciferous veggies play a special role in helping to reduce the risk of lung cancer in smokers. Researchers attribute the effect to isothiocyanates, which slow down the rate of cancer growth.[37]

■ An extract made from the flowers of the cauliflower plant was shown to have both antithrombotic (anticlotting) and cytotoxic properties, highlighting its potential as a safe, low-cost means of achieving cardioprotective and anticancer benefits.[38]

■ Phenethyl isothiocyanate (PEITC), a dietary compound derived from cauliflower and other *Brassica* vegetables, was shown to be toxic to cervical cancer cells in vitro.[39]

See also: Broccoli (page 110), Brussels Sprouts (page 112), Cabbage (page 113)

we love cauliflower

What's not to love? Here's how to buy and enjoy.

■ **USE YOUR HEAD.** Avoid cauliflower if it has brown spots on its ivory (or purple) florets. That means that it's already past its nutritional peak. Choose cauliflower heads that are surrounded by many thick green leaves. These heads are better protected and will be fresher.

■ **STORE WITH CARE.** Store cauliflower with the stem side down to prevent moisture from developing in the floret clusters.

■ **ENJOY IT RAW.** To keep cauliflower's cancer-fighting indoles intact, keep it out of the heat, advises Dr. Michnovicz, MD, PhD, president of the Foundation for Preventive Oncology in New York City. Your best bet is either eating it raw or cooking it quickly in a steamer, wok, or microwave, he says. Boiling is the worst way to cook this crucifer. Submerging cauliflower in the hot, boiling water will cause it to lose about half of its valuable indoles, he says.

■ **STEAM IT RIGHT.** Steaming cauliflower releases the maximum amount of sulforaphane. But be sure to cut cauliflower into large (not small) pieces before you steam it. Larger pieces equal smaller surface area exposed. The greater the surface area exposed, the more nutrients can leach out.

Though many of us know that a broth-based soup is the healthier choice, many of us favor a comforting, creamy soup. One way to get rid of the guilt of eating such a rich soup is to substitute pureed veggies, like cauliflower, for that heavy cream. Gather some of your favorite veggies, and make sure to add some starches for that creaminess factor, then sauté them to bring out the flavor. Add enough liquid, either water or a low-sodium broth, to cover and let them simmer. For the smoothest texture, blend them in your blender until they're smooth.

fennel

If you combine fennel's use in traditional as well as modern medicine, it may just be the world's most widely used herbal plant. It's been used to treat more than 40 disorders and is antimicrobial, antiallergenic, antiviral, anti-inflammatory, antimutagenic, analgesic, fever-reducing, antispasmodic, antithrombotic, apoptotic, cardioprotective, chemomodulatory, antitumor, hepatoprotective, hypoglycemic, hypolipidemic, stress-reducing, antiflatulence, sleep-enhancing, libido-enhancing, lactation-enhancing, and memory-enhancing. It's even been used to treat both diarrhea and constipation![40] One of its most popular uses is as a digestive aid; it's been used since ancient Roman and Egyptian times to treat indigestion, bloating, poor appetite, and flatulence.[41] Fennel contains calcium, iron, phosphorous, magnesium, manganese, zinc, selenium, vitamin K, vitamin C, and folate and is a natural source of estrogen. It can be eaten raw or cooked, and its seeds, bulb, stalks, and leaves are all edible. Let's take a look at some of the recent studies on *Foeniculum vulgare*.

- In India, it's customary to chew fennel seeds after a meal to aid in digestion and freshen your breath. Now research has found another benefit: Chewing fennel seeds after eating is a great way to increase salivary pH, which prevents demineralization of enamel and has an anticavity effect.[42]

- In postmenopausal women, fennel seed extract has been shown to suppress bone resorption by modulating mature osteoclasts, prevent the decrease of bone mass, and enhance bone strength. These effects were observed in vitro as well as in vivo in women who took 30 or 100 mg a day of fennel seed extract for 6 weeks. These results highlight fennel's role as a natural way to prevent bone loss in postmenopausal osteoporosis.[43]

- A randomized, placebo-controlled trial on 125 infants found that fennel seed oil emulsion relieved colic in 65 percent of the infants.[44]

- There is evidence that fennel tea can decrease hunger, reduce food intake, and promote feelings of fullness. A study of overweight women who drank fennel tea before a meal demonstrated these effects, suggesting that fennel may have a role as a low-cost, easy means of appetite control. (Fenugreek tea had a similar effect.)[45]

- In a 3-month study of 80 women, a 30 mg fennel supplement was shown to relieve nausea and weakness associated with premenstrual syndrome (PMS) and to reduce the duration of menstrual periods if used consistently. In this study, the women took the fennel supplement every 4 hours beginning 3 days before menstruation and continuing until the 5th day.[46]

- A skin cream containing 4 percent fennel extract improved skin moisture, roughness, scaliness, smoothness, and wrinkles.[47]

greens

One of the most oft-repeated bits of health advice is to "eat dark, leafy greens." So what's the big deal about greens, and which plants exactly *are* dark, leafy greens? Spinach and kale are likely the first examples that come to mind, and while these delicious, cancer-fighting, cardio-protective, antioxidant-rich, bone-health-supporting veggies are excellent examples of why dark, leafy greens are healing foods powerhouses, there's a whole world of greens to sample. Technically, broccoli and members of the cabbage family can fall into this category, but as those cruciferous vegetables have their own entries, here we'll focus on true "greens," or edible plant leaves. We're talking amaranth leaves, arugula, beet greens, chard (Swiss and rainbow), chickweed, chicory, collard greens, dandelion greens, endive, escarole, lettuces (butter, green leaf, iceberg, red leaf, and romaine), mustard greens, red clover, turnip greens, watercress . . . and yes, spinach and kale.

super-charge your meals

Take one gulp of your kale smoothie and can't stomach the rest? We may have another way for you to sneak in the nutritional benefits of this dark, leafy green. Try throwing it into one of your favorite soups. The kale will wilt down and have a somewhat similar texture to spinach.

Dark, leafy greens have earned their reputation as superfoods because they're strongly associated with a reduced incidence of a wide range of chronic diseases. In fact, the Centers for Disease Control and Prevention (CDC) recently ranked a variety of fruits and vegetables according to their nutrient and phytochemical content, and dark, leafy greens far and away came out on top. Specifically, they contained the most nutrients identified as having public health importance: potassium, fiber, protein, calcium, iron, thiamin, riboflavin, niacin, folate, zinc, and vitamins A, B_6, B_{12}, C, D, E, and K. Who was the win-

getting the most from your greens

With the exception of residents of the Southern states, Americans as a rule aren't all that familiar with cooking greens. Those of us who live in other areas of the country throw them in salads and maybe put them on sandwiches. But why limit yourself to raw leaves? Greens are very easy to cook once you know a few tricks.

- TRIM THE STEMS. While the leaves are often surprisingly tender, the stems on leafy greens can be unpleasantly tough and should probably be discarded or used in vegetable stock. Before cooking greens, separate the leaf from the stem by running a sharp knife alongside the stem and center rib.

- MAKE SURE YOUR GREENS ARE CLEAN. Since the leafy greens grow close to the ground, and the frilly leaves readily capture the dirt and grit, it's important to wash all parts of greens thoroughly. The easiest way is to fill the sink or a large bowl with cold water and swish the greens around, allowing any dirt or sand to sink to the bottom. When the greens are clean, transfer them to a colander to drain.

- CUT THICK GREENS INTO RIBBONS. When cooking thick greens like kale or Swiss chard, it's helpful to cut them into ribbons, or small pieces. This will help them cook more quickly and become tender.

- BOIL THEM QUICKLY. The easiest way to prepare greens is to submerge them briefly in boiling water. Drop the greens in a cup of boiling water, cover, and cook for about 4 minutes, or until tender. You can then sauté them more quickly, if desired, for certain stir-fries and other recipes.

Smoothies are one of the easiest ways to add healing foods to your diet, especially dark, leafy greens. With just the right balance of the two, you won't even taste that cup of kale or spinach added to your shake! Want an extra sneaky nutritional punch? Toss in a tablespoon or two of flaxseeds or chia seeds.

---

ner overall? Watercress,[48] that humble water plant that should be upgraded from garnish to main dish. To see which dark, leafy greens join watercress as nutrient-dense veggies, see "The CDC's Top 20 Powerhouse Fruits and Vegetables" on page 122.

We'll look at research on specific greens below, but first, a few general observations. Typically, the darker the green, the higher the phytonutrient content—thus kale or collards will provide far more healing food power than iceberg lettuce. All greens are exceptionally low in calories, fat, sodium, cholesterol, carbs, and sugar and exceptionally high in fiber and water content. Vitamin and mineral content and potency vary somewhat by each specific green, but generally, most any dark, leafy green will be a great source of vitamins A, C, and K and folate, a B vitamin that promotes cardiovascular health and helps to prevent cancer, especially of the breast, cervix, lung, and pancreas.[49] Other notable nutrients in dark, leafy greens are manganese, iron, copper, potassium, and even cal-

cium; those who don't eat meat and/or dairy products have long looked to dark, leafy greens as a dietary source of calcium. Nonlactating adults should get 1,000 to 1,200 mg of calcium per day,[50] and dark, leafy greens get you well on your way: Just 1 cup of chopped frozen collard greens contains 357 mg of calcium (1 cup of fresh chopped collards contains 268 mg), 1 cup of cooked amaranth leaves contains 276 mg of calcium, and 1 cup of cooked spinach contains 245 mg of calcium.[51] Let's turn our attention to the many other health benefits these superfood veggies offer.

- A recent metastudy based on data from nearly 1.7 million people found an inverse relationship between consumption of green, leafy vegetables and risk of bladder cancer: Every 0.2 serving increment of leafy greens is associated with a 2 percent decrease in bladder cancer risk.[52]

- Frequent consumption of green, leafy vegetables is associated with a reduced incidence of lung, esophageal,

the cdc's top 20 powerhouse fruits and vegetables

"Powerhouse" fruits and vegetables are the foods most strongly associated with reduced chronic disease risk. To be considered a powerhouse fruit or vegetable in the ranking system conducted by the Centers for Disease Control and Prevention (CDC), a food had to provide, per 100 calories, 10 percent or more of the daily value of 17 nutrients with public health importance: potassium, fiber, protein, calcium, iron, thiamin, riboflavin, niacin, folate, zinc, and vitamins A, B_6, B_{12}, C, D, E, and K. Nutrient density scores ranged from 10.47 to 122.68; for ease of interpretation, scores were capped at 100. Here are the CDC's top 20 powerhouse foods, along with their nutrient density scores.[53] Leafy greens are best in class.

FOOD	NUTRIENT DENSITY SCORE
Watercress	100.00
Chinese cabbage	91.99
Chard	89.27
Beet greens	87.08
Spinach	86.43
Chicory	73.36
Leaf lettuce	70.73
Parsley	65.59
Romaine lettuce	63.48
Collard greens	62.49
Turnip greens	62.12
Mustard greens	61.39
Endive	60.44
Chives	54.80
Kale	49.07
Dandelion greens	46.34
Red peppers	41.26
Arugula	37.65
Broccoli	34.89
Pumpkin	33.82

Source: Adapted from: J. Di Noia, "Defining Powerhouse Fruits and Vegetables: A Nutrient Density Approach," *Preventing Chronic Disease* 11 (2014): 130390.

nasopharyngeal, breast, skin, and stomach cancer.[54]

▪ Dietary nitrate has been shown to exert a range of beneficial vascular effects, including reducing blood pressure, inhibiting platelet aggregation, improving endothelial function, enhancing exercise performance, protecting against ischemia-reperfusion injury, and reducing arterial stiffness, inflammation, and intimal thickness (a marker of atherosclerosis). Dark, leafy greens are among the best sources of vegetable dietary nitrate. The highest content is found in arugula, followed by spinach, lettuces, radishes, beetroot, and Chinese cabbage.[55]

▪ A long-term study based on data from nearly 75,000 people found that, out of all vegetables, green, leafy vegetables were the most protective against stroke.[56]

▪ Likewise, it's been well established that fruit and vegetable intake is associated with a reduced risk of coronary heart disease, and green, leafy vegetables are particularly protective.[57]

▪ The same holds true for type 2 diabetes (T2D): Fruit and vegetable consumption is associated with a reduced risk of developing T2D, and green, leafy vegetables are particularly effective. A study based on more than 424,000 people, including 24,013 cases of T2D, found that every 0.2 serving per day increase in green, leafy vegetables resulted in a 13 percent lower risk of T2D.[58]

▪ Raw cruciferous vegetables are the major dietary source of isothiocyanates, natural phytochemicals that are lauded for their cancer-fighting effects. In a chemical analysis of the isothiocyanate yield of various cruciferous vegetables, mustard greens were the clear winner, with 61.3 µmol per 100 g. Cabbage came in a distant second with 31.7 µmol, and in third place was Brussels sprouts, at 9.6 µmol.[59]

▪ An isothiocyanate called erucin is present in large quantities in arugula, kohlrabi, and Chinese cabbage. In an in vitro study, erucin was found to be effective at inhibiting cell proliferation of breast cancer cells.[60]

mushrooms

One could easily write a book on edible mushrooms, one of the most abundant, variegated, and complex foods on the planet. There are more than 2,000 types of edible mushrooms, but only a fraction of those are commonly eaten. In the United States, some of the most popular types are common white button mushrooms, portobellos, cremini ("baby bellas"), oysters, chanterelles, morels, and shiitake mushrooms, but any attempt to highlight a few 'shrooms is sure to miss someone's favorite. As Americans have become more enamored with these edible fungi, varieties such as enokis, porcini, and the large, richly flavored hen-of-the-woods have become easy to find in local supermarkets.

Mushrooms have been used for thousands of years for their medicinal effects, and it could be said that modern research is only just catching up to this powerful healing food, but more than 100 medicinal effects have been identified already.[61] Before we turn to the research, mushrooms deserve special mention as an excellent source of vitamin D. Vitamin D is difficult to obtain through dietary means—our main source is sun exposure—and mushrooms are one of the very few plants that generate vitamin D when exposed to sunlight. Mushrooms are also a good source of vitamin C, vitamin E, B vitamins, selenium, potassium, riboflavin, niacin, protein, and fiber.

■ Mushroom polysaccharides from the beta-glucan family have been shown to exert an anticancer effect by enhancing cellular immunity. Numerous studies have shown that mushroom consumption is associated with a decreased risk of breast cancer, and vitamin D_2 may be responsible for this effect. Further studies have shown that various mushroom extracts can suppress proliferation of breast cancer cells. Other cancers that have been shown to be susceptible to mushroom compounds include bladder, cervical, colorectal, endometrial, liver, lung, ovarian, prostate, pancreatic, and skin cancers, as well as leukemia.[62]

■ Mushrooms exhibit significant antioxidant effects because of bioactive compounds such as polyphenols, polysaccharides, vitamins, carotenoids, and minerals. Thus they're a readily available, natural means of reducing oxidative stress and inflammation, and they help prevent a range of conditions associated with an excess of reactive oxygen species, including metabolic disease, cardiovascular disease, Alzheimer's disease, Parkinson's disease, premature aging, and various cancers.[63]

■ The reishi (or lingzhi) mushroom, which has been used as a medicinal plant in Asian countries for more than 4,000 years, is such a powerful healing food that it's known as the "mushroom of immortality." Indeed, its health benefits are so extensive that you can see why it earned its name. Reishi mushroom extract exerts antibacterial, antiviral, and antifungal properties. Compounds from the reishi mushroom have exhibited an antitumor effect in various cancers, including breast, liver, and gastric cancer, as well as leukemia. Reishi mushrooms also exhibit anti-inflammatory, antioxidant, hypoglycemic, cholesterol-lowering, and immune-boosting effects. They've been shown to help heal ulcers, prevent angiogenesis (the growth of new blood vessels) in cancer cells, inhibit androgen-mediated diseases, and protect your liver.[64]

■ In a study of 73 obese people who substituted mushrooms for red meat for 1 year, those on the mushroom diet lost more pounds and a greater percentage of body weight; achieved a lower body mass index, waist circumference, and percentage of total body fat; had lower systolic and diastolic blood pressure; and saw improvements in their lipid profiles and inflammatory markers.[65] Perhaps not surprisingly, then, one study showed that mushroom consumers are less likely to be overweight or obese and less likely to have metabolic syndrome.[66]

■ In a study on the effect of mushrooms on the immune system, 51 healthy adults ate either 50 or 100 grams of dried shiitake mushrooms every day for 28 days. Blood tests revealed no significant difference between the serving sizes, so researchers pooled the data. After 28 days, subjects experienced a marked increase in several interleukins (which stimulate immune response) and tumor necrosis factor alpha (which regulates immune cells), as well as a decrease in macrophage inflammatory protein-1 alpha (a marker of inflammation).[67]

onions

Onions are generally grouped into two categories: green onions (scallions) and dry onions, which include common bulb onions such as yellow, red, white, and Vidalia. Whatever the type, onions are extremely versatile when it comes to culinary use. Red onions and scallions in particular are delicious eaten raw, and onions can be sautéed, frizzled, fried, grilled, pickled, baked, and used in a nearly endless variety of dishes. These members of the *Allium* genus are one of our best dietary sources of the powerful flavonoid quercetin, which acts like an antioxidant and has multiple cardioprotective, anti-inflammatory, and antiallergy effects. Other compounds in onions have exhibited anticancer effects, antiplatelet activity, antithrombotic activity, antiasthmatic activity, antibiotic effects,[68] and cholesterol-lowering effects. A high intake of onions and their close cousin, garlic (*Allium sativum*), has been associated with a decreased risk of cancers of the oral cavity, pharynx, larynx, esophagus, colon and rectum, endometrium, ovary, and stomach.[69]

■ Obese women who took a 100 mg capsule of onion peel extract every day for 12 weeks experienced significantly reduced waist and hip circumferences by the end of the study. Plasma reactive oxygen species (ROS) levels were lower, while superoxide dismutase (SOD) activity was higher, indicating onion peel extract's antioxidant capabilities. The beneficial effects are thought to be due to the high levels of quercetin found in onion peel.[70]

■ In an 8-week study of obese or overweight women with polycystic ovary syndrome, consuming raw red onions was found to lower total and LDL cholesterol. The effect was greater in those who consumed more onions: 40 to 50 grams twice a day if overweight or 50 to 60 grams twice a day if obese.[71]

■ Adults with moderately high cholesterol were divided into two groups: one group drank 100 ml of onion juice daily for 8 weeks, and the second group drank a placebo. By the end of the study, the onion group experienced significantly decreased waist circumference, total cholesterol, and LDL cholesterol. Further, the quercetin-rich onion juice increased their total antioxidant capacity and prolonged the lag time of LDL oxidation.[72]

get caught eating onions

We should all be eating more onions. To get the most nutrients from your daily dose, eat several different kinds. Red and yellow onions and shallots have the highest flavonoid content, while white onions have the least.

SAVE YOUR BREATH. If the fear of having horrific halitosis is keeping you from enjoying the health benefits of onions, here's a freshening tip. Eat a sprig of fresh parsley. This will help neutralize the sulfur compounds before they turn into offending breath. A breath freshener made with parsley seed oil can also help.

peppers, bell

The term "bell pepper" is often used interchangeably with "sweet pepper," though according to some sources bell peppers are a type of sweet pepper, while others insist that they're two different peppers entirely. To make things more confusing, some people use terms like "sweet bell pepper" or "sweet red pepper." Note, too, that there are peppers whose official name always includes "sweet," such as sweet banana peppers and sweet cherry peppers—and these are distinctly different from bell peppers. And are you ready for your mind to be completely blown? Peppers of any type are actually fruits, not vegetables. But we're including peppers in our Vegetables section because that's how they're most often thought of when it comes to culinary use and grocery store shelving.

While all peppers are members of the *Capsicum* genus, the peppers we're talking about here contain zero capsaicin, the compound that gives chile peppers their kick. Bell peppers boast a range of colors, from white to chocolaty brown, and they all taste fresh and range in sweetness, but they're not spicy. Depending on their color, they'll have slightly different nutritional profiles. Green peppers are a potent source of vitamin C and a good source of fiber and vitamins A, B_6, and K. Red peppers are also a potent source of vitamin C, but they contain greater amounts of vitamin A, quercetin, and luteolin, and they're a good source of fiber, vitamin B_6, and folate. Yellow and orange peppers are similar to red pepper in terms of nutrients. Purple bell peppers will have a higher anthocyanin content than the other varieties, as well as high levels of vitamins A and C. All peppers have zero sodium, cholesterol, and fat and contain very few calories. They're delicious eaten raw or cooked, though there is some evidence that cooking peppers enhances their phenolic content.

- Increased consumption of vitamin C–rich foods, including bell peppers and broccoli, has been correlated with a decreased risk of prostate cancer.[73]

- Bell peppers are an abundant source of the flavonoids quercetin, luteolin, and apigenin, as well as flavonoid glycosides, which exert antioxidant, anti-inflammation, and antiallergy effects.[74]

- A combination of beta-carotene and lutein from pepper fruits exhibited a photoprotective effect and may help prevent skin carcinogenesis.[75]

peppers, chile (hot peppers)

Like their bell pepper cousins, chile peppers are actually fruits, and they're members of the genus *Capsicum*. But these guys, also referred to as hot peppers, deliver up a strong dose of spice. And it turns out that the same substances that give them their piquant punch—chemicals called capsaicinoids—lend them their healing power. Perhaps counterintuitively, one of the most celebrated healing effects of hot peppers is their ability to relieve pain. There are different theories as to how capsaicin works as an analgesic, but some believe that it depletes neurons of "substance P," a neurotransmitter that plays a role in creating the sensation of pain. Another is that it decreases cutaneous sensitivity and reduces pain by "defunctionalizing" pain receptors.[76] However it works, it's certainly effective: The topical application of capsaicin (in the form of creams, lotions, or patches) has been shown to relieve the pain of arthritis, diabetic neuropathy, HIV-associated neuropathy, psoriasis, postoperative neuralgia, peripheral inflammation, nerve injury, migraine, chronic back pain, and intractable pain associated with cancer.[77]

Familiar varieties include jalapeño, habanero, cayenne, poblano, serrano, and bird's eye chile peppers. But as Americans have grown bolder (and more curious), they've branched out into sampling some of the hottest members of the chile pepper family, whose names alone tell you what you're in for: devil's tongue, Naga Viper, Trinidad scorpion, ghost pepper. The world's hottest chile pepper, the Carolina Reaper, was developed right here in the United States. But don't worry—you need not set your mouth on fire to reap the healing benefits of hot peppers. The varieties you can find in your local market deliver plenty of capsaicinoids, and 100 g of fresh chiles contains about 240 percent of the recommended daily value of vitamin C.[78] They're also a good source of vitamin A and vitamin B_6. The capsaicin in chile peppers has exhibited antioxidant, anti-inflammatory, anticancer, hypolipidemic, cholesterol-lowering, and cardioprotective effects.[79] Let's look at some of the research on the healing effects of these fruits that sting.

- A metastudy based on 2,050 participants examined the use of herbal medicines for low-back pain and found that cayenne cream was the most effective for relieving pain.[80]

- Capsaicin is also delivered intranasally as a treatment for nonallergic rhinitis. In a review of four studies involving 302 people with nonallergic rhinitis, capsaicin was shown to be effective in relieving some nasal symptoms, such as nasal blockage and sneezing. Further studies are required to assess the efficacy of different dosages of capsaicin on a range of rhinitis severities.[81]

■ Capsaicin exhibits antibacterial and antiviral activity. It's been shown to be effective against common human pathogens such as *Streptococci*, *Escherichia coli* (commonly known

the 411 on hot peppers

Cooking with hot peppers is like riding a Harley. You have to do it very carefully.

"Approach hot peppers with respect," says Bill Hufnagle, author of *Biker Billy Cooks with Fire*. To use hot peppers without getting burned, follow these Hufnagle tips:

■ PROTECT YOUR HANDS. When you're cooking with very hot peppers—"anything hotter than a jalapeño," Hufnagle says—put on a pair of disposable plastic gloves. (If you have sensitive hands, you may want to wear gloves even when you're working with milder peppers.) When you're done, thoroughly rinse the tips of the gloves with soapy water before taking them off to avoid transferring the pepper oil to your fingers. Then immediately wash your hands, says Hufnagle.

■ USE PLENTY OF SOAP. Chile oil sticks to the skin and water alone won't get it off. You need to use plenty of soap as well. "You might want to wash your hands more than once, depending on the kind of pepper you were working with and how much of it you handled," says Hufnagle.

■ PROTECT AGAINST PEPPER DUST. When grinding or crushing dried hot peppers, wear a dust mask and goggles. "The dust can get in your throat and eyes," says Hufnagle.

■ CRUSH THEM BY HAND. It may be convenient to grind dried hot peppers in a blender or coffee grinder—but you won't appreciate the aftershocks. "How thoroughly can you wash a coffee grinder or blender, anyway?" says Hufnagle. "If you use them to grind peppers, you're going to have some nice hot spicy coffee—or milkshakes." At the very least, you may want to consider getting a separate grinder to use on dried hot peppers only.

as *E. coli*), *Klebsiella pneumoniae*, *Staphylococcus*, *Helicobacter pylori*, and others.[82]

■ Capsaicin inhibits acid secretion, stimulates alkali and mucus secretion, and stimulates gastric mucosal blood flow, all of which help to prevent and heal gastric ulcers.[83]

■ Chile peppers can play a role in weight loss and weight management. Capsaicinoids have been shown to accentuate the impact of calorie restriction, increase energy expenditure, curb appetite, and help to prevent regaining weight after weight loss.[84]

■ We saved the best for last: Remarkably, a population-based cohort study that examined data from more than 487,000 people found that regularly eating spicy foods was inversely associated with . . . death! Compared to those who ate spicy food less than once a week, those who said yes to spice six or seven times a week showed a 14 percent lower risk of death from any cause. Researchers also looked at different causes of death, and they observed inverse associations between spicy food consumption and deaths due to cancer, ischemic heart diseases, and respiratory diseases. In this study, fresh and dried chile peppers were the most commonly used spices.[85]

sauerkraut

Sauerkraut, German for "sour cabbage," gets its own entry apart from cabbage because of the powerful health benefits that come from the fermentation process, not the least of which is sauerkraut's high probiotic content. Salt and sometimes various spices are added to cabbage to make sauerkraut, but essentially, sauerkraut is finely shredded cabbage that has been fermented by *Lactobacillus* bacteria. It's eaten as a side dish; as an ingredient in stews, soups, and casseroles; as a topping to other dishes; and, perhaps most famously, as an essential ingredient in the Reuben sandwich. Fermented cabbage was eaten as far back as the 4th century BCE,[86] and sauerkraut is becoming more popular in America as its reputation as a health food grows. Sauerkraut is rich in vitamin C and vitamin K, and it's a good source of fiber, iron, and manganese. Both the sauerkraut and its brine, sometimes referred to as kraut juice, contain high levels of probiotics, though the probiotics are killed by cooking or heating, so if at all possible, eat your sauerkraut cold and unpasteurized. Some people find that drinking kraut juice is easier on their digestive systems than eating the cabbage, which can cause gas.

- Sauerkraut contains compounds called isothiocyanates, which are produced during the fermentation process.[87] Isothiocyanates have been extensively studied for their anticancer potential and have been found to prevent cancer by altering carcinogen metabolism; inhibiting tumor progression, cell proliferation, and cell progression; inducing cancer cell death; and inhibiting cell signaling pathways in various types of cancer.[88]

- Cabbage and sauerkraut juices have exhibited strong chemopreventive activity against human breast cancer.[89] (Other studies of sauerkraut and its juices have demonstrated a chemopreventive effect against kidney and liver cancer in animal models.)[90] The effect is explained in part by cabbage's ability to inhibit aromatase expression; aromatase inhibitors stop the production of estrogen, which can stimulate the growth of hormone-receptor-positive breast cancer cells.[91]

- Lactic acid bacteria have been used to treat diarrhea, inflammatory bowel disease, and food allergies, and new evidence demonstrates that these bacteria may have a role in preventing colorectal cancer, the third-leading cause of cancer deaths worldwide.[92] Sauerkraut, with its high *Lactobacillus* and fiber content, may provide extra protection against deadly colorectal cancer.

- There's also evidence that probiotic-rich foods such as sauerkraut can have an anxiety-relieving effect. In one study, 710 young adults completed questionnaires on fermented food consumption, neuroticism, and social anxiety. Researchers found that in those who tended toward neuroticism, a higher consumption of fermented foods, including sauerkraut, resulted in fewer symptoms of social anxiety.[93]

sea vegetables and seaweeds

The health benefits of marine plants have already become a hot topic in the health and wellness community, and you'll be hearing more about this incredibly rich source of healing in the years to come. Seaweeds and sea vegetables are rich in phenolic compounds that are not available in land plants, and their sheer quantity makes them attractive as an eco-friendly and nearly limitless source of food and medicine. Seaweed especially can grow at terrific rates; seaweed farming has been practiced for centuries in Asia and is becoming increasingly popular in the United States as the public becomes more aware of seaweed's health benefits. Both the variety and the taste of plants sourced from the ocean can take a little getting used to. But you probably already know more than you think about sea plants. If you've eaten sushi, you've had nori (sea lettuce), the seaweed "wrapper" used in sushi rolls. Kombu is the thinly cut seaweed commonly added to miso soup. Carrageenan is a food additive sourced from seaweed that you'll find in many products, including plant milks, yogurt, ice cream, and salad dressings; agar, sourced from algae, is used in desserts and as a vegetarian substitute for gelatin. Kelp, a variety of brown algae, and spirulina, a type of blue-green algae, are already popular as health foods. Other examples of sea plants that you'd find at Asian markets and health food stores include dulse, hijiki, arame, and sea palm.

So why are sea vegetables so healthy? Nutritional profiles differ according to the type of plant, but generally they provide iodine, vitamin A, vitamin C, vitamin K, manganese, protein, and fiber. Sea lettuce and nori deserve a special mention for their high levels of vitamin B_{12}, making them the only vegetarian sources of this essential nutrient that is more often found in animal products.[94] Brown seaweed and algae also contain a unique class of phytonutrients called fucoidans, a sulfated polysaccharide that has shown a range of health benefits, including anti-inflammatory, cardioprotective, antiviral, and anticancer effects. Eating seaweed on a daily basis has been associated with a reduced risk of cardiovascular disease, hyperlipidemia, breast cancer, and type 2 diabetes.[95] There is much more to learn about the benefits of foods from the sea.

■ Fucoidan from brown algae and seaweed has demonstrated a range of anticancer effects, including the suppression of growth, a decrease in metastasis, the inhibition of angio-

super-charge your meals

Seaweed has a unique taste and texture that can be a challenge to get used to, so start off small when adding it into your meals so that you don't miss out on all the nutritional benefits. Try dried, ground varieties of different seaweeds to use in seasoning your favorite dishes.

genesis (the growth of new blood vessels), and the induction of cell death. In vitro studies have shown its anticancer effects against breast cancer, colon cancer, lung cancer, and lymphoma.[96]

■ Seaweed can help prevent and manage type 2 diabetes. Polysaccharides and seaweed's high dietary fiber content can promote satiety, thereby reducing blood glucose levels and insulin sensitivity. Seaweed's fiber, monounsaturated fats, and polyunsaturated fats help mitigate the inflammatory response due to hyperglycemia and obesity. Seaweed is also able to reduce the rate of carbohydrate digestion and absorption and to stimulate a hormone that triggers insulin secretion.[97]

■ Spirulina has been shown to reduce total cholesterol, LDL cholesterol, and triglycerides and to boost HDL cholesterol.[98]

■ Sea vegetables have such a positive health profile that some researchers are not only advocating for their consumption as whole foods, they're also advocating using them as additives to reduce the damage caused by unhealthy foods such as the fast foods, bakery goods, and snacks that comprise a large part of the Western diet. With their high dietary fiber, more nutritious form of potassium salt (rather than conventional sodium salt), nutrient density, and ability to boost antioxidant capacity, sea plants are excellent functional foods, in their whole forms or as nutrient-boosting additives.[99]

■ Studies have shown that blue-green algae, which contains an abundance of bioactive components, including plant sterols and carotenoids, can lower total cholesterol and triglycerides. It also reduces inflammation by inhibiting nuclear factor-kappa beta activity and reducing the production of proinflammatory cytokines. Further, blue-green algae inhibits lipid peroxidation and exerts free radical scavenging activity. The multitude of blue-green algae's health benefits make it an effective tool in the prevention of metabolic, inflammatory, and cardiovascular diseases.[100]

soy products

Soy products include whole soybeans (also known as edamame), tofu (soybean curd), and soy milk; fermented soy products such as tempeh, natto, miso, and soy sauce; and foods such as soybean oil and soybean flour. Soy is used to make an astonishing number of food products—everything from veggie burgers to soy nut butter to hydrolyzed vegetable protein to soy cheese to yogurt. As is the general rule for all foods, the less processed, the better. So look for whole food (such as edamame) or lightly processed (such as tofu) soy options. Many people find that fermented soy products are easier to digest than unfermented, as well. Another thing to keep in mind with soy is that the vast majority of soy products in the United States come from genetically modified soy, so if you want to avoid GMO (genetically modified organism) products, be sure and buy organic, non-GMO soy.

Frozen edamame is a rich source of vitamin K, manganese, and folate and a good source of fiber and protein. Fresh soybeans are rich in protein, manganese, vitamin C, and folate and are a good source of fiber, calcium, iron, magnesium, phosphorous, potassium, and thiamin. Tofu is rich in protein, calcium, phosphorous, copper, manganese, and selenium and is a good source of fiber, magnesium, zinc, and thiamin. All soy is rich in isoflavones, which act as phytoestrogens and confer a number of health benefits, including a lower risk of osteoporosis, heart disease, some cancers, and some menopausal symptoms. The main isoflavones in soy are genistein and daidzein.

- Obese women who consumed 80 g of soybeans a day for 12 weeks experienced significant improvements in weight, BMI, waist circumference, and sagittal abdominal depth (belly fat).[101]

- High-protein (26 g) soy snacks consumed in the afternoon were shown to reduce appetite and led to fewer high-fat and high-sugar snacks in adolescents. Beneficial outcomes to mood and cognition were also observed.[102]

- Postmenopausal women who ate fermented soybeans daily for 6 months experienced lower total cholesterol and a significant increase in progesterone.[103]

super-charge your meals

Tofu and other soy products provide a lot of protein. Though soy has become a more popular ingredient, many are still afraid to add it to their foods. Supercharge a breakfast scramble by adding diced tofu along with other healthy ingredients.

about tofu

You've seen tofu in the produce section of your supermarket. But how do you eat this pale, spongy stuff?

Almost any way you want. The advantage of tofu is that while it has little taste of its own, it takes on the flavor of whatever it's cooked with. You can use it with meats and in soups, vegetable dishes, and even desserts.

There are two main types of tofu, firm and soft. Which one you buy depends on how you're going to use it.

- FIRM TOFU has had much of the water removed, giving it a solid consistency. It's usually used when you want the tofu to keep its shape, as in recipes for stir-fries, casseroles, or mock meatballs.

- SOFT (ALSO CALLED SILKEN) TOFU contains more water than the firm variety, giving it a soft, creamy texture. It's usually used for making dips, salad dressings, and desserts.

Both types of tofu should be rinsed with cold water before using. If you're not planning to use the tofu immediately after opening the container, or if you buy it fresh from an open container at an Asian market, rinse it daily and keep it submerged in fresh water. You can also keep it frozen.

After rinsing, press out excess water with your hands or by placing the tofu between several layers of paper towels and pressing with your palm. Removing the excess water will help the tofu maintain its shape during preparation.

- Epidemiological studies have shown that a high consumption of soy products is associated with lower incidence of hormone-mediated cancers, including breast and prostate cancer. Genistein, one of the primary isoflavones in soy products, has been shown to inhibit carcinogenesis as well as angiogenesis, the uncontrolled proliferation of blood vessels involved in cancer growth, invasion, and metastasis.[104]

See also: Milk (Plant-Based) (page 12)

sweet potatoes

Although sweet potatoes and yams are often thought of as interchangeable and are sold under either name, they're actually two distinct vegetables. True yams are drier and starchier, and they're relatively difficult to find in the United States. (Yes, those yams you've been buying for Thanksgiving are probably orange sweet potatoes.) Most importantly, sweet potatoes are nutritionally superior to yams, with roughly 100 times the vitamin A, more protein, more vitamin C, fewer calories, and a lower glycemic index. They're also, by the way, nutritionally superior to white potatoes. While sweet potatoes actually have a slightly higher carbohydrate content, they contain more fiber and calcium and have a lower glycemic load than white potatoes. In addition to the nutrients listed above, sweet potatoes are also an excellent source of manganese and a good source of fiber, potassium, vitamin B_6, and lutein. Sweet potato leaves are edible and highly nutritious, providing antioxidants, protein, fiber, and minerals, especially potassium, phosphorous, calcium, magnesium, iron, manganese, and copper.[105]

- Sweet potato protein has been shown to exert a powerful antiproliferative and antimetastatic effect against colorectal cancer cells.[106]

- In in vitro studies, extracts made from purple-fleshed sweet potatoes have been shown to inhibit the growth of breast cancer, gastric cancer, and colon cancer.[107]

- An ointment made from white sweet potato flour was shown to speed cutaneous wound healing. Further, suspensions made from white sweet potato flour prevented ethanol-induced gastric ulceration, while in

power pairs
sweet potatoes and cayenne pepper

Spicy sweet potato fries can do more than satisfy a craving for some crunch: Sprinkling some cayenne pepper or chili powder on orange foods rich in beta-carotene, like sweet potatoes and butternut squash, enhances vitamin A absorption. Go ahead and dig into those fries![108]

one potato, two potato, sweet potato

Sweet potatoes come in all shapes and sizes, so don't be surprised the veggie touted by that name at your supermarket looks a little different from month to month. Sweet potatoes can have skin that's white, yellow, orange, red, or even purple. Inside, the flesh may be yellow or deep orange. But don't call it a yam—true yams are grown in South America, the Caribbean, and Africa. They have brown or black outer skin and flesh that's off-white, purple, or red and tastes sweeter than that of a sweet potato. Most "yams" sold in US supermarkets are really sweet potatoes.

Because they are cured (meaning they are kept in high humidity and temperatures for about a week and a half) by growers before they are shipped to market, sweet potatoes are excellent keepers and will stay fresh for about a month after you bring them home from the store. It's important, however, to store them carefully to prevent them from going bad.

- **KEEP THEM COOL.** Sweet potatoes should be stored in cellars, pantries, or basements, where temperatures are 45°F to 55°F. (Don't put them in the refrigerator, since this shortens their shelf life.) When sweet potatoes are stored at room temperature, they'll keep for about a week.

- **STORE THEM DRY.** Sweet potatoes will spoil once they get wet. That's why it's best to store them dry, then wash them only when you're ready to start cooking.

- **TREAT THEM GENTLY.** Sweet potatoes spoil quickly when they get cut or bruised, so don't buy them if they look damaged. At home, treating them gently will help ensure their longevity.

- **BAKE A BIG BATCH.** Baked sweet potatoes will keep in the refrigerator for 7 to 10 days. To bake, scrub the potatoes, dry them, and pierce the skins in several places. Place them on a baking sheet covered with aluminum foil (to catch dripping juices) and bake at 350°F for about 1 hour. Any leftovers can be reheated in the microwave oven or mashed with trans-fat-free margarine (buy a brand that's low in saturated fat, too) and a dab of brown sugar for a quick side dish later in the week.

vitro experiments showed that crude extracts were able to scavenge free radicals.[109]

■ An in vitro study showed that purple sweet potato extract exhibited anti- lipogenic, anti-inflammatory, and lipolytic effects on fat cells. It also showed free radical scavenging and reducing activity.[110]

whole grains

barley

Barley is a cereal grain with a nutty flavor and chewy texture. It's famous as an ingredient in soups, but you can use it any way that you'd use rice or you can eat it as a hot cereal. Barley is also used in several beverages, including beer, whiskey, wine, tea, malted milk drinks, and barley water. A good source of fiber, manganese, molybdenum, and selenium, this ancient grain is a low-GI food and, like oats, is very rich in beta-glucans, polysaccharide soluble fibers known for their cholesterol-lowering, glucose-regulating, and immune-supporting effects. It also has a high antioxidant capacity due to the presence of phenolic compounds such as flavonols, benzoic acid, and cinnamic acid.[1] With its high fiber content and complex carbohydrates, barley prevents constipation and lowers cholesterol. It does contain a small amount of gluten, so if you're looking for gluten-free grains or cereals, try amaranth, buckwheat, millet, or quinoa, instead.

barley for beginners

Unlike rice and wheat, which are quite mild, barley has a robust, slightly pungent taste that complements highly flavored dishes like lamb stew or mushroom soup. But you prepare it in much the same way as other grains by mixing it with water and letting it simmer, covered, until the kernels are tender. Here are a few additional tips.

- **PLAN FOR EXPANSION.** One cup of dried barley will expand to about four times that amount during cooking, so be sure to use a pan that is slightly oversized.
- **GIVE IT TIME TO TENDERIZE.** Hulled barley is extremely tough and slow to cook, so it should be soaked overnight before cooking. Pearl barley, on the other hand, has had the tough outer husk removed and doesn't require soaking.
- **USE IT AS AN ADD-IN.** Even properly prepared barley is somewhat chewy, so it's rarely served as a side dish. Most cooks prefer to make barley ahead of time, then add it to soups or stews.

- Barley beta-glucans have been found to improve the growth of probiotic microbes and enhance their performance, even after exposure to in vitro digestive tract simulation.[2]

- A study of healthy adults who added either whole wheat flour or whole grain barley pasta containing 3 grams (g) of beta-glucans to their diets examined the probiotic and bacterial effects after 2 months of intervention. *Lactobacilli* and short-chain fatty acids both increased significantly, while levels of bacterial pathogens decreased.[3]

- In an in vitro study, green barley extract exhibited antiproliferative activity against leukemia and lymphoma cells.[4]

- A study of adults who ate boiled barley kernels as part of their evening meal found that barley helped regulate blood glucose, increased the release of glucagon-like peptide-1, decreased hunger and thus the number of calories consumed over the subsequent two meals, and reduced fasting free fatty acids the next morning. (When higher, fasting free fatty acids may indicate type 2 diabetes.)[5]

See also: Oats (page 142)

buckwheat

Don't let the name fool you: Buckwheat is not a wheat, and even though it's listed here in the Whole Grains section, it's not technically a grain, either! Buckwheat is an edible fruit seed that's related to rhubarb and sorrel. It's referred to as a pseudocereal because like true cereals (such as barley and wheat) it's rich in complex carbohydrates, and it can be eaten in a similar manner. But buckwheat is not a grass like true cereals are, and it is naturally gluten free.

The hulled seeds (groats) of buckwheat are used to make hot breakfast cereals (like porridge or farina), and sprouted buckwheat groats are becoming increasingly popular food items. Buckwheat flour is used to make noodles, pancakes, crackers, breads, and other baked goods, and even tea, honey, beer, and whiskey. Buckwheat has an amazing nutritional profile. It's rich in protein, fiber, iron, magnesium, phosphorous, potassium, zinc, copper, selenium, riboflavin, niacin, and pantothenic acid, and it's also a good source of manganese, thiamin, vitamin B_6, and folate. Buckwheat is also a source of health-promoting bioactive compounds such as cholesterol-lowering sterols, D-chiro-inositol (shown to help treat polycystic ovary disease), antioxi-

cooking buckwheat

Unlike wheat, buckwheat has no gluten, a protein with a gluelike consistency. Without gluten to hold the grain together, "buckwheat will turn to mush unless you precook it," says Clifford Orr, director of the Buckwheat Institution in Penn Yan, New York. Here's what he advises.

- Put the buckwheat in a hot skillet, and toss gently for 3 to 5 minutes. This expands and strengthens the outer skin, which will help it stay intact during the simmering process.

- If you're using kasha (the roasted form of buckwheat) that's been cracked, toss it with an egg white before adding it to the pan. The albumen in the egg will help keep it firm. Uncracked kasha, however, can be cooked without the egg.

- Transfer the buckwheat to a saucepan, and add 2 cups of water for each cup of buckwheat. Always begin with boiling water, which will seal the outer surface and help the buckwheat hold its shape during cooking.

- Simmer the buckwheat, covered, until all the water and the kernels are tender. Cracked kasha will take 8 to 10 minutes, and whole will require 10 to 12 minutes.

dant phenolic acids (caffeic, gallic, and chlorogenic), and the flavonoid quercetin. Consider these additional discoveries research has uncovered.

- Buckwheat is one of the very best food sources of rutin, a flavonoid that has exhibited anti-inflammatory, antidiabetic, antiatherosclerotic, cholesterol-lowering, and anticarcinogenic properties.[6]

- In vitro, flavonoids, polysaccharides, lectins, phenylpropanoids, and proteins from buckwheat have shown anticarcinogenic activity against a wide range of cancer cells, including liver cancer, leukemia, cervical cancer, and breast cancer.[7]

- Studies have confirmed buckwheat's blood-pressure-lowering power; its various bioactive compounds, including quercetin and rutin, have strong angiotensin converting enzyme (ACE) inhibitory activity, which relaxes blood vessels.[8]

- Buckwheat honey improves the symptoms of the common cold and can treat a chronic cough.[9]
- Peptides from buckwheat proteins have demonstrated antiplatelet activity on a molecular level, highlighting buckwheat's potential as an antithrombotic functional food.[10]

oats

Oats are a cereal grain. The myriad types of oats you find in stores all start with the whole, unprocessed kernels, called groats. From there, hulled groats result in whole oat groats or just whole oats, which are harder to find in stores than the other varieties and take a long time to cook. Steel-cut oats are whole oat groats that have been chopped with a steel blade; the smaller size cuts down on the cooking time. The variety called rolled oats is probably more familiar to Americans, and these are sometimes referred to as whole oats or as old-fashioned oatmeal. Rolled oats are oat groats that have been steamed and then rolled into flakes. Rolled oats can be further processed into quick or instant, which dramatically cuts down on their cooking time. Anything from the whole oat groats on down can be eaten plain, usually as a hot breakfast cereal, and oats and oat flour are commonly used in baked goods. All forms of oats are high in fiber, particularly the polysaccharide fiber known as beta-glucan, and all forms of oats are famous for their ability to lower cholesterol.

- Oats are the only source of avenanthramides, a group of antioxidants that, in addition to anti-inflammatory activity, have been shown to exert cardioprotective benefits.[11]
- A metastudy of trials on the effect of oat or barley beta-glucans on acute glycemic response found that oat and barley foods containing at least 4 g of beta-glucan and 30 to 80 g of available carbohydrates can significantly reduce postprandial blood glucose. This study included both

super-charge your meals

Though oats are a healing food all on their own, it doesn't mean once in awhile you can't switch them out for another healing food, such as quinoa. This sweet substitution may be a gentle way to try quinoa, if you aren't familiar with it. Instead of the typical oatmeal crumb on top of your fruit dessert, try using red quinoa for the same crunchy—and healthy—texture.

Oats are among the easiest foods to cook. Just add one part oatmeal to two parts water, cover, simmer for 20 to 25 minutes, depending on the cut, and serve. Here are a few ways to change both the texture and the taste of oats to suit your personal preference.

■ **CREAM THEM WITH MILK.** Cooking oats in milk instead of water yields a much creamier porridge, which some people prefer to the firmer, water-cooked variety.

■ **MAKE THEM COARSER.** If you prefer your oats with a firm, slightly coarse texture, chefs advise adding the oats to water that's already boiling rather than mixing them with cold water and raising the heat.

■ **CHANGE THE TASTE.** To add extra flavor to oats, you can eliminate the water or milk altogether and cook them in apple, pear, or peach juice. Since the sugars in fruit juices can readily scorch and give the cereal a slightly burnt taste, make sure that you use a heavy bottomed pan or use a double boiler over a slow, steady heat, and watch the time carefully.

whole grains and processed foods containing oats or barley, but the positive glycemic response was greater for whole grains.[12]

■ Oatmeal has long been used as a natural means to treat itchy and/or inflamed skin. Studies have shown that colloidal oatmeal (finely ground oats), either applied topically or added to a warm bath, can soothe itchiness and heal skin injuries or conditions. It's recommended for atopic dermatitis, psoriasis, eczema, and other skin ailments, and it even provides some measure of UV protection.[13]

■ Oats exhibit anti-inflammatory and antioxidant actions. In one study, oats were shown to inhibit tumor necrosis factor alpha–induced nuclear factor-kappa beta activation (very generally, cell death caused by cancer) by up to 27.5 percent.[14]

■ Oats and oatmeal can help with weight management by increasing satiety and improving appetite control. In a study of volunteers who ate either oatmeal or a cold breakfast cereal, oatmeal resulted in a greater increase in fullness, greater reduction in hunger, less desire to eat, and less food intake.[15] These effects were also observed using instant oatmeal.[16]

See also: Barley (page 139)

quinoa

Quinoa is one of the most popular of the "ancient grains." One of the main reasons people have flocked to quinoa is that it's one of the very few plant-based complete proteins. That means it contains all of the essential amino acids. Like buckwheat, quinoa is a pseudocereal and is naturally gluten free. The three most widely cultivated varieties are red, black, and white quinoa; quinoa flakes and flour are also available. Besides being a good vegetarian source of protein, quinoa is also very rich in manganese, and it's a good source of fiber, magnesium, and phosphorous. It also contains a number of phenolic com-

get the most from your grain

While wheat, rice, and other grains are all prepared in similar ways, quinoa is smaller and more delicate and must be treated a little bit differently. Here's what chefs advise.

- WASH IT WELL. As quinoa grows, it develops a natural, protective coating called saponin, which sometimes has a bitter taste. To wash away the residue, rinse quinoa before you start cooking.

- WATCH THE TIME. Quinoa cooks more quickly than other grains, and because of its delicate texture, it can get twice as mushy when you overcook it. To get the proper consistency, bring 2 cups of water to a boil,

add 1 cup of quinoa, and reduce the heat to low. Cook, covered, for 10 to 15 minutes, or until the grains are tender but still slightly crunchy and all the liquid has been absorbed.

- USE A LITTLE, GET A LOT. Some folks balk at the price of quinoa, which is quite a bit more expensive than other grains. But because it plumps up a lot during cooking—up to four times its original volume—a little goes a long way.

pounds (such as quercetin, vanillic acid, ferulic acid, and gallic acid) that display high antioxidant activity. Darker quinoa has been observed to have higher phenolic concentrations and antioxidant activity than lighter varieties,[17] and a higher antioxidant content means a better ability to fight cell-damaging free radicals and prevent inflammation. If you aren't convinced yet, consider the research.

- In a 4-week study of overweight, postmenopausal women, one group consumed 25 g of quinoa flakes daily while the other group consumed the same amount of corn flakes. At the end of the study, those in the quinoa group experienced a reduction in total cholesterol and LDL cholesterol and an increase in glutathione, an antioxidant that can prevent free radical damage.[18]
- An in vitro study found that quinoa leaf extract exhibited a number of anticancer effects against prostate cancer. Researchers hypothesized that quinoa leaves could exert a chemopreventive (cancer-fighting) and anticarcinogenic effect due to their high content of phenolic acids (including ferulic, sinapinic, and gallic acids), kaempferol, isorhamnetin, and rutin.[19]

sorghum

You may be more familiar with sorghum if you were raised in the southern United States, and even then you may know it as sorghum molasses rather than a protein- and iron-rich whole grain. Sorghum is gaining traction as the new "wonder grain" in town, even though it's actually an ancient grain that's been around for millennia. Sorghum is more eco-friendly than many crops because it requires less water. Add to that its gluten-free status and robust nutritional profile, and you have all the makings of the next big superfood. One study even found that high-tannin sorghum bran (which is available in health food stores) was higher in antioxidants than blueberries, strawberries, plums, grapes, watermelon, and oranges.[20] Sorghum can be used in any of the ways you'd use rice, barley, or quinoa, and sorghum flour and sorghum bran can be used in baked goods. Sorghum is a hearty grain with a nutty flavor and it boasts a high soluble fiber content, which makes it effective at preventing or treating constipation and promoting satiety. It's high in tannins, anthocyanidins, plant sterols, and phenolic acids.

- Sorghum is emerging as a diabetes-friendly food: Sorghum-based products have a lower glycemic load than their comparable wheat- or rice-based foods, and a lower glycemic load helps decrease postprandial blood glucose levels.[21] Studies have also shown that eating at least two servings of whole grains a day reduces your risk of type 2 diabetes.[22]

▪ Eating sorghum is an excellent way to add more heart-healthy, gluten-free whole grains to your diet.

Research studies have consistently shown that those who eat a lot of whole grains have a lower risk of cardiovascular disease, type 2 diabetes, and some cancers.[23] And in a meta-analysis that examined the association between whole grain consumption and stroke, researchers found that those who eat a lot of whole grains also enjoy a significantly reduced risk of stroke.[24]

2

conditions

The greatest wealth is health.
—*Virgil*

You don't need to spend a fortune on drugs and preventive care, the antidotes to a wide range of our most common ailments lay right in your kitchen. The power of food goes well beyond satisfying hunger—food can heal serious conditions like cancer, dementia, and high blood pressure. Turn the page to see how combining rich ingredients can cure over 100 conditions, and completely restore your well-being.

acid reflux

Acid reflux occurs when the ring of muscle connecting your esophagus to your stomach (known as the lower esophageal sphincter, or LES) doesn't close completely after food passes through it, or when your LES opens more often than it should. When this valve malfunctions, stomach acid can spill into your esophagus, triggering the familiar symptom of heartburn. Acid reflux can cause a variety of uncomfortable symptoms in addition to heartburn, including nausea, bloating, bloody or dark stools, unexplained weight loss, chronic hiccups, or a feeling of having something stuck in your throat. If you experience the symptoms of acid reflux more than twice a week, doctors describe it as acid reflux disease, or what's sometimes known as gastroesophageal reflux disease (GERD).

People suffering from acid reflux disease or GERD should be assessed by their doctors in order to rule out a hiatal hernia or other underlying cause. But there are food-based interventions anyone can start right away to get quick relief.

To put out the fire of heartburn, opt for low-acid foods with a pH value of 5 or higher. (The higher the pH number, the lower the acid content. Lemon juice, for example, has a pH of 2, while egg whites have a pH of up to 9.)[1] Foods such as bananas, brown rice, melons, oatmeal, and whole grain bread made from unprocessed flour are all low in acid. For protein, avoid all fried foods and instead eat lean fish or poultry that's grilled, poached, steamed, or baked, and make sure to remove the skin to cut down on the fat content, which can worsen acid reflux. Organic tofu and egg whites, with pH values of 7 and 8, respectively,[2] are good vegetarian sources of low-acid protein.

As for specific foods, both traditional wisdom and the latest research agree that ginger, fennel, licorice, and chamomile can be your sour stomach's best friends. Ginger has long been established as an antinausea and antivomiting remedy, safe even during pregnancy, but it also has anti-inflammatory properties.[3] Try skipping the onions and garlic in your next stir-fry and include grated fresh ginger, instead. Stir powdered ginger into your bowl of oatmeal for a double dose of acid reflux relief, or flavor fish, lean poultry, or tofu with ginger. Ginger tea is readily available in most grocery stores, and with zero caffeine, it won't trigger acid reflux and won't keep you up at night.

Fennel has been shown to soothe nausea, ease stomach pain, and act as an anti-inflammatory, as well.[4] Add fresh, raw, thinly sliced fennel to salads, or munch on slices for a snack or an after-dinner digestive. But fennel is also great cooked and, like ginger, fennel can be consumed as a tea. You can also chew dried fennel seeds after a meal to aid digestion and prevent bloating, gas, and gastrointestinal (GI) irritation.

Licorice has been shown to stimulate the production of gastric mucus, which lends a protective coating to your esophagus, stomach lining, and any existing ulcers, making your digestive tract more resistant to irritating stomach acid.[5] Most of us associate licorice with the pungent and overly sweet black candy—licorice is 50 times as sweet as sugar!—but you can add licorice to your diet more healthfully by chewing on licorice root or drinking licorice root tea. The tea is readily available at health food stores and large supermarkets, or DIYers can steep 1 to 5 grams of dried licorice root in boiling water and drink the tea up to three times a day to soothe the pangs of acid reflux.[6] Proceed with a dose of caution, though: The active ingredient in licorice, glycyrrhizin, comes with a host of possible side effects, especially at high doses or when used long term. Pregnant or breastfeeding women should avoid

common triggers for acid reflux

1. Spicy foods
2. Citrus foods, including grapefruit, lemons, limes, oranges, and tomatoes
3. Alliums, such as garlic, onions, and shallots
4. Fatty and/or fried foods
5. Acidic drinks, such as coffee or high-acid juices (such as citrus juices)
6. Alcohol
7. Chocolate
8. Caffeine
9. Mint

licorice entirely, as should anyone with heart, liver, or kidney disease; a hormone-sensitive cancer; erectile dysfunction; or diabetes. Licorice also has the potential to interfere with many medications.[7] A form of licorice from which the glycyrrhizin has been removed, called deglycyrrhizinated licorice or DGL, is available as an herbal supplement and has far fewer potential contraindications than the whole food. In any form, if you plan to include licorice regularly in your self-care routine, it's best to consult with a health-care provider.

In contrast, chamomile is considered generally safe, though some sources advise against taking it during pregnancy because of reports of miscarriage.[8] An ancient remedy for relieving heartburn, indigestion, ulcers, and general stomach upset, chamomile has been shown to neutralize gastric acidity and help dispel gas and relax intestinal muscles.[9] Chamomile tea is the primary way to include this delightfully floral herb in your diet, and for some people, it has the added benefit of enhancing sleep. Chamomile tea bags are available at most supermarkets, or you can brew your own by steeping the flowers for 10 to 15 minutes.

Finally, don't underestimate the power of water to help with acid reflux. Drinking water (preferably filtered) flushes stomach acid down where it belongs.

See also: Gastritis (page 290), Heartburn (page 322), Indigestion (page 345)

acne

Acne, that familiar bane of adolescence, can crop up at any time, especially if you're stressed, experiencing a hormonal fluctuation, changing your diet or skin-care routine, or are simply prone to breakouts. Some people experience breakouts in response to specific foods, and these triggers can be highly idiosyncratic. The most commonly cited trigger foods for acne are chocolate, spicy foods, dairy (it's highly inflammatory), sugar (especially the processed sugar found in many candies and prepackaged desserts), and carbohydrate-rich foods (bread, chips, rice cakes, and pasta). Because insulin and a hormone called insulin-like growth factor have been found to increase sebum, the oil produced by your skin's sebaceous glands,[1] foods with a high glycemic index (GI)—those leading to a spike in glucose and insulin levels—deserve a special mention when it comes to acne prevention. High-GI foods include white bread and bagels, white rice, white potatoes, pretzels, saltine crackers, instant oatmeal, melons, pineapple, and any sugary dessert or candy. In one study, subjects who followed a low-GI diet for 10 weeks experienced significant improvement in acne, reduced size of sebaceous glands, and decreased inflammation.[2]

In fact, the latest dermatological research confirms that acne is primarily an inflammatory disease.[3] The high-glycemic carbs, dairy products, sugars, and saturated fats common to the Western diet spark an inflammatory response that results in increased sebum production and an overgrowth of *Propionibacterium acnes*, the bacteria that causes acne.[4] The inflammation-acne cycle works like this: Oxidative stress—a state of imbalance in which cell-damaging free radicals start to outnumber your antioxidant defenses—lowers the oxygen content of sebum, creating a more hospitable environment for *P. acnes*. As the bacteria proliferate, further inflammation occurs, resulting in the angry red bumps and whiteheads we all know so well. Studies have indicated that people with chronic acne have lower levels of antioxidants and higher levels of inflammatory chemicals than people with healthy skin.[5]

The key, then, is to interrupt the inflammatory cycle with a two-pronged approach: Eat to decrease inflammation and eat to increase antioxidants. To ward off inflammation, stay away from those high-GI foods and turn to foods rich in omega-3s, which are anti-inflammatory. Sardines are anti-inflammatory powerhouses: One 3.5-ounce serving contains 1.5 grams of omega-3 fatty acids.[6] Salmon and other cold-water fatty fish (such as mackerel, herring, tuna, halibut, and trout) are also great choices for inflammation-fighting omega-3s. For vegetarian sources of this essential fatty acid, go for walnuts, flaxseeds, or chia seeds; flaxseed oil and walnut oil are also good sources. Then, to get the antioxidants your body needs for healthy skin, eat berries. Strawberries, blackberries, and cranberries are packed with free radical–neutralizing antioxidants. Other excellent fruit and vegetable sources of antioxidants include papayas, cherries, broccoli, plums, and raw peppers. Ginger and turmeric are among the spices with the highest levels of antioxidants, and grape juice, cranberry juice, tomato juice, red wine, and green tea are at the top of the list of antioxidant-rich beverages.[7] Consume grape and cranberry juice in moderation, however: While their antioxidant content is chart-topping, any fruit juice also delivers up a concentrated dose of sugar. You'll also want to opt for an organic, 100 percent juice without additives.

Another great nutrient for your skin is zinc. Zinc has antibacterial properties, and it provides key support to your skin's oil-producing glands. Studies have also found that people with acne have lower levels of zinc than people with clear, healthy skin. The winning food here? Oysters. They're the very best dietary source of zinc, with over 500 percent of your daily requirement in fewer than 60 calories.[8] Other foods high in zinc are beef, turkey, pumpkin seeds, sesame seeds, fortified cereals, and wheat germ.

Finally, to top off your antiacne diet, consider fermented dairy products. While regular dairy is inflammatory and can exacerbate acne and other skin conditions, the fermentation process converts lactose to lactic acid, which has been found to increase skin thickness and promote collagen production. Emerging research has found that fermented dairy products, such as plain yogurt (make sure it has active cultures), kefir, and lassi, can have beneficial effects on your skin. They can be applied directly to your skin to reduce inflammation and consumed for their antimicrobial and anti-inflammatory benefits. Eating yogurt seems to be more effective than applying it topically to treat acne and atopic dermatitis (eczema), as the probiotics exert a healthy effect on your gut microbiome.[9] Much of the latest research highlights the link between a healthy gut and healthy skin. So your most powerful antiacne tool yet may be a bowl of yogurt with berries and chia seeds!

adrenal exhaustion/
adrenal fatigue

Adrenal exhaustion, also referred to as adrenal fatigue, adrenal apathy, or adrenal fatigue syndrome, is not currently recognized as a medical diagnosis by the established medical community, but among the health-care professionals who diagnose and treat it—and the people who suffer from it—the theory is that chronic, long-term stress overstimulates your adrenal glands, leaving them overworked, exhausted, and unable to produce sufficient hormones. Perhaps the distinguishing symptom of the syndrome is a persistent feeling of fatigue that cannot be assuaged by adequate sleep; many sufferers report needing caffeine or other stimulants to "get through the day" or to complete tasks. Other common symptoms include body aches, frequent headaches, sleeping difficulties, difficulty thinking clearly, mild depression, salt and/or sugar cravings, decreased libido, gastrointestinal problems, hair loss, hot flashes, low blood pressure, increased susceptibility to infection, abrupt weight loss, weight gain, difficulty losing weight, and general weakness—a wide array, thanks to the adrenal glands' crucial role in supporting many bodily functions.

In addition to prolonged exposure to stress, adrenal exhaustion can also be triggered by an infection or illness, exposure to pollutants or toxic chemicals, or any situation that is especially taxing to your body, such as a major surgery, recurrent illness, malnutrition, or an addiction problem. Adrenal fatigue is diagnosed with a blood or saliva test that measures hormone levels. Again, conventional medicine does not recognize the legitimacy of these tests or the diagnosis, but alternative and complementary practitioners have accumulated a great deal of wisdom on how to treat adrenal fatigue syndrome. A healthy diet designed to support the adrenals is crucial for restoring and maintaining adrenal health.

Tricia Pingel, NMD, author of *Total Health Turnaround*, emphasizes the importance of a varied, well-balanced diet because your body needs a *synergy* of nutrients. To treat adrenal fatigue, it's far more beneficial to focus on nutrients than on calories. "If you strictly look at calories," says Dr. Pingel, "you can easily miss proper nutrition. For example, you could eat an entire plate of kiwi or broccoli for the same calories as half a Snickers bar. So which is better for you? Which provides your body with more nutrient density? One of the biggest mistakes that many dieters make is eating 'diet foods' that are lower in calories and fat, but also lower in nutrients. It takes nutrients to break down fat, carbohydrates, and protein. You will not succeed at long-term weight management if you are malnourished." In her book, Dr. Pingel provides her full adrenal health nutrition plan and tells you how to customize it to your stage of adrenal fatigue, but here are a few highlights that apply to anyone suffering from adrenal fatigue.

- Stay hydrated. Every day, drink at least half of your body weight in ounces of water. This means that a 150-pound person should drink at least 75 ounces of water per day. Some home-brewed herbal tea is okay, as well.

- Don't skimp on calories. Starving your body will worsen your adrenal fatigue. If your body isn't getting the nutrients it needs, it will store fat in an attempt to keep up its energy reserves. The goal of dietary therapy for adrenal fatigue is to eat a varied, nutrient-rich diet so your body has the fuel it needs to get through the day. "Your diet should be predictable to your body but variable to your palate," says Dr. Pingel. This means you should eat at regular intervals each day.

- Instead of three large meals, eat five or six small meals a day. Make sure they're comprised of whole foods such as fresh fruits and vegetables, whole grains, and proteins.

- Eat gluten-free grains. They're your best option because gluten affects insulin sensitivity, plus gluten-free grains such as amaranth, buckwheat, brown or wild rice, oats, quinoa, and spelt have a higher nutritional and mineral content than other grains.

- Get your protein from beans, GMO-free tofu, lentils, nuts, organic chicken, organic eggs, wild-caught fish, and wild game meats. Get the majority of your protein from plant-based sources, and eat no more than 3 ounces of meat, poultry, or seafood twice each week. "The key is to focus on plants as your primary source of food intake and supplement with other macronutrients," Dr. Pingel says.

- Processed, prepackaged foods are not a healthy choice for anyone, but artificial sweeteners, dyes, additives, and preservatives put more stress on your body and worsen adrenal fatigue, so avoid these food items.

- Eliminate dairy from your menu. Cow's milk is highly inflammatory and can exacerbate many gastrointestinal problems, and it's possible to get all the calcium and vitamin D you need from dark, leafy greens; nuts and nut milks; tofu; fish and fish oil; and mushrooms.[1]

See also: Anxiety (page 165), Depression (page 232), Fatigue (page 266), Hair Loss (page 304), Lightheadedness (page 368), Thyroid Disease (page 429)

allergic rhinitis (hay fever)

One of the few downsides of springtime, up to 60 million Americans suffer from the familiar constellation of symptoms that indicate seasonal allergic rhinitis, more commonly known as hay fever: itchy, watery, and/or red eyes; runny nose; headache; sneezing; nasal congestion; itching in the nose or throat; cough; and dark circles under the eyes (known as allergic shiners). Though many of its symptoms mimic those of the common cold, hay fever is caused by an allergen, rather than a virus. Hay fever also does not cause a fever, while a cold usually does, and the nasal discharge from hay fever is clear and watery, rather than the thick, yellow mucus that is a sign of infection. The most common cause of allergic rhinitis is pollen, but it can be caused by any allergen you breathe in, such as pet dander, dust, or mold. Food allergies can also cause some of the same symptoms as allergic rhinitis.

Though there's no cure for allergic rhinitis, the condition passes once the allergen is removed. That said, the symptoms can be severe, and prolonged hay fever can lead to sinusitis or an ear infection and can worsen asthma or other lung conditions. The most common treatment for hay fever is antihistamines, but severe allergic rhinitis may be treated with corticosteroids or allergy shots.

There's evidence that honey can supercharge the effect of antihistamines. Researchers studied allergy sufferers for 8 weeks. Each participant received a daily dose of 10 milligrams (mg) of loratadine (Claritin) for 4 weeks, but the case group ingested 1 gram (g) of honey (20 g = 1 tablespoon) per kilogram of body weight daily for 4 weeks. (So a person who weighed 150 pounds, or 68 kilograms, would have consumed about 3.5 tablespoons of honey per day.) Participants' allergy symptoms were recorded at the start of the study, at 4 weeks, and at 8 weeks. At week 4, both groups showed improvement in symptoms, but at week 8, only the group that had received the "honey treatment" showed a significant improvement in allergic rhinitis symptoms. What's more, their results lasted an entire month after the study concluded.[1] It's not unreasonable to expect, then, that for at least some seasonal allergy sufferers, honey alone is enough to alleviate some symptoms. Honey is also a great natural remedy for a dry cough: Honey coats and soothes your throat, stopping that persistent tickle that's associated with seasonal allergies. It has been shown to decrease inflammation of mucous membranes, and it has an antioxidant effect.[2] Try 1 tablespoon of honey up to three times a day for an easy, inexpensive way to suppress a cough.

The flavonoid quercetin is a natural antihistamine and anti-inflammatory.[3] While human studies on quercetin's antiallergy effects are limited, in test tubes, it has stopped the production of histamine, and in mice, it significantly reduced nasal symptoms such as sneezing and inflammation of nasal passages.[4] Food and beverage sources high in quercetin include apples, citrus fruits, onions, dill, cilantro, fennel, kale, cranberries, chokecherries, tea, and red wine. But capers take the prize here, with a whopping 234 mg of quercetin per 100 g of raw capers, or 173 g of quercetin in 100 g of canned capers.

Another natural antihistamine is curcumin, the active phenolic compound in turmeric. It protects against allergies by suppressing mast cell histamine release.[5]

A study on the protective effect of antioxidants against allergic rhinitis found that a high level of carotenoids was associated with a lower incidence of allergic rhinitis. Carotenoids are the yellow, orange, and red pigments synthesized by plants, and the six this study focused on were alpha-carotene, beta-carotene, lycopene, lutein/zeaxanthin, canthaxanthin, and cryptoxanthin.[6] Good food sources of carotenoids include pumpkin; squash; peppers; carrots; tomatoes; tangerines; sweet potatoes; and dark, leafy greens.

There's also emerging evidence that probiotics can help with the symptoms of allergic rhinitis and can even prevent allergies. In one small study, researchers exposed volunteers with a history of allergic rhinitis to grass pollen and then gave them a probiotic preparation consisting of the common bacterial strains *Lactobacillus acidophilus* and *Bifidobacterium lactis.* The treatment significantly reduced nasal itching and the percentage of white blood cells in nasal fluid.[7] An earlier study found that fermented milk with the *L. paracasei* strain decreased nasal itching and congestion in allergic rhinitis sufferers.[8] Yet another study compared the effects of the *B. lactis* strain on people with a history of allergic rhinitis. (Notably, this trial was "conducted during the peak of the pollen season.") One group of volunteers received *B. lactis* every day for 8 weeks; the other received a placebo. Concentrations of cytokines were significantly lower in the probiotic group at the end of the study, and nasal symptom scores and markers of allergic activity were far lower in the probiotic group in the second month.[10]

The active compound in licorice, glycyrrhizin, has been shown to prevent inflammation of the nasal mucous membranes.[11] Licorice products are available in licorice root tea, liquid extracts, capsules, and tablets, and you can also chew licorice root. Pregnant or breastfeeding women should avoid licorice entirely, as should anyone with heart, liver, or kidney disease; a hormone-sensitive cancer; erectile dysfunction; or diabetes. Glycyrrhizin raises blood pressure and comes with a host of possible side effects, especially at high

doses or when used for the long term. Licorice also has the potential to interfere with many medications, among them blood pressure medications, MAO inhibitors (a common type of antidepressants), ACE inhibitors and diuretics, insulin, oral contraceptives, warfarin (Coumadin), digoxin, and corticosteroids.[12]

An Australian study of more than 156,000 middle-aged adults examined dietary patterns and occurrence of asthma as well as a dual diagnosis of asthma and hay fever. Researchers found that, for men and women, diets generally high in meat appeared to be risk factors for asthma and hay fever. More specifically, diets marked by greater consumption of poultry, seafood, and red and processed meats raised the risk for women, and diets marked by greater consumption of red meat, processed meat, and cheese raised the risk for men.[13]

One last thing to keep in mind if you have hay fever is a phenomenon called oral allergy syndrome (OAS), which is often mistaken for a true food allergy. If you have OAS and hay fever, an allergic reaction occurs in your mouth when you eat certain foods that contain proteins similar to pollen—this is called cross-reactivity. For example, ragweed pollen cross-reacts with bananas and melons, so people with a ragweed allergy may react to bananas, cantaloupes, watermelon, or honeydew. People with a grass allergy may also have an allergic reaction to celery, peaches, melons, oranges, and tomatoes. Cross-reactivity can also occur in people with a birch pollen allergy or a natural rubber latex allergy. For more information on OAS and to see a full list of foods that can trigger it, see the Web site of the Asthma and Allergy Foundation of America (www.aafa.org), and if you suspect OAS, follow up with your health-care provider. With the correct diagnosis, you'll know which foods to avoid. It's estimated that about one-third of allergic rhinitis sufferers also experience OAS, and about 2 percent of OAS cases could lead to anaphylaxis.[14]

See also: Asthma (page 174), Coughs (page 220), Hives (page 339)

alzheimer's disease

Alzheimer's disease (AD) is the most common form of dementia, accounting for 60 to 80 percent of dementia cases. It's a long-term neurodegenerative disease that progresses over time, resulting in the loss of memory, impaired social functioning, communication problems, behavioral changes, disorientation, mood swings, loss of bodily functions, and ultimately, death. There is no known cure for Alzheimer's, but medications can improve symptoms. With such grim prospects for those who receive a diagnosis of AD—not to mention the enormous burden that falls on caregivers—there is a global push for research into therapies that can prevent AD, delay its onset, and treat the disease after diagnosis. And with AD rapidly becoming one of the world's most prevalent public health concerns, researchers, health-care providers, and advocates are working tirelessly to make advances.

One thing we know unequivocally is that there are several diseases and disease processes known to be risk factors for developing Alzheimer's. Among them are cardiovascular disease, diabetes, hypertension, neurodegeneration, and overweight and obesity. Vascular disorders greatly increase your risk of Alzheimer's, and hypertension is perhaps the one most closely correlated with the disease.[1] The biggest risk factor for AD, however, is not pathology, but advancing age. Beyond the age of 65, the prevalence of AD nearly doubles every 5 years. By 2050, the number of people over 80 will *triple* its current number, and about half of those over 85 will have Alzheimer's.[2]

Ready for some good news? Here it is: Most of the disease risk factors for AD can be avoided through lifestyle factors and good nutrition—and to a great degree, the problems of aging can, as well. A recent metastudy of all the modifiable risk factors for AD found that the number-one modifiable risk factor is heavy smoking, while the most protective factor is a healthy diet[3]—two factors that are entirely within your control. And even if you have a family history of Alzheimer's, exercise can erase that risk factor. It sounds too good to be true, but numerous studies have proved the cognitive-protective power of exercise. In a study conducted at the Cleveland Clinic, researchers recruited cognitively healthy men and women ages 65 to 89, many of whom had a family history of AD. Genetic testing revealed that about half of the group carried the e4 gene, which increases your risk of developing Alzheimer's. The subjects were divided into four groups based on their e4 status and their exercise habits, and researchers scanned their brains at the outset of the study and again 18 months later. The results? As expected, those without the e4 gene showed little to no shrinkage of the hippocampus, which is a hallmark of the progression of AD. But those with the e4 gene who exercised regularly showed the same results. In effect, even with a high risk for AD, the volunteers who exercised regularly suffered no loss to their hippocampi. Meanwhile, the hippocampi of their sedentary counterparts with the e4 gene shrank by 3 percent. Bear in mind that these changes occurred in just 18 months.[4]

The emerging research on the cognitive-protective power of diet is just as exciting. There is strong evidence showing that an overall healthy dietary pattern—such as the Mediterranean diet, the DASH diet, or the MIND diet— significantly protects against Alzheimer's disease.[5] There are small differences in each of these patterns, but they all recommend a diet that's high in fresh fruits and vegetables,

plant-based proteins, seafood, whole grains, and legumes. In contrast, the typical Western diet, which is high in red meats, saturated fats, fried foods, processed foods, and sugary desserts and drinks, is a direct contributor to dementias of any type.[6] Being overweight at midlife even predicts increased incidence of Alzheimer's disease. Based on a cohort of 1,394 cognitively normal people, 142 of whom developed AD later in life, researchers found that every unit increase in BMI at midlife predicts an earlier onset of AD by 6.7 months.[7] But once again, dietary changes can preserve cognitive function. The MIND diet was associated with a slower decline in cognitive function as assessed in five domains. In those who best adhered to the MIND diet (compared to those with the least adherence), the difference in cognitive decline rates was equivalent to being 7.5 years younger. MIND is an acronym for Mediterranean-DASH Intervention for Neurodegenerative Delay—in other words, it's a combination of the Mediterranean and DASH (Dietary Approaches to Stop Hypertension) diets, with modifications based upon the most compelling findings concerning nutrition and cognitive health. Brain-healthy foods included in the MIND diet include vegetables (especially dark, leafy greens), berries, nuts, olive oil, whole grains, fish, beans, poultry, and wine. Foods that contribute to cognitive decline and are to be avoided, on the other hand, are red meats, fast foods, fried foods, high-fat cheeses, pastries and sweets, and butter and margarine.[8] In a study comparing the Mediterranean diet, the DASH diet, and the MIND diet in 923 participants ages 58 to 98, the evidence showed that the greatest adherence to the MIND diet resulted in a 53 percent reduction in cognitive decline and those who had moderate adherence experienced a 35 percent reduction. This effect was independent of other lifestyle factors and any cardiovascular conditions.[9]

The main source of fat in the Mediterranean diet is extra-virgin olive oil, and recent studies have shown that olive oil's high phenolic content works against Alzheimer's disease by reducing inflammation; activating antioxidant defense; stimulating neurogenesis; and counteracting the disease's effects on the brain, including plaque and tangle aggregation and toxicity.[10] With such an abundance of effects, another study pointed out that natural phenols are a powerful "multitargeting" intervention for neurodegenerative diseases.[11] Natural phenols are also found in red wine, green tea, red berries, and spices, all of which have shown promise in fighting amyloid aggregation on a molecular level.[12]

Green tea can inhibit amyloid beta aggregation and can even alter amyloid beta fibrils to make them less toxic. Amyloid beta is the main component in amyloid plaques, which cause the degradation of neurons in Alzheimer's patients. The active ingredient is epigallocatechin gallate (EGCG), a powerful polyphenol. Want to supersize the effect of EGCG? Eat cold-water, fatty fish such as salmon and mackerel: Fish oil has been shown to increase the bioavailability of EGCG.[13]

There is evidence that long-chain omega-3 fatty acids can slow cognitive decline and prevent the progression of Alzheimer's by alleviating low-grade inflammation—but only in the early stages of cognitive impairment.[14] (And indeed, a recent 4-month study on patients with cognitive impairment or Alzheimer's found that omega-3 supplementation produced no discernible improvements to cognition or mood.)[15] Given that there is widespread acceptance that omega-3s have positive effects on brain structure and cognitive function,[16] omega-3s are recommended more for the *prevention* of Alzheimer's than as a treatment. Food sources of omega-3s include flaxseeds, flaxseed oil, walnuts, walnut oil, chia seeds, sardines, salmon, mackerel, herring, trout, tuna, and halibut. But where long-chain fatty acids lose their

to fight alzheimer's disease, think "comprehensive"

Nutritional interventions are clearly very powerful when it comes to preventing Alzheimer's disease (AD), but it should be noted that the best chances of preventing Alzheimer's involve a comprehensive approach to good health. An article published in *Neurobiology of Aging* in late 2014 summarized the most effective guidelines for AD prevention. By now, most of them will sound quite familiar.

1. Minimize intake of saturated fats and trans fats.

2. Emphasize vegetables, legumes, fruits, and whole grains rather than meats and dairy products.

3. Get enough naturally occurring vitamin E. Studies have found that vitamin E is associated with reduced incidence of Alzheimer's and dementia, but only when it comes from food sources rather than supplements. Good sources include seeds; nuts; dark, leafy greens; whole grains; mangoes; papayas; avocados; and red bell peppers.

4. Make sure you're getting the RDA of vitamin B_{12}, which is 2.4 micrograms per day for adults. Vitamin B_{12} is essential for brain and nervous system health and blood cell formation. Some of the best food sources are clams, mussels, and mackerel, but it's also found in crab, beef, salmon, turkey, chicken, eggs, and dairy products.[17] Sea lettuce and nori deserve a special mention for their high levels of vitamin B_{12}, making them the only vegetarian sources of this essential nutrient that is most often found in animal products.

5. If you take a multivitamin, choose one without iron and copper. Some studies have suggested that excessive iron and copper intake may contribute to cognitive problems.

6. Consider eliminating aluminum, which is found in cookware, baking powder, antiperspirants, and antacids. The connection between aluminum and Alzheimer's is still under investigation, but in large amounts it is a known neurotoxin.

7. Get regular aerobic exercise.

This article also emphasized the importance of getting at least 7 hours of sleep per night for optimal cognitive health, as well as the benefits of performing regular mental activities that promote new learning.[18]

efficacy, the medium-chain fatty acids found in coconut may take over. A recent study pointed out that medium-chain fatty acids are unique in that they are easily absorbed and metabolized by your liver, and they can be converted to ketones. Ketones are an important alternative energy source in your brain and may be beneficial to people who already have memory impairment, as in Alzheimer's disease. Further, the phenolic compounds in coconut can help prevent the aggregation of amyloid beta peptide, potentially inhibiting a key step in AD progression.[19]

Perhaps the newest way medical professionals are thinking of AD is casting it as "type 3 diabetes": There is strong evidence linking insulin resistance and Alzheimer's disease. Insulin resistance has been shown to predict brain amyloid deposition[20] and is associated with lower regional cerebral glucose metabolism, which in turn may predict worse memory performance, increasing your risk for Alzheimer's.[21] And so it's key to avoid sugary desserts and sweets, as well as any foods that can cause a spike in glucose, such as sodas, white sugar, white flour, refined carbs, processed foods, and syrups.

We may have saved the best for last. In an 8-week study on 90 elderly individuals, cocoa flavanols were shown to improve cognitive function, insulin resistance, blood pressure, and lipid peroxidation. Results were best for those who drank a high-flavanol (993 milligrams [mg] per serving) cocoa drink, but those with an intermediate-flavanol (520 mg per serving) drink had improved outcomes, as well.[22] These results echo other studies that have found neuroprotective effects of cocoa flavanols.[23]

See also: Dementia (page 226), Diabetes (page 238), Heart Disease (Cardiovascular Disease) (page 313), High Blood Pressure (Hypertension) (page 327), Insomnia (page 357), Overweight and Obesity (page 396), Stroke (page 423)

anxiety

Anxiety disorders are the most common mental health conditions in the United States, affecting approximately one out of every five people. Ranging from periodic bouts of excessive worry to fear so debilitating it prevents you from performing the routine activities of daily living, anxiety is a serious condition that requires a multifaceted treatment approach that varies according to the individual. Symptoms include nervousness, excessive worry, excessive sweating, shaking, nausea, vomiting, nightmares, insomnia, racing heart, trouble concentrating, irritability, headache, diarrhea, and hyperventilation. Some people with anxiety suffer from phobias or obsessive-compulsive disorder. Others suffer panic attacks, which are brief periods of intense fear and dread accompanied by any of the above physical symptoms but also including disorientation, dissociation (or feeling "removed from it all"), and even fainting. Many of the physical symptoms of a panic attack can be mistaken for symptoms of a heart attack. As debilitating as anxiety can be, there are many options for treatment. Here, we'll focus on the nutritional interventions that can assuage anxiety.

Let's start with some general dietary principles that apply to anyone with a proclivity for anxiety. First, avoid simple sugars and carbohydrates, as well as all processed foods. This is great health advice for anyone, but particularly for anxiety sufferers, as these foods cause a spike in blood sugar followed by an inevitable drop, which in turn causes shakiness, lightheadedness, and weakness—symptoms that are uncomfortably reminiscent of anxiety symptoms. In fact, experiencing these symptoms is distressing enough for some people that it actually triggers a panic attack. Healthier choices include lean, high-protein foods, such as seafood or skinless chicken or turkey, which will keep your blood sugar at a steady level and preclude that constellation of distressing symptoms. Vegetarians can get their protein through eggs, nuts and nut butters, and tofu. When eating carbs, go for complex whole grains such as whole grain bread, stone-ground oatmeal, and the so-called "ancient" grains: quinoa, farro, millet, spelt, and amaranth. The goal is to keep yourself feeling sated and your blood sugar levels steady, which simple carbs and sugars never do.

There is also new evidence that eating an overall healthy diet decreases your odds of both anxiety and depression. In a study of more than 3,800 adults, greater adherence to a lacto-vegetarian diet was found to have a protective effect against anxiety and psychological distress in men and women, and against depression in women. The traditional American diet—in this case, high in meat, salt, legumes, starchy vegetables, poultry, hydrogenated vegetable oils, dried fruits, fish, and organ meats—increased the odds of depression in women and increased the odds of anxiety in both men and women. To lower your chances of psychological disorders, study authors recommended that you increase your consumption of fruits, low-fat dairy, tomato products, and vegetables and you reduce between-meal snacking, high-fat dairy products, chocolate, carbonated drinks, sweets, and desserts.[1] Another study of nearly 300 adults conducted over 9 years found that a higher fruit and vegetable intake was associated with lower odds of both depression and anxiety. These results were true even after researchers controlled for age, gender, income, education, physical activity, chronic illness, and smoking.[2] Part of the credit goes to polyphenols, naturally occurring compounds in plant-based foods that combat oxidative stress, boost mood, and exert neuroprotective properties.[3]

The other general dietary advice for anxiety sufferers concerns caffeine and alcohol. Caffeine, especially at high doses, can leave you feeling jittery and anxious. Adding sugar to caffeinated drinks can increase the effect *and* leave you more vulnerable to that drop in blood glucose levels that leads to shakiness and nervousness. It may be especially important for people with chronic anxiety to avoid the commercial energy drinks that are high in caffeine and added sugars. All this having been said, there is evidence that caffeine can boost mood and improve attention—and there is even evidence that drinking tea can alleviate anxiety. A small study examined the effects of green tea, shaded white tea, and warm water on volunteers as they performed a series of stressful tasks. Researchers measured volunteers' salivary concentrations of chromogranin A (CgA), a marker of autonomic nervous system activity. CgA levels rose in response to the stressful tasks, but drinking tea inhibited the increase. Shaded white tea, which is a type of unfermented and uncured tea, was even more effective than green tea.[4] (Tazo, Bigelow, and Teavana all sell white teas; they're readily available in most supermarkets, as well as in specialized tea stores.) Part of the anxiety-calming effect can be attributed to L-theanine (an amino acid found almost uniquely in tea), which attenuates some of the vascular effects of caffeine, such as elevated blood pressure.[5] L-theanine produces a calming effect on your brain and increases production of the neurotransmitters GABA (gamma-aminobutyric acid) and dopamine.[6] GABA is your body's main inhibitory neurotransmitter and is involved with feelings of calmness and relaxation. Dopamine, which has been called the happiness hormone, plays a role in promoting motivation and feelings of pleasure. Similarly, chamomile, long used as a natural antianxiety treatment, has recently been shown to alleviate comorbid anxiety and depression. Though these studies were done on chamomile extract,[7] it stands to reason that chamomile tea, with its natural theanine content, reduces anxiety.

Anxiety sufferers also need to be careful about alcohol consumption. As a sedative and a depressant, alcohol does have an initial calming effect, but some people find that their anxiety symptoms are worse after the effects of alcohol wear off. Also, self-medicating with alcohol puts the anxiety sufferer at serious risk for an addiction problem. More immediately, alcohol has a dehydrating effect, and it can interfere with sleep. So use caution when it comes to alcohol. One glass of red wine a day for women and two for men is considered heart-healthy, and most medical professionals have no problem with drinking in moderation. If you have any questions or concerns, check with your health-care provider.

With this healthy foundation in place, let's add on by discussing foods and beverages that have a direct effect on mood and that can lessen the experience of anxiety. Some of the most exciting emerging research has to do with probiotics and fermented foods. Study results announced at the 2015 annual meeting of the Society for Neuroscience found that volunteers taking a daily probiotic containing *Bifidobacterium longum* experienced decreased stress and improved performance on memory tasks. Participants perceived less stress, and lower levels of cortisol were observed in their bloodstreams, as well.[8] These results confirm earlier animal studies that showed that probiotics can reduce anxiety.[9]

As more knowledge about the gut microbiota and brain axis accumulates, more studies are being conducted with human volunteers. Fermented foods were found to be especially helpful in those who were prone to social anxiety and neuroticism (a tendency to experience

dietary guidelines
to prevent and assuage anxiety

Controlling anxiety through diet can be achieved by eliminating some foods and adding others.

Limit or Eliminate

- Processed foods
- Alcohol
- Caffeine
- Simple sugars and carbohydrates: white bread, white rice, white pasta, sugary cereals, desserts, and candies

- Saturated fats and omega-9 fats: fats from animal products, including high-fat dairy; canola oil; and sunflower oil

Consume More

- Lean protein: chicken, low-fat dairy, nuts, tofu, and turkey
- White tea and herbal tea: lavender and chamomile
- Probiotics: dark chocolate, kefir, kimchi, miso soup, pickles, probiotic yogurt, soy milk, sauerkraut, and tempeh
- Omega-3 fatty acids: chia seeds, flaxseeds, flaxseed oil, herring, mackerel, salmon, sardines, trout, tuna, walnuts, and walnut oil
- Turmeric
- Foods with vitamin C: acerola cherries (West Indian cherries), broccoli, Brussels sprouts, cantaloupe, cauliflower, gac fruit, grapefruits, guavas, kiwis, lemons, limes, oranges, papayas, parsley, red peppers, strawberries, and tomatoes

- Foods with vitamin B_6: avocados, bananas, brown rice, chicken breast, fish, potatoes, molasses, pistachios, and turkey breast
- Foods with vitamin B_{12}: beef, chicken, clams, crab, dairy products, eggs, mackerel, mussels, nori, salmon, sea lettuce, and turkey
- Iron-rich foods: beef, cashews, chickpeas, dark chocolate, fortified whole grain cereals, kidney beans, lentils, spinach, tofu, tomatoes, and white beans
- Magnesium-rich foods: sesame seeds; sunflower seeds; almonds; cashews; walnuts; oats; dark, leafy greens; seaweed; tofu; whole grains; avocados; and bananas

negative emotions such as nervousness, anger, and depression). Researchers speculate that fermented foods may have an antianxiety effect above and beyond that of probiotic supplements because these foods contain peptides and other chemicals that affect the brain.[10]

Lavender has been used for years for its calming, relaxing, and antianxiety effects and for help in promoting sleep. Normally we think of adding lavender essential oil to a bath or using it in aromatherapy. But there is evidence that lavender taken orally combats anxiety, too. Pure lavender oil, on the other hand, may be toxic and shouldn't be taken orally. One study showed that 80 milligrams (mg) of lavender a day was superior to a placebo in reducing anxiety. Another found that 80 mg of lavender a day was as effective as 0.5 mg of lorazepam (Ativan) in alleviating anxiety in adults with generalized anxiety disorder.[11] Lavender is available as an essential oil; a tea; in capsule form; as an extract; and as whole, dried flowers. It is a common ingredient in soaps, lotions, and bath gels. Sedative medications interact with lavender, so don't combine them. If you're pregnant or breastfeeding, avoid lavender.

Some fascinating studies have been conducted on the role of essential fatty acids in preventing and treating anxiety disorders and mood disorders.[12] A study of more than 7,600 women found that a higher intake of omega-6 fatty acids and linoleic acid was associated with less likelihood of anxiety, while a higher intake of omega-9 fatty acids and oleic acid increased the likelihood of anxiety.[13] Linoleic acid is the predominant type of omega-6 fatty acid; food sources include soybean oil, safflower oil, canola oil, and sunflower oil. Oleic acid is a monounsaturated omega-9 fat found in animal fat from chicken, beef, eggs, sausage, and bacon and in vegetable oils including canola oil and sunflower oil, so you may want to cut down on these foods. A study that monitored medical students during alternating times of low and high stress found that those who received an omega-3 supplement containing EPA and DHA (eicosapentaenoic acid and docosahexaenoic acid) experienced a 20 percent reduction in anxiety symptoms. They also had lower levels of inflammatory markers compared to the students who received a placebo.[14] Recent evidence also shows that curcumin, the active ingredient in turmeric, boosts DHA synthesis, resulting in higher DHA levels in the brain.[15] A small study examined the effect of 30 days of curcumin supplementation in obese individuals and found that curcumin therapy (1 gram per day) produced a significant reduction in anxiety.[16] As black pepper can increase the bioavailability of curcumin by as much as 2,000 percent,[17] combine these two robust spices for an extra mood-boosting effect.

Lastly, let's look at individual nutrients that can help ease anxiety symptoms. Vitamin C has been shown to reduce anxiety, and with its powerful antioxidant properties, it may play a key role in reversing the free radical damage caused by chronic stress.[18]

The B vitamins have long been studied for their ability to regulate mood; vitamin B supplementation has been shown to be effective at improving mood.[19] A deficiency in vitamin B_{12} has been linked to increased psychological distress,[20] and low concentrations of vitamin B_6 and iron have been observed in people suffering from panic attacks. Moreover, vitamin B_6 and iron play key roles in the production of serotonin, and studies have shown that low serotonin is partially responsible for panic attacks.[21]

Magnesium is known to have a relaxing effect, and it promotes melatonin secretion, which can help with a good night's sleep. Symptoms of magnesium deficiency include agitation and anxiety, not to mention insomnia, hyperventilation, and irritability, which are all symptoms of anxiety as well.[22]

arthritis and joint pain

There are more than 100 types of joint diseases that fall under the general term "arthritis," and with more than 50 million Americans affected, arthritis is the number one cause of disability in the United States. Its most common symptoms include pain in the joints, swelling, stiffness, and decreased range of motion. Symptoms can come and go, and they range from mild discomfort to debilitating pain and disfigurement of the affected joint. No matter the type or cause of arthritis, the pain it causes results from inflammation of the affected joint. So your first line of defense in nutritional intervention for arthritis is a diet that prevents and reduces inflammation.

At the forefront of any anti-inflammation diet are the foods rich in omega-3 fatty acids, which come primarily from wild-caught fish, nuts, and nut oils. (Specific recommendations can be found in "Healing Foods to Prevent and Ease Arthritis Pain" on page 173.) The Harvard T. H. Chan School of Public Health recommends eating seafood twice a week to get the omega-3s your body needs.[1] Omega-3s work against inflammation by inhibiting the production of an enzyme called cyclooxygenase (COX), which produces the prostaglandin hormones that spark inflammation.[2]

Other foods that inhibit inflammation are pineapple, pomegranate, and foods that are high in sulforaphane, a naturally occurring chemical that in addition to inhibiting inflammation may block enzymes that are linked to joint destruction.[3] (See "Healing Foods to Prevent and Ease Arthritis Pain" on page 173 for recommendations.)

For beverages, the drink of choice for easing arthritis is green tea. Green tea is bursting with inflammation-fighting antioxidants—especially catechins, flavonoid compounds that stabilize free radicals—but it's the catechin known as epigallocatechin gallate, or EGCG, that makes all the difference for arthritis sufferers. Several studies have demonstrated EGCG's ability to slow cartilage deterioration and protect collagen.[4] Still others have demonstrated EGCG's anti-inflammatory and antiarthritic effects on a cellular level,[5] which makes it a promising treatment for preventing arthritis before it starts, rather than just treating symptoms once they've appeared. One cup of green tea typically provides 60 to 125 milligrams (mg) of catechins,[6] including EGCG, but with such a range and with so many products available on store shelves, *Women's Health* set out to identify which green teas had the most EGCG. The results? At only 10 cents per tea bag, Lipton Green Tea was the most economical choice and boasted 71 mg of EGCG per cup. For a bit more money, Teavana Gyokuro Imperial Green Tea had the highest amount of EGCG of any brew tested, at 81 mg per cup. A 2-ounce package costs $20 per ounce, which yields 12 cups of tea.[7]

From the herbs and spices family, try ginger and turmeric. In a metastudy on the effects of ginger on osteoarthritis, researchers compiled data from 593 subjects and found that those who used ginger rather than a placebo experienced reduced arthritis pain and reduced disability.[8] Ginger is wonderfully versatile and can be consumed in its whole form, as a tea, as a powder, or as an extract, and one study even revealed that it can relieve arthritis pain when used topically. In this study, chronic arthritis sufferers applied a warm ginger compress or patch to the midlumbar region for half an hour. (Each compress was made using 1 gram of ginger powder and purified water.) The results were remarkable: After

1 week of treatment, study participants reported 48 percent less pain and 49 percent less fatigue, and participants' overall health satisfaction scores went from a dismal 80 percent dissatisfied to 70 percent satisfied. Participants were given the option to continue self-treatment at home, and in all subjects, scores in pain, fatigue, function, and overall health showed steady improvement over the 24 weeks of follow-up.[9]

As for turmeric, its active compound, curcumin, has long been touted for its anti-inflammatory and antioxidant effects. In a study of 367 patients with arthritis of the knee, a curcumin extract of 1,200 mg a day was found to be as effective as 1,200 mg of ibuprofen a day—and without the side effects of abdominal pain and discomfort that the ibuprofen users reported.[10] In a recent study on the effect of curcumin on rheumatoid arthritis, patients were divided into three groups: One received curcumin alone, another received curcumin plus a common anti-inflammatory medication, and the third received a placebo. The curcumin group showed the highest percentage of improvement in joint pain, tenderness, and swelling, as well as in their Disease Activity Score, a measure of rheumatoid arthritis activity and progression.[11]

Turmeric has a warm, bitter taste and is most often used in small

∫healing foods
TO PREVENT AND EASE ARTHRITIS PAIN

So often when we think of chronic pain, we think of taking pills. Consider adding these foods to your diet instead.

- Omega-3-rich foods: flaxseeds, flaxseed oil, halibut, herring, mackerel, salmon, sardines, trout, tuna, walnuts, and walnut oil
- Foods that are high in sulforaphane: broccoli especially, but also other cruciferous vegetables such as arugula, bok choy, Brussels sprouts, cabbage, cauliflower, collards, and kale

- Ginger
- Green tea
- Hot peppers
- Pineapple
- Pomegranate
- Red wine
- Tart cherry juice
- Turmeric

---

amounts as a spice to flavor foods. To supercharge the effect of turmeric, combine it with black pepper. Black pepper boosts the bioavailability of turmeric's active ingredient, curcumin, by as much as 2,000 percent.[12] It's no coincidence that traditional curry recipes always include turmeric and black pepper! So to reduce the pain and swelling associated with arthritis, add curry dishes to your menu. (And the hotter the better: Capsaicin, the active agent in hot peppers, has proven anti-inflammatory and analgesic effects and has even been used as a key ingredient in topical arthritis creams.)[13] Better yet, have a glass of red wine with your curry. Curcumin and the resveratrol in red wine naturally inhibit the activation of a transcription factor that triggers inflammatory processes.[14] Fresh turmeric root or its dried, powdered form can easily be added to soups, stews, stir-fries, and scrambled eggs. Turmeric tea is available at health food stores, and many blends also contain ginger, which enhances the taste and amplifies the anti-inflammatory effect.

Not a wine drinker? Go for tart cherry juice. People with osteoarthritis of the knee drank 16 ounces of tart cherry juice a day and experienced less pain, lower high sensitivity C-reactive protein (a marker of inflammation) scores, and improved WOMAC (an assessment of pain, stiffness, and function of the joints) scores.[15]

asthma

Asthma is a chronic inflammatory condition in which airways narrow and swell and produce extra mucus, resulting in difficulty breathing, shortness of breath, wheezing, and coughing. Sometimes asthma symptoms subside on their own, but if they worsen, they result in an asthma attack. Asthma attacks are quite distressing, and untreated, severe asthma attacks can be fatal. The prevalence of asthma is on the rise and at this time there is no known cure, but the disease can be managed through a combination of medication and lifestyle habits such as knowing and avoiding asthma triggers, exercise (as advised by your doctor), and regular medical checkups.

There are also a host of studies that have found promising results when it comes to dietary interventions for asthma. The first line of defense both to prevent asthma and to alleviate symptoms in asthma sufferers is a diet rich in fresh fruits and vegetables. Their powerful antioxidants, known as flavonoids, take center stage here: They possess anti-inflammatory, antiallergenic, antiobesity, and immune-boosting properties.[1] Among the best sources of flavonoids are apples, aronia berries (chokeberries), beans, blueberries, capers, chocolate, coriander, cranberries, currants, dock, elderberries, fennel, grapefruit, hot peppers, juniper berries, kale, kumquats, lovage, onions, oregano, parsley, plums, radicchio, radishes, raspberries (black), red cabbage, red wine, arugula, and serviceberries.[2] (It's also worth noting that the raw forms of many of these fruits and vegetables are higher in flavonoids than the cooked forms.) One study found that individuals who ate apples twice a week were far less likely to have asthma than those in a control group—possibly due to the effect of the natural antihistamine and antiallergenic effects of the flavonoid quercetin.[3] Quercetin's beneficial role doesn't stop there, however. Another study found that quercetin was able to both prevent the constriction of airways and relax the smooth muscles of airways that were already constricted.[4]

Though there are fewer studies on the antioxidant selenium, there is some evidence to suggest that those who consumed a diet high in selenium were less likely to develop asthma.[5] Selenium is found in Brazil nuts, yellowfin tuna, halibut, sardines, shrimp, ham, chicken, cottage cheese, hard-cooked eggs, whole wheat bread, oatmeal, and spinach.[6]

The other nutrients that have been shown to be effective in combating asthma are omega-3 fatty acids. The anti-inflammatory effect of omega-3s has long been established, and researchers believe that omega-3s might influence susceptibility to allergic diseases, including asthma, because they act on immune cells that are involved in the allergic response. In children who are allergic to dairy, higher levels of the omega-3 known as EPA (eicosapentaenoic acid) are associated with a decreased risk of asthma, while higher levels of inflammatory omega-6s are associated with an increased risk of asthma.[7] In fact, the rise of omega-6s in the Western diet—in sources such as corn oil, soybean oil, margarine, and processed foods—along with the decrease in anti-inflammatory omega-3s is thought by many researchers to be the culprit in the rise in asthma cases.[8]

Finally, look to the herb family for asthma relief. Ginger has been shown to trigger a relaxing effect on the smooth muscles of airways, resulting in easier breathing,[9] and the compound known as rosmarinic acid has been shown to have anti-inflammatory and antioxidant effects and to improve allergenic conditions such as asthma and allergic rhinitis.[10] Rosmarinic acid can be found in rosemary, basil, holy basil, lemon balm, marjoram, peppermint, sage, and thyme.

While there is no "asthma diet," there is strong evidence to suggest that the Mediterranean diet has a positive effect on asthma symptoms. Based on the evidence we've reviewed here, this makes perfect sense, as the Mediterranean diet is rich in fresh fruits and vegetables (and thus healthy antioxidants), omega-3s, and many fresh herbs. One study even concluded that a high adherence to the Mediterranean diet resulted in a whopping 78 percent reduction in the risk of uncontrolled asthma. The researchers highlighted the importance of a high intake of fresh fruit and warned against the excessive consumption of alcohol as factors in controlling asthma.[11] To follow the classic Mediterranean diet, plan menus with an abundance of plant-based foods, such as fresh fruits and vegetables, whole grains, nuts, and legumes; eat lean proteins, such as poultry and wild-caught seafood; use healthy fats, such as avocados and olive oil; use herbs and spices to flavor food, rather than salt, butter, or margarine; and drink red wine in moderation. You'll breathe easier on this antiasthma diet knowing that you're giving yourself a host of whole-body benefits.

attention deficit hyperactivity disorder (ADHD)

Attention deficit hyperactivity disorder is a complex neurodevelopmental condition with a host of symptoms and psychosocial implications. It is one of the most common childhood disorders, present in an estimated 11 percent of children in the United States,[1] and it can last into adolescence and adulthood. Our understanding of ADHD is still incomplete but has evolved substantially in the last several years, and a great deal of research has found a link between diet and ADHD—both in the realm of prevention and in the improvement of ADHD symptoms.

Significantly, given the mixed results of various elimination diets, plus the burden of adhering to strict diets for the long term, a 2012 review of the major dietary interventions for ADHD concluded that supplementation to treat known mineral deficiencies, combined with a healthy diet that is rich in seafood, vegetables, fruits, legumes, and whole grain foods, may be the simplest and most effective nutritional intervention for ADHD.[2] A more recent study conducted in Korea supports this conclusion. Researchers studied 96 students with ADHD and 96 controls and found a lower incidence of ADHD in children who ate a healthy diet—in this case, a diet heavy in whole grains, fish, kimchi, and seaweed—and a higher incidence of ADHD in children who ate fast foods and beverages.[3] A study published in the *Journal of Attention Disorders* found similar results: In children who ate a typical Western diet, characterized by high consumption of fats, refined sugars, and sodium and low consumption of omega-3s, fiber, and folate, a diagnosis of ADHD was twice as likely.[4]

Let's look at some of the specifics of a healthy diet. A recent study found that supplementing with omega-3s decreased symptoms of inattention in boys who'd been diagnosed with ADHD—though supplementation had the same effect on the neurotypical group. This finding suggests that omega-3s are beneficial for everyone

healing foods

It's long been known that diet can directly affect symptoms of ADHD. Here are some essential foods to keep in mind.

Foods to Eat

- Seafood: herring, mackerel, salmon, sardines, and tuna
- Flaxseeds and flaxseed oil
- Iron-rich foods: beans; chicken; dark, leafy greens; lean red meat; nuts; oysters; turkey; whole grains; tofu; and sunflower seeds
- Legumes: alfalfa, beans, lentils, peas, and soybeans
- Organic fruits and vegetables
- Nuts, especially walnuts
- Whole grains: quinoa, farro, whole grain breads, and unsweetened whole grain cereals
- Zinc-rich foods: beef, fortified cereals, oysters, pumpkin seeds, sesame seeds, turkey, and wheat germ
- Foods with vitamin D: beef liver, eggs, fatty fish, fortified milk or soy milk, and mushrooms (Also get some sunlight exposure, one of our best sources of vitamin D.)
- Foods with calcium: dairy products (milk, cheese, and yogurt); dark, leafy greens; legumes; and fortified fruit juices

Foods and Beverages to Avoid

- Processed foods
- Fast foods
- Foods with artificial dyes, flavorings, or preservatives
- Sodas or other sugary drinks
- Caffeinated beverages
- Foods that are high in sugar: sugary cereals, desserts, and candies
- Simple carbs: white rice, pasta, white bread, pancakes, and waffles
- Any known food allergen

Dietary Interventions to Consider

- Eliminate gluten. (There is some evidence supporting a link between celiac disease and ADHD.)[5]
- Eliminate common food allergens (dairy, nuts, eggs, chocolate, and shellfish) one at a time to assess their effects.
- Eliminate salicylates: grapes, tomatoes, oranges, potatoes, apples, berries, cherries, all melons, nectarines, peaches, plums, pomegranates, cucumbers, green peppers, radishes, mint, tea, beer, red wine, and aspirin and any product containing aspirin.*

* This is by no means an exhaustive list, and there is mixed evidence for the beneficial effects of a salicylate-free diet. For more on salicylate sensitivities, see http://salicylatesensitivity.com /about/food-guide/.

during general development.[6] Another study found improvements in spelling, attention, hyperactivity, cognitive problems, and oppositional behavior in children with ADHD who added an omega-3 supplement.[7] A metastudy on polyunsaturated fatty acid (PUFA) supplementation in children with ADHD found mixed results but concluded that some of the conflicting evidence was due to methodological differences and that omega-3 supplementation *does* help in treating ADHD symptoms.[8]

Numerous studies have found that ADHD symptoms improve when artificial food colorings are eliminated from the diet.[9] Many people believe that it is no accident that the rise in the use of artificial food colorings—a 500 percent increase in the past 50 years!—mirrors the rise in diagnoses of ADHD.[10]

Though elimination diets such as the Feingold diet and the salicylate-free diet have been the subject of much controversy[11] and may help only a minority of people,[12] it's worth noting that for those people, the benefits are quite real. The most promising evidence points to eliminating artificial food additives, including preservatives and dyes. One metastudy that looked at results of studies from 1976 to 2011 found that as many as 33 percent of children with ADHD could respond positively to a dietary intervention and as many as

8 percent would benefit from the elimination of food dyes.[13] Another recent study concluded that although artificial food dyes are not a cause of ADHD, they worsen symptoms and can actually push a person over the diagnostic threshold for ADHD. Further, noting that exposure to artificial food colors (AFCs) has quadrupled in the last 50 years and that the deleterious effects of AFCs are not confined to ADHD, the authors recommend minimizing exposure to AFCs for *everyone*.[14]

Though results have been mixed, there is also some evidence that eliminating or cutting back on sugar can improve the symptoms of ADHD. If fully eliminating sugar isn't feasible, try your best to decrease your intake. Sugary foods cause a spike in blood sugar levels followed by a sharp decline, which leaves you feeling jittery, irritable, and distracted. Being in a hypoglycemic state can actually cause symptoms that mimic some ADHD symptoms or can exacerbate symptoms that are already present. Keeping sugar to a minimum is also part of the overall healthy dietary pattern that can protect against ADHD and so many other conditions.

As for essential minerals, numerous studies have found an association between iron deficiency and an increased prevalence of ADHD.[15] In one small study, children with a diagnosis of ADHD who received an iron supplement for 12 weeks reported significant improvement in inattention, hyperactive/impulsive behavior, and even restless leg syndrome.[16] A review of several studies on zinc supplementation in children with ADHD found mixed results, though the authors concluded that zinc supplementation *does* improve ADHD symptoms in children who have a zinc deficiency.[17] There is also evidence that those with ADHD are deficient in calcium and vitamin D.[18] These two minerals work hand in hand, as vitamin D helps your body absorb calcium.

See also: Anxiety (page 165), Food Allergies (page 278)

back pain

Back pain hardly needs an explanation—unfortunately, this all too common phenomenon will visit most everyone at some point, and millions of us live with chronic back pain. Back pain can range from a dull ache to sharp, "spiking" pain. It can come on gradually as a result of age, poor posture, pregnancy, stress, or a degenerative disease like arthritis or osteoporosis, or it can strike suddenly as a result of injury, lifting a heavy object, or even sleeping in an awkward position. Back pain is more common as we age and more common among people who are not physically fit.

To prevent back pain, it's important to get regular exercise and adequate rest and to eat to maintain an ideal weight and support vertebrae health. Obesity is one of the top causes of back pain: Extra pounds overtax your vertebrae and the muscles around them, leading to inflammation and strain. (In fact, musculoskeletal pain stemming from obesity can begin as early as childhood,[1] and an elevated body mass index (BMI) is one of the primary risk factors for chronic low-back pain.)[2] If you're overweight, cut out all processed foods and stick with a diet of whole foods that emphasizes fruits, vegetables, whole grains, and legumes, and opt for the healthy fats found in olive oil, avocados, nuts, and flaxseed oil.

To keep your backbone strong, get plenty of calcium and vitamin D. These nutrients can prevent osteoporosis, one of the main contributors to back pain. In a study of patients with lumbar spinal stenosis (also called LSS, a compression of nerves in the spine), more than 74 percent of LSS sufferers were deficient in vitamin D, and those with severe pain had a higher prevalence of vitamin D deficiency.[3] Researchers recommended increased calcium and vitamin D along with traditional medications. Calcium is found in dairy products, fortified cereals (stick with whole grain, sugar-free varieties), and dark, leafy greens. Vitamin D may play an outsize role in preventing and treating back pain: Vitamin D receptors are located in your spinal cord and throughout your nervous system, and vitamin D plays a direct role in pain moderation by making cells less sensitive to pain, exerting an anti-inflammatory effect, stimulating the release of pain mediators, and eliminating toxic metabolites.[4] The main ways to get vitamin D are through direct exposure to sunlight, dietary supplements, and food sources. The foods highest in vitamin D include fish (cod and cod liver oil, herring, oysters, salmon, halibut, mackerel, and sardines), fortified milk and soy milk, eggs, tofu, and mushrooms.[5]

Whatever your weight, eating to avoid inflammation will be key to preventing back pain. Inflamed cartilage between the vertebrae causes pain, stiffness, lack of flexibility, and a decreased range of motion. The main components of an anti-inflammatory diet are fish, lean poultry, fresh fruits and vegetables, sweet potatoes and other tubers, raw nuts, dark chocolate (75 percent cacao or greater), red wine in moderation, coffee and tea, ginger, garlic, turmeric and other spices, and healthy fats such as olive oil or coconut oil.[6] Foods rich in omega-3s are known to decrease inflammation; to get more omega-3s into your diet, eat fatty fish such as salmon, herring, sardines, mackerel, halibut, and tuna. For vegetarian sources of omega-3s, eat walnuts,

walnut oil, flaxseeds, flaxseed oil, and chia seeds.

When back pain does strike, turn to the healing foods that bring natural pain relief. Tart cherry juice has been shown to reduce inflammation, reduce oxidative stress, alleviate muscle soreness, and even prevent muscle damage for those engaged in rigorous exercise. Tart cherries are among the best sources of phenolic compounds, including flavonoids and anthocyanins, which are both powerful antioxidants and anti-inflammatories.[7]

The active compound in turmeric, curcumin, has been found to inhibit inflammation and is in fact so powerful that it may be a viable alternative to NSAIDs (nonsteroidal anti-inflammatory drugs), with the added benefit that it causes no gastrointestinal side effects.[8] To increase the bioavailability of curcumin, combine turmeric with black pepper. Studies have also shown that the resveratrol found in red wine acts as an anti-inflammatory and an antioxidant. It inhibits COX-2, an enzyme that triggers pain and inflammation, in much the same way that a traditional NSAID does—and like turmeric, it does so without causing gastrointestinal side effects. Resveratrol has also been shown to have a protective effect on cartilage.[9]

Finally, studies have found that intramuscular injections of vitamin B_{12} have resulted in a significant decrease in low back pain.[10] Food sources of B_{12} include animal products, such as fish, meat, poultry, eggs, dairy products, or foods containing sea lettuce and nori. At the top of the list are clams and liver, but trout, mussels, mackerel, salmon, crab, and tuna are also good sources of vitamin B_{12}. For vegetarian sources of B_{12}, eat breakfast cereals fortified with 100 percent of the recommended daily allowance.[11]

bladder infections/ urinary tract infections

The term *bladder infection,* also known as cystitis, is often used interchangeably with *urinary tract infection (UTI).* While cystitis is strictly an infection of the bladder, a UTI is an infection of any part of the urinary tract, including the ureters, urethra, bladder, and kidneys. Both conditions occur when bacteria—most often *Escherichia coli,* commonly known as *E. coli*—enter the lower urinary tract. By any name, the symptoms are unmistakable: a burning or stabbing sensation during urination, a frequent urge to urinate, low production of urine, cloudy or bloody urine, and in some cases, incontinence. If bladder infections (or UTIs) go untreated, bacteria can travel up to your kidneys, resulting in potentially serious and permanent damage, and pregnant women run the risk of going into early labor and/or delivering babies with low birth weights.

Many health-care professionals recommend a full course of antibiotics for UTIs because of the risks associated with untreated infections and the potential of bacteria to spread to your kidneys. But antibiotics also kill off the healthy bacteria in your gut, often resulting in an overgrowth of yeast, and those with recurrent UTIs can develop a resistance to antibiotics. Fortunately some of the latest medical research supports the use of low-cost, low-risk food cures to prevent and treat cystitis and UTIs.

Chances are the first healing food you think of when it comes to bladder infections or UTIs is cranberries. Cranberry juice has been the go-to natural remedy for UTIs for many years, as cranberries increase the acidity of urine and prevent bacteria from adhering to cells in the urinary tract. A review of the recent medical literature on the efficacy of cranberries for the prevention and treatment of UTIs, however, reveals mixed results. A 2013 metastudy based on 24 studies with a total of 4,473 participants that examined the role of cranberries in preventing UTIs found that compared with a placebo, water, or no treatment, cranberry in juice, capsule, or tablet form did not reduce the occurrence of UTI.[1] Another metastudy conducted in 2014 identified 11 studies that supported the use of cranberry products (juice, juice cocktail, capsules, or tablets) for the prevention of UTIs. Twelve studies did not demonstrate the effectiveness of cranberry products for UTI prevention. In the end, given the positive study results from some studies and the ease and low cost of cranberry usage, the authors of this study *do* recommend cranberries for the prevention of UTIs, especially in women with recurrent UTIs.[2] Cranberries have also been found to be effective in elderly nursing home residents who are prone to recurrent UTIs and in young and middle-aged women with recurrent UTIs.[3] Cranberry intervention has also been shown to be effective at preventing UTIs after urinary catheterization. In one study, 160 postsurgical patients were randomized to receive either two concentrated cranberry juice capsules twice a day, equivalent to two 8-ounce servings of cranberry juice, or a placebo for 6 weeks after surgery. Cranberry intervention reduced the rate of UTIs by half.[4] Finally, one study examined the effect of dried cranberries on recurrent UTIs, as they contain high concentrations of polyphenols. Twenty women with recurrent UTIs ate one serving (42 grams) of sweetened dried cranberries daily for 2 weeks. The results: Nine of 17 patients (53 percent) reported no UTIs within 6 months of beginning the study, and the average UTI rate per 6 months decreased significantly, from 2.4 to 1.1.[5]

Cranberries seem to be most effective at preventing recurrent UTIs. Opt for the unsweetened, organic, 100 percent juice variety to avoid loading your diet with unwanted sugar and calories. If this is just too much for your taste buds, dilute the unsweetened juice with water. Cranberry supplements can deliver a higher dosage of active polyphenols, as can dried cranberries. With a UTI, it's a good idea to drink as much fluid as possible.

The juice of black chokeberries, also known as aronia berries, has also been studied in relation to UTIs because of its high total phenol content. One study examined the effect of black chokeberry juice given to nursing home residents. Group A, numbering 110 residents, was given 156 milliliters (ml) of juice a day for 3 months, and group B, numbering 126 residents, was given 89 ml for the same period. During the 3-month period of juice drinking, both groups needed fewer antibiotics to treat UTIs. The incidence of UTI was reduced by 55 percent in group A and 38 percent in group B.

There is emerging research that probiotics can be effective at preventing recurrent UTIs. One study compared the effects of oral *Lactobacillus rham-*

nosus and *L. reuteri* with the antibiotic sulfamethoxazole/trimethoprim on the prevention of recurrent UTIs in 252 postmenopausal women. Researchers found that after 12 months of treatment, the average number of UTIs decreased from 7.0 (from the previous year) to 2.9 in the antibiotic group and from 6.8 to 3.3 in the probiotic group. Although the antibiotic was more effective, the probiotic demonstrated efficacy, as well, and can be a valuable add-on treatment for cases of antibiotic-resistant *E. coli*. There was also evidence that the probiotics were more effective at preventing complicated UTIs—women with complicated UTIs experienced an average of 3.4 infections in the probiotic group, as opposed to 4.4 in the antibiotic group over 12 months.[6]

In an in vitro study, the polyphenolic flavonoid luteolin, which is found in broccoli, carrots, celery, chamomile tea, dandelion greens, green peppers, olive oil, oranges, oregano, parsley, peppermint, and thyme, has been shown to be effective at preventing *E. coli* from attaching to and invading bladder cells.

Like probiotics, it can be a valuable treatment in the face of antibiotic-resistant bacteria.[7]

A number of studies have identified food and beverage triggers that make the pain of bladder infections worse. The top offenders show up again and again: alcoholic beverages, carbonated beverages, citrus fruits, coffee, spicy foods, tea, and tomatoes. Artificial sweeteners also increased pain in many subjects, and interestingly, those with the worst pain reported the highest food sensitivities. It's absolutely worth eliminating these trigger foods while a bladder infection is active, and people with recurrent cystitis should consider long-term elimination of trigger foods.[8] Homeopathic practitioners also recommend drinking a baking soda and water solution to help cut down on the burning pain of urination. Add 1 teaspoon of baking soda to an 8-ounce glass of water and drink once or twice a day.

See also: Fungal Infections (General, Yeast Infections, Candidiasis) (page 281)

bronchitis

Bronchitis is an inflammation of the bronchial tubes, or air passages, in your lungs. The condition can be acute or chronic. Acute bronchitis usually develops from a cold or sinus infection that spreads to your lungs, but it can also arise from exposure to pollution, cigarette smoke, or gastroesophageal reflux disease (see Acid Reflux, page 148). Acute bronchitis is characterized by a cough (which often produces mucus), wheezing, sore throat, fever, chest discomfort, and fatigue. It usually lasts a few days but the cough that accompanies it can last for weeks. In contrast, chronic bronchitis is a long-lasting condition that is characterized by a persistent cough that produces mucus, wheezing, shortness of breath, chest discomfort, and, in advanced cases, blue-tinged lips from lack of oxygen and swelling of the feet, ankles, and legs. If you have the symptoms of chronic bronchitis and/or a temperature of less than 95°F or above 104°F, a resting heart rate of more than 125 beats per minute, or a resting breathing rate of 30 breaths per minute or more, seek immediate medical attention.[1] The main cause of chronic bronchitis is cigarette smoking, and indeed, 40 percent of smokers will develop bronchitis at some point during their lifetimes.[2] Prolonged exposure to pollution, secondhand smoke, and dust can also cause chronic bronchitis.

When eating to treat bronchitis, load up on antioxidants to boost your immune system. Dark, leafy greens, such as arugula, broccoli, chicory, collard greens, kale, lettuces, mustard greens, spinach, and watercress, and brightly colored fruits and vegetables such as apricots, beets, berries, cantaloupe, carrots, mangoes, oranges, tomatoes, winter squash, and yellow and orange peppers are excellent sources of immune-supporting vitamins A and C.

To boost the immune-boosting effect, sauté your greens in some olive oil along with minced garlic. Garlic has been shown to prevent the common cold and is a natural antibiotic,[3] and the allicin in garlic reduces inflammation.[4] And though the trade-off is garlic breath, drinking a tea made from steeping fresh garlic cloves gives you a powerful dose of allicin, while the warm liquid soothes your throat and chest and loosens mucus. Ginger tea can work in much the same way, and it has the added benefit of ginger's natural anti-inflammatory and antimicrobial properties.[5] Ginger has been used for centuries to treat coughs, upper respiratory infections, and bronchitis.[6]

Other foods to try are ginseng and mushrooms. Ginseng has been shown to prevent colds and reduce inflammation, and mushrooms contain powerful anti-inflammatory agents.[7] Turmeric, another natural anti-inflammatory, has long been used in traditional Chinese medicine to treat bronchitis.[8]

Cineole is the active component in eucalyptus oil. In one study, 242 patients with acute bronchitis were divided into an experimental group that took a supplement containing 200 milligrams of cineole three times a day for 10 days and a control group that took a placebo. After 4 days of treatment, the cineole group was significantly better than the control group, with a noticeable improvement in coughing fits. Cineole works because it has anti-inflammatory, bronchodilating, and mucolytic (mucus-thinning) properties.[9]

> **BONUS TIP:** The *Moringa stenopetala* plant, also known as the cabbage tree, boasts incredible amounts of vitamins A and C. Native to Africa, this plant can be grown in any warm climate or greenhouse and is a traditional remedy for respiratory problems.[10] The seeds can be eaten, and the leaves may be eaten raw, dried, or cooked. Supplements are available online and in specialty stores.[11]

Other herbs that work: Thyme and primrose in combination have been shown to be an effective treatment for bronchitis in both adults and children, resulting in significantly less coughing[12] and a significantly lower Bronchitis Severity Score.[13] Similar results have been produced by a preparation of thyme and ivy leaf liquid extract, and subjects in this study experienced a 50 percent reduction in coughing 2 days earlier than their counterparts who received a placebo.[14] Ivy leaf extract is a common ingredient in many complementary cough medicines, or you can make your own ivy leaf tea. Add a spoonful of honey for extra cough relief. Not only does honey act as a cough suppressant, it also has natural antimicrobial properties, is full of antioxidants, and boosts your immune system.[15]

A snack eaten in Mexico and long used in traditional medicine has now gained scientific validation for the treatment of cough: Teas and syrups made from the leaves and fruits of the black cherry tree can be used to stop a cough, as can a decoction made from the seeds. The fruits of the black cherry tree are high in antioxidants, and the seeds, which are toasted and eaten as a snack, are high in protein, magnesium, and potassium.[16]

See also: Allergic Rhinitis (Hay Fever) (page 156), Asthma (page 174), Colds (page 214), Coughs (page 220)

bruises

Bruises occur when an impact injury causes capillaries to burst and blood to pool under your skin. Bruises are nearly always harmless and resolve on their own, going through the familiar transition from black-and-blue to yellow-and-green and finally to brown before fading entirely. The main treatment for bruises is patience and maybe an ice pack, if the area is sore or swollen, but research has shown that dietary interventions can speed up the healing process and prevent susceptibility to bruising.

Vitamin K plays a major role in blood clotting and is routinely used to treat bleeding problems and to counteract the effect of too much blood-thinning medication (such as warfarin).[1] Sometimes referred to as "the clotting vitamin," it's found in green vegetables such as Brussels sprouts, broccoli, cabbage, collards, Swiss chard, kale, spinach, mustard greens, turnip greens, lettuces, watercress, and parsley. It's found in smaller amounts in fish, liver, meat, eggs, and fortified cereals.[2]

Deficiencies in vitamin K and vitamin C lead to increased bruising, though vitamin K deficiency is fairly rare. To get more vitamin C, one of the best-known antioxidants, eat fresh fruits and vegetables, especially papayas, bell peppers, tomatoes, any of the citrus fruits (grapefruit, oranges, lemons, and limes), broccoli, Brussels sprouts, strawberries, kiwi, cantaloupe, kale, cabbage, and parsley. Like vitamin K, vitamin C helps strengthen collagen and capillaries, and it prevents easy bleeding. It has the added bonus of increasing iron absorption.

Though human studies are limited, there is evidence that the powerful class of antioxidants known as proanthocyanidins is effective at preventing bruises because it strengthens capillaries and inhibits their permeability, and it stabilizes collagen.[3] Older studies have demonstrated the ability of proanthocyanidins to improve vascular conditions such as varicose veins, venous insufficiency, and capillary weakness; these studies focused on the proanthocyanidins found in grape seeds.[4] Food sources of proanthocyanidins include cranberries, bilberries, black currants, grapes and grape seeds, red wines, black teas and green teas, hazelnuts, pecans, pistachios, and almonds.

burns

There are three basic categories of burns to the skin. First-degree burns involve only the outer layer of skin and result in redness, swelling, and pain. (Most sunburns are first-degree burns; for healing foods specific to sunburn, please see Sunburn on page 427.) Second-degree burns affect the outer and underlying layers of skin; in addition to the symptoms of first-degree burns, these more serious burns are characterized by blistering. Third-degree burns affect all the layers of the skin, as well as the subcutaneous fat, and in some cases even the underlying muscle and bone. With third-degree burns, the skin can be charred or it can take on a white or yellowish color. Because the nerves have been severely damaged, third-degree burns can be painless.

First-degree burns and small second-degree burns are considered minor and in most cases can be treated at home. If a second-degree burn is larger than 3 inches wide, you should see your doctor. Third-degree burns are a medical emergency, and you should seek immediate medical attention for them. People with severe burns are in danger of dehydration and going into shock.

No matter the type of burn, good nutrition plays an enormous role in the recovery process. Nutrition interventions can help ward off infection, speed the healing of skin and tissue, and soothe pain. In the case of a severe burn, nutritional and caloric requirements skyrocket as your body strives to heal, and having a nutritionist or dieti-

cian as part of your care team is highly recommended. Let's look at some of the latest research on dietary treatments for burns.

Honey has long been known to speed the healing of wounds because of its antibacterial, anti-inflammatory, and antioxidant properties.[1] A remarkable study conducted on 150 patients with first- and second-degree burns compared the topical use of honey with the standard treatment of silver sulfadiazine, a prescription antibiotic cream. Each patient had one burn site treated with plain honey and one burn site treated with silver sulfadiazine cream. Wound closure occurred more quickly at the honey-treated sites—after about 13.5 days, compared to nearly 16 days for the burn sites treated with the pre-scription drug cream, and the honey-treated sites healed completely in less than 21 days, compared with 24 days for the prescription drug cream. What's more, 27 patients using the cream tested positive for a common bacterial infection at the burn site, whereas only 6 of the patients who received the honey treatment did, demonstrating honey's natural antibacterial properties.[2] Further, a meta-analysis study on the efficacy of honey for burn treatment confirmed that honey dressings heal partial thickness burns 4 to 5 days faster than conventional dressings.[3] That's fewer infections, less pain, and faster healing—all from an affordable, extremely safe product.

Are some varieties of honey better than others? While the honey already in your pantry has some antibacterial and wound-healing properties, research has shown that manuka honey is the most effective. That's because manuka honey's antibacterial activity is due to an organic compound called methylglyoxal, rather than the hydrogen peroxide that is present in other honeys. Unlike hydrogen peroxide, methylglyoxal is able to withstand substantial wound drainage and still maintain its antibacterial properties.[4] Manuka honey is available in health food stores and through online retailers.

To make your own honey dressing, simply apply a layer of honey evenly to the wound site and cover it with a regular gauze bandage. Alternatively, you can apply honey to the dressing itself and place it over the burned area; use regular bandage tape to keep it in place. Wound dressings should typically be changed daily, though burns that are actively draining will require more frequent changes.

To eat for burn healing, add foods that are rich in antioxidants. Burn trauma can create oxidative stress and the generation of free radicals, endothelial dysfunction (a condition affecting vasodilation and vasoconstriction), and a systemic inflammatory response, and antioxidants can reduce the severity of all of these reactions.[5] Antioxidants have also been shown to reduce the incidence of wound infection, shorten healing time, and even lower the mortality rate of burn patients.[6] Zinc, which has a powerful antioxidant effect, is recommended for burn healing. Zinc levels are known to be significantly lower after burn injuries. In a study conducted on burn patients in Iraq, those who were treated with zinc supplementation experienced less fluid loss and fewer signs of oxidative stress, which led to a decrease in healing time, less eschar formation (dark, leathery patches of dead skin), and a decrease in mortality rate compared to those not treated with zinc. The authors of this study recommend that zinc be taken orally *and* applied topically to burn sites.[7] Zinc-rich foods include oysters, beef, turkey, pumpkin seeds, sesame seeds, fortified cereals, and wheat germ. As for antioxidants generally, any brightly colored fruit or vegetable will be a great source of antioxidants. Examples include citrus fruits; grapes; apples; berries; tomatoes; sweet or hot peppers; any dark, leafy greens; carrots; squash; pumpkin; cauliflower; garlic; ginger; turmeric; onions; and fresh herbs, such as parsley, basil, and oregano. Antioxidants are also found in pecans, almonds, walnuts, hazelnuts, tea, red wine, dark chocolate, and other cocoa products. Pineapple may have a bonus benefit because it contains bromelain, a natural anti-inflammatory.[8]

Don't forget to drink for burn healing, as well. Drink as much filtered water as possible—at least eight glasses a day—and to get in a bit more vitamin C, flavor it with fresh-squeezed lemon or orange juice.

And, contrary to the old wives' tale, do *not* apply butter or oil to burns. There is no evidence that butter or oil speeds the healing of burns, and it, in fact, can delay the healing process by trapping heat in your skin. Interestingly, however, a recent study found that ingesting olive oil can speed healing. In this case, 100 burn patients simply added olive oil to their daily salads and experienced faster healing of their wounds and shorter hospital stays than the placebo group.[9]

See also: Sunburn (page 427)

bursitis

If you've ever experienced bursitis, you may wince just to read the word. Bursitis is a painful condition that occurs when the bursae, the small, fluid-filled sacs that provide cushioning between bones and tendons or muscles around a joint, become inflamed. There are more than 150 bursae in your body, but the most common sites of bursitis are your shoulders, elbows, and hips. Bursitis can occur near any joint that performs frequent, repetitive motion, such as your knees, heels, or big toes. Symptoms include pain, stiffness, swelling, localized warmth, and redness in the affected joint, and flare-ups are common.

As bursitis is an inflammatory condition, you'll want to avoid any food that promotes inflammation and eat foods with natural anti-inflammatory properties. Foods to avoid include red meat, refined or processed foods (including processed meats such as bacon, salami, and hot dogs), fast foods, fried foods, soft drinks, and refined carbohydrates (including pastries, white bread, and white pasta). And while you should make sure you're getting adequate calcium and vitamin D, some people also eliminate or reduce their consumption of dairy products, especially during a bursitis flare-up, as dairy is inflammatory.

As for what to eat, one superfood defense for fighting inflammation is omega-3 fatty acids. Many studies have demonstrated the ability of the omega-3s EPA (eicosapentaenoic acid) and DHA (docosahexaenoic acid) to inhibit the inflammatory response, making them great choices for a host of inflammatory conditions, including bursitis, osteoarthritis, rheumatoid arthritis, asthma, and some inflammatory bowel conditions.[1] Cold-water fish such as salmon, herring, tuna, sardines, and mackerel are among the best sources of omega-3s, but you can also get them from flaxseeds, flaxseed oil, fish oil, chia seeds, walnuts, and walnut oil.

Generally, foods that are high in antioxidants will reduce inflammation by combating the inevitable inflammatory response that accompanies oxidative stress. Any fresh fruit or vegetable is an excellent source of polyphenols, plant metabolites that act as antioxidants. There are more than 8,000 known polyphenols, and the number of foods and beverages rich in polyphenols is far too vast to list, but some common examples include any dark, leafy greens; any type of berry; citrus fruits (and their juices); grapes; red wine; coffee; tea; tomatoes; pears; and cherries.[2] A study that was just released demonstrated the anti-inflammatory power of orange juice, which is rich in polyphenols and antioxidant vitamins. Subjects drank 750 milliliters of 100 percent orange juice daily for 8 weeks. Not only did they experience a significant reduction

eat for any *–itis*: reducing inflammation

Any number of widely available foods can help reduce inflammation. Some can also cause it.

Foods to Eat

- Apples
- Aronia berries (chokeberries)
- Capers
- Cilantro
- Citrus fruits and their juices
- Coffee
- Dark, leafy greens: arugula, kale, spinach, and Swiss chard
- Dark chocolate
- Ginger
- Hot peppers

- Lovage leaves
- Mushrooms
- Omega-3s: salmon, mackerel, herring, sardines, tuna, halibut, trout, flaxseeds, flaxseed oil, walnuts, walnut oil, and chia seeds
- Papaya
- Pineapple
- Tea
- Turmeric (combine with black pepper to increase its effect)

Foods to Avoid

- Fast foods
- Foods containing trans fatty acids
- Foods high in saturated fats
- Foods high in sugar

- High-fructose corn syrup
- Processed foods, including processed meats
- Refined carbohydrates

in inflammation as indicated by a decrease in high-sensitivity C-reactive protein, but they also had lower LDL cholesterol, improved immune function, and higher total antioxidant capacity.[3]

Flavonoids are one of the largest and most researched types of polyphenols, and the flavonoid called quercetin deserves special mention when it comes to bursitis. Quercetin acts like an antihistamine and an anti-inflammatory. Apples contain the highest amount of quercetin found in fruits, but other good sources include dill weed, aronia berries (chokeberries), cranberries, elderberries, juniper berries, cilantro, raw dock (a type of sour wild green), raw fennel leaves, raw kale, onions, hot peppers, arugula, and raw watercress. Capers and raw lovage leaves, however, take the cake in quercetin content, with 172.6 milligrams (mg) of quercetin per 100 grams (g) of canned capers, 233.8 mg of quercetin per 100 g of raw capers, and 170 mg of quercetin per 100 g of lovage leaves.[4]

Pineapple is also highly recommended for bursitis sufferers. Pineapple contains an enzyme called bromelain that reduces inflammation. To get more pineapple into your diet, drink pineapple juice with breakfast, add pineapple to smoothies, include pineapple chunks in fruit salads, or enjoy pineapple chunks or slices for your afternoon snack. Pineapple is also great grilled, so add chunks to kebabs, or throw pineapple rings right onto the grill. Add pineapple chunks to any stir-fry for a delightful tang. One word of caution: Bromelain can increase your risk of bleeding, and the effect is strengthened when combined with turmeric, so if you're on a blood thinner such as Coumadin, consult with your doctor if you're considering bromelain supplements. (The lower amount found in whole foods should not pose a problem.)

To increase the effect of bromelain, combine it with turmeric, a powerful anti-inflammatory. Turmeric's active compound, curcumin, gives it its distinctive yellow color and is responsible for its anti-inflammatory effects. The ways in which curcumin works as an anti-inflammatory are complex and multiform, but one way is by inhibiting the activity of enzymes responsible for inflammation and pain[5] in much the same way that nonsteroidal anti-inflammatory drugs (NSAIDs) do. In one study of patients with rheumatoid arthritis, a highly inflammatory condition, one group of patients received curcumin, a second group received curcumin plus the NSAID diclofenac sodium, and a third group received diclofenac sodium alone. The group that took curcumin alone showed the highest rate of improvement in all areas of assessment: These patients had less pain, their joints were less swollen and tender, and they had lower blood markers of inflammation—with zero side effects.[6] Combining black pepper with turmeric increases its effects.

Another anti-inflammatory spice is ginger, and it pairs wonderfully with turmeric. Like turmeric, ginger acts against inflammation in a manner similar to NSAIDs, and it modulates bio-chemical pathways that are activated in chronic inflammation[7]—all without the gastrointestinal side effects associated with NSAIDs.

Given the powerful anti-inflammatory effects of these foods, the next time you have a bursitis flare-up, your best medicine may be a peppery curry dish with pineapple.

See also: Arthritis and Joint Pain (page 171)

cancer

When it comes to fear-inspiring illnesses, cancer is at the top of many people's lists. The uncontrolled growth of cells known as cancer kills well over 8 million people a year worldwide, and that toll is expected to rise to 13 million by 2030.[1] It's the disease that comes to mind when people think of pain and suffering—not only from cancer itself, but also from radiation and chemotherapy treatments, which can cause a range of distressing side effects. But compare these alarming statistics and scenarios with this powerful medical fact: Fully one-third of cancer deaths are due to just five dietary and behavioral risks.[2]

1. Tobacco use
2. High body mass index (BMI)
3. Low intake of fruits and vegetables
4. Lack of physical exercise
5. Overconsumption of alcohol.[3]

Other leading risk factors for cancer include:

- A family history of cancer
- Increasing age
- Chronic inflammation
- Sun and UV (ultraviolet radiation) exposure
- Exposure to radiation
- Exposure to carcinogenic chemicals or environmental toxins
- Infectious agents such as HPV, HIV, *Helicobacter pylori*, or the hepatitis B or C viruses
- Certain hormones, such as estrogen and progesterone
- Immunosuppression.[4]

A family history of cancer and aging are both obviously beyond our control, but most of these risk factors are avoidable. Of the leading behavioral risk factors, three of them—overconsumption of alcohol, underconsumption of fruits and vegetables, and a high BMI—are directly related to what we eat and drink. Some types of cancer are directly associated with an excess of body fat: postmenopausal breast cancer, colorectal, endometrial, esophageal, gallbladder, kidney, ovarian, pancreatic, and advanced prostate cancers.[5] The American Institute for Cancer Research estimates that eating a healthy diet, staying active, and maintaining a healthy weight could prevent roughly one-third of cancers in the United States, or 340,000 cases a year.[6] The link between dietary factors and an increased risk of many types of cancer really can't be overstated.

The World Health Organization (WHO) has now added processed meats to its list of things that are carcinogenic to humans. This means that any meat prepared by a process of smoking, curing, salting, or adding other chemical preservatives or flavor enhancers (this includes bacon, sausage, ham, hot dogs, pastrami, and any cold cut that has gone through a chemical process) joins carcinogens such as tobacco products, formaldehyde, and mustard gas as an agent known to cause cancer in humans. Red meat—products from beef, lamb, or pork—was categorized as "Probably Carcinogenic to Humans." The WHO has pointed out that agents are placed in categories based on the strength of the evidence behind them, not the level of risk, but the evidence concerning processed meat shows that eating even small amounts on a daily basis, such as one small hot dog, increases your chances of colorectal cancer by 18 percent compared to eating none. There was also a link observed between processed meat and an increased risk of stomach cancer. For red meat, eating 100 grams (g) daily was linked to an 18 percent

increased risk of colorectal cancer. Red meat consumption was also positively linked to an increased risk of pancreatic and prostate cancer. The bottom-line recommendations of the American Institute for Cancer Research are to avoid processed meat (except perhaps on rare occasions) and to limit red meat consumption to 18 ounces per week.[7]

Moreover, the compounds created when meat is cooked at high temperatures (such as when barbecuing) have proven carcinogenic in animal models, and by examining data from 659 renal cell carcinoma patients compared to 699 cancer-free controls, researchers found a link between kidney cancer risk and two compounds known as MeIQx and PhIP, both of which are produced when charring meats.[8]

Not to worry, though—cancer doesn't have us beat yet! There is a great deal of evidence suggesting that a plant-based diet helps prevent cancer. More specifically, plant bioactive compounds such as polyphenols, glucosinolates, and carotenoids have been shown to suppress sustained proliferative signaling, angiogenesis (the growth of new blood vessels that would supply a tumor), and metastasis, as well as promote cancer stem cell apoptosis (cell death).[9] A high intake of fruits and vegetables has been associated with a reduced risk of several cancers, especially cancers of the digestive and respiratory tracts, and evidence suggests that eating a wide variety of fruits and vegetables is advisable for cancer prevention, as the variety of plant bioactive compounds causes a synergistic effect.[10] The Mediterranean diet, which emphasizes antioxidant-rich foods such as fresh fruits and vegetables, olive oil, tea, and red wine in moderation, as well as legumes, nuts, seeds, and lean proteins, has been shown to reduce the risk of colorectal cancer and is associated with lower cancer mortality overall.[11]

Let's turn our attention to specific foods and food groups known to be cancer fighters. Considering that cancer can affect any organ or body tissue, healing foods recommendations for this disease could truly fill a book. While there is no one food or food group that can eradicate cancer, there are plenty of foods that *directly fight cancer.* This is by no means an exhaustive list, but if you maintain an overall healthy dietary pattern and eat a mostly plant-based diet, you've effectively adopted a cancer-fighting diet.

apples

Apples of all types have shown anticancer abilities because of their antioxidant properties and cell cycle control cell (function). They are rich in flavonoids (including the powerful antioxidant quercetin), phenolic compounds, vitamins, and fiber.[12] In a study based on data from more than 10,000 cases of 14 different cancers and about 17,000 controls, people who ate at least one apple a day were found to have a reduced risk of cancers of the mouth and pharynx, colon and rectum, larynx, breast, and ovaries.[13] Pink Lady apples have been shown to be particularly effective at protecting against breast and colon cancer. It's the flavonoids in the apples that inhibit cancer growth, and the more you eat, the greater the cancer-fighting power. Don't peel your apples before eating them: The peel of Pink Lady apples, for example, contains far more antioxidant power than the flesh.[14]

beans

Beans are excellent sources of fiber, which makes them a superfood for preventing colorectal cancer. Preliminary data link bean consumption to a reduced risk of breast and prostate cancer, as well, but research is ongoing.[15] In particular, black bean extract has been shown to inhibit the growth of colon, breast, liver, and prostate cancer cells via apoptosis while leaving normal cells intact.[16] Mung bean extract has demonstrated cytotoxic effects against hepatocellular carcinoma, a common liver cancer, and cervical cancer, the second-most-frequent cancer occurring in females worldwide.[17] A hemagglutinin (a compound that causes red blood cells to aggregate) made from northern red beans was found to exert antiproliferative activity against breast, liver, and nasopharyngeal cancer cells.[18]

berries

As foods that are high in vitamin C, fiber, and antioxidants, berries of any type are potent cancer-fighters. Vitamin C is particularly effective against esophageal cancer, and fiber protects against colorectal cancer.[19] Regular consumption of anthocyanins—the flavonoid phytopigments that give berries their red, blue, or purple color—is associated with a lower risk of cancer generally.[20] And because berry phytochemicals can be absorbed in your mouth as well as in your gastrointestinal tract, they may provide particular chemopreventive effects against cancers of the mouth, esophagus, stomach, colon, and rectum.[21] (Two berries that exhibited particularly strong cytotoxic effects against colon cancer cells are bilberry and chokeberry.)[22] Some berries can even enhance the effect of cancer treatments: Chokeberry extract, for example, increases the effect of the chemotherapy drug gemcitabine.[23]

It seems that berries in any form can help fight cancer—whole, juiced, extracts, or even less common forms, such as dried and powdered. Blueberry powder has been shown to increase natural killer cells,[24] a type of white blood cell that targets tumor cells while leaving healthy cells intact.

The juices of black currants, cranberries, raspberries, and gooseberries all showed antiproliferative effects against stomach cancer in in vitro studies.[25] An anthocyanin-rich berry juice made with grapes and bilberries also inhibited pancreatic cancer cell migration in an in vitro study.[26]

In another in vitro study, an anthocyanin-rich chokeberry extract was shown to inhibit human colon cancer cell growth by 65 percent.[27] An in vitro study has demonstrated that acai berry extract has anti-inflammatory and cytotoxic effects against colon cancer cells.[28] In vitro studies have also shown that anthocyanin-rich blueberry extract has antiproliferative activity against ovarian and cervical cancer cells. Cervical cancer cells were more sensitive: Cell viability decreased from 100 percent to 45.9 percent after 24 hours of exposure to blueberry extract. Likewise, anthocyanins from black currant extract caused decreased cell viability in ovarian and cervical cancer cells but also inhibited growth in liver, melanoma, breast, colon, and prostate cancer cells.[29] Extract from the yellow Himalayan raspberry, which grows in Hawaii and in the southern United States, has shown potent antiproliferative activity against human cervical cancer cells while showing no cytotoxicity to normal cells.[30] Cranberry, black raspberry, and strawberry extracts were all found to exert an antiproliferative effect against human oral cancer in in vitro studies. Both cranberry and black raspberry extract were found to exert anticancer effects against esophageal cancer. A number of berry extracts have also shown anticancer activity against liver cancer cells, including strawberries, blueberries, cranberries, black currants, and bilberries.[31]

carrots

A recent metastudy found that whole carrot consumption is associated with a significant decrease in the risk of prostate cancer.[32] In vitro studies of wild carrot extract demonstrated a significant antiproliferative effect against human breast cancer cells and colon cancer cells, as well as a cytotoxic effect against acute myeloid leukemia cells.[33]

citrus fruits

In a study based on data from more than 10,000 cases of 14 different cancers and about 17,000 controls, researchers found that consumption of four or more citrus fruits a week was associated with a reduced risk of mouth and pharyngeal cancer, esophageal cancer, stomach cancer, colorectal cancer, and laryngeal cancer. Citrus fruits are rich in vitamin C, flavanones, and other compounds with antioxidant, antimutagenic, and antiproliferative properties.[34] A study based on 111 cases of thyroid cancer compared to 115 benign controls found that a high consumption of raw vegetables, persimmons, and tangerines may decrease thyroid cancer risk and help prevent early-stage thyroid cancer.[35] A meta-analysis of 19 studies found that citrus fruit intake could reduce your esophageal cancer risk by as much as 37 percent.[36] A high intake of citrus fruits could also reduce your risk of breast cancer by 10 percent.[37] A meta-study based upon 14 clinical trials concluded that citrus fruit consumption was associated with a reduced risk of bladder cancer.[38]

coffee

One simple cup of black coffee offers a host of anticancer effects. A recent review based on nearly 150 studies lists the following chemopreventive agents in black coffee: antioxidant agents, anti-inflammatory agents, cell proliferation inhibitors, cell cycle progression inhibitors, metastatic growth metabolism modulators, angiogenesis (new blood vessel growth) inhibitors, invasion and metastasis inhibitors, immune cell stimulants, and cytotoxins. Though space doesn't permit a summary of individual studies on coffee's chemopreventive agents, we can point out some of the superstars from coffee's cancer-fighting arsenal. Chlorogenic acids are the most abundant phenolic compounds in coffee. They exert antioxidant and anti-inflammatory effects and can induce DNA damage in cancer cells, inhibit angiogenesis, and trigger cancer cell death. Caffeine also acts as an antioxidant and anti-inflammatory, and it has been shown to induce cell cycle arrest; protect against cirrhosis and hepatic fibrosis, two chronic inflammatory diseases that can lead to liver cancer; and exert in vitro antiproliferation effects against breast cancer, colon cancer, and cervical cancer. Two lipids in coffee, cafestol and kahweol, are reactive oxygen species scavengers and have shown antiangiogenic (preventing new blood vessel formation), antigenotoxic, antiproliferation, antimigration, and cancer cell–death-inducing effects. Melanoidins are produced during the roasting process and exhibit anti-inflammatory and antioxidant effects. Melanoidins have been shown to reduce proliferation and induce cell cycle arrest in colon cancer cells and to induce cell cycle arrest in glioma (the most common brain tumor) cells.[39]

Is there a recommended "dose" of coffee? Science says yes—and there are some additional guidelines to bear in mind, too. First, 750 milliliters (ml) of black coffee a day is recommended to protect against cancer and prevent its progression. That's a little more than three 8-ounce cups per day—or what would translate to four to six cups in a standard-size mug. Second, it's recommended that you use a metal filter to prepare coffee, such as in a French press, rather than a paper filter, as the metal filter releases more caffeine, cafestol, and kahweol. (The paper filter can absorb these compounds.) And third, caffeinated coffee does appear to contain greater levels of cancer-fighting compounds than decaffeinated coffee does.[40] That's not to say that decaf doesn't also confer some health benefits, however. Let's take a look at the research.

Data based on 47,911 men found that those who consumed 6 or more cups of coffee per day—and happily, that's decaf or regular—had a lower adjusted relative risk for prostate cancer compared with non-coffee-drinkers. Researchers speculated that coffee's protective effect against prostate cancer comes from its bioactive compounds and phenolic acids that have potent antioxidant activity and can affect glucose metabolism and sex hormone levels.[41]

In a study of 1,090 patients with breast cancer, moderate (2 to 4 cups a day) to high (5 or more cups a day) consumption of coffee was associated with smaller invasive primary tumors and a lower proportion of estrogen receptor–positive (ER-positive) tumors compared to patients who drank one or fewer cups of coffee per day. Moderate to high consumption was also associated with a lower risk of breast cancer events in tamoxifen-treated patients with ER-positive tumors. Further, caffeine caused impaired cell-cycle progression and enhanced cell death.[42]

There is also some evidence that caffeine can protect against nonmelanoma skin cancers.[43] Researchers using data from a total of 112,897 subjects examined caffeine intake in relation to basal cell carcinoma (BCC), squamous cell carcinoma (SCC), and melanoma. They found that consuming caffeine from any dietary source was inversely related with the risk of BCC and that caffeinated coffee was most effective. Compared to those who drank less than 1 cup of coffee per month, those who drank 3 or more cups a day had the lowest risk of BCC. The effect was slightly greater for women than for men. Researchers did not, however, find an association between caffeine and SCC or melanoma, so your decaf will work just as well to combat those cancer types.[44] In a study of 767 people with a median age of 36—377 with early-onset basal cell carcinoma (BCC) and 390 controls—researchers found that regular consumption of caffeinated coffee plus hot tea was inversely associated with early-onset BCC. Those with the highest levels of caffeine intake over their lifetimes had a 43 percent reduced risk of BCC compared to those who didn't consume caffeine.[45]

Despite its many health benefits, use caution when drinking coffee. Excessive consumption of caffeinated coffee can cause symptoms such as heart palpitations, anxiety, sweating, increased blood pressure, and nausea. And remember that all of the research on coffee you'll read in this book is based on black coffee. While adding sugar and cream doesn't cancel out the health-promoting compounds, it does add saturated fat, calories, and sugar, all of which bring their own unwanted health consequences.

cruciferous vegetables

Regularly consuming crucifers, named for their cross-shaped flowers, is one of the best things you can do for your health. Cruciferous vegetables—such as broccoli, Brussels sprouts, cabbage, cauliflower, and kale—are all members of the Brassica family and are associated with a decreased risk of cancer incidence overall. Their chemoprotective effect comes in large part from the sulfur-containing phytochemicals known as isothiocyanate compounds (ITCs).[46] The ITCs phenethyl isothiocyanate and sulforaphane and the indole called indole-3-carbonol have been shown to induce apoptosis and cell cycle arrest in cancer cells as well as to prevent uncontrolled cellular proliferation and protect against DNA damage.[47] Sulforaphane, which is found in broccoli and cauliflower and is present in high quantities in broccoli sprouts, has been shown to protect against colon cancer, breast cancer, leukemia, bladder cancer, and prostate cancer. In a study on its effect on thyroid cancer, sulforaphane was shown to inhibit thyroid cancer cell proliferation, migration, and invasion and to induce cell cycle arrest and apoptosis.[48]

A recent metastudy found that a high intake of cruciferous vegetables was associated with a significantly decreased risk of pancreatic cancer. This is good news regarding one of our deadliest cancers: Most people die within 6 months of diagnosis, and the 5-year survival rate for pancreatic cancer is less than 5 percent.[49] Cruciferous vegetable intake is also associated with a reduced risk of ovarian cancer, as demonstrated by two metastudies,[50] as well as a reduced risk of bladder cancer,[51] breast cancer,[52] and renal cell carcinoma.[53] Raw broccoli intake has been shown to improve the survival odds of those with bladder cancer.[54] An analysis of several large case-controlled studies found that consuming cruciferous vegetables at least once a week (compared to little or no consumption) led to significantly lower odds for cancer of the mouth and pharynx, breast, kidney, colon and rectum, and esophagus. In this particular analysis, there was also some evidence of lower odds of stomach, liver, pancreatic, laryngeal, endometrial, ovarian, and prostate cancer with eating cruciferous vegetables at least once a week.[55]

dark, leafy greens

In a recent study on the protective effects of fruits and vegetables against bladder cancer, the most common cancer of the urinary tract, dark, leafy greens came out on top as the most effective. Based on data from 14 cohorts with 17 studies including 9,447 cases of bladder cancer, researchers concluded that every 0.2 increase in daily servings of dark, leafy greens was associated with a 2 percent decrease in bladder cancer risk. Dark, leafy greens identified from these studies include spinach, kale, mustard greens, chard greens, romaine lettuce, and leaf lettuce.[56] Another study found that a higher consumption of fruits and vegetables was associated with a 54 percent decreased risk of squamous cell carcinoma, a protective effect due mostly to dark, leafy greens, including spinach, Swiss chard, spring onions, and lettuce.[57] Additionally, an observational study found that subjects who ate dark, leafy greens at least three times per week had a decreased risk of cutaneous melanoma.[58]

flaxseeds and flaxseed oil

Flaxseed is one of the richest sources of alpha-linolenic acid (ALA), dietary lignans, and a lignan precursor called secoisolariciresinol diglucoside (SDG). Animal and human studies have shown the preventive role of SDG against breast, lung, and colon cancer as a result of its strong antiproliferative, antioxidant, antiestrogenic, and/or antiangiogenic activity.[59] Flax contains up to 800 times more lignans than other plant foods, and flax lignans have shown the ability to reduce the growth of tumors, especially in hormonesensitive cancers such as breast, endometrium, and prostate.[60] Like any fiberrich food, flaxseeds help to prevent

colorectal cancer.[61] Flaxseeds and flaxseed oil should be kept refrigerated.

garlic

Garlic has been proven protective against colorectal cancer, esophageal cancer, stomach cancer, and renal cancer.[62] In a study based on data from more than 10,000 cases of 14 different cancers and about 17,000 controls, researchers found that a high consumption of garlic and onions resulted in a significantly decreased risk of cancers of the mouth and pharynx, esophagus, colon and rectum, larynx, endometrium, and ovary. A high consumption of garlic was associated with a decreased risk of kidney cancer.[63]

grapes and grape juice

The stilbene polyphenol resveratrol, which is found in grapes and grape juice (and fermented grape juice, i.e., wine), has antioxidant, anti-inflammatory, and anticancer properties. It's been shown to inhibit cancer cell proliferation in several types of cancers, including breast, liver, skin, prostate, lung, and colon cancer.[64] Anthocyanidins, which are found in abundance in grape juice and red wine, have been associated with a 57 percent reduction in the risk of esophageal adenocarcinoma and esophageal squamous cell carcinoma and a decreased risk of mortality for gastric adenocarcinoma.[65]

herbs and spices

According to a study in the *International Journal of Epidemiology*, consuming four or more herbs regularly provides up to a 60 percent reduced risk of melanoma. In this particular study, the herbs included were parsley, rosemary, sage, and basil, and fresh rosemary had the greatest effect.[66] In in vitro studies, rosemary extract has exhibited antitumor effects on breast cancer, liver cancer, prostate cancer, small cell lung cancer, and leukemia.[67] Holy basil extract has been shown to inhibit the proliferation, migration, and invasion of pancreatic cancer cells and to induce apoptosis in vitro.[68] In vitro studies have also shown that thyme extract inhibits proliferation, migration, and invasion of colorectal cancer cells; it also decreases adhesion to fibronectin and increases colon cancer cell death.[69] Extracts of oregano and bay leaf were found to exert anticancer effects against cervical cancer cells in vitro.[70]

Curcumin, the active compound in turmeric, has been extensively studied for its anticancer effects and has been shown to play a chemopreventive role in multiple cancers, including leukemia and lymphoma, gastrointestinal cancers, genitourinary cancers, breast cancer, ovarian cancer, head and neck squamous cell carcinoma, lung cancer, melanoma, neurological cancers, and sarcoma.[71] The evidence suggests that curcumin suppresses tumor initiation, promotion, and metastasis[72] and also suppresses transcription factor nuclear factor-kappa beta, a central protein in many types of cancer.[73] It's been shown to target colon cancer stem cell growth[74] and to protect against skin cancer by diminishing skin-related oxidative stress and suppressing inflammation.[75] Curcumin has also shown antiproliferative and apoptosis-inducing activity in prostate cancer cells.[76]

If curcumin has one weakness, it's low bioavailability. So whenever possible, combine turmeric with black pepper, which increases the bioavailability of curcumin by as much as 2,000 percent.[77]

honey

In vitro studies have shown that honey can induce apoptosis (cell death) in bladder, breast, colon, liver, lung, leukemia, melanoma, oral squamous, osteosarcoma, and renal carcinoma cancer cells. In a human trial, average honey consumption of 4.2 g per day was positively associated with apoptosis of gastric cancer cells.[78] Other in vitro studies have demonstrated honey's anticancer effect in endometrial cancer cells, cervical cancer cells, human non-small cell lung cancer cells, and prostate cancer cells. It has the ability to be highly cytotoxic to cancerous cells but nontoxic to normal cells.[79] Honey is also a source of vitamins, trace elements, amino acids, and protein. Its flavonoids and phenolic compounds have demonstrated anti-inflammatory, antioxidant, antiproliferative, antitumor, antimetastatic, and anticancer effects.[80] Its anticancer abilities occur through several mechanisms, including cell

healthy habits for cancer prevention

- Do not smoke or use tobacco products.
- Do not eat processed meat.
- Eliminate trans fats from your diet. They're linked with many ill effects on health, and research has shown an association between trans fats and an increased risk of breast cancer, nonaggressive prostate cancer, gastric adenocarcinomas, and colorectal adenomas.[81]
- Limit consumption of red meat to no more than 18 ounces per week.
- Eat more fresh fruits and vegetables. There's really no upper limit here!
- Opt for whole grains over refined and complex carbohydrates over simple.
  - For example, instead of products using white flour or dishes made with white pasta or white rice, go for brown rice, quinoa, barley, buckwheat, millet, whole oats, bulgur, sorghum, or farro, as well as products made with whole wheat flour.
- Eat more fiber. Foods high in fiber include whole grains; beans; fruits; dark, leafy greens; legumes; nuts; and seeds.
- If you drink alcohol, do so in moderation.
- Reduce your sugar intake. High-sugar diets promote carcinogenesis by increasing insulin production, increasing oxidative stress, and causing weight gain.[82]
- Stay active by getting at least half an hour of moderate exercise daily.
- Aim for a body mass index (BMI) of between 18.5 and 24.9. A standard BMI calculator can be found here: www.nhlbi.nih.gov/health /educational/lose_wt/BMI/bmicalc .htm.

cycle arrest, cell apoptosis, activation of the mitochondrial pathway, modulation of oxidative stress, inflammation reduction, modulation of insulin signaling, and inhibition of new blood vessel growth in cancer cells.[83]

mushrooms

Mushroom extracts have demonstrated in vitro antitumor effects, due in part to polysaccharides that enhance cellular immunity. Research based on human clinical trials has demonstrated the protective effect of edible mushrooms against breast, cervical, endometrial, gastric, and ovarian cancers. The most promising data thus far appear to demonstrate an inverse relationship between mushroom consumption and breast cancer.[84] Grifolin, a secondary metabolite isolated from the mushroom *Albatrellus confluens*, a North American mushroom with a cabbagelike taste, has been shown to inhibit cell growth and induce cell cycle arrest in multiple cancer cell lines. Neoalbaconol, another compound obtained from *A. confluens*, has been shown to regulate cell metabolism and inhibit cancer cell growth.[85]

nuts

A study of 97 patients with breast cancer and 104 control subjects found that a high consumption (at least 1 ounce once a week or more) of peanuts (though they're not tree nuts, they were included in this study), walnuts, or almonds significantly reduced their risk of breast cancer by two to three times.[86] In a study of 75,680 women, those who consumed 1 ounce of nuts two or more times a week experienced a significantly reduced risk of developing pancreatic cancer. (Total nut consumption was defined as peanuts plus other nuts.)[87] Nut consumption is also associated with a lower risk of death from cancer, heart disease, or death from any cause.[88]

olive oil

In a metareview of 19 studies, people who had the highest olive oil consumption had a 34 percent lower likelihood of developing any type of cancer compared to people with lower olive oil consumption.[89] A long-term study of the Mediterranean diet supplemented with extra-virgin olive oil demonstrated this dietary pattern's effectiveness for the primary prevention of breast cancer. Based on data from more than 4,150 participants, the observed rates of breast cancer per 1,000 person-years were 1.1 for the Mediterranean diet with extra-virgin olive oil, 1.8 for the Mediterranean diet with nuts group, and 2.9 for a control group that was advised to reduce dietary fat.[90]

omega-3s

The anti-inflammatory power of omega-3 fatty acids has been well established, highlighting their potential to prevent cancers initiated by chronic inflammatory disease. Examples of inflammation-related illnesses linked with cancer include *Helicobacter pylori* infection and stomach cancer, hepatitis B or C viruses and liver cancer, human papillomavirus (HPV) and cervical cancer, and inflammatory bowel diseases and colorectal cancer. Though research based on human trials is still ongoing, a number of studies have demonstrated that omega-3 polyunsaturated fatty acids (PUFAs) have a protective effect against colon and colorectal, breast, liver, and prostate cancer. Further, eating a lower omega-6 to omega-3 ratio plays a positive role in cancer prevention.[91] Omega-6s, which are typically overconsumed in the Western diet, are found in vegetable oils such as safflower, canola, grape seed, sunflower, soybean, sesame, and corn oil. Omega-3s are found in cold-water fish such as salmon, herring, mackerel, tuna, sardines, and trout and in walnuts and flaxseeds and their oils. Flaxseed, which is exceptionally high in the omega-3 fatty acid alpha-linolenic acid, inhibits the formation of breast, colon, lung, and skin tumors and reduces human estrogen receptor–positive breast tumors.[92]

Other studies have shown that omega-3s, especially eicosapentaenoic acid and docosahexaenoic acid (EPA and DHA), inhibit cancer by affecting cancer cell replication, cell cycle, and cell death. Omega-3 polyunsaturated fats (PUFAs) have shown anticancer activity against breast, colorectal, gastric, prostate, and pancreatic cancer, as well as leukemia.[93] A recent study that examined omega-3 intake and endometrial cancer found that the highest omega-3 intake compared to the lowest intake was associated with a 15 to 23 percent reduction in endometrial cancer risk—but the effect was only observed in normal weight women (women with a BMI lower than 25).[94]

onions

Consuming seven or more servings of onions per week has been shown to be protective against esophageal cancer. Onion consumption is also associated with a reduced risk of developing brain cancer.[95] In a study based on data from more than 10,000 cases of 14 different cancers and about 17,000 controls, a high consumption of garlic and onions resulted in a significantly decreased risk of cancers of the mouth and pharynx, esophagus, colon and rectum, larynx, endometrium, and ovaries.[96]

pomegranate

This fruit's juice, peel, and oil have been shown to possess anticancer activities, including interference with tumor cell proliferation, cell cycle, invasion, and angiogenesis.[97] Other mechanisms that have been reported include induction of apoptosis, inhibition of DNA damage, exertion of anti-inflammatory activity, and inhibition of metastasis.[98] A recent in vitro study examined the effect of pomegranate peel extract on several different cancer cells, including non-small cell lung, breast adenocarcinoma, ovarian, and prostate adenocarcinoma. In all of the cancer cell lines, pomegranate extract reduced cell viability to values below 40 percent, even at the lowest dose of 5 micrograms per milliliter. Breast adenocarcinoma cells were the most responsive to pomegranate's antiproliferative effects.[99] Pomegranate has also shown in vitro anticancer effects against bladder cancer, colon cancer, liver cancer, skin cancer, gliomas (the most common brain tumors), and leukemia. Pomegranate's anticancer effect is thought to be due to its high content of polyphenols, including ellagitannins, ellagic acid, and other flavonoids

such as quercetin, kaempferol, and luteolin glycosides. It has shown promise both as a dietary preventive means to reduce the onset of tumors and as an anticancer treatment, especially if used at the higher dosages found in supplements.[100]

sea vegetables

Dieckol, a bioactive compound of the brown algae *Ecklonia cava,* has been shown to induce apoptosis in ovarian cancer cells and to suppress tumor growth.[101] Fucoidan, a fucose-containing sulfated polysaccharide derived from brown seaweeds, has shown antiproliferative, antiangiogenic, and anticancer properties in vitro. Among the many types of cancer cells for which fucoidan has exhibited an anticancer effect are colon, leukemia, gastric adenocarcinoma, lung carcinoma, prostate, liver, and breast. In animal models, fucoidan has shown antiangiogenic effects, as well as inhibition of tumor growth.[102]

In an in vitro study, researchers found that antioxidant-rich polyphenols from five different types of brown algae reduced pancreatic cancer cell viability, inhibited pancreatic cancer cell proliferation, and induced apoptosis in pancreatic cells.[103]

Sea cucumbers, which are actually marine animals in the same family as sea urchins and starfish, have long been a part of Chinese, Korean, Japanese, and Indonesian cuisine and medicine. There are at least 1,250 known species of sea cucumber. They are rich in protein and are known to possess antimicrobial, antioxidant, antiangiogenic, anti-inflammatory, immunomodulatory, and antitumor properties. Research on the anti-cancer properties of sea cucumbers is still under way, with much of the work focused on their unique bioactive compounds. A hot water extract of the species *Stichopus japonicus* was reported to significantly inhibit proliferation, decrease cell viability, induce apoptosis, and produce cytotoxicity in colon cancer cells. Frondoside A, a glycoside isolated from the sea cucumber *Cucumaria frondosa*, was shown to have an antiproliferative effect on cervical cancer cells, leukemia cells, and pancreatic cancer cells. In an animal model, Frondoside A, along with the chemotherapy drug gemcitabine, shrank pancreatic tumors. Alone, it's been shown to inhibit lung and breast cancer cell proliferation, and in an animal model, injections of Frondoside A were found to shrink lung cancer tumors. Animals treated with Frondoside A showed a reduction in breast cancer tumor volume of about 87 percent, compared to controls. Extracts from three sea cucumbers (*Holothuria leucospilota, H. scabra,* and *S. chloronotus*) exerted an antiproliferative effect on non-small cell lung cancer cells and cervical cancer cells.[104]

Studying the health benefits of eating sea cucumbers and sea vegetables is one of the most exciting areas of cancer research. Seaweeds are an excellent source of vitamins A, B_1, B_{12}, C, D, and E; riboflavin; niacin; pantothenic acid; and folic acid. They're also rich in minerals such as calcium, potassium, phosphorous, and sodium. Their amino acid content is well balanced, containing most of the essential amino acids needed for life and health. They have more than 54 trace elements required for the human body's physiological functions, and they're present in quantities greatly exceeding those in vegetables and other land plants. And with microflora and microalgae alone constituting more than 90 percent of the oceanic biomass, there's nearly endless potential for the development of new therapies to prevent and treat cancer.[105]

Examples of edible sea vegetables include nori, kombu, kelp, wakame, arame, hijiki (hiziki), agar, Irish moss, dulse, sea lettuce, and chlorella. Sea vegetables are available at large grocery stores, health food stores, Asian markets, online, and through independent purveyors.

tea

A study from Greece found that regular consumption of herbal teas protected against thyroid cancer as well as thyroid diseases. Chamomile tea was the winner, but sage tea and Greek mountain tea (made from the leaves of the *Sideritis* plant and also known as shepherd's tea) also had a cancer-protective effect. Those who'd been chamomile tea drinkers for 30 years reduced their risk of thyroid cancer by nearly 80 percent.[106]

The polyphenols in green and black tea, namely EGCG (epigallocatechin gallate) and theaflavin, have been shown to inhibit cell proliferation in prostate cancer cells.[107] In vitro studies have shown tea's protective effects against cancer of the breast, skin, lung, and gastrointestinal tract, as well. The data suggest that tea yields better results as a preventive measure or during early-stage cancers.[108]

tomatoes

Lycopene, a carotenoid with potent antioxidant properties, is especially effective for prostate cancer because it can reach higher concentrations in prostate tissue than in other tissues. Lycopene extracted from tomatoes— as well as gac fruit, watermelon, pink grapefruit, pink guavas, red carrots, and papayas—has been shown to be effective in prostate cancer prevention and treatment.[109] Consuming a large amount of tomatoes has also been shown to be protective against colorectal cancer.[110] Cooked tomatoes actually provide more lycopene than fresh.

whole grains

Whole grains have been shown to be protective against colorectal cancer. In contrast with refined grains, which preserve only the endosperm, whole grains retain the germ and bran, which are rich in substances with cancer-fighting properties, including fiber, antioxidants, and phytochemicals.[111] Consumption of whole grains more than seven times a week also results in a reduced risk of breast cancer.[112]

cold sores

Also known as fever blisters, cold sores are a viral infection resulting in small, fluid-filled blisters on or around the mouth. Often the blisters cluster together; after they break, a crust forms over the blister. Cold sores usually heal on their own after 10 to 14 days. Cold sores are caused by the highly contagious herpes simplex virus (HSV-1), which is similar to but not the same as HSV-2, the virus that causes genital herpes. It's estimated that at least half of the adult population has been exposed to HSV-1, though some people show no signs of infection. Antiviral medications can shorten the duration of the blisters, but currently there is no known cure for cold sores.

Some people with recurring cold sores have found that certain foods trigger outbreaks. Among the most common triggers are chocolate, peanuts, sunflower seeds, meat, yogurt, and cheese. Others cite menstruation, illness, stress, and fatigue as cold sore triggers.

To prevent *and* treat cold sores, increase your zinc intake. One study found that zinc levels in people with active cold sores were significantly lower than in people in the convalescent phase of the illness and that both groups had significantly lower levels of zinc than people who'd never experienced cold sores.[1] To get more zinc in your diet, eat oysters, shellfish, crab, shrimp, lean turkey, grass-fed beef, lima beans, pinto beans, miso, green beans, pumpkin seeds, or sunflower seeds.

Generally, healing foods for cold sores include foods that can strengthen your immune system as well as foods that have been shown to have antiviral properties. Vitamin C has been shown to be effective at suppressing the replication of the HSV-1 virus.[2] Use caution when eating foods high in vitamin C if you have active cold sores, however, as many of these foods are acidic and can irritate blisters and lesions. The best nonacidic sources of vitamin C include broccoli, asparagus, potatoes, red and green peppers, cantaloupe, and dark, leafy greens. Foods that are higher in vitamin C (but also higher in citric acid) include citrus fruits (oranges, limes, lemons, grapefruit, and pineapple), tomatoes, kiwifruit, berries, and mangoes.

The plant flavonoid quercetin works in much the same way; like ascorbic acid, quercetin can inhibit the replication of viruses, including herpes simplex 1. Apples, capers, lovage, onions, parsley, red wine, tea, berries, and olive oil are all high in quercetin. A recent study of quercetin and resveratrol, a plant polyphenol, found that these two antioxidants can inhibit HSV-1 production and even protect against possible cellular damage to neurons triggered by the virus.[3] Sources of resveratrol include red wine, grapes, dark chocolate, and blueberries.

Finally, there is some evidence that honey and royal jelly, a honeybee secretion, have inhibitory effects on HSV-1.[4] As honey is known to aid in wound healing, there may be value in taking a double dose of honey for cold sores: Eat honey to stop viral production and apply it to cold sores to speed healing.

colds

It's not called "the common cold" for nothing: Each year, adults typically come down with two or three colds, and it's not unusual for children to get eight or more. That totals up to more than one billion colds annually in the United States alone. Colds are caused by many different viruses, but human rhinoviruses are the most common. Typical symptoms include sore throat, runny nose, congestion, cough, fever, muscle aches, and sneezing. Colds usually last 7 to 10 days.

To prevent colds *and* to cut down on the duration of a cold if you do get one, increase your zinc intake.[1] Zinc has been extensively researched for its cold-fighting power, and it's one of the most effective food cures for this all too common condition. Zinc is most effective when taken within 24 hours of symptom onset. One recent study found that the optimal dose was 80 milligrams (mg) a day.[2] This study examined zinc lozenges, but there are whole foods with high concentrations of zinc: Canned eastern oysters contain more than 77 mg of zinc per 3-ounce serving, and wild cooked eastern oysters contain nearly 67 mg. Braised beef contains more than 15 mg of zinc per 5 ounce steak, while an 8.5 ounce turkey breast contains about 13 mg.[3] Both sesame and pumpkin seeds contain about 10 mg of zinc per 100 gram (g) serving.[4]

Clinical trials have also revealed vitamin C's effectiveness at preventing colds, reducing their duration, and reducing symptoms.[5] Vitamin C is found in abundance in citrus fruits and fruit juices, as well as in a variety of other types of produce (see "Healing Foods for the Common Cold" on the opposite page).

Mushrooms have a proven antiviral and anti-inflammatory effect. The shiitake mushroom has been used for hundreds of years to treat the common cold, and recent scientific evidence supports its efficacy.[6] Consumption of as little as 5 g of shiitake mushrooms a day has been shown to boost immune function and lower inflammation.[7]

Licorice extract has been shown to be effective against infection of HRSV, or human respiratory syncytial virus, one of the most common causes of upper respiratory illness. It works by preventing HRSV from attaching to and entering host cells and by stimulating the production of interferons, your body's natural antiviral defense mechanisms.[8] Interestingly, ginger has been shown to have the same effect against HRSV, but only in its raw, rather than dried or processed, form.[9] Many people swear by garlic for preventing colds, though the clinical evidence is mixed. In a study of 146 people, however, those who took a daily garlic supplement for 3 months had 24 occurrences of the common cold, whereas the placebo group experienced 65 colds. The garlic group's colds also lasted about 1 day less than the placebo group's.[10] Even with the mixed evidence, garlic's power as an antibacterial and antiviral is well established, so garlic does make the cut for a healing food for the common cold. There is also evidence suggesting that raw, crushed garlic may be more effective than cooked, as cooking decreases

ʒhealing foods
FOR THE COMMON COLD

They say feed a cold and starve a fever. Foods with these vitamins and minerals will help stave off a cold. Should you come down with one, "feed" it with these healthy beverages and yogurt.

To Prevent Colds

- Vitamin C: oranges, limes, lemons, grapefruit, citrus fruit juices, tomatoes, bell peppers, chile peppers, broccoli, kale, strawberries, guavas, papayas, cantaloupe, kiwifruit, acerola cherries (West Indian cherries), gac fruit, and raspberries
- Vitamin D: fatty fish such as salmon, tuna, and mackerel; fish liver oil; eggs; mushrooms; fortified fruit juices: tofu; fortified milk; and soy milk
- Zinc: oysters, beef, turkey, pumpkin seeds, sesame seeds, fortified cereals, and wheat germ

- Garlic (especially raw garlic)
- Green tea
- Honey
- Licorice, licorice extract, and licorice tea
- Mushrooms
- Probiotics: yogurt

To Treat Colds

- Zinc
- Garlic tea
- Ginger
- Green tea
- Honey
- Licorice
- Probiotics: yogurt

garlic's allicin levels. If you just can't stand the pungency of raw garlic, try steeping a clove or two to make garlic tea. You'll get the health benefits of garlic plus the throat-soothing effect of a warm drink.

There is also some evidence that honey can prevent the common cold and shorten its duration. In one study, high school students who ate 10 g of honey per day experienced fewer colds than students in the control group. Researchers noted that the effect was strongest after 6 weeks, suggesting a cumulative protective effect.[11]

There is also evidence that probiotics can protect against the common cold. In one study, children who drank a fermented milk drink containing *Lactobacillus casei* for 90 days experienced a reduction of 0.6 upper respiratory infections per 100 days.[12] A study of children in Mexico City who received probiotic drops for 90 days produced similar results: The 204 children who received the placebo developed upper respiratory tract infections, while only 93 of the children who received a probiotic containing *Lactobacillus reuteri* came down with respiratory infections. Perhaps even more fascinating, the benefit remained after the children stopped taking the probiotic. In a 3-month follow-up, 197 children in the placebo group developed colds, while only 129 of

the children who'd taken the probiotic did. The children who'd taken the probiotic also had significantly fewer cases of diarrhea and used fewer antibiotics.[13] And in a metastudy on the effects of probiotics containing strains of *Lactobacillus* and/or *Bifidobacterium* on respiratory infections in children and adults, researchers found that subjects experienced significantly fewer days of illness, a shorter duration of colds by an average of 1 day, and fewer missed days from school or work.[14]

Numerous studies have demonstrated that vitamin D lends a protective effect against respiratory infections by boosting immunity, and low levels of vitamin D have been shown to increase susceptibility to respiratory infections. According to the results of one metastudy, people who supplemented with vitamin D experienced respiratory tract infections at a rate of 21.7 percent, while those who did not had an infection rate of 30.1 percent.[15] You can boost your vitamin D through food sources (see "Healing Foods for the Common Cold" on page 215) and can also get it from sun exposure. The amount of time you should spend in the sun for adequate vitamin D production depends in part on your complexion. Fair-skinned people may only need to spend 15 to 20 minutes outdoors, while those with darker complexions can spend as much as 2 hours. Obviously, you don't want to become sunburned, so err on the side of caution. Your doctor or dermatologist can give you recommendations based on your skin tone.

What about beverages? In addition to the well-known advice to drink orange juice (or other citrus fruit juices), try green tea. Green tea has been shown to have antiviral and anti-inflammatory properties. EGCG (epigallocatechin gallate), a catechin antioxidant found in abundance in green tea, is even able to kill the influenza virus.[16]

See also: Allergic Rhinitis (Hay Fever) (page 156), Coughs (page 220), Influenza (page 352), Sore Throat (page 417)

constipation

The medical definition of constipation is three or fewer bowel movements a week. Stools can be hard, dry, and painful to pass, and constipation can cause pain, abdominal bloating, loss of appetite, and nausea. This common condition affects nearly everyone at some point, and it usually resolves on its own with no long-term effect.

The most common causes of constipation are not getting enough fiber in your diet, a lack of physical exercise, and changes in routine or eating habits, such as dieting or traveling. A lack of adequate fluid intake can exacerbate constipation by making your stool harder and more difficult to pass. Pregnancy can cause temporary constipation, as can some medications, an illness, and having surgery, and aging increases your chances of experiencing constipation. In less likely scenarios, chronic constipation can be a sign of a more serious illness such as inflammatory bowel disease, or it can be associated with other serious illnesses, such as diabetes, hypothyroidism, or neurodegenerative conditions such as Parkinson's disease. But constipation is usually a temporary and ultimately harmless condition that can easily be remedied by dietary changes.

Healing foods for constipation include anything that's high in fiber: fruits (blueberries, dates, prunes, apricots, raisins, apples, pears, and grapes); green, leafy veggies (kale, spinach, Brussels sprouts, broccoli, and cabbage); legumes (lentils, beans, and split peas); and whole grains (oatmeal, barley, bulgur, quinoa, whole grain breads, and cereals). Fiber unquestionably increases the frequency of bowel movements and in most cases softens stool, making it easier to pass.[1]

Standard guidelines for recommended daily fiber intake are often based upon age and gender. But the latest evidence agrees that the more accurate metric is determined by calorie intake. According to this guideline, you should be eating 14 grams (g) of fiber per 1,000 calories. Thus, regardless of age, gender, or weight, if you eat 2,000 calories per day, you should be getting at least 28 g of fiber. By either standard, a whopping 90 percent of Americans do not get enough fiber; the average intake is only 15 g per day.[2] We know the whole foods groups that are highest in fiber—fruits, vegetables, legumes, and whole grains—so let's look at how we can reach an adequate intake by way of some healing foods.

Most any type of bean is an excellent source of dietary fiber. One cup of roasted soybeans contains more than 30 g of dietary fiber, cooked navy beans contain 19 g, and boiled adzuki or kidney beans both contain almost 17 g of fiber per cup. Cooked split peas contain just over 16 g of fiber per cup, and lentils pack in 16 g per cup. Fruit is another excellent source of fiber. In addition to more well-known sources, such as blueberries and avocados, which both contain 16 g of fiber per cup, the little-known mammy apple, also known as the South American apricot, boasts an impressive 25 grams of fiber per fruit. In the United States, mammy apples are grown in Florida and Hawaii. If you can't find mammy apples, go for raw passion fruit, which contains the same amount of fiber per cup. But raw choke-cherries win the prize here: 1 cup of raw chokecherries contains nearly 31 g of dietary fiber. Thus, with one serving, you exceed your daily recommended intake of fiber for a 2,000-calorie diet, and you get that with only 250 calories, plus a good dose of vitamin C and calcium.[3] You can also try baking with whole grain flours. Carob flour contains 41 g of fiber per cup, rye flour contains 31 g, and wheat flour contains 21 g.[4] To sneak more fiber into any meal, add chia seeds, which contain almost 10 g of fiber per ounce. Chia seeds can be sprinkled onto oatmeal (whole oats are a good source of fiber in themselves, with more than 8 g per cup), onto yogurt, onto salads, and into smoothies and baked goods.[5]

Finally, there's a great deal of emerging research on the benefits of probiotics for overall digestive health. A recent metastudy on probiotics and constipation found that probiotics reduced the amount of time it took stool to move through the gut by more than 12 hours, increased bowel movements by an average of 1.3 per week, and improved stool consistency. The probiotic that was most effective was *Bifidobacterium lactis,* which is present in many commercially available yogurts, probiotic milk drinks, and probiotic supplements.[6] In a study on nursing home patients, daily consumption of a fermented milk drink containing a *Lactobacillus* strain resulted in less constipation *and* less diarrhea.[7] A study on people with chronic constipation found that drinking kefir, a probiotic fermented milk drink, increased bowel movements, improved stool consistency, and decreased the use of laxatives.[8] Kefir is widely available in most supermarkets and comes in a variety of flavors.

coughs

Coughing is your body's way of removing foreign substances and irritants from your airways and getting mucus out of your lungs and upper airways. Some coughs are due to obvious but removable irritants such as smoke, dust, or air pollutants. Coughs associated with allergies, respiratory infections such as the common cold or bronchitis, or even more serious conditions such as COPD can be treated. If a cough lasts more than 2 weeks and/or does not respond to treatment, you should see your doctor to determine the cause.

There are two types of cough remedies: suppressants (antitussives) and expectorants. Suppressants do just what you'd expect—suppress a cough—and expectorants work to thin and loosen mucus so it can be expelled through coughing. Among suppressants, the queen bee of natural food remedies is, you guessed it, honey. Honey has been used since ancient times to soothe the throat and calm an irritating cough.[1] One of the most effective methods for ingesting honey for a cough is in tea sweetened with honey. Honey dissolved in warm water can be just as effective, as can simply eating a spoonful of honey as needed. One study on children found that plain honey was more effective at suppressing a nighttime cough than an over-the-counter cough syrup.[2] Honey is safe for people ages 12 months and older, and taking 2.5 milliliters of honey before bedtime can decrease coughing and enhance sleep.[3] Another study on adult men found that honey decreased inflammation of mucous membranes and had an antioxidant effect.[4] One rather unusual study found that a combination of honey and coffee is a more effective means of treating persistent cough than a steroid. In this study, researchers created a jam-like paste using about 21 grams (g) of honey

BONUS TIP: In a small but persuasive new study, subjects found improvement in cough symptoms from a surprising source: losing weight. Researchers found a high correlation between a high-fat, high-calorie diet and coughing—probably because of the high incidence of gastroesophageal reflux disease (GERD), which often produces coughing—in those who are overweight.[5] Lose the weight, lose the GERD, lose the cough!

and 3 g of instant coffee; volunteers consumed this mixture three times a day for 1 week for quick cough relief.[6]

Other food cures for cough include licorice, eucalyptus, and ginger—all of which are common ingredients in herbal cough syrups and remedies. The glycyrrhizin in licorice stimulates saliva production and induces a more frequent swallowing reflex, which helps to suppress a cough.[7] The active ingredient in eucalyptus oil, cineole, has been shown to decrease coughing fits in people with acute bronchitis. Cineole has anti-inflammatory, bron-chodilating, and antimucus effects,[8] and it has even been shown to suppress coughs by acting on the area in the medulla responsible for the cough reflex.[9] In addition to eucalyptus, cineole is found in ginger, cinnamon, sage, peppermint, rosemary, and spearmint. Ginger has long been a folk remedy for upper respiratory infections, bronchitis, and cough.[10] It works because it has both anti-inflammatory and antibacterial effects.

See also: Allergic Rhinitis (Hay Fever) (page 156), Bronchitis (page 186), Colds (page 214)

dandruff

Also known as seborrhea, dandruff is a very common condition affecting up to half of all adults. Health-wise, it is not a serious condition, but the flaking, dead skin cells that shed from your scalp can create embarrassment and social awkwardness. The most common cause of dandruff is dry skin, though occasionally it can be caused by other conditions, such as psoriasis, a fungal infection, or an allergic reaction; it can also occur as a reaction to chemotherapy. The most common treatment is a medicated antidandruff shampoo, though corticosteroid creams that reduce inflammation and antifungal creams are sometimes used, as well.

When dandruff results from a fungal infection, the most likely culprit is a ubiquitous yeast called *Malassezia*. *Malassezia* can live on your skin and cause inflammatory reactions resulting in skin diseases, including eczema and dandruff. (Dandruff shampoos work in large part because they contain an antifungal agent to help eradicate *Malassezia*.) *Malassezia* is thought to be responsible for dandruff in billions of people.[1] Some of the most effective food treatments for dandruff are able to moisturize dry skin as well as fight *Malassezia*. Apricot seed oil, available online and at health food stores, moisturizes dry skin and also has antifungal properties.[2] Lemongrass oil works in just the same way, and a shampoo made with 2 percent lemongrass oil has been found to be effective against the *Malassezia*

fungus.[3] Asparagus root extract is also effective in eradicating *Malassezia,* and it has an anti-inflammatory effect, as well.[4] The topical application of oils containing essential fatty acids can also make a difference—and some of these are probably already in your pantry. Olive oil and coconut oil both have a moisturizing effect, but sunflower seed oil may be the winner when it comes to overall skin health. Sunflower seed oil has been shown to increase the linoleic acid content of the skin, reduce water loss, reduce skin scaliness, and improve skin barrier recovery.[5]

Proving once again that it can be used for virtually anything, honey has been used as a topical treatment for dandruff. In a study of patients experiencing scaling, itching, and hair loss, patients applied a solution of 90 percent honey, 10 percent water to seborrheic lesions every other day for 4 weeks. Itching and scaling disappeared within a week. Skin lesions were healed within 2 weeks, and subjects reported an improvement in hair loss. Treatment was continued for 6 months in the experimental group while a control group used a placebo. None of the patients who continued using honey experienced a relapse of symptoms, while 12 out of 15 people in the placebo group had a relapse 2 to 4 months after discontinuing treatment.[6] One of the reasons honey works to treat dandruff is that it's an antifungal: It's able to fight off the *Malassezia* fungus.[7]

decreased libido

The waning of sexual drive is most often due to perfectly normal factors, rather than pathology. Many things can have a negative impact on libido, including relationship troubles, stress, anxiety, depression, inadequate rest, illness, recovering from illness or surgery, childbirth, and the normal aging process. Decreased libido can also result from medical conditions such as cardiovascular disease, diabetes, high blood pressure, obesity, metabolic syndrome, or neurodegenerative disorders. What we're focusing on here is decreased libido in otherwise healthy adults.

A few general guidelines first: As you'll see from the health conditions that have a negative impact on libido, there is ample evidence that staying physically active[1] and eating a whole-foods, plant-based diet, such as the Mediterranean diet, can keep your sex drive high.[2] This makes intuitive sense, as a healthy body means you have ample bloodflow, plenty of energy and stamina, and no dysfunction to compromise sexual desire or sexual performance. As chronic stress is known to decrease sexual desire,[3] you can also eat to reduce stress and anxiety. (See Stress on page 419.)

To eat for increased libido specifically, you'll need to become acquainted with a signaling molecule called nitric oxide (NO). It doesn't sound sexy until you realize that nitric oxide is a vasodilator, meaning that it causes blood vessels to expand. Without an adequate amount of NO, men can't get erections and women can't become engorged and lubricated. (Viagra works because it enhances NO-mediated vasodilation.) While there are no whole-food sources of NO, what Mother Nature does serve up is an amino acid called L-arginine, the precursor to nitric oxide. L-arginine is a common ingredient in many supplements designed to increase libido and enhance sexual pleasure. Among the foods highest in L-arginine are sesame seeds, soy protein, crustaceans (lobster, shrimp, crab, and crayfish), spinach, seaweed, chicken breast, turkey breast, walnuts, and egg whites.[4]

And guess what improves the bioavailability of nitric oxide? Chocolate! Though chocolate is famous for its aphrodisiac properties, those effects have yet to be clinically proven. But chocolate does improve absorption of nitric oxide and it can boost mood because of its phenylethylamine content, which can help to put you in *the* mood.[5]

A mineral that plays a role in libido is zinc, as it is essential for testosterone production. Even a mild zinc deficiency can cause lower serum testosterone levels,[6] and testosterone has a direct impact on sexual desire for both men and women. One study found that men with normal levels of testosterone had significantly higher levels of zinc than men with low testosterone.[7] In a study of 560 healthy women ages 19 to 65, sexual desire was positively correlated with levels of free testosterone (testosterone that's unattached to proteins) and androstenedione,[8] a steroid that's converted to testosterone. Excellent food sources of zinc include oysters, chicken, crab, beans, oatmeal, yogurt, pumpkin seeds, sesame seeds, sunflower seeds, and pine nuts.

Another healing food for waning libido is the Peruvian plant called maca, which is part of the *Brassica* (mustard) family. In a study of women whose sex drives had been negatively impacted by antidepressants, 12 weeks of maca root supplementation (3 grams a day) resulted in an improvement in sexual function—most likely because maca boosted testosterone levels. Interestingly, the women who were postmenopausal experienced the greatest improvement.[9] Numerous studies have been done on maca and sexual function, though most were conducted on mice.

While a review of the few studies done on humans did show a positive effect, further research is needed.[10]

There is some evidence that ginger can act as an aphrodisiac by increasing testosterone—not to mention sperm count, viability, and motility—suggesting that it may play a beneficial role in fertility, as well.[11]

Red clover extract has been found to boost libido in women—and to provide additional benefits. Postmenopausal women were assigned to take either an 80 milligram supplement of red clover extract or a placebo for 90 days. The women in the experimental group reported better moisture, texture, and overall condition of their skin; an improvement in scalp hair; and improvements in mood, libido, sleep, and tiredness.[12]

Finally, increased folic acid has been shown to improve hot flashes and some of the other symptoms of menopause,[13] which can lead to increased sex drive. Folic acid (vitamin B_9), the synthetic form of folate, is found in supplements and fortified foods. Folate is the natural form of vitamin B_9, and it can be found in avocados; asparagus; beans; broccoli; Brussels sprouts; citrus fruits; dark, leafy greens; eggs; grains; and seafood.[14]

See also: Erection Problems, Erectile Dysfunction (page 263); Infertility (page 348); Stress (page 419)

dementia

Dementia is a general term that refers to a decline in mental function that interferes with everyday living and relationships. Sometimes used interchangeably with "senility," true dementia is diagnosed when changes to two or more brain functions—for example, memory loss and a decline in language skills—occur without a loss of consciousness. Though some loss of memory is to be expected as we grow older, dementia is *not* a natural consequence of aging.

There are many causes of dementia, including Alzheimer's disease (AD, which accounts for up to 70 percent of dementia cases), frontotemporal dementia, Huntington's disease, and Creutzfeldt-Jakob disease. These types of dementia are permanent, but treatment can improve symptoms and slow their progression. Other types of dementia and dementia-like symptoms may be treatable, depending on the nature and severity of the cause. Examples from this category include vascular dementia (dementia resulting from damage to the blood vessels, including stroke), traumatic brain injury, infections, a reaction to a medication, metabolic disorders, a brain tumor, or malnutrition.

Symptoms of dementia vary according to the cause of the problem and which part of the brain is affected. In general, they include memory loss, apathy, depression and other changes in mood, impaired communication skills, behavior changes, poor judgment, inability to focus and pay attention, and disorientation (including getting lost going to familiar places). As dementia progresses, these symptoms worsen, and people eventually have trouble swallowing, walking, and performing basic self-care; in the latter stages of dementia, round-the-clock care is required. The World Health Organization estimates that by 2040 there will be more than 81 million cases of dementia worldwide.[1]

Though there is some evidence that nutritional interventions can slow the progression of this condition, our healing foods recommendations are, by and large, based on what to eat and drink to *prevent* dementia. Diet and exercise do have an enormous impact on decreasing the risk of any type of brain impairment, as well. Let's take a look at the lifestyle factors you can take advantage of to make your brain as healthy as it can be.

First, the basics: Don't smoke; maintain a healthy weight; get regular exercise; and ensure that your blood pressure, blood sugar, and cholesterol levels are within acceptable ranges. You'll notice that these are the basic recommendations for general health and wellness—and that's no accident. Your brain is part of a vast, highly connected system, and having it functioning at optimal levels depends on good nutrition and a constant blood supply. Midlife obesity increases your risk of late-onset Alzheimer's disease, and diabetes is a known risk factor for AD.[2] Being overweight or obese has been shown to increase the risk of brain atrophy, white matter changes, AD, and late-onset dementia.[3] There is also strong evidence showing that people with dementia are far more likely to suffer from additional diseases and general ill health than their healthy counterparts. In a study that compared nearly 900 patients with vascular dementia to a control group, VaD (vascular dementia) sufferers were 12.6 times more likely to have a cerebrovascular disease, 4.6 times more likely to have atherosclerosis, nearly three times more likely to experience heart failure, and almost twice as likely to have atrial fibrillation. What's more, VaD sufferers had more septicemia, injuries, lung diseases, and urinary diseases than controls did.[4] The best evidence confirms that a heart-healthy diet is the best diet for your brain, as well.

In fact, many of the latest studies on nutrition and cognitive health

healthy insight

A small study on rosemary showed that 750 milligrams of dried rosemary powder had a significant positive effect on speed of memory. Though the study pool was small at 28 volunteers, they were ages 65 to 90, the group most at risk for memory loss. Further, this dosage of rosemary is the amount found in normal culinary use, so it's easy to get an adequate amount of rosemary for brain health. Higher dosages actually caused impairment of memory and mood.[5]

specifically recommend the heart-healthy Mediterranean diet.[6] In one study, researchers followed people with an average age of 67 for 4 years. One group was asked to follow the Mediterranean diet and supplement with 1 liter of olive oil per week; another to follow the Mediterranean diet and supplement with 30 grams a day of nuts; and a third group that served as a control was advised to reduce fat intake. The results were striking: The olive oil group saw an improvement in cognitive function and the nuts group experienced a significant improvement in memory, but the group following a low-fat diet experienced overall cognitive decline and a decline in memory.[7] In a metareview of human studies on the link between diet, cognitive decline, and dementia, the research overwhelmingly supports the Mediterranean diet for a reduction in cognitive decline, dementia, and Alzheimer's.[8] In yet another study of overall diet and dementia, researchers compared what they termed a "prudent" diet with a typical Western diet. A total of 2,223 dementia-free participants age 60 or younger were followed for up to 6 years. Not surprisingly, the highest adherence to the prudent diet resulted in the lowest levels of mental decline, and the highest adherence to the Western diet resulted in the highest levels of mental decline. What, in brief, are the

components of these respective diets? The prudent diet was significantly higher in fruits, vegetables, legumes, low-fat dairy products, whole grains, fish, poultry, and water, while the Western diet was significantly higher in fruit juice, potatoes, trans fats, medium- or high-fat dairy products, red meat, sweets, sodas, and beer.[9] Sound familiar? The prudent diet is essentially the Mediterranean diet.

One of the latest overall diet plans to protect against cognitive decline is the aptly named MIND diet. MIND is an acronym for Mediterranean-DASH Intervention for Neurodegenerative Delay—in other words, it's a combination of the Mediterranean and DASH (Dietary Approaches to Stop Hypertension) diets, with modifications based upon the most compelling findings on nutrition and cognitive health. High blood pressure and stroke are known risk factors for dementia. Even in people who've never had a stroke, the presence of risk factors for stroke (such as hypertension) causes greater cognitive decline and vastly increases the chances of dementia.[10] Hypertension alone is one of the most powerful risk factors for Alzheimer's disease,[11] making DASH diet food choices a wise addition to an antidementia strategy. Brain-healthy foods recommended in the MIND diet include vegetables (especially dark, leafy greens), berries, nuts, olive oil, whole grains, fish, beans, poultry, and wine. Foods that contribute to cognitive decline, on the other hand, include red meat, fast foods, fried foods, high-fat cheeses, pastries and sweets, butter, and margarine. To test the MIND diet's effectiveness, researchers assessed cognitive change in 960 volunteers over an average of 4.7 years. The results? The difference between those who got the top scores in the MIND diet and those who received the lowest scores was equivalent to a 7.5-year age difference.[12]

Now let's look at some of the individual nutrients that can play protective roles. Flavonoids, a large family of bioactive compounds synthesized by plants, exhibit powerful cognitive benefits. Flavonoids are found in a variety of fruits, vegetables, and legumes, as well as in tea, red wine, and even chocolate. A 6-year study on flavonol (a class of flavonoids) consumption in more than 10,000 middle-aged adults found that greater flavonol intake resulted in greater benefits to cognitive function— and the lower the flavonol intake, the more rapid the decline in cognitive function. The results were consistent for the three main flavonols in the diet, myricetin, kaempferol, and quercetin. Researchers credit these flavonols' antioxidant properties, along with their ability to reduce inflammation and

associated cytokine release, with their neuroprotective benefits.[13] These flavonols are found in a wide variety of fruits and vegetables (see "Boost Your Brainpower: Healing Foods to Prevent Dementia" on page 230).[14]

Flavonoids also prevent dementia by improving vascular function; researchers speculate that improvements in cognitive function after consuming flavonoids is due in part to the ability of flavonoids to increase cerebral bloodflow.[15] In a study on cocoa flavonols, 90 elderly individuals were divided into three groups and assigned to drink a high-, intermediate-, or low-flavonol cocoa beverage daily for 8 weeks. All of the groups saw an improvement in cognitive function, but those who drank a high- or intermediate-flavonol cocoa beverage fared the best, performing significantly better on verbal tests and a test that measures executive function and cognitive processing speed. What's more, those in the high- and intermediate-flavonol groups experienced a significant improvement in blood pressure, insulin resistance, and lipid peroxidation.[16]

Data from the long-term Nurses' Health Study found that eating blueberries and strawberries can delay cognitive aging by as much as 2.5 years—and the greater your intake of these berries, the slower the cognitive decline.[17] Berries are

boost your brainpower: healing foods to help prevent dementia

We know that certain nutrients affect cognitive ability. Here are some foods that contain those good vitamins and minerals, and some foods to avoid.

Eat More . . .

- Natural, plant-based foods
- Dark, leafy greens: arugula, broccoli, spinach, cabbage, kale, dandelion greens, mustard greens, and collard greens
- Foods with beta-carotene: apricots, asparagus, broccoli, carrots, grapefruit, kale, onions, peppers, plums, pumpkin, squash, spinach, sweet potatoes, and watercress
- Vitamin C–rich foods: lemons, limes, grapefruit, oranges, tomatoes, guavas, and papayas
- Vitamin D–rich foods: salmon, mackerel, tuna, sardines, eggs, mushrooms, tofu, fortified milk, and fortified juice
- Vitamin E–rich foods: almonds, hazelnuts, peanuts, sunflower seeds, spinach, and wheat germ

- Berries, especially blueberries and strawberries
- Extra-virgin olive oil
- Nuts
- Whole grains: amaranth, brown rice, bulgur, quinoa, whole oats, millet, and barley
- Beans
- Lean poultry
- Seafood (two or three times a week): herring, salmon, mackerel, sardines, and tuna
- Herbs and spices: chili powder, oregano, paprika, parsley, and rosemary
- Black and green tea
- Red wine (in moderation)
- Cocoa and dark chocolate

Limit or Eliminate . . .

- Red meat and meat products
- Butter
- High-fat cheeses
- Pastries and other sweets
- Fried foods

- Fast foods
- Processed foods
- Any trans fat: margarine, anything with partially hydrogenated oil
- Soft drinks and sodas

rich in flavonoids, especially anthocyanins, which give red and blue fruits their colors.

As for individual vitamins, a study on people ages 60 to 75 found that a combined treatment of vitamin E, vitamin C, and beta-carotene showed increased cognitive function over a treatment of vitamin E and vitamin C alone. The combination treatment also reduced levels of amyloid beta and elevated levels of estradiol, both of which are closely associated with cognitive dysfunction and dementia.[18] Beta-carotene is the yellow or orange pigment found in fruits and vegetables such as carrots, but this powerful antioxidant, which your body converts to vitamin A, can also be found in other vegetables and many herbs and spices.

Vitamin D deficiency has also been associated with brain structural abnormalities, cognitive decline, and dementia. A study of 382 people with an average age of 75.5 found that 26.2 percent had deficient levels of vitamin D (less than 12 ng/ml) and 35.1 percent had insufficient levels (12 to 20 ng/ml). Vitamin D levels in those with dementia were significantly lower than in those who were cognitively normal or even those who had mild cognitive impairment at the start of the study. What's more, those who were deficient in vitamin D declined 2.5 times faster in two domains of cognitive function: episodic memory and executive function. About 60 percent of the study participants were found to have inadequate levels of vitamin D. One other interesting note about this study was that African-American and Hispanic participants had significantly lower levels of vitamin D than Caucasian participants, suggesting that skin pigmentation plays a direct role in vitamin D absorption from sunlight.[19]

See also: Alzheimer's Disease (page 160), Depression (page 232), Diabetes (page 238), Heart Disease (Cardiovascular Disease) (page 313), High Blood Pressure (Hypertension) (page 327), Overweight and Obesity (page 396), Stroke (page 423)

depression

Depression is a very serious mental health condition that affects some 350 million people worldwide.[1] Occasional sadness and periodic episodes of feeling "blue" or "down in the dumps" are normal parts of life, but depression is an altogether different phenomenon. Symptoms of depression can vary greatly from person to person, but some of the typical signs include diminished interest in or pleasure taken from activities; a change in sleeping habits; feelings of hopelessness, worthlessness, and/or excessive guilt; loss of energy; difficulty concentrating or making decisions; and suicidal ideation and/or a suicide attempt. Depression can develop slowly over weeks or come on quite suddenly.

There is strong evidence that the quality of your diet directly affects your mental health[2] and that any sort of "depression diet" mirrors a heart-healthy diet. (This entry includes the most current research, and there's a lot of it, so please be sure to review " Eat Your Way Out of Depression: Mood-Boosting Foods" on page 234 for a complete list of specific healing foods.) Research has revealed a link between depression, metabolic disorders, and cardiovascular disease: Insulin sensitivity, chronic inflammation, and endothelial dysfunction (a vasodilation and vasoconstriction condition) are all present in those with depression and cardiovascular disease. Moreover, chronic inflammation and endothelial dysfunction interfere with the production of brain-derived neurotrophic factor (BDNF),[3] a protein that plays a key role in neuronal growth and long-term memory. Studies have shown that a decrease in BDNF levels increases susceptibility to depression, anxiety, and bipolar disorder.[4] There are also numerous studies that show that depression and cardiovascular disease (CVD) go hand in hand: Those with CVD tend to be more depressed than their healthy counterparts, and people with major depression exhibit an increased incidence of major CVD risk factors, including overweight and obesity, metabolic disorder, reduced heart rate variability, impaired vascular function, and higher incidence of chronic inflammation. CVD patients with depression even have a higher incidence of mortality and morbidity than those without depression.[5]

One longitudinal study confirms the

link between healthy dietary patterns and a reduced incidence of depression. This study analyzed data from 15,093 participants for an average period of 8.5 years; all participants followed either the Mediterranean diet, the Pro-Vegetarian Dietary Pattern (PDP), or the Alternative Healthy Eating Index-2010 (AHEI-2010). All of these dietary patterns emphasized fruits, vegetables, legumes, nuts, and seafood, and they all placed restrictions on red meat and sweets. High or even moderate adherence to these diets resulted in significantly less incidence of depression, with the Mediterranean and PDP diets being more effective.[6] Likewise, a study of 9,255 Seventh-day Adventists, who are traditionally vegetarian, found that eating vegetables, fruits, legumes, nuts, and olive oil was associated with a positive effect on mood, while eating sweets, sodas, and fast foods detracted from that positive effect. These results were determined after controlling for a number of factors, including age, gender, ethnicity, body mass index (BMI), education, sleep patterns, exercise, total caloric intake, and alcohol intake.[7] Similarly, a study of nearly 300 adults found that a higher fruit and vegetable intake was associated with lower odds of both depression and anxiety. In this study, researchers controlled for age, gender, income, education, physical activity, chronic illness, and smoking.[8]

In contrast, the typical Western diet, which is high in red meat, saturated fats, sweets, and processed foods, has been associated with a significant increase in depression. A fascinating study examined the impact of the Western diet on the hippocampus, a part of the brain specifically linked to depression. Depressed people have lower hippocampal volumes, though antidepressants can increase hippocampal volume and increase neurogenesis. Aging, stress, inflammation, and oxidative stress also decrease the size of the hippocampus. In this study, researchers found that the healthier the diet, the greater the left hippocampal volume, and conversely, the less healthy the diet (characterized by the Western diet), the smaller the hippocampal volume. The healthy dietary pattern was characterized by the consumption of fresh vegetables, salad, fruit, and grilled fish, and the Western diet was characterized by the consumption of red meat, fried foods, and soft drinks.[9]

A 7.2-year study of more than 3,500 people ages 65 and older without depression found that following the Mediterranean diet was associated with a reduced likelihood of developing depressive symptoms. For those who adhered best to the diet—with the highest consumption of whole grains, vegetables, fruits, olive oil, fish, and legumes and a lower consumption of meats and high-fat dairy—the annual rate of developing depressive symptoms was 98.6 percent lower than for those whose dietary patterns were least like the Mediterranean diet. Interestingly, the participants with the lowest adherence to the Mediterranean diet had lower caloric intake and alcohol consumption, but their red meat consumption was in excess of the acceptable target by 360 percent.[10]

Let's not allow the Mediterranean diet to hog the spotlight, though: The typical Japanese diet has also been associated with a lower prevalence of depression. A study based upon the Furukawa Nutrition Study concluded that a diet characterized by a high consumption of vegetables, fruits, mushrooms, seaweeds, soybean products, potatoes, fish, and green tea and a low intake of rice resulted in fewer depressive symptoms. The study was conducted on more than 2,000 people ages 19 to 69.[11]

eat your way out of depression: mood-boosting foods

We joke about eating a pint of ice cream when we're feeling low. In fact, plenty of feel-good foods exist that really can boost your mood or stave off the blues before they hit.

Eat More . . .

- Omega-3-rich seafood, especially fatty fish such as salmon, mackerel, tuna, sardines, trout, halibut, and herring (at least two or three times a week)
- Fish oil
- Fresh, brightly colored fruits and vegetables
- Dark, leafy greens: arugula, broccoli, collard greens, kale, mustard greens, spinach, and Swiss chard
- Foods rich in selenium: seafood, brown rice, mushrooms, Brazil nuts, eggs, and spinach

- Foods rich in vitamin B$_{12}$: clams, mussels, mackerel, crab, eggs, poultry, low-fat dairy products, and fortified cereals
- Foods rich in zinc: oysters, beef, turkey, pumpkin seeds, sesame seeds, fortified cereals, and wheat germ
- Foods rich in vitamin D: mushrooms, fatty fish, eggs, tofu, low-fat dairy products, fortified juice, fortified milk, and soy milk
- Seaweed
- Soybean products, including tofu, miso, tempeh, and natto

One of the reasons these diets are so protective against depression is that they have a high omega-3 content. Omega-3s have been used therapeutically for many psychiatric conditions, including depression, anxiety, bipolar disorder, and obsessive-compulsive disorder. In a metastudy of omega-3 polyunsaturated fatty acids (PUFAs), PUFA supplementation was found to have beneficial clinical effects for those with major depressive disorder, bipolar disorder, and those with depressive symptoms.[12] Why is it so effective? Research is ongoing, but mounting evidence demonstrates that a proinflammatory state can give rise to depression, and omega-3s reduce inflammation.

We do know that societies with a higher intake of fish have a lower prevalence of depression and mood disorders. Conversely, patients with a major depressive disorder show lower levels of PUFAs, which are found in abundance

- Berries, especially blueberries and strawberries
- Extra-virgin olive oil
- Nuts: walnuts, Brazil nuts, and almonds
- Nut oils
- Flaxseeds and flaxseed oil
- Legumes: lentils, peas, and beans
- Whole grains: brown rice, bulgur, whole oats, quinoa, barley, and millet

- Spices: turmeric, cinnamon, ginger, cloves, nutmeg, and saffron
- Herbs: parsley, lemongrass, rosemary, sage, thyme, and fennel
- Black and green tea
- Coffee
- Red wine (in moderation)
- Cocoa and dark chocolate
- Water

Limit or Eliminate . . .

- Red meat and meat products
- High-fat dairy products
- Pastries and other sweets
- Refined carbohydrates
- Fried foods

- Fast foods
- Processed foods
- Sodas
- Excessive alcohol consumption

in seafood. Depressed individuals also have higher levels of inflammatory biomarkers, and proinflammatory cytokines can actually cause depression. Anti-inflammatory PUFAs are effective not only against depression but also against several inflammatory-related physical illnesses, and they are safe enough for pregnant women and children.[13] PUFAs also attenuate oxidative stress mechanisms, which protect against depression. A study of 51 older adults at risk for depression compared one group who received omega-3 supplementation for 12 weeks with a group that received a placebo. The placebo group had increased markers of oxidative stress, resulting in a worsening of depressive symptoms. Omega-3s directly affect these markers and thus protect against depression.[14] Another study of adults with major depressive disorder who had not responded to standard antidepressants found that 12 weeks of EPA (eicosapentaenoic acid, a type of long-chain fatty acid) supplementation resulted in significantly higher response rates (53 percent) compared to a placebo (29 percent), with marked improvement in mood, anxiety, insomnia, libido, and suicidal tendencies. A meta-analysis of 19 studies on omega-3 PUFAs and depression found that omega-3s were effective at treating people with a diagnosis of major depressive disorder as well as those with no

formal diagnosis but with depressive symptoms.[15]

There are a few key mineral deficiencies that are associated with an increased risk of depression. In a study of 300 women, those who had the lowest selenium intake were found to be three times more likely to develop a major depressive disorder.[16] Lower vitamin D levels have been associated with a higher incidence of depression,[17] as well as worse depressive symptoms.[18] Evidence of the effectiveness of vitamin D in preventing or treating depression has been mixed,[19] but there is some evidence indicating that vitamin D supplementation in those who are depressed can improve symptoms.[20]

Vitamin B_{12} and zinc deserve a special mention because a deficiency in these vital nutrients can actually *cause* symptoms of depression and anxiety. If vitamin B_{12} deficiency becomes extreme, it can even lead to paranoia, delusions, impaired gait, memory loss, cognitive impairment, and jaundice. Those at higher risk for a vitamin B_{12} deficiency include vegetarians, people over 50, and those with conditions that hinder nutrient absorption, such as Crohn's disease or celiac disease. A study of depressed patients compared those who took an antidepressant to those who took an antidepressant as well as a vitamin B_{12} supplement (1,000 micrograms [mcg] injected once a week). After 3 months of treatment, 100 percent of the antidepressant plus B_{12} group showed a reduction in depressive symptoms, while only 69 percent of the first group saw improvement.[21] The average adult needs 2.4 mcg of B_{12} a day, and as this is a vitamin your body can't make on its own, you have to get it from food. It's estimated that 3.2 percent of adults over the age of 50 have a serious vitamin B_{12} deficiency, and up to 20 percent have a borderline deficiency. As for zinc, a zinc deficiency is commonly associated with depression and has been linked to an increased severity of depressive symptoms; moreover, some of the symptoms of zinc deficiency itself are depression, confusion, and behavioral disturbances.[22] In studies that examined the role of zinc supplementation along with standard antidepressants, zinc significantly lowered depression scores.[23]

Both coffee and green tea have been shown to protect against depression. Part of their antidepressive effect can be attributed to the polyphenols found in these drinks. Polyphenols have been shown to affect a wide array of mechanisms in your brain, exerting a positive effect on cognitive function, synaptic plasticity, mood, and neuronal function. In a study of 537 people ages 20 to 68, those who drank 4 or more cups of green tea a day had a 51 percent lower prevalence of depressive symptoms than those who drank only 1 cup a day. Those who drank 2 or more cups of coffee a day also had less depression than those who drank 1 cup or less.[24] Similarly, a study on an elderly population—1,058 individuals age 70 and over—found that those who drank 4 or more cups of green tea a day experienced a 44 percent lower prevalence of depressive symptoms than those who drank 1 or fewer cups per day.[25] In addition to coffee and tea, polyphenols are also found in plant-based foods such as fruits and vegetables, as well as in spices and wines.[26]

But don't discount the power of plain water! One study found that greater water intake was associated with more favorable mood states. The study adjusted for variables including exercise and consumption of caffeine, protein, carbohydrates, and fat. Those with the highest water intake had the best outcomes for tension, depression, vigor, anger, and confusion, plus the highest total mood scores.[27] In another study, when those who normally drank 2.5 liters of water a day were restricted to 1 liter, their moods deteriorated. They reported a decrease in contentedness, calmness, vigor, and positive emotions. Meanwhile, when those who normally drank only 1 liter a day increased their water consumption to 2.5 liters a day, they reported a significant decrease in fatigue and confusion, along with less sleepiness.[28] Even mild dehydration can have a deleterious effect upon mood,[29] so drink up!

diabetes

There are two main kinds of diabetes mellitus, both of which cause blood glucose to rise to unhealthy levels. In type 1 diabetes, the pancreas produces very little or no insulin, the hormone that converts sugar, starches, and other foods into energy. People with type 1 diabetes must manage their blood sugar levels with insulin injections. With type 2 diabetes (T2D), your body makes insulin, but it does not use it properly, or it produces insufficient insulin. This condition is known as insulin resistance. Type 2 diabetes can often be managed through good nutrition, maintaining a healthy weight, and regular exercise, though some people with T2D need an oral medication and/or insulin injections, as well. (A third type of diabetes, gestational diabetes, occurs during pregnancy and usually resolves once the baby is delivered.) The cumulative effect of having too much glucose in your blood can cause serious health problems, including cardiovascular disease, stroke, neuropathy, increased susceptibility to infection, blindness, and kidney failure. (In fact, diabetes is the leading cause of blindness and kidney failure in adults.)[1] The World Health Organization estimates that in 2012, diabetes was the direct cause of 1.5 million deaths.[2] Total deaths from diabetes are expected to rise by 50 percent over the next 10 years.[3]

Despite these frightening facts and statistics, type 2 diabetes (which accounts for more than 90 percent of cases) is highly preventable. Most cases of type 2 diabetes can be avoided with simple lifestyle changes that obviate the risk factors: Maintain a healthy body mass index (BMI) through regular exercise and good nutrition, and don't smoke. If you're eating right, exercising regularly, and not smoking, chances are very good that you won't have a problem with hypertension, obesity, high triglycerides, or low HDL cholesterol, all of which can directly contribute to the development of T2D. Additionally, there are healing foods that can prevent the onset of T2D and help manage both types of diabetes. (See "Antidiabetic Eating and Drinking" on page 242 for specific foods.)

There is substantial evidence that a diet rich in whole grains protects against diabetes,[4] while a diet rich in simple, refined carbohydrates increases your risk. One study that followed more than 70,000 women for 24 years found that a high-starch, low-fiber, and high-starch-to-cereal fiber diet was associated with an increased risk of T2D. Total fiber, cereal fiber, and fruit fiber were all inversely associated with T2D.[5] Another study found that whole grain consumption is associated with a 20 to 30 percent reduction in your risk of developing T2D. Credit goes in large part to whole grains' phytochemicals, which act as antioxidants and have the power to mitigate the oxidative stress and systemic inflammation that play a part in the development of T2D.[6]

Similarly, there is also substantial evidence indicating polyphenols—micronutrients found in fruits, vegetables, tea, and wine—are effective at preventing diabetes. Polyphenols have powerful antioxidant properties, and they've been shown to improve glucose regulation and enhance insulin secretion. In a study on flavonoids, a class of polyphenols, researchers found that each two-and-one-half–fold increase in flavonol intake was associated with a 26 percent lower incidence of type 2 diabetes, and each two-and-one-half–fold increase in flavan-3-ol intake was associated with an 11 percent lower incidence of T2D. The top sources of flavonols and flavan-3-ols in this study were tea, apples, and pears; bananas also provided flavan-3-ols.[7]

In a study of nearly 2,000 women, half of them postmenopausal, higher anthocyanin and flavone intake was associated with significantly lower insulin resistance. Study participants also showed significantly lower markers of chronic inflammation, which is linked to cardiovascular disease, and higher levels of adiponectin, a protein that helps regulate glucose levels. The anthocyanin and flavone sources in this study? Berries, grapes, oranges, pears, peppers, and wine.[8]

Believe it or not, there's also evidence that cocoa is effective in treating T2D. A metastudy involving almost 1,300 patients found that a variety of chocolate or cocoa products created a significant reduction in serum insulin levels.[9] Sound too good to be true? Not if you remember that cocoa is full of polyphenols. A recent article in the *Journal of Agriculture and Food Chemistry* offered a survey of seven studies done on chocolate and/or cocoa and diabetes. Though the studies ranged in size, among the positive outcomes were improved endothelial function (vasodilation and vasoconstriction), reduced insulin resistance, and reduced total cholesterol. And in the studies that monitored weight, no weight gain was reported, despite the extra calories chocolate or cocoa provided. The study authors concluded that 20 to 45 grams (g) of chocolate per day can safely be added to the diets of people with diabetes.[10]

Guess what else has been associated with a decreased risk of type 2 diabetes: coffee. The long-term Nurses' Health Study and Health Professionals Follow-Up Study, which followed nearly 42,000 men and well over 84,000 women over a period of years, found that long-term coffee consumption resulted in a significantly lower risk of T2D.[11] A 2015 study also found that coffee consumption was associated with a lower risk of T2D—as well as a lower risk of obesity and metabolic syndrome.[12] If you're wondering whether caffeinated and decaffeinated coffee are both effective, you're not alone: Researchers found that both regular joe and decaf significantly lower the risk of T2D, but the amount does count. Six cups per day (decaf or regular) confers the most benefit, resulting in a 33 percent lower risk of developing T2D. What's at work here? Research is still ongoing, but the authors of this study speculate that chlorogenic acid, a phenolic compound and a major component of coffee, has a lot to do with it. Chlorogenic acid has been shown to reduce blood glucose concentrations and reduce glucose absorption in the intestines. It also reduces oxidative stress and liver glu-

cose output. Other coffee components that may play a role include lignans, quinides, trigonelline, and magnesium.[13] Bottom line? Coffee lovers, drink up!

Tea drinkers, however, aren't left out. The Women's Health Study found that women who drank up to 4 cups of tea a day had a 30 percent lower risk of developing T2D than non-tea-drinkers, and a Japanese study found that those who drank up to 4 cups of green tea a day had a 33 percent lower risk of T2D. Another study on green tea found that after 12 weeks of green tea consumption, people with T2D experienced a decrease in insulin and an increase in glycated hemoglobin (HbA1c) levels.[14] There is also some evidence indicating that the South American tea known as yerba maté has positive effects on insulin resistance.[15]

In a study on dairy products and diabetes, low-fat dairy was shown to have an inverse association with the development of type 2 diabetes—and this was especially the case with fermented low-fat dairy products, including yogurt. This study was based on 4,127 subjects, including 892 cases of diabetes, who were followed for 11 years. Those who had a greater intake of low-fat fermented dairy products—mostly consisting of yogurt—had a 24 percent decreased risk of developing diabetes compared to those who did not eat yogurt. Other low-fat fermented dairy products this cohort consumed were unripened cheeses such as cottage cheese and fromage frais.[16]

There is also evidence that some spices protect against diabetes. Fenugreek has long been used to treat diabetes and is one of the most popular nonpharmacological treatments. These pungent seeds, a staple of Asian cuisine, have been found to reduce glucose and glycated hemoglobin (HbA1c) levels.[17] In one study, researchers compared the effect of a meal without fenugreek to a meal with 15 g of ground fenugreek in type 2 diabetics. In 17 of the 21 participants, there was a significant reduction in postprandial glucose after the fenugreek-enriched meal.[18] A study that was just released followed prediabetic men and women ages 30 to 70 for 3 years. Sixty-six participants ingested 5 g of fenugreek powder twice a day before meals; they were compared to 74 age-matched controls. By the end of the study period, the control group had a 4.2 times greater chance of developing diabetes than the fenugreek group did. The group that ate fenugreek also had a significant reduction in fasting plasma glucose, postprandial plasma glucose, and LDL cholesterol, while insulin increased.[19]

Turmeric has been a treatment for diabetes in Ayurvedic and traditional Chinese medicine for thousands of years, and it (and its active compound, curcumin) has since been studied extensively in animals.[20] Much more research is needed with human subjects, but promising results are already emerging. In a study of 240 prediabetic adults, one group received a curcumin supplement while the other group received a placebo for 9 months. At the end of the study, 16.4 percent of the subjects had converted to type 2 diabetes, but none in the curcumin group had. The curcumin group also showed better beta cell function, a lower level of insulin resistance, and higher adiponectin, a protein involved in regulating glucose levels.[21] A large metastudy on research published from 1998 through 2013 on curcumin and hyperglycemia and insulin resistance found that curcumin reduces blood glucose and HbA1c levels and has insulin sensitizer effects.[22]

Cinnamon is another widely used traditional antidiabetic remedy. Clinical trials have produced varying results,[23] while a metastudy that was just released found an improvement in glycemic control in patients who were prediabetic, those who had high HbA1c levels, and, perhaps most fascinatingly, in those who were receiving cinnamon as their sole diabetes therapy.[24]

Tulsi, also known as holy basil or

Ocimum sanctum, has been shown to decrease glucose levels and improve blood pressure and lipid profiles.[25] And in a study of male non-insulin-dependent diabetics, a combination of holy basil and neem leaf powder (up to 2 g per day) resulted in a significant decrease in a range of diabetic symptoms, including excessive thirst, excessive urination, excessive eating, fatigue, sweating, burning sensation in the feet, itching, and headache.[26] Holy basil is available as a whole food, but also in powder form, in capsules, as an extract, and as an essential oil. It's easily found at supermarkets and drugstores (as is

antidiabetic eating and drinking

The very best way to prevent type 2 diabetes and even to reverse it is to follow an overall healthy dietary pattern that supports whole-body health. Such a diet will follow certain basic guidelines.

- Increase your consumption of fresh fruits and vegetables, legumes, nuts, and whole grains.

- Try to get most of your protein from plant-based sources such as beans, soy products, nuts and nut butters, and whole grains. Eat seafood or fish two or three times a week.

- In the best-case scenario, eliminate consumption of foods and beverages that are high in saturated fats and sugars. This includes red meat, fried foods, desserts, pastries, sodas, and sugary baked goods. If you can't eliminate these foods entirely, then strictly limit them.

- Eliminate all processed foods and trans fats.

- Engage in regular physical activity. Adults should aim for a *minimum* of 150 minutes of moderate aerobic activity per week.

- Consume alcohol in moderation: one serving per night for women, two for men. Red wine has the biggest benefit, with the highest flavonoid content, making it a good choice.

- Diabetics and prediabetics: Avoid foods with a high glycemic index (GI), which can cause a spike in blood glucose levels. High-GI foods include white bread and bagels, white rice, white potatoes, pretzels, saltine crackers, instant oatmeal, melons, pineapple, and any sugary dessert or candy.

neem, a tree native to India and the Indian subcontinent), and it's been used as a medicinal plant for thousands of years. Clinical trials have shown its efficacy at treating an impressive range of health conditions, and it has antibacterial, antiviral, and anti-inflammatory properties.[27]

Ginger has been shown to improve insulin sensitivity and reduce total cholesterol, triglycerides, and some markers of inflammation in people with type 2 diabetes.[28] In one study, diabetic patients were given either a placebo or capsules containing 1 g of ginger three times a day for 8 weeks. The ginger

In addition to these overall healthy guidelines, here are a few foods and beverages that have a supercharged antidiabetic effect.

Whole Foods

- Whole grains: wheat, barley, bulgur, buckwheat, rye, oats, amaranth, millet, quinoa, teff, brown rice, and wild rice
- Flavonoid-rich foods: apples, aronia berries (chokeberries), arugula, beans, blueberries, capers, cranberries, currants, dock, elderberries, fennel, garlic, grapefruit, grapes, hot peppers, juniper berries, kale, kumquats, lovage, onions, oranges, parsley, plums, radicchio, radishes, raspberries, red cabbage, serviceberries, and tomatoes
- Pears
- Bananas
- Beans
- Dark chocolate and other cocoa products
- Fermented, low-fat dairy products: yogurt, cottage cheese, and kefir
- Bitter melon

Spices and Herbs

- Turmeric
- Fenugreek
- Cinnamon
- Bay leaves
- Ginger
- Sage
- Holy basil (tulsi)
- Milk thistle

Beverages

- Coffee
- Green tea
- Yerba maté
- Red wine

group showed an average decrease of 10.5 percent in fasting blood glucose levels. HbA1c also fell, and insulin resistance was significantly improved in the ginger group.[29]

A small study of 40 people with type 2 diabetes demonstrated that bay leaves reduced glucose levels and improved lipid profiles. For 30 days, subjects took capsules containing 1, 2, or 3 g of ground bay leaves. After 30 days, glucose fell for all three groups that consumed ground bay leaves. It fell by 21 to 26 percent; total cholesterol decreased 20 to 24 percent, LDL cholesterol fell 32 to 40 percent, and HDL cholesterol (the "good" cholesterol) increased 29 and 20 percent in the groups receiving 1 and 2 g of bay leaves, respectively. Triglycerides also decreased 34 and 25 percent in groups consuming 1 and 2 g of bay leaves, respectively. There were no significant changes in the placebo group.[30]

Type 2 diabetes patients who were given sage leaf extract three times a day for 3 months experienced lowered fasting glucose, HbA1c, total cholesterol, triglycerides, and LDL cholesterol, and higher HDL cholesterol.[31] Sage is available as a whole food and in crushed or powdered form, and also as a tea.

Finally, silymarin, or milk thistle, has demonstrated beneficial effects on several diabetic complications, including diabetic neuropathy (nerve damage brought on by diabetes), diabetic nephropathy (kidney damage brought on by diabetes), and nonalcoholic steatohepatitis (a type of liver disease), mainly by means of its antioxidant properties. It has exhibited hypoglycemic, antilipidemic, and anti-obesity properties, as well.[32]

diarrhea

Occasional diarrhea, caused by a virus or bacteria, stress, a reaction to a medication, or simply a food that doesn't agree with you, is not uncommon and usually resolves within 48 hours. Most of the time diarrhea can be treated at home, but if it doesn't clear up within 2 or 3 days or is accompanied by a high fever or blood in your stool, see your health-care provider. Chronic diarrhea, which is diarrhea that lasts for more than 4 weeks, should also be evaluated by your health-care provider, as it is a hallmark of many gastrointestinal illnesses. The other common cause of chronic diarrhea is a food intolerance or food allergy. In this case, eliminating the food (or food group) from your diet is the safest way to avoid diarrhea. (For more on food sensitivity, intolerance, and allergies, see Food Allergies on page 278.)

The two main things you want to watch out for with diarrhea are dehydration and any food (in addition to allergy or sensitivity triggers) that will exacerbate the condition. This means that while you have diarrhea you should avoid foods that are fried, acidic, high in fat, spicy, greasy, or high in fiber. It's also a good idea to avoid caffeinated beverages, as caffeine can stimulate your digestive system, and artificial sweeteners, as they have a laxative effect on some people. Eliminate alcohol while you have diarrhea, as alcohol has a dehydrating effect. Other foods to consider eliminating are dairy products, which are highly inflammatory and can exacerbate diarrhea even if you're not lactose intolerant. The exception here is probiotic dairy such as yogurt or kefir, which we'll discuss below.

To stay hydrated, drink plenty of clear liquids. Filtered water is an excellent choice, but a quick and easy solution to replacing the electrolytes your body loses when diarrhea strikes is to sip a salt-sugar-water solution. Known as oral hydration therapy or oral hydration salts, this ultrasimple and low-cost treatment is so effective that it made the World Health Organization Model List of Essential Medicines.[1] To make your own solution, stir 6 teaspoons of sugar and ½ teaspoon of salt into 5 cups of water[2] and drink this solution throughout the day. For a less potent but better-tasting home remedy, you can drink diluted juice for sugar and clear broth for its salt content. The goal is to stay hydrated and to replace the electrolytes lost to frequent elimination.

Much of the emerging research on healing foods for diarrhea is on probiotics, with evidence demonstrating their efficacy for both the prevention *and* treatment of this condition. In an article based on two metastudies, researchers found that probiotics can reduce the duration of diarrhea and prevent it in many cases (including antibiotic-induced diarrhea and diarrhea caused by rotavirus).[3] A study based on children found that a daily probiotic containing *Lactobacillus reuteri* significantly reduced the frequency and duration of episodes of diarrhea. This study followed the children during 3 months of supplementation and an additional 3 months without the probiotic. In addition to the antidiarrheal benefit, the children also had significantly fewer cases of upper respiratory infections, less absenteeism from school, and less antibiotic use. Though slightly less potent after the probiotic intervention, the protective effects lasted into the 3 months of follow-up.[4] A metastudy that examined results from a total of more than 8,000 subjects found that probiotics shortened the duration of diarrhea as well as stool frequency in acute infectious diarrhea.[5] Common food sources of probiotics include kefir, yogurt, cheese, tempeh, natto, buttermilk, kimchi, sauerkraut, soy milk, and olives.

Studies have also shown that the low-FODMAP diet can be helpful in reducing diarrhea. Developed to help people suffering from irritable bowel syndrome (IBS), FODMAP is an acronym for fermentable oligosaccharides, disaccharides, monosaccharides, and polyols. FODMAPs are short-chain carbohydrates that are poorly absorbed in your small intestine and are quickly fermented by bacteria in your gut. Especially in those with IBS, high-FODMAP foods can produce gas, bloating, abdominal pain, diarrhea, and/or constipation. The low-FODMAP diet is quite comprehensive, with many dozens of foods to eliminate or reduce, so this healing foods method is probably "too much medicine" for a simple case of acute diarrhea. But if your diarrhea is chronic or you receive a diagnosis of IBS, the low-FODMAP diet can be a long-term means of treatment. (See Irritable Bowel Syndrome on page 360 for more information and for a list of common high-FODMAP foods to avoid.)

One all-natural remedy for diarrhea that is less well known is diosmectite, a natural clay. Clay has been used as an antidiarrheal in traditional and complementary medicine for years, but modern research has proven its efficacy, as well. Studies have shown that it's effective at treating infectious diarrhea and preventing intestinal damage,[6] and in a study of acute childhood diarrhea, 3 to 6 grams of clay per day was found to significantly decrease the duration of diarrhea and speed the cure rate. (It was found effective against all types of diarrhea except that caused by dysentery.)[7] Another study found it particularly effective at treating diarrhea caused by rotavirus.[8] And in a small pilot study, natural clay was found to be effective at treating cancer-related diarrhea.[9] Further research is needed, but results are promising. If you want to try natural clay, it's best to purchase it from a health food store or other certified dealer and ensure that it's for internal use so you can be sure it's not contaminated with lead, cadmium, other heavy metals, or environmental toxins.

See also: Irritable Bowel Syndrome (page 360)

diverticulitis

Diverticula are small, bulging pouches that form within your bowel wall; the presence of these pouches is known as diverticulosis. These pouches most often occur in your large intestine, but they can form in your small intestine, as well. It's estimated that at least half of Americans age 60 and older have diverticulosis (the presence of these pouches) and will never experience problems. But in about 20 percent of cases, these small pouches become inflamed, resulting in the painful condition known as diverticulitis.[1] The causes of diverticulitis are not entirely clear. For years, conventional wisdom was that a diet lacking in sufficient fiber was the main culprit, but more recent studies are challenging this assumption. The recommendation to avoid eating nuts, seeds, and corn (including popcorn) has also been found to be baseless, as nuts and seeds do *not* increase the risk of diverticulitis or diverticular bleeding.[2] Risk factors proven to increase the chances of developing diverticulitis include aging, obesity, smoking, lack of exercise, and the use of steroids, opiates, or nonsteroidal anti-inflammatory drugs (such as Aleve or Naprosyn). There is evidence that a BMI of over 30 nearly doubles your chances of developing diverticulitis, and having a family member with diverticulitis also increases your risk.[3] Whatever the cause, diverticula can remain asymptomatic for years, and then, with little or no warning, cause abdominal tenderness and pain (especially after a meal), nausea and/or vomiting, fever, gas, bloating, and/or a change in bowel habits—some people experience constipation, others diarrhea.

So what can we eat to prevent this painful condition or treat it if it occurs? As some medical professionals still recommend a high-fiber diet (25 to 40 grams of fiber a day) to prevent diverticulitis, and as adequate fiber intake prevents a host of other health concerns, we're including it on our list of healing nutritional components for this condition. So load up on cruciferous vegetables such as kale, spinach, lettuces, arugula, and chard, and eat whole grains, beans, and fruits, especially prunes, apricots, apples, raisins, and dates. Adequate fluid intake also helps prevent constipation, which can irritate your colon.

Though research is limited, there is

some evidence that vitamin D can protect against diverticulitis. Noting that a higher incidence of hospitalizations for diverticulitis coincided with a trend toward less ultraviolet (UV) light exposure (the result of greater awareness about skin cancer), researchers decided to investigate. Using data collected over nearly 20 years, researchers identified 9,116 patients with asymptomatic diverticulosis and 922 patients with diverticulitis that required hospitalization. Those with diverticulosis had significantly higher levels of vitamin D than patients who developed diverticulitis. Likewise, patients with higher levels of vitamin D had a much lower risk of uncomplicated diverticulosis becoming diverticulitis.[4] UV exposure is the most effective way to get vitamin D, but food sources include salmon, tuna, fish oils, mushrooms, and eggs. Smaller amounts of vitamin D are found in beef liver, cheese, and other dairy products.[5]

As obesity is one of the prime risk factors for developing diverticulitis, it's important to eat to maintain a healthy weight. So in addition to eating the high-fiber foods mentioned above, avoid fried foods, processed foods, foods that are high in saturated or trans fats, sodas, and sugary desserts, and limit your consumption of red meat.

If you do experience an attack, switch to a clear liquid diet until your symptoms subside; drink water or herbal teas, and eat clear soups or broths. When your health-care provider says it's safe to resume eating whole foods, eat foods that can fight inflammation, such as wild-caught seafood (salmon, mackerel, tuna, herring, sardines, and halibut), walnuts, flaxseeds, and/or flaxseed oil. Foods rich in vitamin C can also help: citrus fruits; papayas; bell peppers; hot peppers; mangoes; tomatoes; kiwifruit; cantaloupe; dark, leafy greens; and parsley. Finally, turmeric, ginger, pineapple, and green tea all have powerful anti-inflammatory properties.

See also: Constipation (page 218), Irritable Bowel Syndrome (page 360), Overweight and Obesity (page 396)

dry eyes

Dry eyes can range from an occasional irritating condition to daily red, itchy, gritty-feeling, and/or burning eyes. Sometimes fluctuating visual disturbances can occur, and symptoms are often worse in the evening. When these symptoms persist, sufferers are said to have dry eye syndrome or dry eye disease. Dry eye syndrome is a result of a chronic lack of lubrication and moisture on the surface of your eye, which causes inflammation of the ocular surface. There are many causes for this lack of moisture, including aging, wearing contact lenses, taking certain medications, living in a dry climate, exposure to pollutants, and insufficient blinking. Less common causes of dry eyes include systemic diseases such as lupus, rheumatoid arthritis, and Sjögren's syndrome. The go-to treatment for dry eyes is lubricating eye drops; over-the-counter drops or stronger prescription versions are readily available. But what about food and beverage remedies?

First and most obviously, sufficient hydration is essential to preventing dry eyes. Water is best, but herbal teas and 100 percent fruit juices are okay, too. Remember that alcohol can have a dehydrating effect, causing or exacerbating the symptoms of dry eyes. Though it's often said that coffee and other caffeinated drinks can be likewise dehydrating, studies in fact reveal caffeine to be a surprising cure for dry eyes. One study compared the effect of a caffeinated beverage to plain water. Tear secretion was measured at 45, 90, 135, and 180 minutes after treatment and was found to be higher in the caffeine group at 45 and 90 minutes after ingesting caffeine. Conclusion? Caffeine stimulates tear production, though the effect may wear off after 90 minutes.[1] Another study found that caffeine increases tear volume. Specifically, tear volume was 0.08 mm greater in those who ingested caffeine than in those who had a placebo.[2] At first glance 0.08 mm doesn't seem like a lot, but it's volumes to dry eye sufferers!

Foods containing omega-3 fatty acids can also improve dry eye symptoms. (Some commercial eye drops even contain fish oil.) In a study of dry eye patients who supplemented with omega-3s compared to those who received a placebo, 65 percent of the patients in the omega-3 group experienced an improvement in symptoms after 3 months, while only 33 percent of the placebo group did. The omega-3 group scored significantly better on the TBUT (tear break-up time) test, which measures the time between the last blink and when the first dry spot appears in tear film.[3] Omega-3 fatty acids have also been found effective in treating dry eyes specifically caused by extended computer use[4] and in dry eyes caused by contact lens wearing.[5] Cold-water fish such as salmon, sardines, sablefish, halibut, cod, and herring are excellent sources of omega-3s. Eat these fish three times a week to get your omega-3s. For a vegetarian source of omega-3s, eat walnuts, flaxseeds, or flaxseed oil. Use flaxseed oil to make salad dressings, or grind flaxseeds and sprinkle them onto salads or into smoothies. Ground flaxseeds can also be used in baking. Any food containing omega-3s can increase lubrication and reduce inflammation.

There also seems to be a correlation between vitamin D deficiency, dry eyes, and impaired tear function,[6] so to increase your vitamin D intake, eat fatty fish, cheese, eggs, beef, mushrooms, or fortified milk (dairy, soy, or nut). The best source of vitamin D is sunlight, but make sure to wear shades when you're out, as bright sun can exacerbate symptoms of eye irritation.

Though fairly rare, the condition called xerophthalmia causes dry eyes and other ocular symptoms as a result of a vitamin A deficiency. Vitamin A's role in promoting good vision has long been established, so making sure your vitamin A intake is adequate is a good idea for healthy vision all around. It can help improve night vision, reduce eye inflammation, and reduce dry eye symptoms. Food sources of vitamin A include beef liver, fish and fish oils, sweet potatoes, spinach, carrots, cantaloupe, sweet peppers, mangoes, black-eyed peas, apricots, broccoli, eggs, and fortified milk and cereal.[7]

See also: Allergic Rhinitis (Hay Fever) (page 156)

dry mouth

Dry mouth, also known as xerostomia, is characterized by the feeling that there is not enough saliva in your mouth. Your tongue and the inside of your mouth can feel rough and dry, and if dry mouth continues, your lips can become cracked. Severe dry mouth can interfere with your ability to chew, swallow, enjoy food, wear dentures, and talk, and it can lead to halitosis and tooth decay. (The American Dental Association recommends regular use of a fluoride toothpaste and mouthwash to prevent dental caries in people with dry mouth. Prescription-strength fluoride gels or in-office fluoride therapy may be indicated, as well.)[1]

In the vast majority of cases, dry mouth is a temporary nuisance that will resolve on its own. Nervousness, blocked nasal passages that cause you to breathe through your mouth, snoring, and many medications can cause dry mouth, as can chemotherapy and tobacco use. But if it becomes a chronic problem, dry mouth may indicate an underlying condition such as anxiety, depression, or malnutrition. Sjögren's syndrome, an autoimmune disorder in which your white blood cells attack your body's moisture-producing glands, causes dry mouth, along with dry eyes, fatigue, and joint pain. Chronic dry mouth can also be a symptom of anemia, diabetes, HIV/AIDS, a hormone disorder, or cancer of the salivary glands. If you're suffering from persistent dry mouth and/or dry mouth along with any other new symptoms, see your doctor for an evaluation.

When dry mouth occurs, avoid crunchy, spicy, or acidic foods, as well as foods that are excessively dry, such as crackers, bread, and toast. Also avoid carbonated and caffeinated drinks, which can irritate your mouth and cause further dryness.

Easy remedies for temporary dry mouth include increased hydration (beyond just drinking water, you can let ice chips dissolve in your mouth), chewing sugarless gum, or sucking on sugarless hard candy. (These latter two stimulate saliva flow.) Other conventional treatments include alcohol-free mouthwashes designed to relieve dry mouth, oral sprays, salivary stimulants, and saliva substitutes. Acupuncture, medications, and gene therapy have been tried as well, with varying success.[2]

Chewing on foods with a high water content is a highly effective way to stimulate saliva and hydrate your mouth. So keep celery sticks, apple slices, cucumber slices, water chestnuts, fennel slices, grapes, bell pepper slices, watermelon chunks, or strawberries handy. Sugar-free popsicles, smoothies, yogurts, soups, and broths are also good choices for moisture-rich foods that can be easy to eat when you have dry mouth.

And though it wasn't as effective as a commercial oral spray, marshmallow root has been shown to be effective at relieving dry mouth. Patients with abnormally low salivation took marshmallow root four times a day and experienced symptom relief.[3] If you're looking for a safe, all-natural way to combat dry mouth, marshmallow root is an excellent option.

See also: Halitosis (page 307), Tooth Decay (page 435)

dry skin

Dry skin is a very common condition that is rarely serious. Much of the time it's caused by environmental factors such as cold or dry weather; sun exposure; long, hot showers; or central heating. Other common causes are chlorinated pools, detergents and soaps, certain vitamin deficiencies, dehydration, and skin conditions such as psoriasis, eczema, and atopic dermatitis. Less commonly, persistent dry skin that does not respond to moisturizers and other simple treatments can be an indication of a more serious condition, such as diabetes or hypothyroidism. Consult your doctor or dermatologist if dry skin lasts for more than 2 weeks and doesn't respond to at-home treatments, if dry skin is severe enough that it's widespread and accompanied by cracking or bleeding, if it develops suddenly, or if sudden dry skin is accompanied by itching.

The first line of defense in preventing and treating dry skin is proper hydration. Water is the obvious choice, though surprisingly, there's actually mixed evidence on the role of drinking water in keeping your skin moisturized. Several studies have questioned the oft-repeated advice to "drink eight 8-ounce glasses of water a day"[1] for moisturized skin. But a recent study published in the journal *Skin Research and Technology* found a clear relation between water intake and skin water content—as long as the volunteers were drinking large amounts of water. Study participants who drank a "water overload" of 2 liters per day for 30 days *in addition to their regular water consumption* all experienced a significant increase in both superficial and deep hydration of their skin.[2] Even with the mixed evidence, it's undoubtedly a good idea to stay hydrated for skin health and health overall. Good choices include filtered water, herbal teas, decaffeinated green tea, and 100 percent fruit juices (though drink these in moderation because of their high sugar content).

For healing foods for dry skin, recent research has revealed a connection between the health of your skin and the health of your gut. When something goes amiss in your intestinal environment, gut bacteria produce metabolites known as phenols. Phenols also naturally occur in foods such as fruits and vegetables, but the phenols produced by gut bacteria can collect in your skin and cause epithelial cells to lose their moisture—resulting in dry, scaly, itchy skin. So what prevents this entire process? The answer came from an unexpected source. A study on women who were experiencing abnormal bowel movements found that they also exhibited a high frequency of dry skin. Daily consumption of *Bifidobacterium* fermented milk and galacto-oligosaccharides, a type of commercially available prebiotic, decreased phenol production and prevented dry skin.[2] Other studies have shown the moisturizing effect of probiotics. One clinical trial examined the effect of *Lactobacillus plantarum* on women ages 41 to 59 with dry skin and wrinkles. Sixty-one volunteers received a daily probiotic for 12 weeks, and 49 served as controls. At week 12, there was a significant increase in skin water content in the faces and hands of the probiotic group, and there was less transepidermal water loss. What's more, the probiotic group experienced a significant reduction in wrinkle depth, better skin gloss, and a 22 percent improvement in skin elasticity by week 12.[4] A large metastudy done on infants and breastfeeding mothers found that probiotics were effective at preventing atopic dermatitis in children and decreasing its severity; *L. rhamnosus* was most effective for

long-term prevention. Atopic dermatitis, a form of eczema, results in dry, itchy, and inflamed skin. This study also found that prebiotics and black currant seed oil were effective in preventing atopic dermatitis.[5] Probiotics work for adults, too: Adults with atopic dermatitis who took *L. salivarius* and *B. breve* for 12 weeks experienced a significant improvement in symptoms.[6]

Certain nutrients can help prevent or treat dry skin. Vitamin A, niacin (vitamin B_3), essential fatty acids (omega-3s and omega-6s), and vitamin E all support skin health. A deficiency in vitamin A leads to dry, rough skin, and low levels of niacin can cause dermatitis and scaling.[7] Food sources of vitamin A include sweet potatoes; carrots; dark, leafy greens; squash; dried apricots; red peppers; mangoes; and tuna. Food sources of niacin include coffee, breakfast cereals, mushrooms, tuna, mackerel, salmon, peanuts, green peas, sunflower seeds, and avocados. A deficiency in essential fatty acids leads to dry, scaly skin and a greater loss of epidermal moisture.[8] A 12-week study on flaxseed oil and borage oil supplements found that, compared to a placebo, both oils reduced roughness and scaling, decreased epidermal moisture loss, and reduced inflammation.[9] Vitamin E is crucial for healthy skin and is the most abundant lipophilic antioxidant found in skin. A group of molecules rather than a single compound, vitamin E's main form in your body is alpha-tocopherol. Among other things, it helps protect your skin against UV rays and acts as an anti-inflammatory.[10] Good sources of vitamin E include almonds, hazelnuts, peanuts, spinach, sunflower seeds, and wheat germ. There are also numerous topical vitamin E creams used to treat dry skin, but use these with caution, as they can cause acne breakouts in some people.

For fast, topical relief for dry skin, there are several healing foods to try. Topical treatment with virgin coconut oil was found to be superior to mineral oil for soothing dry, itchy skin resulting from atopic dermatitis.[11] Avocado oil and grape seed oil can penetrate your skin,[12] leading to deep moisturization and improving the appearance of dry skin upon application. Other topical treatments that can be found in your kitchen pantry include olive oil, almond oil, and flaxseed oil—any of these can be applied directly to your skin for dry skin relief, though make sure to rub in any oils well to prevent them from staining your clothes. And of course, last but not least, an oatmeal bath is a tried-and-true method for soothing dry, itchy skin. For quick relief, add 1 cup of colloidal oatmeal (oatmeal that has been finely ground so it will dissolve in water) to a warm bath. Soak in an oatmeal bath for 15 to 20 minutes twice a day, and make sure the water is just warm, not hot, as hot water can dry skin further. (If you don't have colloidal oatmeal on hand, you can finely grind regular oats in a food processor.)

See also: Allergic Rhinitis (Hay Fever) (page 156), Dandruff (page 222), Eczema (page 259), Hives (page 339), Psoriasis (page 410)

earache

Earache can occur in one or both ears, and it can be quite painful. Earache is far more prevalent in infants and children than in adults and is usually caused by a type of ear infection called otitis media, or an infection in the middle ear. Ear infections occur when fluid becomes blocked and accumulates in your eustachian tubes. Many ear infections are preceded by a cold or sinus infection, but other causes of blockages include allergies, exposure to cigarette smoke or other pollutants, and swollen tonsils. Symptoms of otitis media may include earache, ringing in your ears, difficulty hearing, congestion and/or runny nose, or fever. Ear infections usually clear up on their own, but see your doctor if the pain is severe, if pus or blood drain from your ear, or if you experience dizziness or hearing loss. Other sources of earache are blockages in your ear (such as from earwax), jaw pain, wisdom teeth problems, changes in air pressure, or an injury to your ear.

To avoid infection of any type, keep your immune system supported with antioxidants and an adequate intake of vitamins and minerals. Flavonoids, found in abundance in fruits and vegetables, possess anti-inflammatory and immune-boosting properties.[1] Among the best sources of flavonoids are apples, aronia berries (chokeberries), arugula, beans, blueberries, capers, chocolate, coriander, cranberries, currants, dock, elderberries, fennel, garlic, grapefruit, hot peppers, juniper berries, kale, kumquats, lovage, onions, oregano, parsley, plums, radicchio, radishes, raspberries (black), red cabbage, red wine, and serviceberries.[2] There is evidence showing an association between middle ear infections and deficiencies in vitamin A and zinc.[3] Vitamin A is also known to decrease the incidence of ear infection and subsequent hearing loss.[4] Foods that are high in vitamin A include sweet potatoes; pumpkins; carrots; squash; liver; dark, leafy greens;

BONUS TIP: Though there are no studies on humans, studies on rats have shown that basil oil is an effective treatment for otitis media.[5] Basil oil is a popular home remedy for earache. To make your own basil oil, grind fresh basil leaves and add olive or tea tree oil, then heat the mixture. Pour it through a fine sieve or cheesecloth placed over a small glass bowl to remove the leaves. Dispense 4 or 5 drops of warm (not hot) basil oil into the affected ear.

cantaloupe; sweet red peppers; tuna; mangoes; and dairy products. Food sources for zinc include oysters, wheat germ, chicken, crab, beans, oatmeal, yogurt, sunflower seeds, pumpkin seeds, and pine nuts. Food sources for the rest of the immune-supporting nutrients include almonds; bananas; barley; beans; berries of any variety; Brazil nuts; cantaloupe; carrots; chickpeas; citrus fruits; dark, leafy greens; garlic; hazelnuts; lean poultry; mackerel; papayas; peppers of any variety; quinoa; salmon; squash; sweet potatoes; tuna; and yogurt.

To treat an earache topically, try white vinegar or apple cider vinegar. Dilute equal parts vinegar—known to be a potent antibacterial—and water, and put 3 or 4 drops in the ear to treat infection.[6] "Vinegar therapy" has even been shown to clear up a stubborn chronic *Pseudomonas* ear infection in as little as 3 weeks. In that particular case, the patient used a 2 percent vinegar solution twice a day, allowing the drops to stay in place for 15 minutes at a time and then draining them out.[7]

Oil made from extracts of the mullein plant has been shown to have antibacterial, anti-inflammatory, and analgesic properties, and to be effective at treating acute otitis media.[8] Mullein oil is often combined with garlic to enhance the effect; both are common ingredients in herbal and natural eardrops used to treat pain and infection.[9]

eczema

Also known as dermatitis, eczema is characterized by an itchy, red, inflamed rash that can appear anywhere on your body, but it usually appears on your neck, wrists, ankles, and anyplace that bends, such as behind your knees or along your inner elbows. (The National Eczema Association considers atopic dermatitis a more severe form of eczema.) Eczema affects some 30 million Americans. In addition to the red rash, eczema sufferers experience dry, sensitive skin; severe itching; scaling; rough or leathery patches; localized swelling; and oozing or crusting. The causes of eczema are not entirely clear, though it tends to run in families, and there is a strong association between eczema and allergies. Flare-ups occur in response to certain triggers, among them food allergens. This can happen either when you eat the food or when you come into contact with it. We'll cover a lot of ground in this entry, so be sure to check out "Healing Foods for Eczema" on page 261 for lists of specific foods to prevent and soothe eczema flare-ups.

Some of the most promising emerging eczema research has to do with early intervention. Pregnant and breastfeeding mothers who consume probiotics significantly decrease the chances that their babies will develop eczema,[1] and infants given probiotics are at a substantially lower risk for developing eczema, especially if they're given a mixture of probiotics.[2] A large metastudy done on infants and breastfeeding mothers found that probiotics were effective at preventing atopic dermatitis in children and in decreasing its severity; *Lactobacillus rhamnosus* was most effective for long-term prevention. This study also found that ingestion of prebiotics and black currant seed oil was effective at preventing atopic dermatitis and that alpha-linolenic acid reduced its severity.[3] A study of 40 infants newly diagnosed with eczema found that symptoms significantly improved in those who received a probiotic supplement.[4] Probiotics work for adults, too: Adults with atopic dermatitis who took *L. salivarius* and *Bifidobacterium breve* for 12 weeks experienced a significant improvement in symptoms.[5] Probiotics are found in yogurt and fermented foods (see page 261). Alpha-linolenic acid can be found in flaxseeds and flaxseed oil, canola oil, walnuts and walnut oil, pumpkin seeds, soybeans and soybean oil, and tofu.

But probiotics aren't the only healing foods for eczema prevention. In a study of more than 3,200 children ages 6 to 7, children were less likely to develop eczema if they ate fruits and pulses (lentils, chickpeas, and dried beans) three or more times a week. Dairy products (such as milk and butter) and rice were also negatively associated with eczema.[6] A study comparing dairy and nondairy beverage consumption also found a protective role in dairy: Children with eczema who drank more milk had less severe symptoms than those who didn't.[7]

Vitamin D supplementation has been advised for eczema sufferers,[8] and lower levels of vitamin D have been seen in those with eczema compared to those without, which may help explain the protective role of dairy products. Vitamin D has also been shown to influence immune system regulation, suppress skin inflammation, and improve skin barrier function.[9] Perhaps it's no surprise, then, that many eczema sufferers notice improvement after sun exposure. Of course, sun exposure should be limited so as to prevent sunburn, and those with extremely sensitive skin should be especially mindful of the effects of sunlight, as well as heat.

Another study found markedly lower levels of the antioxidant vitamins A, C, and E; the macro minerals sodium, potassium, and calcium; and the trace minerals zinc and iron in eczema sufferers than in nonaffected controls. This study also found greater lipid peroxidation—the process by which free radicals attack lipids, resulting in cell damage—in those with eczema. Study authors concluded that there is a strong association between eczema and elevated lipid peroxidation and depleted levels of the above nutrients.[10] Most people do *not* need to add sodium to their diets, but doing so is as simple as adding a small amount of salt to a meal. Himalayan crystal salt is one of the best options because it's loaded with essential minerals, and it's less burdensome to your kidneys and cardiovascular system than regular sodium chloride. See the opposite page for foods rich in the vitamins and minerals mentioned above.

Before you hit the grocery store or farmers' market, you'll need to take into account any food triggers or sensitivities that can cause eczema flare-ups. Numerous studies have uncovered a link between food sensitivities and eczema.[11] The most common food triggers that cause eczema flare-ups are wheat, nuts, seeds, dairy products, eggs, and soy products. If you have eczema, you should pay careful attention to your skin's response to these common triggers and eliminate or vastly reduce the foods that aggravate your skin.

Because eczema is characterized by inflamed skin, it also makes sense to avoid foods that cause inflammation and

For relief of dry, itchy skin, here are foods to eat and foods to avoid.

Foods to Eat (assuming they are not triggers for you)

- Foods high in probiotics: yogurt, sauerkraut, kimchi, tempeh, miso soup, sour pickles, sourdough bread, kefir, and some soft cheeses

- Antioxidant-rich and anti-inflammatory foods: apples; aronia berries (chokeberries); beans; blackberries; blueberries; capers; cherries; coriander; cranberries; currants; dark chocolate; dock; elderberries; fennel; garlic; grapefruit; hot peppers; juniper berries; kale; kumquats; dark, leafy greens; lovage; olive oil; omega-3-rich fish (salmon, mackerel, herring, tuna, halibut, trout, and sardines); onions; oregano; parsley; plums; radicchio; radishes; raspberries; red cabbage; red wine; strawberries; and tomatoes

- Food sources of vitamin A: sweet potatoes; carrots; dark, leafy greens; squash; dried apricots; red peppers; mangoes; and tuna

- Food sources of vitamin D: low-fat dairy products (fortified milk, yogurt, and cheese), eggs, fish, fish oil, tofu, mushrooms, fortified juice, fortified soy milk, and nut milks

- Food sources of vitamin E: almonds, hazelnuts, peanuts, sunflower seeds, spinach, and wheat germ

- Potassium-rich foods: sweet potatoes, tomato products, beet greens, beans, yogurt, clams, halibut, soybeans, tuna, winter squash, cod, bananas, spinach, dried peaches, dried apricots, prunes, cantaloupe, milk, honeydew melon, lentils, oranges, and carrot or prune juice

- Calcium-rich foods: dairy products and dark, leafy greens

- Zinc-rich foods: oysters, wheat germ, sesame seeds, pumpkin seeds, fortified cereals, and beef

- Iron-rich foods: dark, leafy greens; beef; sunflower seeds; molasses; dark chocolate; nuts; and tofu

- Food sources of niacin: coffee, breakfast cereals, mushrooms, tuna, mackerel, salmon, peanuts, green peas, sunflower seeds, and avocados

- Foods containing quercetin: apples, citrus fruits, aronia berries, black currants, grapes, capers, blackberries, blueberries, onions, parsley, sage, tea, and red wine

Foods to Avoid

- Dairy products
- Eggs
- Nuts
- Seeds
- Soy products
- Wheat products

to eat foods that prevent or calm inflammation. As a rule, avoid proinflammatory foods such as processed foods, refined foods, fast foods, foods containing trans fats, sodas, and red meat. Curcumin, the active agent in turmeric, has a powerful anti-inflammatory effect,[12] and combining turmeric with black pepper increases its potency. Pineapple is also recommended because of its anti-inflammatory and analgesic enzyme bromelain.[13] Quercetin, a naturally occurring flavonoid, may be a beneficial treatment for eczema, as it has been found to inhibit histamine and inflammatory cytokine release, and in two pilot trials, it significantly decreased contact dermatitis and photosensitivity.[14]

Honey has been used as a topical treatment for atopic dermatitis (the most severe form of eczema), seborrheic dermatitis, and psoriasis. In a study of patients experiencing scaling, itching, and hair loss, patients applied a solution of 90 percent honey and 10 percent water to seborrheic lesions every other day for 4 weeks. Itching and scaling disappeared within a week. Skin lesions were healed within 2 weeks. Treatment was continued for 6 months in the experimental group, while a control group used a placebo. None of the patients who continued using honey experienced a relapse of symptoms, while 12 out of 15 of the placebo group had a relapse 2 to 4 months after discontinuing treatment.[15]

Finally, because people with eczema tend to be prone to dry skin, further healing foods all include nutrients that can help with overall skin health and with preventing or treating dry, irritated skin. A deficiency in vitamin A leads to dry, rough skin, and low levels of niacin can cause dermatitis and scaling.[16] A deficiency in essential fatty acids leads to dry, scaly skin and a greater loss of epidermal moisture.[17] A 12-week study on flaxseed oil and borage oil supplements found that, compared to a placebo, both oils reduced roughness and scaling, decreased epidermal moisture loss, and reduced inflammation.[18] Vitamin E is crucial for healthy skin and is the most abundant lipophilic antioxidant found in skin. A group of molecules rather than a single compound, vitamin E's main form in your body is alpha-tocopherol. Among other things, vitamin E helps protect your skin against ultraviolet (UV) rays and acts as an anti-inflammatory.[19] There are numerous topical vitamin E creams used to treat dry skin, but use these with caution, as they can cause acne breakouts in some people.

See also: Allergic Rhinitis (Hay Fever) (page 156), Dry Skin (page 254), Food Allergies (page 278)

erection problems, erectile dysfunction

The most basic definition of erection problems is difficulty getting or maintaining an erection. Different iterations of erectile problems branch out from there: Some men may not be able to get an erection at all; others may not be able to get an erection that's firm enough for intercourse, while others may lose their erection prematurely. Erection problems are very common, and they often subside without treatment. But when erection problems become an ongoing concern, they're classified as erectile dysfunction (ED). Erection problems can affect any man at any age, but they become more common with age. The causes of erectile problems can be physical or mental, and up to 85 percent are due to a physical cause.

The key to remember when eating to improve erectile problems is that many erectile dysfunction problems result from poor bloodflow to the penis. Thus any diet that supports vascular health will also help with erectile problems. Not to mention that it will have the added benefit of substantially decreasing your risk of high blood pressure, high cholesterol, cardiovascular disease, and obesity. In a study of 236 men with metabolic syndrome, researchers found that an astonishing 96.5 percent had erectile dysfunction. Further, 39.6 percent reported decreased libido, 22.7 percent experienced premature ejaculation, and 4.8 percent had delayed ejaculation.[1] One of the most well-studied and effective heart-healthy diets is the Mediterranean diet, which emphasizes fresh fruits and vegetables; whole grains; lean protein sources, such as seafood and skinless poultry; legumes; nuts; seeds; red wine in moderation; and extra-virgin olive oil as the main source of fat. The Mediterranean diet also discourages consumption of red meat, trans fats, processed foods, fast foods, sugary desserts, and sodas.

Beyond this overall healthy dietary pattern, we can single out a few foods that deserve special mention for their potential healing effect for erectile problems. A signaling molecule called nitric oxide (NO) plays a key role in your ability to get and maintain an erection.

Nitric oxide is a vasodilator, meaning it causes blood vessels to expand; without adequate nitric oxide, erections aren't possible. (It's worth mentioning that Viagra works because it enhances NO-mediated vasodilation.) While there are no whole-food sources of nitric oxide, foods do provide an amino acid called L-arginine, the precursor to nitric oxide. L-arginine is a common ingredient in many supplements designed to increase libido and enhance sexual pleasure. Among the foods highest in L-arginine are sesame seeds, soy protein, crustaceans (lobster, shrimp, crab, and crayfish), spinach, seaweed, chicken breast, turkey breast, walnuts, and egg whites.[2]

A favorite food of many, chocolate improves the bioavailability of nitric oxide. Though chocolate is famous for its aphrodisiac properties, those effects have yet to be clinically proven. But chocolate does improve absorption of nitric oxide and it can boost mood because of its phenylethylamine content.[3] Dark chocolate has also been shown to increase nitric oxide production due to its flavonol content.[4]

Another food that plays a role in nitric oxide production is beets. Beets are a rich source of nitrates, which are converted into nitric oxide, and beets have been shown to improve endothelial function (vasodilation and vasocon-striction).[5] Dietary nitrates have been linked to a range of beneficial vascular effects, and remember that you want to eat to improve vascular function in order to improve erectile function. Other healthy food sources of nitrates include arugula, spinach, lettuces, radishes, Chinese cabbage, turnips, green beans, leeks, onions, cucumbers, carrots, garlic, and peppers.[6]

Though evidence in human trials is slim, some men have reported improvement in erectile dysfunction after drinking pomegranate juice.[7] In animal studies, pomegranate juice or extract has been shown to improve bloodflow, smooth muscle relaxation, and erectile response. Notably, the authors of one of these studies observed that long-term consumption of antioxidants appears to improve erectile dysfunction by protecting nitric oxide bioavailability.[8] If you're following a Mediterranean-style diet, you'll get plenty of antioxidants. Antioxidants are found in abundance in brightly colored fruits and vegetables, red wine, chocolate, tea, and coffee.

There are many herbs and supplements that claim to boost sexual desire and improve erections, but most of them lack scientific support. One that does show efficacy in clinical trials, however, is panax ginseng. Researchers reviewed data from six clinical trials containing data from a total of 349 men.

They found that ginseng significantly improved erectile function compared to a placebo over 4 to 12 weeks. Overall, 58 percent of men experienced improvement in some aspect of sexual function.[9] Another study had 69 men with mild to moderate erectile dysfunction take either a placebo or red ginseng extract powder for 8 weeks. After 8 weeks, all of the men who'd used ginseng reported improvements in erectile function, sexual desire, orgasmic function, intercourse satisfaction, and overall satisfaction.[10]

Lastly, recent evidence shows that a deficiency in folic acid is to blame for some cases of erectile dysfunction and premature ejaculation. Researchers examined serum levels of folic acid in 42 men with erectile dysfunction, 36 with premature ejaculation (PE), 25 men with both ED and PE, and 30 healthy men who served as controls.

They found that while there were no significant differences in levels of sex hormones in any of the men, folic acid levels were significantly lower in the men with ED and/or PE than in the controls. Thus, folic acid supplementation may be an effective therapy for men experiencing sexual dysfunction.[11] Folic acid, also known as vitamin B_9, is the synthetic form of folate and is found in supplements and fortified foods. Folate is the natural form of vitamin B_9 and is found in foods such as avocados; asparagus; beans; broccoli; Brussels sprouts; citrus fruits and juices; dark, leafy greens; eggs; grains; seafood; and spinach.[12]

See also: Anxiety (page 165), Decreased Libido (page 224), Depression (page 232), Diabetes (page 238), Heart Disease (Cardiovascular Disease) (page 313), High Blood Pressure (Hypertension) (page 327), High Cholesterol (page 334), Overweight and Obesity (page 396), Stress (page 419)

fatigue

More than just tiredness or the feeling of drowsiness after not sleeping well, fatigue is a state of chronic, extreme weariness. Think of exhaustion, or a total lack of energy. Fatigue is a normal response to life events such as stress, insomnia, extended physical activity, a temporary illness such as a cold or flu, or surgery. Fatigue is also associated with chronic pain, and it can be a side effect of certain medications, including blood pressure medications, cold and cough medicines, diuretics, and steroids. When fatigue doesn't subside after proper sleep, good nutrition, and/or the cessation of illness or a short-term medication, it's advisable to see your doctor. Fatigue is distressing on its own, making the activities of daily living difficult and burdensome, but chronic fatigue can be a sign of serious illness.

Because the causes of fatigue are so numerous and so varied, it's not possible to create a one-size-fits-all antifatigue diet. But the best overall dietary pattern to prevent common deficiencies in minerals and vitamins that can cause fatigue is the Mediterranean diet or one of its close cousins. That is to say, a diet characterized by high consumption of a wide variety of fresh fruits and vegetables; moderate to high consumption of whole grains; high consumption of legumes (lentils and beans) and nuts; protein sources that are primarily plant based, with additional protein from lean fish and poultry and little to no red meat; a limited intake of high-fat dairy products; the use of olive oil as the primary cooking oil and fat source; low to moderate consumption of red wine; limited intake of sugar and sweets; and elimination of processed or fast foods and trans fats.

Modifications can be made to this general dietary pattern based upon your geographical location, the season, and your taste preferences. But sticking to the basics of a healthy dietary framework highly increases your chances of getting the proper amounts of all the nutrients you need for optimum health and energy. From there, you can supplement additional healing foods according to your specific needs. According to the Centers for Disease Control and Prevention (CDC), the most common vitamin deficiencies in the United States are vitamin B_6, iron, vitamin D, and vitamin

C. (Vitamins B_{12}, A, E, and folate are also common deficiencies but are far less prevalent than these top four.)[1] Interestingly, fatigue is a known symptom of deficiencies in vitamin B_6, iron, and vitamin C, and muscle weakness is a symptom of vitamin D deficiency.

The recommended daily allowance of vitamin B_6 for adults through age 50 is 1.3 milligrams (mg) a day. After age 50, men should get 1.7 mg a day and women 1.5 mg a day. Breastfeeding mothers should consume 2.0 mg a day. Some of the best food sources of vitamin B_6 are salmon, russet potatoes, turkey, chicken, avocados, spinach, bananas, dried plums, hazelnuts, and fortified breakfast cereals.[2]

To get more iron in your diet, eat oysters, clams, tuna, eggs, shrimp, spinach, molasses, lentils, brown rice, raisins, prunes, kidney beans, tofu, or cashews. One of the best sources of iron, of course, is red meat, especially chicken or beef liver. Red meat can be consumed in small quantities, especially if your iron levels are quite low. But a vegetarian, heart-healthy source that tops red meat in iron content is raisin bran cereal; some versions contain as much as 18 grams of iron.[3]

Sunlight exposure is your primary means of getting vitamin D, and though increasing awareness of the harmful effects of UV rays has led more people to use sunscreen, it has also inadvertently contributed to less vitamin D absorption. Food sources of vitamin D include dairy products, eggs, fish and fish oil, mushrooms, and fortified orange juice.[4]

Vitamin C is found in an abundance of whole foods and beverages. The top sources include acerola cherries (West

healthy insight

Radix puerariae, otherwise known as kudzu, the invasive vine that has overtaken large parts of the American South, has been shown to be an effective antifatigue agent in mice models.[5] Kudzu root is an established remedy in traditional Chinese medicine and is used in complementary medicine.[6] Use caution if you're considering kudzu, however: Human studies are limited, and kudzu has known interactions with birth control pills, anticoagulants, methotrexate, and tamoxifen. Also be aware that kudzu contains caffeine, and it has the potential to lower blood sugar.

Indian cherries) and their juice, guavas, dried lychees, currants, oranges and orange juice, grapefruit and grapefruit juice, peaches, kiwifruit, papayas, apples, persimmons, strawberries, pineapples and pineapple juice, kumquats, lemons, and limes.[7] Vitamin C can also be found in tomatoes, sweet red peppers, broccoli, potatoes, and spinach.[8] Vitamin C strongly enhances your body's ability to absorb iron.

Perhaps the key thing to remember about fatigue is that it is not a disease in and of itself but rather a symptom of some underlying cause. Thus additional healing food recommendations would be based upon treatment of the particular condition that's causing the fatigue. Treating the underlying condition treats the fatigue.

Many people wonder about specific foods or beverages that can boost energy or confer an antifatigue effect. First, the best course of action is to rely on an overall healthy diet that gives you the benefit of a *synergy* of nutrients. Rather than overloading on a single food or nutrient, your body works best when the fuel you're giving it is varied.[9] Second, avoid the temptation to rely on caffeine and sugar to fight fatigue. The boost you get from coffee and tea comes from their stimulant effect, and once that wears off, you may feel even more lethargic. Attempting to use sugar as a fatigue fighter is even more dangerous. You may feel an uptick in energy shortly after eating sugar, but it's short-lived, and the well-known "sugar crash" leaves you feeling even worse than before. More importantly, sugar consumption is associated with an elevated risk for a laundry list of health problems: cardiovascular disease, type 2 diabetes, cancer, tooth decay, and weight gain, to name just a few. Third, the majority of studies on antifatigue agents have been conducted on mice, and though results are promising, it's simply not known exactly how these agents would play out in human trials. With these precautions in mind, there is some evidence indicating an antifatigue effect from the following foods and nutrients.

Resveratrol, the well-known polyphenolic compound in red wine, grapes, blueberries, bilberries, cranberries, peanuts, and cocoa, has been shown to combat fatigue and improve exercise performance in mice.[10]

A study of curcumin's effect on mood in 60 healthy adults ages 60 to 85 found that curcumin significantly improved mood, cognitive function, and general fatigue.[11]

The lion's mane mushroom has antifatigue effects—and this healing food has been studied in humans. This mushroom, long a part of Asian cuisine,[12] has anti-inflammatory, antioxidative, and immune-boosting properties and is available in the United States in Asian markets, some specialty foods stores, and, increasingly, at farmers' markets.

Garlic has been extensively studied in humans, and it's been shown to improve physical fatigue, fatigue due to cold, and general fatigue. The most effective form seems to be aged garlic extract.[13]

Please note: *Chronic fatigue syndrome (CFS) is different from the symptom of fatigue as described in this entry; though the healing foods for fatigue will have some beneficial effect for sufferers of CFS, because CFS is a multisymptom, systemic disorder that affects individuals in vastly different ways, people with CFS should be under the care of their health-care providers before trying any of the suggestions here. Please also see Fibromyalgia on page 272, as it shares some of the same symptomatology, and thus recommendations, as CFS.*

See also: Adrenal Exhaustion/Adrenal Fatigue (page 153), Bronchitis (page 186), Depression (page 232), Diabetes (page 238), Fibromyalgia (page 272), Influenza (page 352), Insomnia (page 357), Lupus (page 370), Menopause (page 381), Motion Sickness (page 386), Muscle Cramps (page 388), PMS (Premenstrual Syndrome) (page 404), Pneumonia (page 407), Shingles (page 413), Sinusitis (page 415), Stress (page 419), Thyroid Disease (page 429)

fibrocystic breasts

At least 50 percent of women of childbearing age experience fibrocystic breasts. Fibroadenomas—masses of fibrous tissue—can feel firm, smooth, and rubbery to the touch. Cysts are fluid-filled sacs within the breast that feel like a round, movable lump. Cysts can be tender to the touch. Fibrocystic breast condition, also sometimes referred to as benign breast disease, is the most common benign breast condition and can occur any time after menstruation begins, though it rarely occurs after menopause. It most often occurs in women ages 30 to 50. This noncancerous condition is characterized by breast lumps that can change according to normal monthly hormonal fluctuations. Some women experience pain, tenderness, and/or swelling in their breasts, especially just before their periods.

Fibrocystic breasts are quite normal and the condition itself is no cause for concern; the conversion of fibroadenomas to a malignancy is quite rare.[1] The biggest risk associated with fibrocystic breasts, however, is that the condition can make it more difficult to detect potentially cancerous lumps. This is all the more reason women should conduct monthly self-exams and be aware of the baseline texture and feel of their breast tissue. If new or unusual lumps occur, if lumps are particularly painful, if you experience discharge from a nipple, dimpling of your skin, or unexplained bruising on your breast, contact your doctor.

For years the standard nutrition advice was to reduce or eliminate caffeine, but more recent studies have found no association between caffeine and fibrocystic breasts. And though a high body mass index (BMI) *is* associated with an increased risk of breast cancer, it is not correlated with benign fibrocystic breasts.[2]

As for the latest evidence concerning healing foods and fibrocystic breasts, a study of 258 women with fibrocystic breasts and 1,035 control women analyzed a wide array of nutritional data. Researchers found a lower incidence of fibrocystic breasts in women who had high intakes of daidzein and genistein. Daidzein and genistein are soy isoflavones that can be found in soybeans, tofu, tempeh, and miso. They also found a lower risk of fibroadenomas with a higher intake of EPA and DPA (eicosa-pentaenoic acid and docosahexaenoic acid), fatty acids found in fatty fish and fish oil.[3] A slightly older study conducted by many of the same researchers found that increased fruit and vegetable intake was associated with a significantly lower risk of developing fibroadenomas. Other protective factors included the use of oral contraceptives, having been through natural menopause, an increasing number of live births, and moderate exercise. Notably, women who performed heavy physical activity in their twenties increased their risk of developing fibrocystic breasts. In this study, researchers singled out sesame oil and lychees as being particularly protective.[4]

Finally, if you're the parent or grandparent of a young girl, this last paragraph is for you. There is a great deal of evidence that a girl's dietary and lifestyle habits during preadolescence and adolescence, when her breasts are still developing, have a direct impact on later breast health. Alcohol consumption during adolescence can predispose a woman to fibrocystic breasts,[5] while adequate consumption of beta-carotene (found in lettuces, kale, spinach, carrots, peppers, mustard greens, pumpkin, sweet potatoes, and squash) can significantly reduce the risk.[6] Adequate vitamin D intake during adolescence exerts the same protective effect.[7] Yet another study found that a higher intake of vegetable oils, vitamin E, fiber, and nuts and a lower intake of red meat, animal fats, and alcohol during adolescence were associated with a significantly reduced risk of benign breast disease. Researchers highlighted apples and peanuts as being particularly protective: Girls who ate one to three apples a month had a 40 percent reduced risk of benign breast disease, and those who ate at least one serving of peanuts a week had about one-third the risk of developing benign breast disease as girls who ate less than one serving a month.[8] These results provide further confirmation that healthy eating patterns should start as early as possible. They'll last a lifetime.

fibromyalgia

Fibromyalgia is a complex, chronic illness that is not yet fully understood. It causes achiness and pain throughout your body that lasts for 3 months or more; debilitating fatigue, even with proper rest; swelling; and tenderness. It is often accompanied by anxiety and/or depression. Fibromyalgia can be difficult to diagnose, but one of its distinguishing features is tenderness and pain at specific points on your neck, shoulders, back, arms, legs, and hips. For unknown reasons, it disproportionately affects women: Some 80 to 90 percent of cases are in women. Other fibromyalgia symptoms include headaches, dry mouth, hypersensitivity to cold and heat, concentration and/or memory problems, irritable bowel syndrome, an increased severity of PMS, restless leg syndrome, muscle stiffness, and numbness or tingling in your hands and feet. There is no cure for fibromyalgia, but with proper rest, regular medical care, stress management, and good nutrition, sufferers experience an improvement in symptoms as well as a decrease in their number of flare-ups. Medications are also used to manage symptoms and reduce pain.

To help manage the symptoms of fibromyalgia through nutrition, it's a good idea to tend to your overall dietary pattern. Evidence shows that fibromyalgia sufferers tend to have a poorer diet than their healthy counterparts.[1] One study compared 45 fibromyalgia patients with 25 age-matched controls and found that those with fibromyalgia had significant oxidative DNA damage, lower enzyme antioxidant activity, diminished total antioxidant capacity, and deficiencies in key nutrients, such as zinc. Significant correlations were found between oxidative DNA damage and

mental health symptoms and between zinc deficiency and physical symptoms.[2] Being overweight also worsens symptoms, leading to more pain, greater fatigue, worsened sleep quality, and higher incidence of mood disorders such as depression and anxiety.[3]

To boost your antioxidant intake, plan your meals around fresh fruits and vegetables. Just a few sources of antioxidants include pineapple, berries, tomatoes, red grapes, red cabbage, kale, spinach, arugula, onions, apples, broccoli, soybeans, apricots, beets, cantaloupe, carrots, mangoes, oranges, winter squash, yellow and orange peppers, green tea, coffee, red wine, dark chocolate, cocoa, and papayas. Planning meals with fruits and vegetables as the focal point rather than as a side dish can also significantly help with weight reduction. To increase your zinc levels, eat oysters, wheat germ, chicken, crab, beans, oatmeal, yogurt, sunflower seeds, pumpkin seeds, and pine nuts.

There is also a connection between fibromyalgia and iron. One study showed that fibromyalgia patients had lower ferritin levels than a control group and that having a serum ferritin level of less than 50 ng/ml caused a six-and-one-half–fold increased risk of developing fibromyalgia. A different study found no relationship between iron and fibromyalgia, but as low iron is one common cause of fatigue, we are including iron-rich foods in our recommendations. For healthy sources of iron, eat lean poultry; oatmeal; potatoes; seafood; beans; dark, leafy greens (kale, spinach, arugula, etc.); Swiss chard and any type of green (mustard, collard, turnip, etc.); peas; dried fruits (prunes and raisins); and blackstrap molasses in small quantities. Vitamin C increases the absorption of iron and is one of our most powerful antioxidants, as well. Great food choices for vitamin C include citrus fruits; bell peppers; broccoli; dark, leafy greens; guavas; hot peppers; kiwis; mangoes; papayas; and tomatoes.

One nutrient that shows up again and again in research studies on fibromyalgia is vitamin D. A deficiency in vitamin D has been linked to chronic pain and to musculoskeletal pain.[4] In one study, 71 percent of chronic pain patients had a vitamin D deficiency and another 21 percent had insufficient vitamin D.[5] In those with fibromyalgia, low vitamin D also seems to intensify the perception of pain.[6] As vitamin D levels tend to be significantly lower in those with fibromyalgia, one study hypothesized that elevating vitamin D would alleviate pain. Thirty fibromyalgia patients were randomized to a treatment group of vitamin D_3 supplementation or a control group. Evaluation was performed at 20 weeks and again in another 24 weeks. The treatment group all experienced a significant reduction in pain.[7] Vitamin D even plays a role in the anxiety associated with fibromyalgia: Fibromyalgia sufferers who are deficient in vitamin D (with levels less than 25 nmol/l) are far more prone to anxiety and depression than those with normal or even insufficient levels of vitamin D.[8] As there is increasing evidence that vitamin D deficiency is more common worldwide than we once thought, and as boosting vitamin D levels is a low-cost means of treatment, many health-care professionals recommend it for fibromyalgia sufferers. Sunlight exposure is the primary means of getting vitamin D. Food sources of vitamin D include dairy products, eggs, fish and fish oil, mushrooms, tofu, and fortified juices or milks.[9]

Now, what about what *not* to eat if you have fibromyalgia? One of the areas under exploration is the excitotoxin elimination diet. Excitotoxins are types of chemicals (usually amino acids) that overstimulate neuron receptors. Researchers have hypothesized that excitotoxins play a role in the central sensitization that is prevalent in many fibromyalgia cases, leaving people with greater sensitivity to pain. At high concentrations, excitotoxins can lead to neuron death. The two most common food sources of excitotoxins are not foods at all, but additives: monosodium glutamate (MSG) and the artificial sweetener aspartame. A very small study conducted some years ago found that fibromyalgia patients who eliminated MSG alone or MSG and aspartame from their diets experienced a complete or nearly complete remission of symptoms.[10]

In a more recent study, people with fibromyalgia and irritable bowel syndrome (IBS) were placed on a 4-week diet that eliminated MSG and aspartame. Eighty-four percent of those who completed the diet experienced more than a 30 percent reduction in symptoms. Researchers then took those who'd responded well to the elimination diet and placed them on a 2-week double-blind trial that alternated MSG consumption and consumption of a placebo. The results? Eating MSG resulted in a significant return of symptoms overall, and more specifically, a worsening of fibromyalgia severity and a decreased quality of life in regard to IBS symptoms.[11] However, a study that looked at the effect of the excitotoxin elimination diet on a single symptom of fibromyalgia—pain— found no clinical difference between those who eliminated MSG and aspartame and those who served as controls.[12] Though the evidence is conflicting, it appears that some fibromyalgia patients experience remarkable improvement after eliminating MSG and aspartame, so it's certainly worth a try. Remember that MSG can show up on labels in many different forms, including anything with the word "glutamate," "glutamic," or "hydrolyzed." MSG also occurs naturally in foods such as tomatoes, seaweed, some cheeses, and proteins. Aspartame is a different story in that it is purely artificial. It's most often found in diet soft drinks, but it can show up in candies, chewing gum, syrups, jellies, low-fat yogurts, and breath mints.

There is also emerging evidence on the role of gluten in fibromyalgia. A small study (with 20 participants) put fibromyalgia patients without celiac disease on a gluten-free diet and found, as researchers put it, "remarkable clinical improvement." This study is ongoing, but the average follow-up period for the gluten-free diet at the time of publication was 16.4 months. The results? All patients experienced a significant improvement in chronic, widespread pain, and 15 patients were pain-free. Fifteen patients returned to work or normal life. The three patients who'd used opioids for pain control discontinued their medications. Two patients went into complete remission from psoriatic arthritis and spondyloarthritis. Finally, when eight patients went back to eating gluten, their symptoms returned—but ceased again once they returned to a gluten-free diet. Researchers concluded that nonceliac gluten sensitivity is a treatable underlying cause of fibromyalgia syndrome.[13]

A much larger study compared celiac-like symptoms in those with fibromyalgia to healthy controls and to those with an established gluten intolerance. Researchers found that every celiac symptom, with the exception of anemia, was significantly more extreme in patients with fibromyalgia. The findings of this study as well as others suggest that a subgroup of fibromyalgia patients have either celiac disease or nonceliac gluten intolerance[14] and that eliminating gluten can be beneficial, especially with improving the gastrointestinal (GI) symptoms that are commonly associated with fibromyalgia.[15] Research is ongoing, but as with the excitotoxin elimination diet, the existing results are persuasive. One of the challenges of treating fibromyalgia is that symptoms can vary greatly from individual to individual—and so can treatment options. For fibro sufferers with GI complaints, eliminating gluten certainly seems worth a try.

See also: Adrenal Exhaustion/Adrenal Fatigue (page 153), Anxiety (page 165), Depression (page 232), Irritable Bowel Syndrome (page 360), Overweight and Obesity (page 396), Thyroid Disease (page 429)

flatulence

The accumulation and expulsion of intestinal gas is a normal biological process, but excessive flatulence can cause bloating, abdominal discomfort, and embarrassment. The typical person passes gas between 10 and 20 times a day. If you're experiencing excessive flatulence, the good news is that simple changes to your diet are the easiest and quickest ways to prevent or remedy painful and problematic gas.

In this case, one of the most effective remedies is the most obvious: Avoid foods that cause gas. Beans are notorious for producing gas, and simply saying no to beans and bean dishes will prevent the production of gas. Dairy products also give plenty of people trouble, and flatulence after eating dairy products may be a sign of lactose intolerance.[1] Other top offenders include carbonated drinks, onions, broccoli, cauliflower, wheat and wheat products, and fatty foods such as pan-fried or deep-fried items. For most people, the best course is to note which foods consistently cause flatulence and then avoid those foods and beverages, or at least reduce consumption of them.

If you're looking for a diet to reduce gas, this may be the *sole* case in which the Mediterranean diet is not recommended. A low-flatulogenic diet is restricted to foods low in fermentable residues, which are known to increase gas production. In a study of a low-flatulogenic diet versus the Mediterranean diet, the test diet reduced the number of times subjects passed gas per day by 54 percent. It also significantly reduced abdominal distension and enhanced digestive well-being.[2] In addition to the "top offender" foods mentioned above, a typical low-flatulogenic diet omits Brussels sprouts, celery, carrots, raisins, and bananas.

People with excessive flatulence have also benefited from the low-FODMAP diet. FODMAP is an acronym for fermentable oligosaccharides, disaccharides, monosaccharides, and polyols. In brief, FODMAPs are short-chain carbohydrates that are poorly absorbed in your small intestine and are quickly fermented by bacteria in your gut. As the inevitable by-product of the fermentation process is gas, it makes sense to avoid high-FODMAP foods. The full list of high-FODMAP foods is far too long to list here,[3] but in brief, they are:

Foods High in Fructose

apples

artichokes

asparagus

cherries

fruit juices (any processed food made with high-fructose corn syrup)

honey

mangoes

peaches

pears

sugar snap peas

watermelon

Lactose

Butter

Ice cream

Milk

Soft cheeses

Yogurt

Oligosaccharides

artichokes

asparagus

barley

beans

beetroot

Brussels sprouts

cabbage

chickpeas

chicory

chicory drinks

fennel

garlic

inulin (a common food additive)

leeks

lentils

okra

onions

peaches

peas

persimmons

pistachios

rye

shallots

soy products

watermelon

wheat

Sugar Alcohols (known as polyols)

sorbitol

xylitol (found in apples, apricots, avocados, blackberries, cherries, lychees, nectarines, pears, plums, prunes, cauliflower, mushrooms, snow peas, and any food containing an artificial sweetener)

Echoing the list of "top offenders" above, according to the low-FODMAP diet, onions, garlic, and wheat products are to be avoided entirely, if possible.

The full list of foods to avoid on the FODMAP diet is quite extensive, but the good news is that, in most cases, the diet is a temporary measure to be followed for 6 to 8 weeks, or until flatulence symptoms subside. People with IBS may, under the guidance of their doctors, wish to follow the FODMAP diet for extended periods of time.

See also: Constipation (page 218), Diarrhea (page 245), Irritable Bowel Syndrome (page 360)

food allergies

An allergic reaction to food occurs when your body mistakenly identifies a food as a threat and attacks it, just as it would in the case of a bacteria or virus. More specifically, in response to the allergen your immune system overreacts and releases large quantities of immunoglobulin E (IgE), an antibody that triggers the release of histamine and other chemicals, which in turn trigger the allergic reaction. A food allergy is distinguished from a food sensitivity or intolerance by that immune system reaction; food intolerances, in contrast, occur in your digestive system because your body is unable to break down a particular food. While the symptoms of food intolerance can mimic the mild symptoms of a food allergy (and both can make you feel miserable), the former is not a life-threatening condition, while the latter has the potential to be, even if the person is exposed to trace amounts. If you suspect a food allergy, it's a good idea to see an allergist who can give you specific guidelines suited to your unique needs and advise you on your ongoing care.

While there are at least 160 known food allergens, just eight foods account for fully 90 percent of food allergies: milk, eggs, peanuts, tree nuts, soy, wheat, fish, and shellfish. In the United States, the FDA requires any food product that contains even trace amounts of these eight allergens to be labeled accordingly.

The symptoms of a food allergy can be as mild as a rash or itching or as extreme as a potentially lethal reaction called anaphylaxis. Mild symptoms of an allergic reaction include rash; hives; eczema; itching of your mouth, throat, or ear canal; nausea or vomiting; sneezing; runny nose and/or nasal congestion; dry cough; diarrhea; abdominal pain; or an odd taste in your mouth. More severe symptoms that can indicate an anaphylactic reaction include swelling of your lips, tongue, face, or throat; wheezing or difficulty breathing; faint pulse; dizziness; reduced blood pressure; a sense of dread or impending doom; and loss of consciousness. These symptoms usually occur very quickly after the food is consumed. Many people with severe food allergies keep an epinephrine auto-injector (for example, an EpiPen) with them at all times; prompt treatment with epinephrine can save your life. Always treat an anaphylactic reaction as a medical emergency, even if your symptoms subside after receiving epinephrine. It's a good idea to get a medical evaluation, as some patients experience a second wave of symptoms hours or even days later.

Food allergies are on the rise in developed nations—and reactions are becoming more severe. While at this time it's unclear why and there is no known cure, researchers are making great strides in ways to prevent and treat allergies, and in some cases children do "grow out of" their allergies, especially if the allergen is milk or eggs. Other therapies under investigation include producing genetically engineered plants that can produce hypoallergenic foods, molecular manipulation of foods to reduce allergenicity,[1] gradual exposure to progressively higher doses of the allergen to induce desensitization to it (oral, sublingual, or epicutaneous immunotherapy), anti-IgE antibodies,[2] vaccines, probiotic and prebiotic supplementation, and traditional Chinese medicine (TCM) herbal therapy.[3]

Some of the most promising advancements have been made in the area of peanut allergy through the landmark LEAP (Learning Early About Peanut Allergy) study. Researchers demonstrated that very early introduction of peanuts in infants who are at high risk of peanut allergy can prevent the development of the allergy. More than 600 babies between 4 and 11 months old with severe eczema, egg allergy, or both were put into two groups on the basis of

a preexisting sensitivity to peanuts: one group with a positive reaction to a skin-prick test, the other with no measurable reaction. They were then randomized either to consume a peanut-containing snack at least three times a week up until the age of 5 or to avoid peanuts altogether. Of the 530 children who initially had a negative reaction to the skin-prick test and avoided peanuts, 13.7 percent went on to develop a peanut allergy by the time they were 5. But of the children who were exposed to peanuts early, only 1.9 percent developed a peanut allergy. Among the 98 children who initially had positive test results, the prevalence of peanut allergy was 35.3 percent in the avoidance group and 10.6 percent in the consumption group. This translates to an 86.1 percent relative reduction of peanut allergy in the first group and a 70 percent relative reduction in the second group. These are extraordinary results with life-changing potential—especially considering that peanut allergy is the leading cause of anaphylaxis and death associated with a food allergy.[4] Based upon the LEAP data, the American Academy of Pediatrics now recommends that high-risk infants should be exposed to peanuts between 4 and 11 months of age. An allergist or physician with training in allergic diseases can help parents implement these recommendations and monitor their child's care.[5]

Many people wonder if there is a way to prevent allergies, especially as adults who have food allergies have a roughly 65 percent chance of passing them on to their children. There is evidence demonstrating the protective effect of breastfeeding. One study found that children diagnosed with a food allergy before the age of 2 had been introduced to solid foods earlier (at less than 16 weeks of age) and were less likely to be receiving breast milk when cow's milk was introduced. The study supports allergists' recommendations to breastfeed infants for 4 to 6 months, with continued breastfeeding thereafter, and provides evidence that continued breastfeeding while solids are introduced, as well as delaying solids until at least 17 weeks, reduces the odds of developing food allergies.[6] There is also evidence suggesting that prenatal consumption of probiotics and prebiotics, plus postnatal supplementation up to the age of 2, offers some protection against food allergies and eczema. Supplementation for children up to age 4 is effective for those at high risk of allergy, and this study found that *Lactobacillus rhamnosus* was most effective.[7]

Even with these remarkable strides, the primary way to manage food allergies remains strict avoidance of trigger foods, even in small amounts. This can be a significant burden on individuals and families, but there is a great deal of research under way, and the general public is more knowledgeable than ever on how to meet the needs of allergy sufferers at schools, restaurants, workplaces, and the grocery store. Until science finds a cure, people with food allergies can manage symptoms through food avoidance, medications (antihistamines for mild reactions, epinephrine for severe ones), and/or, with the help of an allergist, possible immunotherapy. People with multiple food allergies can benefit from following set dietary guidelines such as the MEWS diet (a diet free of milk, eggs, wheat, and soy). If you have a food allergy, it's also a good idea to get periodic evaluations to make sure that you're not deficient in certain vitamins and minerals that you may not be getting through your diet; calcium and vitamin D are concerns for those who are on a milk-free diet, for instance. A certified nutritionist can help you modify your diet to meet your nutrient needs. Finally, there may be some relief available through the healing foods that treat other allergic conditions, such as eczema and allergic rhinitis, as long as there is no allergy or food sensitivity to those foods.

See also: Allergic Rhinitis (Hay Fever) (page 156), Asthma (page 174), Eczema (page 259), Hives (page 339)

fungal infections (general, yeast infections, candidiasis)

There are more than 20 types of *Candida* yeast that can cause fungal infections, the most common of which is *Candida albicans*. *Candida* yeasts are naturally occurring organisms that live on your skin, in your gut, and in your mucous membranes. Normally *Candida* species don't cause infection. But when something occurs to cause *Candida* overgrowth—such as antibiotics that kill off the beneficial bacteria keeping *Candida* in check—candidiasis results, bringing a host of distressing symptoms. The term "yeast infection" is often used to denote a vaginal yeast infection, but candidiasis can affect most any part of your body—including your entire body, which is known as systemic candidiasis or invasive candidiasis. Other common sites of yeast infection include your mouth (oral thrush), throat, gastrointestinal tract, nails, ears, nose, and penis. A yeast infection can also occur in your navel or within skin folds. Jock itch, ringworm, athlete's foot, and diaper rash are all forms of yeast infection. *Candida* thrives in any environment that's warm and moist.

People with compromised immune systems, such as those with HIV/AIDS, diabetes, mononucleosis, or patients receiving chemotherapy, are at an increased risk for yeast infections. Other risk factors include stress, hormone replacement therapy, pregnancy, and the use of oral contraceptives, antibiotics, or corticosteroids.

Signs and symptoms of a yeast infection depend on the part of your body that is affected. Thrush causes a telltale growth of white patches on your tongue and the insides of your cheeks. A vaginal yeast infection causes severe itching, a cottage-cheese-like discharge, redness, and irritation. On the penis, a yeast infection can cause a rash or red, scaly patches and itching. Yeast infections on skin surfaces cause a red, flat rash; itching or burning; and sometimes nearby pimples or patches of rash called satellite lesions. If candidiasis spreads throughout your gastrointestinal system it can cause painful ulcers, nausea, and vomiting. Invasive candidiasis can cause fever and chills that don't improve with antibiotic therapy. Symptoms as diverse as bloating, gas, constipation, diarrhea, joint pain, fatigue, headaches, sinus problems, depression, and anxiety may occur.[1] Left unchecked, invasive candidiasis will affect multiple organ systems, and the condition can be fatal. The standard treatment for yeast infections is antifungal medications. Some can be applied directly to the affected area, such as for thrush or vaginal yeast infections. Oral medications such as fluconazole can also be prescribed, and for serious or systemic infections, antifungals can be given intravenously.

Fortunately, there are many healing foods that can prevent and treat overgrowth of *Candida,* both as part of a diet and as topical agents. Many health-care providers recommend a low-carbohydrate, low-sugar diet to combat candidiasis, as *Candida* yeast feed on sugar in any form. In addition to added sugar, you can eliminate fruits, starchy vegetables, legumes, and grains for 2 to 3 weeks to help slow and reverse *Candida* growth.[2] Some health-care providers also recommend temporarily eliminating alcohol, yeast, aged or processed cheeses, processed or smoked meats, peanuts, pistachios, black tea, coffee, and vinegar, as they exacerbate candidiasis by compromising immunity,

producing toxins, and damaging intestinal flora, or because they contain molds.[3]

Apple cider vinegar is the exception. It's a frequently recommended antifungal in homeopathic and complementary medicine. Recently, apple cider vinegar was shown to be an effective antifungal agent against the *Candida* species responsible for denture stomatitis (inflammation of the gums).[4]

Sesame oil, safflower oil, and olive oil are effective at inhibiting the growth of *Candida albicans.* In an in vitro study comparing the three, sesame oil was the most effective.[5]

Cranberry extract and cranberry juice were shown to exhibit an antiadhesion effect against *C. glabrata*, suggesting its efficacy as an oral thrush treatment.[6]

Clove and cassia cinnamon have been shown to inhibit *Candida* growth.[7]

Persian shallot (*Allium hirtifolium*) was shown to be highly effective against *C. albicans.*[8] Another study demonstrated that shallot demonstrated antifungal activity against 33 different species of *Candida.*[9]

In a small study of HIV-positive and HIV-negative women, probiotic yogurt inhibited *Candida* colonization in both groups.[10] In a study of women with vaginal candidiasis, 207 were given an oral and vaginal antifungal medication; a second group of 209 received the same treatment but added 10 applications of a vaginal probiotic. Clinical complaints persisted after treatment in nearly 80 percent of the first group, but only in 31.1 percent of the probiotic group. Thus probiotic treatment increases therapy efficacy and could prevent a relapse.[11] In a study of 276 elderly patients, eating a probiotic cheese resulted in reducing the risk of high yeast counts by 75 percent, suggesting that probiotic intervention can be effective in controlling oral *Candida*.[12]

Garlic has long been used as an antifungal in traditional and complementary medicine, and many fungi have been shown to be sensitive to garlic, including *Candida (Torulopis) glabrata, Trichophyton, Cryptococcus, Aspergillus, Trichosporon*, and *Rhodotorula*. Allicin and ajoene are the active antifungal agents in garlic, and fresh garlic is more effective than aged or freeze-dried garlic extracts.[13] In home remedies, crushed garlic is added to coconut oil or tea tree oil and applied directly to the affected area. Coconut oil has anti-fungal properties (next column), and it can soothe skin and decrease itchiness. Tea tree oil also works as a fungicide; is active against *C. albicans* as well as many other yeasts, dermatophytes, and other filamentous fungi; and has antiseptic and antimicrobial properties.[14]

Virgin coconut oil is an effective antifungal. In an in vitro study, coconut oil was shown to be active against *C. albicans* at 100 percent concentration when compared to fluconazole. Study authors concluded that especially in light of emerging drug-resistant *Candida* species, coconut oil should be used as an antifungal treatment.[15]

In vitro studies have also shown that EGCG (epigallocatechin gallate), the major catechin in green tea, is superior to fluconazole and flucytosine against dermatophytosis (fungal infection of the skin) caused by various fungi, including *Candida* and *Trichophyton rubrum* species.[16] Another in vitro study examined the effects of 23 teas and tea catechins, including EGCG, upon six different strains of fungi, five of them *Candida* species. All of the teas exhibited antifungal activity against *C. glabrata*. Several were effective against *C. albicans*, and one green tea was active against *C. parapsilosis*, but the most potent effect was seen against *C. glabrata*.[17]

An in vitro study demonstrated powerful antifungal properties of the antioxidant hydroxytyrosol against *C. albicans*. Hydroxytyrosol is found in olive oil and olive leaves.[18]

See also: Dandruff (page 222), Fungal Infections (Nails) (page 284), Vaginitis (page 442)

fungal infections (nails)

Fungal nail infections, also known as onychomycoses, are common maladies of the fingernails and toenails. They occur when a fungus enters through a small crack in your nail or an opening in the surrounding skin. Infection is more common in toenails than in fingernails, and symptoms include nail discoloration, thickened nails, and nails that become ridged and brittle and that crack easily. The most common cause of onychomycosis is a group of fungi called dermatophytes, which can cause fungal infections of the nails, skin, and hair, but yeasts and non-dermatophyte molds can cause onychomycosis as well. Whatever the cause, fungal nail infections are often difficult to cure, requiring up to a year for the affected nail to return to its normal appearance, and the most common treatments are oral or topical antifungal medications.

A review of food-based treatments for nail fungus revealed a great many home remedies, but there are few peer-reviewed research trials to demonstrate their efficacy. There is, however, strong emerging research on topical applications of essential oils derived from edible plants. Because their active compounds have such a low molecular weight, they're able to easily penetrate the nail plate and reach the fungus responsible for infection. Essential oils are a safe topical treatment, and some types have been shown to be superior to standard oral antifungal medications.[1] An overview of some of the most effective essential oils follows.

- Clove oil was shown to be an effective fungicidal for several types of fungus that cause onychomycosis, including *Candida*.

- Tea tree oil, also known as melaleuca oil, has been shown to have an antifungal effect against *Candida*, and tea tree oil nanocapsules have been shown to have an antifungal effect against the *T. rubrum* fungus.

- Thyme oil is one of the strongest essential oil antimicrobials. Thyme oil has even been shown to have antifungal effects against fluconazole-resistant *Candida*. In a study of 39 patients with onychomycosis,

60 percent saw improvement and 15 percent were cured after using a solution of thyme oil in chloroform topically for at least 3 months.

- Lavender oil has been shown to be effective against more than 40 strains of fungus that cause onychomycosis, including dermatophyte fungi and *Candida.*

- Eucalyptus oil has strong antifungal activity against many fungi and yeasts.[2] Interestingly, it is a major ingredient in Vicks VapoRub, which is a favored home remedy for nail fungus. In a study of 18 people who used Vicks VapoRub daily for 48 weeks, five people were cured of nail fungus by the end of the trial and 10 had partial clearance. Three showed no change.[3]

- Oregano oil has also been shown to be protective against at least 15 strains of fungi, including *C. albicans* and *T. rubrum.* Oregano oil was superior to tea tree oil and lavender oil against *T. mentagrophytes.*

- Sage oil is effective against many strains of fungi and yeast, including *T. rubrum* and *T. mentagrophytes.*[4]

- Myrrh oil has been shown to have powerful antifungal effects and is a recommended topical treatment for fungal infections of the skin and nails.[5]

- Turmeric oil has long been used as an antifungal and is especially effective against *T. rubrum.* Further, it has antioxidative and anti-inflammatory properties.[6]

- Garlic's antifungal effects have been extensively documented. The topical application of garlic oil is highly recommended for the treatment of nail fungus, but a longtime folk remedy recommends applying crushed raw garlic or crushed garlic sautéed in olive oil to the affected nails. There is scientific evidence to back this up: Crushing garlic yields allicin, a sulfur compound that's responsible for most of garlic's health benefits.[7]

> **BONUS TIP:** Though clinical evidence is lacking, we feel we'd be remiss if we didn't mention a few time-honored home remedies for nail fungus. Many people swear by apple cider vinegar (ACV): Mix ACV and water in equal parts and soak the affected nails for 30 minutes a day. Dry your nails thoroughly afterward. This treatment should be done for several weeks. Some people also add 1 tablespoon of ACV to water and drink it to speed healing.
>
> White vinegar is also an option, and some people have found that it works faster than ACV. Mix one part white vinegar with two parts water, and soak the affected nails for 15 to 20 minutes a day.
>
> Other home remedy food cures include the topical application of lemon juice, coconut oil, or a paste made from baking soda and water.

- The antifungal effect of shallot oil is also well established, and for some strains of fungus, shallot oil is more effective than miconazole.[8]

- Pomegranate skin extract has been shown to have potent antifungal activity against the dermatophytes *T. mentagrophytes, T. rubrum, Microsporum canis,* and *M. gypseum.*[9]

- Bergamot essential oil has been shown to have both antibacterial and antifungal properties and is effective against *Candida* species.[10]

Finally, one study examined the effects of 26 plant-derived essential oils against four common dermatophyte fungi: *M. canis, Epidermophyton floccosum, T. rubrum, and T. mentagrophytes.* Four essential oils emerged on top with the strongest antifungal activity: apricot oil, almond oil, olive oil, and peppermint oil. Combining these four oils had the strongest fungicidal effect.[11] The results of this last study open up many treatment possibilities for nail fungus: As all of the oils listed here have clinically proven antifungal effects and their potency increases in combination, you can mix and match at will or have a compounding pharmacy prepare a customized essential oil combination for you.

gallstones

Gallstones are small pieces of solid material that form in your gallbladder. They can be as small as grains of sand or as large as golf balls. The gallbladder, a small, pear-shaped organ under your liver, stores cholesterol-rich bile, an alkaline fluid that's released into your intestines after you eat to help break down fat. Most gallstones are made of cholesterol, with the remainder being pigment stones made of the liver enzyme bilirubin. Some gallstones cause no symptoms and do not require treatment, but if a gallstone lodges in a bile duct and blocks the flow of bile, it can result in intense abdominal pain. If you experience sudden, intense pain in your abdomen (especially after eating a fatty meal), a fever with chills, or jaundice (yellowing of your skin and the whites of your eyes), seek medical attention immediately. Nausea and vomiting can also be associated with a gallbladder attack, as can clay-colored stools. Eating a diet that's high in fat and cholesterol and low in fiber significantly increases your risk of gallstones, as does being overweight (especially if your weight is concentrated in your abdomen). Other factors that raise the risk of gallstones are diabetes, experiencing rapid weight loss (3 or more pounds per week), pregnancy, high triglycerides, low HDL ("good") cholesterol, and having a family history of gallstones. Your risk of gallstones increases with age, and they're more common in women.

In some cases gallstones subside on their own, but the standard treatments for gallstones are medications to dissolve the stones (which can take months) or cholecystectomy, the surgical removal of the gallbladder. A procedure known as lithotripsy, in which sound waves are aimed at the gallstones to break them into pieces, is also available, followed by medication to dissolve the pieces.

When it comes to eating for gallbladder health, it's all about prevention. A study of 101 women with gallstone disease and 204 healthy controls revealed a healthy and an unhealthy dietary pattern associated with gallstone disease. The healthy dietary pattern included eating lots of vegetables, fruits, low-fat dairy products, vegetable oil, nuts, whole grains, legumes, fruit juice, fish, and spices, plus a low salt intake. The unhealthy dietary pattern was characterized by a high intake of refined grains, tea, sugar, red meat, solid fat, soft drinks, baked potatoes, snacks, processed meats, high-fat dairy products, eggs, salt, pickled foods, and sauerkraut, and a low coffee intake.[1] On the subject of coffee alone, there has been mixed evidence in its role in preventing gallstones. But a recent metastudy that examined data from more than 227,749 people, including 11,477 cases of gallstone disease, found a positive association between coffee consumption and a reduced risk of gallstones. The effect was more pronounced in women than in men, and it was dose-dependent: The more coffee participants drank, the lower their risk of gallstones.[2] A healthy diet that is low in fat and high in fiber is the first line of defense in preventing gallstones and, along with proper exercise, will obviate most of the risk factors for developing gallstones.

Obesity increases the amount of cholesterol in bile, which can contribute to gallstone formation. But if prolonged fasting and/or rapid weight loss occur, your liver secretes extra cholesterol into bile, which increases your risk of gallstones. One study compared two groups undergoing rapid weight loss through a calorie-restricted diet of 520 to 800 calories a day for 5 weeks. The first group ate a fiber-rich diet while the second group ate a protein-rich diet. After 5 weeks, the first group lost an average of just over 24 pounds, and the second group lost an average of nearly 25 pounds. But the fiber-rich group showed significant benefits for the prevention of biliary sludge accumulation, which leads to gallstones.[3] Healthy, high-fiber foods include fruits (blueberries, chokeberries, strawberries, dates, prunes, apricots, raisins, apples, pears, and grapes); dark, leafy greens (kale, spinach, Brussels sprouts, and broccoli); legumes (lentils, beans, and split peas); whole grains (oatmeal, buckwheat, barley, bulgur, quinoa, and whole grain breads and cereals); and seeds (flaxseeds and chia seeds).

A diet that is higher in fat also protects against gallstone formation during rapid weight loss, as fat stimulates gallbladder contractility. In a metastudy of 13 trials totaling 1,836 patients undergoing weight loss through dieting or bariatric surgery, those whose weight-reducing diets were higher in fat (19 to 30 percent) experienced a reduced incidence of gallstones compared with a diet lower in fat (3 to 5 percent).[4] It's important, however, to opt for healthy fats, such as polyunsaturated fats that come from seafood, walnuts, and flaxseeds, or monounsaturated fats that come from avocados and olive oil.

Beyond this, there are certain foods that can stimulate your gallbladder to empty. (Gallstones are more likely to form when your gallbladder doesn't empty completely or often enough.) The rate of emptying varies greatly from person to person, but generally, the higher the fat content, the faster the rate of emptying. In a recent study comparing the effects of various foods on gallbladder emptying, the largest gallbladder volume change (42 percent) occurred in response to fat. Curcumin, the active compound in turmeric, caused a gallbladder volume change of 23 percent, coffee caused a gallbladder volume change of 22 percent, and tea, 18 percent.[5] Homeopathic practitioners recommend dandelion greens, red beets and beet tops, and sauerkraut and sau-erkraut juice to improve bile flow, but clinical research is inconclusive. In animal models, artichoke leaf extract has been shown to increase bile flow.[6]

Black radish has been shown to lower cholesterol, and its main secondary metabolite, glucosinolates, can decrease hepatic cholesterol levels, leading to the prevention of cholesterol gallstones. Black radish juice has been shown to dissolve gallstones in animal models.[7] Silymarin, or milk thistle, has long been used for the treatment of liver and gallbladder diseases, and it exhibits antiobesity and lipid-reducing properties that can help prevent gallbladder disease.[8] Milk thistle is available in the form of capsules, a liquid extract, and a tincture, and some forms can be used to brew tea.

gastritis

Gastritis has been used as a catchall term that refers to many ailments of the upper abdomen, but strictly speaking, gastritis is inflammation of your stomach lining. Typical symptoms include a gnawing or burning pain in your abdomen, nausea, vomiting, and a feeling of fullness in your upper abdomen after eating. Gastritis can occur suddenly and be short-lived, or it can persist over an extended period. Gastritis that lasts for many years is called atrophic gastritis, and this condition destroys stomach mucosa and eventually results in problems such as peptic ulcers, malnutrition from malabsorption problems, and even gastric cancer. There's a long list of factors that could cause gastritis or predispose you to it, including infection (bacterial, fungal, viral, or parasitic), alcohol use, cigarette smoking, stress, radiation, food allergies or sensitivities, autoimmune disorders, and the use of certain drugs, including cocaine and NSAIDs (nonsteroidal anti-inflammatory drugs) such as ibuprofen. Most often, gastritis can be attributed to long-term use of NSAIDs that irritate your stomach lining, or a bacterium known as *Helicobacter pylori*. Indeed, *H. pylori* acquired in childhood is the number one cause of chronic gastritis worldwide.[1] A fairly rare type of gastritis known as autoimmune gastritis occurs when your body develops antibodies to parietal cells (essential to the digestive process) and their components. Autoimmune gastritis leads to a vitamin B_{12} deficiency and pernicious anemia, and it is a risk factor for gastric cancer.

The most effective treatment for common gastritis is to identify the cause of the inflammation and eliminate it. Keeping track of any foods that consistently cause irritation is key; once you can identify these foods you should eliminate them from your diet. Typical food irritants include alcohol and acidic foods and beverages (such as citrus juices, citrus fruits, carbonated beverages, and coffee). Other common irritants include cigarette smoking and NSAIDs. All of these substances should be eliminated for the duration of gastritis symptoms, if not permanently.

But there are food and drink interventions you can add to your diet to help prevent the occurrence of gastritis or to reduce its duration. There is a long list of foods that have been shown to inhibit the growth of *H. pylori,* including barberry, pumpkin and pumpkin seeds, quince and quince juice, apples, arugula, mulberry leaves, Indian gooseberries, pomegranates, turmeric, grape skins and grape seeds, probiotics of the species *Lactobacillus* (found in many probiotic yogurts and also in kimchi, sauerkraut, miso, and tempeh), broccoli, cranberry juice, and hot peppers.[2] For more on these specific foods, see Ulcers (Peptic) on page 439.

In this section, we'll focus on healing foods that have exhibited the ability to reduce gastric inflammation. Nuclear factor-kappa B (NF-κB) is a proinflammatory signaling pathway. Apigenin, a flavonoid that's present in high levels in parsley and celery, was found to inhibit NF-κB activation, thus reducing the inflammatory response. Other dietary components that were shown to suppress NF-κB activation in *H. pylori* infection are curcumin, the active compound in turmeric, and capsaicin, the active compound in chile peppers.[3] Clinical trials have demonstrated curcumin's ability to reduce the symptoms of dyspepsia and ulcerative colitis, to inhibit intestinal spasms and ulcer formation, and to protect the gastrointestinal (GI) tract through its natural anti-inflammatory properties.[4] Ginger,

like turmeric, has anti-inflammatory properties and has long been used to treat gastrointestinal conditions.[5] Fennel has been shown to soothe nausea, ease stomach pain, and act as an anti-inflammatory.[6] Both ginger and fennel can be consumed as a tea, or you can chew dried fennel seeds after a meal to aid digestion and prevent bloating, gas, and GI irritation. Licorice may be even more effective, as it's highly effective in combating *H. pylori* and it stimulates the production of gastric mucus, which lends a protective coating to your esophagus, stomach lining, and any existing ulcers, making your entire digestive tract more resistant to irritating stomach acid.[7] Use caution with licorice, however: The active ingredient in licorice, glycyrrhizin, comes with a host of possible side effects, especially at high doses or when used long term. Do not eat licorice root if you are pregnant or breastfeeding or if you have heart, liver, or kidney disease; a hormone-sensitive cancer; erectile dysfunction; or diabetes. Licorice also has the potential to interfere with many medications, among them blood pressure medications, MAO antidepressants, ACE inhibitors, and diuretics; insulin; oral contraceptives; warfarin; digoxin; and corticosteroids.[8] A form of licorice from which the glycyrrhizin has been removed, called deglycyrrhizinated licorice, or DGL, is available as an herbal supplement and has far fewer potential contraindications than the whole food. In any form, if you plan to include licorice regularly in your self-care routine, it's best to consult a health-care provider. In contrast, chamomile has a similar effect but is considered generally safe, though it should also be avoided during pregnancy. An ancient remedy for relieving heartburn, indigestion, ulcers, and general stomach upset, chamomile has been shown to neutralize gastric acidity and help dispel gas and relax intestinal muscles.[9]

See also: Acid Reflux (page 148), Heartburn (page 322), Indigestion (page 345), Ulcers (Peptic) (page 439)

gingivitis

Gingivitis is inflammation of the gums (gingiva) characterized by bleeding gums, swelling, halitosis, receding gums, and gums that have taken on a red or purple hue. Gums can also appear shiny and be tender when touched. As gingivitis progresses it leads to periodontitis, an inflammatory disease that damages tissue and causes progressive loss of the bone supporting your teeth, which ultimately results in the loss of teeth. Gingivitis is caused by plaque formation below the gumline that leads to infection. The primary and most effective way to avoid gingivitis is to engage in proper dental hygiene. That means brushing at least twice a day with a soft-bristle brush, flossing at least once a day, and seeing your dentist for a professional cleaning and checkup every 6 months.

Far more than just a gum condition, gingivitis has been associated with an increased risk for several serious conditions, including heart disease, stroke, diabetes, and lung disease. Periodontal disease can make diabetes more difficult to manage, as well. Bacteria from infected gums can travel throughout your body, causing systemic infection. Gingivitis can even lead to premature birth and giving birth to a baby with a low birth weight.

Research has shown that there is a connection between vitamin C (ascorbic acid) and periodontal health. A deficiency in vitamin C leads to gingivitis as well as scurvy and bleeding gums. But increasing vitamin C consumption is an easy and highly effective means of reversing gingival damage due to deficiency and stimulating gingival cell growth.[1] Vitamin C is found in a wide variety of fruits and vegetables, including citrus fruits; tomatoes; papayas; bell peppers; broccoli; dark, leafy greens; pineapple; kiwifruit; mangoes; berries; cantaloupe; acerola cherries (West Indian cherries); gac fruit; and watermelon.

The other vitamin that plays a crucial role in preventing and treating gingivitis is vitamin D. One 3-month study found that vitamin D supplementation improved gingivitis scores in direct proportion to the amount administered. Vitamin D significantly reduced inflammation in all three treatment groups, but the group that received 2,000 international units

(IU) had the most improvement in gingival scores and experienced improvement earlier than groups that received 1,000 or 500 IU of vitamin D.[2] Another study evaluated the association between calcium and vitamin D levels and oral health in 106 women. A deficiency in calcium was observed in 59 percent of the women and a deficiency in vitamin D in 71 percent. Further, 72 percent consumed soft drinks on a daily basis. With these risk factors in place, it's not surprising, then, that 100 percent of the study participants exhibited signs of gingivitis. The one-third of the group with the highest number of caries (cavities) had significantly lower calcium and vitamin D levels than the other women, as well as significantly higher protein intake, daily consumption of soft drinks, plaque scores, and sugar intake compared to the rest of the women.[3] To increase vitamin D levels, get safe exposure to sunlight, and eat foods such as dairy products, cod liver oil, eggs, fish and shellfish, mushrooms, and tofu. To boost your calcium, eat dairy products; dark, leafy greens; nuts; salmon; soy milk; almonds; tofu; black-eyed peas; green peas; baked beans; and oranges.[4] Avoid foods that are high in sugar, especially soft drinks.

Probiotics have also proven effective at treating gingivitis. In one study, 59 patients with moderate to severe gingivitis were divided into three groups: Two received different strains of *Lactobacillus reuteri* and one group received a placebo. After 2 weeks, plaque fell significantly in both of the probiotic groups, and gum health improved, as well.[5] And in a rather unusual study, 28 volunteers with healthy gingiva (gums) drank a probiotic milk drink daily for 4 weeks; a control group was not given a probiotic food or drink. After 2 weeks, they were asked not to brush their teeth for the remaining 14 days of the study period. All the participants experienced increased inflammation after they ceased brushing, but the probiotic group had significantly lower clinical indications of gingivitis. Researchers concluded that probiotics reduce the effects of plaque-induced gingival inflammation.[6] Probiotics are found in many fermented foods, including yogurt, kimchi, kefir, tempeh, natto, sauerkraut, and pickles.

In cases where you're unable to brush after eating, chewing sugar-free gum is recommended. It's been shown to help clear away plaque, and in a study of 220 participants who did not brush the teeth of their lower jaw but did chew a sugar-free gum five times a day for 10 minutes, chewing gum improved gum health.[7]

Curcumin, the active ingredient in turmeric, has been used in a number of cleaning agents to combat gingivitis. In one study, curcumin gel was shown to be effective in the prevention of plaque and gingivitis, though it should not be used as a substitute for regular brushing with toothpaste. Curcumin is effective for periodontal health because it exhibits antioxidant, anti-inflammatory, antiviral, antibacterial, antifungal, and antiseptic properties.[8] Massaging teeth and gums with roasted, ground turmeric has been shown to eliminate pain and swelling, and using a paste twice a day made from 1 teaspoon of turmeric, ½ teaspoon of salt, and ½ teaspoon of mustard oil provides relief from gingivitis and periodontitis.[9]

A mouthwash containing a 2 percent green tea extract was found to be effective at reducing plaque and bacteria on the gums.[10] But green tea may be far more effective when it's consumed. A metastudy of the use of green tea in periodontal health determined that drinking green tea regularly is beneficial due to its polyphenolic content, especially the amino acid theanine, and catechins, which have antioxidant properties.[11] Green tea protects against bacterial-induced dental caries and eradicates halitosis through the modification of sulfur components. Oral cavity oxidative stress (when your body has difficulty counteracting the presence of free radicals in your

mouth) and inflammation may likewise be reduced.[12]

A number of food extracts have been shown to combat gingivitis, as well. In regard to the gingivitis-associated bacteria *Actinomyces naeslundii* and *Prevotella intermedia*, extracts of cranberry, shiitake mushroom, raspberry, Guinness beer, green tea, black tea, and red chicory all showed antibacterial activity.[13] Other foods that have exhibited in vitro antibacterial activity in regard to *Streptococci* strains, which contribute to periodontal disease, are apples, red grape seeds, red wine, nutmeg, caraway seeds, coffee, chicory, and mushrooms. In vivo anticaries activity has been shown by cranberry, licorice root, myrtle extract, garlic extract, cocoa extracts, and propolis (a honeybee product).[14]

Oil pulling has been shown to reduce the presence of *Streptococcus mutans*,[15] the main cause of tooth decay and dental plaque,[16] and many people experience a teeth-whitening effect, as well. Oil pulling is simply the practice of swishing an edible oil—such as sunflower, sesame, olive, or coconut oil—in your mouth for 10 to 15 minutes. It works by "pulling" bacteria and other disease-promoting microorganisms from your mouth and should be followed with normal brushing. Studies using sunflower oil and sesame oil have demonstrated the efficacy of oil pulling to treat plaque-induced gingivitis. One study had 60 subjects with plaque-induced gingivitis try oil pulling using coconut oil for 30 days, in addition to their regular oral hygiene routines. Gingival indices were measured at days 1, 7, 15, and 30. A statistically significant decrease in plaque and gingival indices was noticed from day 7 onward, and the scores continued to decrease during the period of study.[17]

See also: Dry Mouth (page 252), Halitosis (page 307), Tooth Decay (page 435)

glaucoma

Glaucoma is a group of diseases that damage the optic nerve. It is the leading cause of blindness worldwide and can occur in one or both eyes. There is no cure for glaucoma and treatments are designed to slow the progression of the disease, so regular optical exams are essential for early detection of glaucoma and preserving vision. The major antagonist in glaucoma is eye pressure. When fluid doesn't drain from your eye properly it builds up, exerting increasing pressure on your optic nerve.

There are conventional treatments for glaucoma but no cure, so healing foods for this condition are foremost about prevention and secondarily about helping to slow glaucoma's progression. A recent metastudy found that flavonoids help improve visual function in patients with glaucoma and slow loss of vision. Flavonoids are plant-based polyphenols found in many foods and in particular in berries, citrus fruits, dark chocolate, red wine, and tea. They're thought to protect against oxidative stress in retinal ganglion cells and to improve ocular bloodflow. What's more, flavonoids appear to exert a beneficial effect in a short period of time (6 months or less).[1] The flavonoid resveratrol, found in wine, grapes, peanuts, pistachios, berries, chocolate, and cocoa, has been shown to protect against vascular dysfunction in the retina, exert an antioxidant effect, and induce bloodflow elevation, which could prevent vascular damage and death of optic nerve cells in patients with glaucoma.[2] As oxidative stress has been shown to play a role in the pathogenesis of primary open-angle glaucoma (OAG) and primary angle-closure glaucoma (the two most common types), and as levels of vitamins C and E have been found to be lower in the aqueous humor (fluid of the eye) of glaucoma patients,[3] antioxidant flavonoids are certainly recommended.

In a study of 584 African-American women, 77 were found to have a diagnosis of glaucoma in at least one eye. Women who ate three or more servings of fruit or fruit juices a day were 79 percent less likely to develop glaucoma than women who ate less than one serving a day. Eating collard greens or kale more than once a week decreased the odds of glaucoma by 57 percent compared to women who ate greens less than once a month. This study also identified some specific foods that had a particularly protective effect against glaucoma: fresh oranges, fresh peaches, collard greens, kale, spinach, and carrots. These foods are high in vitamin A, vitamin C, and carotenoids, all of which are known to be beneficial for eye health.[7]

A study of more than 3,500 people looked at the roles of specific nutrients in the origin of open-angle glaucoma (OAG). The most common form of glaucoma, OAG occurs when fluid passes out of your eye too slowly and damages your optic nerve, even though the drain-age angle is open. Over a mean follow-up period of 9.7 years, 91 participants developed OAG. Compared to the participants without glaucoma, OAG patients had a lower intake of beta-carotene, retinol equivalents (vitamin A), vitamin B_1 (thiamin), and vitamin B_{12} and a higher intake of magnesium and vitamin E. After excluding data taken from those who took supplements, researchers concluded that people with a high intake of retinol equivalents (vitamin A) or vitamin B_1 have a twofold lower risk of OAG compared to those with a low intake of these nutrients, and people with a high intake of magnesium have a threefold increase in risk of OAG compared to those with a low intake.[8] Good food sources of vitamin A and beta-carotene, a precursor to vitamin A, include eggs; whole milk; cheese; carrots; sweet potatoes; pumpkin; apricots; melon; and dark, leafy greens. Sources of vitamin B_1 (thiamin) include whole grain cereals, long-grain rice, trout, tuna, mussels, acorn squash, and black beans. If you want to reduce your magnesium intake, avoid or cut back on foods such as ground beef, chicken breast, soy milk, nuts, avocados, baked potatoes, instant oatmeal, kidney beans, and bananas.

Research has also revealed a connection between omega-3 and omega-6 essential fatty acids and glaucoma. In a large, multiyear study, researchers tracked the dietary habits of 17,128 volunteers for an average of 8.2 years. At the outset of the study all volunteers were glaucoma-free, but by the end there were 156 cases of glaucoma. While there was no association between glaucoma and these two fatty acids individually, the ratio of omega-3s to omega-6s made a difference:

Subjects with the highest omega-3-to-omega-6 ratio intake showed a 91 percent increase in their risk of developing glaucoma. For subjects 40 years old and older, those with the highest omega-3-to-omega-6 fatty acid ratio intake had a 143 percent increase in their risk of developing glaucoma.[9] Simply put, *increase* your intake of anti-inflammatory omega-3s by eating foods such as salmon, mackerel, herring, sardines, tuna, walnuts, walnut oil, flaxseeds, and flaxseed oil, and *decrease* your intake of proinflammatory omega-6s by reducing or eliminating vegetable oils such as safflower, canola, grape seed, sunflower, soybean, sesame, and corn oil. Another study found an association between a low intake of fatty fish and walnuts and primary open-angle glaucoma, suggesting a protective effect from omega-3s.[10]

See also: High Blood Pressure (Hypertension) (page 327)

gout

Gout is a type of inflammatory arthritis caused by a buildup of uric acid in your blood. Uric acid is created when your body breaks down purines, which are naturally occurring compounds found in your body and in almost all foods. Excess uric acid leads to the formation of uric acid crystals, known as urate, that accumulate in the lubricating synovial fluid around joints. If you picture tiny sandspurs in your synovial fluid you're not far off, and you can see why gout is so terribly painful. The condition is marked by severe pain, redness, swelling, tenderness, and warmth in any joint, but most commonly in the big toe. Gout attacks decrease in severity over a few days and usually subside completely within 10 days. Chronic gout can occur if uric acid levels remain elevated, eventually leading to joint damage. Hyperuricemia, the state of having too much uric acid in your blood, increases your risk of heart disease, kidney disease, high cholesterol, high blood pressure, and diabetes.

To lower your risk of painful gout attacks, maintain a healthy weight (being overweight increases your risk of gout) and stay hydrated. Sufficient hydration helps flush uric acid out of your body. Copious amounts of water and herbal teas are the best choices for gout sufferers, and sweetened sodas should be eliminated. High-fructose corn syrup is high in purines and leads to the production of uric acid, which increases your risk of gout. Some researchers have cited the rise in consumption of high-fructose corn syrup as the cause of the rising incidence of gout in the United States.[1] You should also limit your alcohol intake, as having more than two drinks a day increases your risk of a gout attack, and steer clear of beer entirely, as it's high in purines. If you're wondering about your morning joe habit, there's good news for you: A number of studies have shown that coffee actually reduces uric acid levels, increases insulin sensitivity, and enhances renal urate excretion. The more coffee you drink, the lower your risk of gout—and that's true for decaf and regular.[2]

As for foods, you'll need to significantly reduce if not eliminate any foods that are high in purines. At the top of the list are meats. (In fact, some doctors say the single best thing you can do to prevent gout is to eat less meat.) Some of the foods highest in purines are listed in "Healing Foods for Gout Prevention."

One study conducted a cross-sectional analysis of nutrition and serum uric acid in 12,765 subjects. Lower levels of uric acid were found in people who consumed more carbohydrates, calcium, and vitamin B_2, while a higher fat intake was associated with a higher concentration of uric acid. More specifically, a high intake of dairy products, high-fiber bread, cereals, and fruits was

healing foods
FOR GOUT PREVENTION

It seems obvious, but it's true that consuming simple foods and beverages will help you avoid a painful affliction that we have long associated with well-fed royalty. Here are some good foods (and drinks) for people with gout and some others to avoid.

Foods to Eat and Drink

- Foods rich in vitamin C (omitting those that are highest in fructose): bananas; oranges; tomatoes; blueberries; strawberries; dark, leafy greens; kiwifruit; cranberries; blackberries; and papayas
- Cherries and cherry products (juice, extract)
- Coffee
- Low-fat dairy products: skim milk, yogurt, and low-fat cottage cheese
- Water

Foods to Avoid

- High-purine foods: sardines, liver, beef, ox, bacon, wild game, dried mushrooms, brewer's yeast, chicken, duck, anchovies, crab, fish roe or caviar, herring, mackerel, trout, sardines, shrimp, and meat products such as stocks and gravies
- Beer
- Excessive alcohol consumption of any type
- Any food or beverage with high-fructose corn syrup (HFCS), especially sodas and processed foods sweetened with HFCS

Foods to Limit

- Foods that are high in fructose: applesauce, honey, fruit juices, canned fruits, watermelon, dates, apples, raisins, dried figs, mangoes, and pears
- Foods that contain moderate amounts of purines: asparagus, broccoli, cauliflower, oats, mushrooms, spinach, lentils, peas, and lima beans

associated with lower uric acid, while a high intake of meat, eggs, beer, and liquor (but not wine) was associated with elevated levels of uric acid.[3] A study of more than 9,000 people found that those with gout (13.8 percent) had higher body mass indices (BMIs), triglycerides, total cholesterol, and LDL cholesterol, as well as larger waist circumferences, than those without gout. They also had lower HDL cholesterol. Further, those with gout had a significantly lower intake of vegetables and dairy products and a higher intake of alcohol. Vitamin A, vitamin B_2, vitamin C, fiber, folate, and calcium were all lower in the group with gout, as well.[4] All of these results suggest that gout sufferers tend to have an overall poorer diet than those who don't develop gout.

Some people wonder if they should reduce or eliminate vegetables that contain a moderate or high level of purines, but the health benefits of these foods are undisputed. Further, some studies have concluded that purines from vegetable sources do not contribute to elevated uric acid levels[5] and that vegetables are beneficial for preventing gout because they reduce insulin resistance.[6] For these reasons, we're including high- or moderate-level vegetables in our list of foods to limit, rather than avoid. For gout prevention, it's far more important to eat a healthy, balanced diet and eliminate the meat-based sources of purines, as well as any form of high-fructose corn syrup.

Much research has been done on the protective role of vitamin C for gout, with conflicting results. Some studies found no benefit,[7] while others found a modest benefit at best,[8] and still others demonstrated that vitamin C clearly lowered uric acid levels.[9] A review of some of the very latest studies, however, reveals overwhelmingly positive results in terms of vitamin C's ability to lower uric acid levels, so we do recommend vitamin C as a gout-prevention tool.[10]

Now what about specific foods that can prevent gout attacks? The best individual healing food for gout is cherries. A large metastudy concluded that eating cherries results in fewer gout attacks. Interestingly, two servings of cherries per day had a better effect than one, and three servings had a better effect than two—but the trend didn't continue for those who ate four or more servings a day. Further, this study concluded that whole cherries, rather than cherry extract, were more effective for preventing gout.[11] Another study had 633 gout sufferers record information about their gout attacks and their exposure to risk factors for 1 year. Researchers found that in the 2 days leading up to a gout attack, cherry intake resulted in a 35 percent lower risk of gout attack compared to no cherry intake; in this study, cherry extract intake produced similar results. When cherry intake was combined with the use of allopurinol (a drug that decreases uric acid in the blood), risk of gout attacks was 75 percent lower.[12]

Low-fat or skim milk and yogurt are also recommended to reduce serum uric acid and gout flare-ups. People who drink milk one or more times a day have been shown to have lower serum uric acid levels than those who drink no milk, and those who eat yogurt at least every other day have been shown to have significantly lower uric acid levels than those who eat no yogurt.[13]

hair loss

Unless you've hit the genetic jackpot, you can expect to experience androgenetic alopecia, or the common male- or female-pattern baldness that is part of the normal aging process and affects some 80 million people in the United States.[1] It's normal to shed anywhere between 50 and 150 hairs a day, but as we age, both men and women experience a higher rate of shedding hair, a slower rate of hair growth, and thinning in individual strands of hair. In both sexes, hair loses color and the scalp becomes increasingly visible. In typical male-pattern baldness, a hormone known as dihydrotestosterone (DHT) inhibits the supply of nutrients to your hair follicles, resulting in shrinking follicles and thinner, finer hair that eventually doesn't grow back at all.

For normal hair loss associated with aging, is it possible to turn back the hands of time through dietary changes? A number of studies have indicated that the main nutritional causes of hair loss are a lack of protein, iron, essential fatty acids, and/or zinc. (There is also some evidence that deficiencies in vitamin A, selenium, and biotin result in hair loss, though studies have reached varying conclusions.)[2] So it makes sense that the first nutritional course in preventing hair loss, whether it's an inherited condition or brought on by environmental conditions, is to make sure you're not deficient in these vital nutrients.

Hair is a protein fiber (the same is true for nails), so you'll need protein to grow hair and to keep existing hair strong. Protein is also required to pro-duce keratin, a key structural component in hair. To pack in the protein, lean meats are a fine choice—one roasted turkey breast contains a whopping 255 grams (g) of protein[3]—but nuts and nut butters, eggs, black beans, kidney beans, pinto beans, and chickpeas are also excellent sources of protein. Chopped walnuts contain about 9 g of protein per ½ cup,[4] and all the beans listed here, including chickpeas, contain about 41 g of protein per cup.

Marine proteins, however, may be especially effective at treating hair loss. This is because in addition to protein, many types of seafood contain abundant amounts of zinc, iron, and fatty acids. A 2012 study of women with female-pattern hair loss (FPHL) found that women who took a marine-based supplement experienced a 125 percent increase in scalp hair after 180 days,[5] and a 2015 study on an extra-strength form of the same supplement produced even more impressive results: Volunteers saw a 32 percent increase in hair after 90 days of treatment and less hair shedding after hair washing.[6] To get similar results through whole foods, the best types of seafood for hair growth are salmon, which contains omega-3 fatty acids that keep your hair conditioned, and oysters and clams, both packed with zinc and iron. Vegetarian sources of omega-3s include nuts (especially walnuts); flaxseeds; flaxseed oil; and dark, leafy greens.

Female-pattern hair loss is reported to affect more than 50 percent of women over the age of 50. Some of the most promising research on reversing FPHL has recently been released in the *Journal of Cosmetic Dermatology*. Subjects in this study received a nutritional supplement containing omega-3 and omega-6 essential fatty acids and antioxidants for 6 months. More specifically, they consisted of 460 mg fish oil, 460 mg black currant seed oil, 5 mg vitamin E, 30 mg vitamin C, and 1 mg lycopene. The results were overwhelmingly positive: After 6 months, 89.9 percent of subjects reported a reduction in hair loss, 86.1 percent reported an improvement in hair diameter, and 87.3 percent reported an improvement in hair density.[7] To achieve similar results, choose foods high in omega-3s, such as cold-water fish (salmon, herring, mackerel, sardines, and trout), walnuts, and flaxseeds. Most people don't need to add omega-6s to their diet, but sources of this fatty acid include vegetable oils such as safflower, canola, grape seed, sunflower, soybean, sesame, and corn oil. Antioxidants are found in abundance in fresh fruits and vegetables and also in tea, coffee, red wine, and cocoa. Sources of antioxidants include pineapple, berries, tomatoes, red grapes, red cabbage, kale, spinach, arugula, onions, apples, broccoli, soybeans, apricots, beets, cantaloupe, carrots, mangoes, oranges, winter squash, yellow and orange peppers, green tea, dark chocolate, and papayas.

A recent study has shed light on the role of iron in hair loss. A total of 210 patients with either female- or male-pattern hair loss were compared to 210 healthy controls without hair loss. Patients' serum ferritin concentrations—an indirect indicator of iron levels—were significantly lower in the women with FPHL, at about 49 micrograms per liter (mcg/l) compared to nearly 78 mcg/l in the women with no hair loss. In men, 22.7 percent of the MPHL patients had iron levels below 70 mcg/l, while none of the healthy age-matched males did. These results show a strong correlation between iron and hair loss, especially in premenopausal FPHL.[8] In another study that looked at the roles of iron and vitamin D_2

in female hair loss, researchers found similar deficiencies: Those with hair loss had significantly lower iron and vitamin D_2 levels than age-matched controls.[9] Iron-rich foods include prunes, oatmeal, spinach, potatoes, raisins, and blackstrap molasses. To increase your absorption of iron, eat foods that are rich in vitamin C, such as citrus fruits; bell peppers; broccoli; dark, leafy greens; guavas; hot peppers; kiwifruit; mangoes; papayas; and tomatoes. For vitamin D, eat dairy products, cod liver oil, eggs, fish and shellfish, mushrooms, and tofu.

Zinc seems to be a super nutrient when it comes to preventing and treating hair loss. Researchers compared the zinc levels of 50 people with hair loss due to alopecia areata to 50 healthy controls and found that all of the alopecia patients had significantly lower zinc levels. Further, the lower the zinc level, the worse the alopecia in terms of severity, duration, and resistance to therapies.[11] Another study examined the serum zinc and copper levels in 312 men and women experiencing hair loss. No matter the cause of the hair loss, all subjects had significantly lower zinc levels than controls. (Copper levels were not significantly different.)[12] A study of women who experienced hair loss after surgery found that low levels of zinc and iron are good predictors of hair loss. Fortunately, zinc supplementation can stop hair loss in the majority of these cases.[13] And, given that hair loss is one of the hallmarks of zinc deficiency, it makes sense to increase your intake of this vital nutrient. Food sources of zinc include oysters, walnuts, spinach, eggs, sunflower seeds, green peas, wheat germ, oatmeal, and chickpeas.

As for healing foods you can apply topically, though there are a great many home remedies out there (among them onion juice, garlic, lavender oil, licorice root, and green tea), clinical trials on these treatments are lacking. Coconut oil, however, has been shown to protect hair against protein loss,[14] and rosemary oil has been shown to increase hair growth comparable to minoxidil (Rogaine)—and with less scalp itching.[15]

BONUS TIP: A recent study found that a supplement containing *Cistanche tubulosa* (a desert plant used in traditional Chinese medicine) and *Laminaria japonica* (an edible brown seaweed) promoted hair growth in people with mild to moderate hair loss. After 16 weeks of supplementation, volunteers saw a 13 percent increase in hair density and a 27 percent increase in hair diameter. The supplement was also effective at treating scalp inflammation and dandruff.[10]

See also: Adrenal Exhaustion/Adrenal Fatigue (page 153), Dandruff (page 222), Lupus (page 370), Thyroid Disease (page 429)

halitosis

The main cause of halitosis, or bad breath, is the breakdown of food particles in your mouth. As any organic compound breaks down it releases an odor, and when food particles become lodged between your teeth, in your gums, or on the rough surface of your tongue, bad breath is inevitable. Most halitosis subsides after routine brushing and flossing. Mouthwash can temporarily alleviate halitosis by killing the bacteria that cause bad breath, but mouthwash also contains alcohol and other harsh chemicals that many people want to avoid.

We all know the foods that cause bad breath—garlic, onions, fish (especially tuna), coffee, and horseradish are among the worst offenders. But are there foods that can alleviate this embarrassing condition and leave your mouth feeling *minty* fresh?

You guessed it—mint and peppermint are among the best halitosis-busting food remedies. Drinking mint tea with your meal lends your mouth a fresh taste and aroma and washes away food particles that can cause bad breath. For even more potency, chew on mint leaves. Mint is easy to grow in a kitchen garden, and you can munch on a leaf or two throughout the day as needed, and especially after meals.

Another quick fix is to munch on any unprocessed food that's crunchy and relatively low in sugar—we're talking celery, apples, water chestnuts, bell peppers, radishes, or carrots. These foods scrub your teeth and stimulate saliva production, cleansing your mouth of any leftover food particles that might stick around and cause bad breath.

Other food and beverage remedies combat bad breath on the microbial level by ridding your mouth of the bacteria that causes halitosis. Black and green tea are especially effective. The polyphenols in tea prevent the growth of bacteria that can cause bad breath, and they cut down on the bacteria's production of foul-smelling by-products.[1]

The probiotics found in yogurt inhibit bad breath for exactly the same reason. A Japanese study found that volunteers with halitosis who ate 3 ounces of yogurt twice a day had decreased levels of hydrogen sulfide, a compound that causes halitosis.[2] Several more recent studies also found that probiotics can prevent the proliferation of odor-causing bacteria in your mouth.[3] Though these studies used probiotic lozenges or supplements, it stands to reason that foods containing probiotics, such as yogurt and fermented foods, can achieve similar results. Probiotic mouthwashes, lozenges, and gums are now readily available for the treatment of halitosis. A halitosis remedy that may sound strange to Western ears is the age-old Indian custom of oil pulling. Oil pulling is simply the practice of swishing an edible oil—such as sunflower, sesame, olive, or coconut oil—in your mouth for 10 to 15 minutes. It works by "pulling" bacteria and other disease-promoting microorganisms from your mouth and should be followed up with normal brushing. In one study, one group swished with sesame oil for 10 to 15 minutes per day for 14 days, while the control group swished with a normal mouthwash for 1 minute per day for 14 days. The results? Oil pulling was just as effective as the oral mouthwash at combating bad breath, and the group who tried oil pulling actually reported higher satisfaction in a self-assessment of their breath.[4] Oil pulling has also been shown to reduce the presence of *Streptococcus mutans*,[5] the main cause of tooth decay and plaque in the mouth,[6]

and many people experience a teeth-whitening effect, as well. With its bevy of benefits, oil pulling can be an excellent way to promote overall oral health without using the harsh chemicals found in conventional mouthwashes.

Halitosis is a common condition that can be remedied through simple food and beverage interventions and regular oral hygiene. But if it persists, it can be a sign of an underlying condition; it's not uncommon to experience halitosis as a result of sinusitis, bronchitis, tonsillitis, thrush, postnasal drip, periodontal disease, or even the common cold, for example. Research has also shown a clear association between halitosis and gastrointestinal complaints such as GERD (gastroesophageal reflux disease) and *Helicobacter pylori* infection.[7] But the good news in all of these cases is that treating the underlying condition gets rid of the halitosis. If you experience halitosis that develops rather suddenly or that does not respond to treatment and proper dental hygiene, see your doctor for a diagnosis and treatment plan.

See also: Acid Reflux (page 148), Gastritis (page 290), Gingivitis (page 293), Tooth Decay (page 435)

headaches/migraines

There are dozens of potential causes of headaches and migraines, and there are many types of headaches. But every type falls into one of the two overarching categories of *primary* or *secondary* headaches. The healing foods suggestions below apply to primary headaches. Most secondary headaches are far more serious medical events—some with life-threatening causes—and should be treated by a doctor.

A primary headache isn't a symptom of some other condition but a condition in and of itself. Examples include tension headaches; cluster headaches, which are recurring, severe headaches that occur on one side of your head; migraines; chronic daily headaches, or recurring headaches of unspecific origin; and trigeminal autonomic cephalalgia (TAC), a type of headache that occurs on one side of your head in the trigeminal nerve area and produces accompanying symptoms such as a drooping eyelid, eye watering, or a runny nose. (TACs include cluster headaches as well as other subtypes, such as paroxysmal hemicrania.) Primary headaches can be triggered by many potential causes—far too many to list here. Some of the more common triggers are stress, insomnia, hormonal changes, certain medications, red wine and beer (usually in response to the sulfite content in these beverages), caffeine, nitrates (commonly found in processed foods), MSG, various food sensitivities, and skipping meals.

Secondary headaches, on the other hand, are symptoms of an underlying condition. Again, there are multiple causes, from the innocuous and short-lived "ice cream headache" all the way to a severe headache that arises from an emergency event such as a brain aneurysm or carbon monoxide poisoning.

One of the first food-related treatments for a headache or migraine is to identify and eliminate the responsible food trigger. Common culprits are monosodium glutamate (MSG), sulfites (found in beer, wine, and processed foods such as meats, fish, fruits, and vegetables preserved with sulfites), caffeine, chocolate, aged cheeses, fermented foods, potato chips, nuts, and tomato products. There are many other foods that trigger headaches in people;

the key is to keep a food diary and note which food or foods consistently cause a headache. One study found that those who adopted a vegan diet for 4 weeks experienced less pain, less headache intensity, and fewer headaches during the study period. (Subjects also lost an average of 8 pounds and saw their total cholesterol fall by 14 mg/dl and their LDL cholesterol fall by 9 mg/dl.) Researchers speculate that the improvements could be due to any of the following factors: (1) a common trigger food, such as meat or dairy, was eliminated; (2) meats increase inflammation, and eliminating meat decreased neurogenic inflammation and neurogenic vasodilation; (3) plants, on the other hand, are high in antioxidants and anti-inflammatory compounds, and they decrease inflammation; (4) weight loss has been shown to reduce pain and lessen the frequency of headaches; and (5) plant-based diets can lower blood pressure and induce hormonal changes, which can favorably reduce headache symptoms.[1] Bottom line? If you suffer from chronic headaches or migraines, these results make a persuasive case for reducing the amount of meat in your diet, or even eliminating it entirely, and increasing your fruit and vegetable intake.

One trigger to note in particular is a naturally occurring compound called tyramine that's produced by the break-down of the amino acid tyrosine. Tyramine is found in your body, and it's produced in foods as a result of fermentation, aging, or spoilage; its levels increase as foods age. It's such a common trigger of headaches and migraines that the National Headache Foundation has created the Low Tyramine Headache Diet. Their full recommendations can be found at www.headaches.org, but generally, the diet advises migraine sufferers to avoid aged, dried, fermented, pickled, salted, or smoked meat products; aged cheeses; fermented vegetable products such as miso, olives, pickles, sauerkraut, soy sauce, and teriyaki sauce; vegetables such as broad beans, fava beans, and snow peas; all nuts and nut products; most alcoholic beverages; and food additives or ingredients such as brewer's yeast, hydrolyzed or auto-lyzed yeast, meat extracts, meat tenderizers, MSG, nitrates, nitrites, seasoned salt, and yeast and yeast extracts.[2]

But what can you consume to prevent headaches or treat them? The American Academy of Neurology and the Canadian Headache Society have recommended the following nonpharmacological means to prevent migraines: butterbur, riboflavin, magnesium, and coenzyme Q_{10} (CoQ_{10}).[3] Butterbur, a plant in the sunflower family, has been studied extensively and shown to be effective at preventing migraines, but it should be used with caution because it has the potential to damage your liver.[4] Riboflavin is found in foods such as milk or soy milk, spinach, and red meats, and magnesium is found in sesame seeds; sunflower seeds; almonds; oats; dark, leafy greens; avocados; and bananas. CoQ_{10} is a naturally occurring compound in your body and is found in high amounts in beef (especially beef liver), herring, rainbow trout, mackerel, sardines, peanuts, pistachios, sesame seeds, broccoli, cauliflower, oranges, strawberries, eggs, and soybean oil.

Research just out shows that omega-3 fatty acids can decrease the frequency of migraines. This study analyzed data from 105 migraine sufferers, ages 15 to 50, and found that lower intakes of both DHA (docosahexaenoic acid) and EPA (eicosapentaenoic acid) were associated with more frequent migraine attacks.[5] Put another way, increasing DHA and EPA consumption results in fewer migraines. Another study of chronic headache sufferers found that an increase in omega-3s along with a concurrent decrease in omega-6s led to fewer headaches per month and a significant decrease in psychological distress, as well as improvements in overall well-being.[6] To increase your omega-3 intake, eat wild-caught, cold-water fish such as salmon, herring, halibut, mackerel, sardines, and tuna; flaxseeds and flaxseed oil; walnuts; dark, leafy greens; and chia seeds. To decrease omega-6s, eliminate or cut back on certain vegetable oils (safflower, canola, grape seed, sunflower, soybean, sesame, and corn) and sunflower seeds.

B vitamins also play a role in headache and migraine prevention and treatment. Riboflavin (vitamin B_2) has been used to reduce the frequency of migraine headaches.[7] Doses of 200 or 400 milligrams (mg) a day have been found to be effective at reducing headache frequency, intensity, and duration.[8] Riboflavin is found in milk, eggs, malted barley, almonds, beef liver, mackerel, salmon, chicken, broccoli, spinach, asparagus, mushrooms, whole wheat bread, cheese, and yeast.

A study on pyridoxine—a form of vitamin B_6—found that consuming an additional 80 mg of pyridoxine a day led to a significant decrease in headache severity and the duration of a headache attack. It did not, however, find that vitamin B_6 decreased the frequency of attacks.[9] Some of the best food sources of vitamin B_6 are salmon, russet potatoes, turkey, chicken, avocados, spinach, bananas, dried plums, hazelnuts, beans, papayas, oranges, cantaloupe, fortified breakfast cereals, pistachios, and sunflower seeds.[10]

Another nutrient, magnesium, has been shown to be effective at preventing headaches. Evidence shows that those who suffer from cluster headaches and migraines have lower magnesium levels than those who don't.[11] One study showed that migraine attack frequency was reduced by more than 41 percent in those who received magnesium supplementation.[12] The best food sources of magnesium are dairy products, oatmeal, bran flakes, asparagus, beets, peas, broccoli, bananas, almonds, sesame seeds, cashews, Brazil nuts, sunflower seeds, peanuts, and walnuts.

Finally, one of the simplest headache cures is . . . to eat. Hypoglycemia, or having an abnormally low blood sugar level, has triggered headaches and migraines in people.[13] To prevent a hypoglycemia-induced migraine, don't skip meals, and if you're trying to lose weight, do so gradually rather than by resorting to "crash" diets—you'll have better success with keeping the weight off, too. Eat smaller, more frequent meals to avoid hypoglycemia, and eat plant-based proteins (tofu, nuts, nut butters, beans, legumes, and seeds), complex carbohydrates and fiber (buckwheat, barley, bulgur, whole oats, whole grain breads, quinoa, and farro) to stay full longer and keep blood sugar levels stable.

heart disease (cardiovascular disease)

Heart disease is the number one cause of death worldwide, accounting for more deaths than all types of cancer combined. It's responsible for 17.3 million deaths per year, and this number is expected to grow to more than 23.6 million by 2030.[1] Heart disease, also known as cardiovascular disease (CVD), encompasses several types of heart and vascular conditions, among them coronary artery disease, heart attack (myocardial infarction), congestive heart failure, congenital heart disease, atrial fibrillation, peripheral artery disease, hypertensive heart disease, rheumatic heart disease, and stroke. Coronary artery disease (CAD) is the most common type of heart disease in the United States.

The risk factors for any type of heart disease are smoking, overweight and obesity, high LDL ("bad") cholesterol, high blood pressure (hypertension), physical inactivity, excessive alcohol consumption, diabetes, poor nutrition, and chronic stress. Your risk of heart disease increases as you age, and those with a family history of heart disease are at an increased risk, as well. As with the related conditions hypertension, type 2 diabetes, and stroke, a great many of the risk factors for heart disease can be ameliorated or outright eliminated through lifestyle changes. In this section, we'll discuss nutritional interventions that can prevent and even reverse heart disease, but be sure to check out "Eat and Drink for Your Heart's Content" on page 318 for a handy list of specific healing foods.

Several key risk factors for cardiovascular disease—hypertension, poor diet, overweight and obesity, high cholesterol, diabetes, and excessive consumption of alcohol—are all related to nutrition. There is overwhelming evidence that a Mediterranean-style diet high in fruits, vegetables, whole grains, seafood rich in polyunsaturated fatty acids (PUFAs), seeds, legumes, nuts, and dairy products, and that features little or no red meat, sweetened beverages, desserts, and saturated fats supports cardiovascular health.[2] There is just as much evidence showing that the opposite dietary pattern greatly contributes to cardiovascular risk factors and leads directly to cardiovascular disease. Processed food and trans fats should be avoided entirely.

Further, in the Mediterranean diet, the primary source of added fat comes from monounsaturated olive oil, which has been shown to decrease C-reactive protein and interleukin-6 (both markers of inflammation) in the endothelium and to increase vasodilation and vasoconstriction.[8] The Mediterranean diet also encourages wine in moderation for cardiovascular benefits.[9] (The American Heart Association defines drinking in moderation as no more than two drinks per day for men and no more than one for women.)[10] Wine consumption has been found to increase longevity overall.[11] Noting that the Mediterranean diet has long been associated with lower incidence of cardiovascular disease, a recent study of nearly 33,000 women set out to examine its effect on more specific types of CVD. Researchers found that better adherence to a Mediterranean diet was associated with a lower risk of heart attack, heart failure, and ischemic stroke.[12] Another recent study that focused upon 7,447 people at high risk of cardiovascular disease found that the Mediterranean diet reduced the risk of major cardiovascular events by approximately 30 percent overall. In this study, participants followed a Mediterranean diet supplemented with either olive oil or nuts, and the average follow-up period was 4.8 years.[13]

One of the most well-researched and universally agreed upon heart-healthy food groups is dark, leafy greens. Michael Miller, MD, professor of cardiovascular medicine, epidemiology, and public health at the University of Mary-

BONUS TIP: The Role of Stress in Cardiovascular Disease Risk factors such as smoking and a lack of regular physical activity tend to get the spotlight, but chronic stress and psychological distress are now identified as risk factors for heart disease.[3] People suffering from prolonged stress can experience sizable and/or prolonged increases in heart rate and blood pressure, leaving them more susceptible to hypertension, heart attack, and premature death by heart disease.[4] Regular exercise is an excellent way to relieve stress, but also consider adding meditation, deep breathing, a spiritual practice, "downtime" spent with friends, and therapy. Also, consider adding tai chi or yoga to your regular exercise routine. Tai chi has been found to be effective at decreasing resting blood pressure and resting heart rate and cardiac output and enhancing cardiovascular endurance,[5] though it's gentle enough even for patients with coronary heart disease and chronic heart failure.[6] Yoga, in addition to its relaxation effects, has been shown to lower blood pressure, improve body weight and body mass index, and even lower cholesterol.[7] For nutritional interventions that can help beat stress, please see Anxiety (page 165) and Stress (page 419).

land School of Medicine and author of *Heal Your Heart: The Positive Emotions Prescription to Prevent and Reverse Heart Disease,* recommends three servings a day of green vegetables. "Green vegetables protect our blood vessels and maintain their youth and vitality by releasing cardioprotective chemicals," he says. "For example, arugula, Swiss chard, and mesclun are high in nitrate, a chemical that's converted to nitric oxide. Other green vegetables, such as asparagus, broccoli, and green beans, are rich in the powerful antioxidant lutein, and high blood levels of lutein are associated with increased levels of physical activity, which are a by-product of lutein's positive effect on mood and behavior—and therefore on energy level. Celery also contains the chemical 3-n-butylphthalide, which was recently shown to reduce blood pressure by 5 to 10 mmHg in adults with mild hypertension." Dr. Miller also added that Brussels sprouts, collards, and kale contain sulforaphane and anthocyanins that have been shown to protect against heart damage in animal models. "The bottom line," says Dr. Miller, "is to eat three servings a day of your favorite greens and lower your risk of a heart attack or stroke by 25 percent or more."

Epidemiological studies have shown that eating a flavonoid-rich diet reduces your risk of heart disease. Flavonoids are a large family of bioactive compounds synthesized by plants. There are more than 5,000 known flavonoids and more are sure to be discovered. One study looked specifically at the role flavonoids play in inflammation. Based upon 2,375 participants, researchers found that higher anthocyanin and flavonol intakes resulted in a reduction in inflammation scores by 73 and 42 percent, respectively, when flavonoids were classed into five major categories. Higher anthocyanin intake was consistently associated with lower inflammation scores across all markers of inflammation, whereas higher flavonol intake was associated with lower cytokine and oxidative stress biomarker concentrations. When researchers conducted a food-based analysis, the foods that made the biggest difference in inflammation scores were apples, pears, strawberries, and red wine.[14]

The most well-known flavonoids are perhaps quercetin and catechin, which have been studied extensively for their cardioprotective benefits. Quercetin can be found in apples, berries, broccoli, capers, citrus fruits, cocoa powder, cranberries, dill, fennel, lingonberries, onions, red wine, and tea. It has been shown to lower blood pressure,[15] improve endothelial function (vasodilation and vasoconstriction), improve dyslipidemia (elevated LDL or low-level HDL), decrease oxidative stress (very simply put, when free radicals cause cell damage), inhibit atherogenesis (plaque formation in the arteries), and exert an anti-arrhythmic effect, meaning it works to correct an irregular heartbeat.[16] Catechins can be found in tea, black grapes, blackberries, broad beans, red wine, cherries, raspberries, strawberries, apricots, apples, pears, and chocolate, but it's epigallocatechin gallate (EGCG), the most abundant catechin in tea, that's considered to be the most effective bioactive component for lowering cholesterol. EGCG can also improve endothelial function and has even been shown to reverse endothelial dysfunction and improve vasodilation in people with coronary artery disease.[17] A metareview of long-range studies on the effect of tea consumption on cardiovascular disease found that both black and green tea protect against heart disease. Green tea significantly reduced total cholesterol and blood pressure, and black tea reduced LDL cholesterol and blood pressure.[18]

Dairy products appear to have a protective effect upon cardiovascular health. One study monitored 2,512 men every 5 years for an average of 22.8 years. Researchers found that compared to the lowest intakes of dairy consumption, those with the highest intakes had reduced arterial stiffness. For the men who had the highest rates of milk consumption, systolic blood pressure was 10.4 mmHg lower than that of men who had the lowest milk consumption. With the exception of butter, which increased insulin, triglycerides, total cholesterol, and diastolic blood pressure as consumption increased, dairy products did not have detrimental effects on arterial stiffness or metabolic markers.[19]

Nuts, with their unique combination of unsaturated fatty acids and bioactive compounds such as L-arginine, fiber, healthful minerals, vitamin E, phytosterols, and polyphenols,[20] are a powerhouse healing food when it comes to protecting against cardiovascular disease. Nuts lower cholesterol and exert a positive effect on oxidative stress, inflammation, vascular reactivity, blood pressure, abdominal fat deposits, and metabolic syndrome. Regular nut consumption was associated with a 50 percent reduced risk of diabetes and a 30 percent reduced risk of cardiovascular disease. Stroke was reduced by nearly half in those who ate a Mediterranean diet along with a daily serving of nuts (15 grams [g] of walnuts and 7.5 g of hazelnuts). What's more, regular nut consumption does not appear to contribute to weight gain.[21] A study of walnuts and cardiovascular health assigned 40 subjects to a walnut-enriched diet (43 g a day) and then a Western-style diet or vice versa, each for 8 weeks and separated by a 2-week washout period. Compared with the control diet, the walnut diet significantly reduced non-HDL-cholesterol and apolipoprotein B, the main protein component of lipoproteins, after adjusting for age, gender, body mass index, and diet sequence. This helps explain why regular nut consumption decreases coronary heart disease risk.[22]

Omega-3 polyunsaturated fatty acids (PUFAs) should be a mainstay of any cardioprotective diet. They're found mainly in cold-water fish but also in walnuts, cod liver oil, and flaxseed oil. Omega-3 fatty acids have anti-inflammatory, antiarrhythmic, and antithrombotic (anti-blood-clot) effects. They improve endothelial function by enhancing the vasodilatory effect of nitric oxide and by decreasing free radical production, and they inhibit the formation of atherosclerotic plaques. Omega-3s lower total cholesterol and triglycerides and decrease the production of apolipoprotein B (a component of LDL or "bad" cholesterol). Overall, omega-3s have been shown to significantly reduce the risk of sudden death caused by cardiac arrhythmias and death from any cause in patients with coronary heart disease.[23]

Now, if all of this sounds too good to be true, consider some of the clinical evidence.

■ In the DART study, 2,033 men who'd suffered a heart attack (cardiac infarction) were followed for 2 years. One group was instructed to increase their fish intake to achieve daily EPA (eicosapentaenoic acid) and DHA (docosahexaenoic acid) consumption of approximately 900 milligrams (mg), and the control group received no specific instructions. The intervention group experienced a 29 percent reduction in all-cause mortality and the incidence of reinfarction was reduced by 32 percent.[24]

■ Another study that focused on 11,323 heart attack survivors assigned one group to take 850 mg of EPA and DHA daily; the control group did not receive any intervention. Omega-3 supplementation significantly reduced risk of death from any cause by 28 percent after only 4 months, mainly because the risk of sudden cardiac death fell by 45 percent. Even better, the results remained significant for the whole 3.5-year duration of the study. In a group of 3,494 heart failure patients, one group received 850 mg of omega-3 fatty acids daily and 3,481 received a placebo. Omega-3s reduced the risk of death from any cause by 9 percent and hospitalization for cardiovascular reasons by 8 percent.[25]

(continued on page 320)

eat and drink for your heart's content

It's not news that you can help your heart by eating right. Here are the latest guidelines.

General Recommendations

- Eat an overall healthy diet, such as the Mediterranean diet or a similar heart-healthy diet, such as the DASH (Dietary Approaches to Stop Hypertension) diet, MIND (Mediterranean-DASH Intervention for Neurodegenerative Delay) diet, Nordic diet, or traditional Japanese diet.

- Emphasize fresh fruits and vegetables, especially citrus fruits and dark, leafy greens.

- Get your protein from omega-3-rich seafood, plant-based proteins such as soy products, nuts, nut butters, and occasional lean poultry. Eliminate or drastically reduce your consumption of red meat.

- Eliminate all trans fats—anything that contains hydrogenated vegetable oils. Watch out for hidden sources of trans fats, such as commercially prepared baked goods or fast foods.

- Eat whole grains, legumes, nuts, and seeds.

- Drink alcohol in moderation. Red wine may be the best form of alcohol for heart health, as it's rich in resveratrol and anthocyanins.

- Limit consumption of sugary desserts and beverages.

Beverages That Support Cardiovascular Health

- Beetroot juice (to lower blood pressure)
- Black tea
- Coffee
- Fruit juices, in moderation
- Green tea
- Fermented beverages: kefir and kombucha
- Red wine: up to two glasses per day for men; one glass per day for women
- Water

Foods That Support Cardiovascular Health

- Apples
- Apricots
- Asparagus
- Berries: strawberries, blueberries, cranberries, blackberries, and lingonberries
- Broccoli

- Capers
- Celery
- Cherries
- Citrus fruits: oranges, limes, lemons, grapefruit, and tangerines
- Cocoa products
- Dark chocolate
- Figs
- Garlic
- Grapes, black or red
- Greens: amaranth, arugula, mesclun, Swiss chard, collard greens, Brussels sprouts, kale, spinach, and dock
- Herbs and spices: cayenne pepper, parsley, oregano, sage, black cumin, and basil
- Legumes: lentils, chickpeas, peanuts, green beans, split peas, adzuki beans, black beans, broad beans, and kidney beans
- Low-fat dairy products: milk and cottage cheese
- Nuts: Brazil nuts, walnuts, almonds, pistachios, and hazelnuts
- Olive oil
- Onions
- Pears
- Peppers: sweet, bell, chile, and jalapeño
- Pineapple
- Poultry: lean chicken and turkey
- Seafood, two or three times per week: salmon, halibut, mackerel, herring, sardines, trout, and tuna
- Seaweed/spirulina
- Shellfish: crab, lobster, mollusks, and shrimp
- Seeds: flaxseeds, chia seeds, pumpkin seeds, and sunflower seeds
- Soy products: soybeans, tofu, and tempeh
- Tomatoes and tomato products
- Whole grains: barley, buckwheat, bulgur, quinoa, farro, whole grain breads, whole oats, millet, unsweetened whole grain cereals, and wheat germ
- Yogurt and fermented dairy products

Foods and Beverages to Avoid or Reduce

- Foods that are high in sodium
- Processed foods
- Fried foods
- Any food containing trans fats
- Refined foods, including refined carbohydrates
- Alcohol, in excess (more than two drinks per day for men or more than one for women)
- Sodas or other sweetened beverages

■ Another study found that a higher EPA/AA (arachidonic acid) ratio was associated with a lower prevalence of coronary artery disease, as well as with improvements of triglyceride metabolism, HDL cholesterol metabolism, and systemic inflammation.[26] EPA is a type of polyunsaturated fatty acid found in abundance in fish and fish oils. Flaxseeds, walnuts, and canola oil all contain ALA, or alphalinolenic acid, which your body converts to EPA. AA is a polyunsaturated omega-6 fatty acid. The typical Western diet is known to be far too high in omega-6 fatty acids, which are found in vegetable oils such as corn oil, safflower oil, soybean oil, palm oil, cottonseed oil, hempseeds, and hempseed oil. While omega-3s reduce inflammation, omega-6s promote inflammation. Research indicates that the Western diet has an omega-3 to omega-6 ratio of anywhere from 1 to 15 to 1 to 16.7. For cardiovascular health, the ratio should be 1 to 4 or better.[27]

■ A study that followed 84,628 women and 42,908 men for 24 to 30 years found that a higher intake of polyunsaturated fatty acids (PUFAs) and carbohydrates sourced from whole grains was associated with a significantly lower risk of coronary heart disease. Carbohydrates from refined starches and added sugars increased the risk of coronary heart disease. Further, replacing 5 percent of energy intake from saturated fats with the equivalent energy intake from PUFAs, monounsaturated fatty acids, or whole grain carbohydrates was associated with a 25 percent, 15 percent, and 9 percent lower risk of coronary heart disease, respectively.[28]

A study on protein intake and cardioprotective amino acids (arginine, cysteine, glutamic acid, glycine, histidine, leucine, and tyrosine) found that a higher intake of these nutrients resulted in lower systolic blood pressure, mean arterial pressure, and pulse-wave velocity (a measure of arterial stiffness). Researchers also found that a higher intake of protein from vegetable sources was associated with lower central blood pressure and augmentation index, another measure of arterial stiffness. Researchers concluded that increasing your intake of these seven amino acids is a relatively easy way to reduce your cardiovascular risk.[29] These cardioprotective amino acids come from a wide array of food sources, including those we've listed on page 318.

Certain herbs and spices also have cardioprotective benefits. Capsaicin, the phytochemical that lends spiciness to chile peppers, jalapeño peppers, and cayenne pepper, has been found to boost metabolism and promote vasodilation.[30]

Capsaicin is also associated with a lower prevalence of obesity.[31] Capsaicin are found in sweet peppers as well, though in lower amounts. Basil, with its high polyphenolic content, is an effective anti-inflammatory, and in animal models it has been shown to protect against and treat hyperlipidemia and to lower blood pressure. Oregano can provide vascular benefits by alleviating nitrative stress and has been shown to decrease markers of inflammation.[32] Flavonoids purified from parsley have been shown to inhibit platelet aggregation and to decrease adherence to collagen by more than 75 percent.[33] Sage has been shown to lower serum total cholesterol, triglycerides, LDL cholesterol, and VLDL cholesterol (very low-density lipoprotein) and to increase HDL cholesterol (high-density lipoprotein).[34] Black cumin has been shown to lower blood pressure, LDL cholesterol, and triglycerides; improve fasting glucose; and decrease oxidative stress.[35]

Finally, if you're hankering for a heart-healthy dessert, look no further than dark chocolate, which improves endothelial function and is associated with improved cardiovascular health. One study sought to examine the effects of cocoa and dark chocolate on the augmentation index, which is a measure of vascular stiffness and vascular tone.

For 4 weeks, participants consumed 37 g a day of dark chocolate and a sugar-free cocoa beverage; controls consumed a low-flavonol chocolate bar and a cocoa-free beverage. The cocoa treatment increased the basal and peak diameter of the brachial artery by 6 percent and basal bloodflow volume by 22 percent. Substantial decreases in arterial stiffness occurred—but only in women.[36] A more recent study on 100 healthy adults ages 35 to 60 examined the effects of consuming 450 mg of a cocoa drink. After 1 month, when compared to the control group, the flavonol-rich cocoa drink increased flow-mediated vasodilation (a way to measure arterial response) and HDL ("good") cholesterol and decreased blood pressure, arterial stiffness, and total and LDL ("bad") cholesterol. By applying the Framingham Risk Score, researchers found that cocoa flavonol predicted a significant lowering of 10-year risk for coronary heart disease, myocardial infarction, cardiovascular disease, and death from coronary heart disease and cardiovascular disease.[37] And all of these results were for women *and* men.

See also: Anxiety (page 165), Diabetes (page 238), High Blood Pressure (Hypertension) (page 327), High Cholesterol (page 334), Overweight and Obesity (page 396), Stress (page 419), Stroke (page 423)

heartburn

The term "heartburn" is half correct: It is a burning pain that occurs in your chest, just behind your breastbone. But heartburn does not affect your heart; rather, the pain occurs in your esophagus when your lower esophageal sphincter doesn't close properly, allowing stomach acid to move up into your esophagus. Heartburn usually occurs after eating, and it can worsen when you're lying down or bending over. Being overweight, smoking, and stress can increase the risk of heartburn and make symptoms more intense. Heartburn is also common during pregnancy.

The food triggers for heartburn are identical to the food triggers for acid reflux, and indeed some people use these two terms interchangeably. But technically, heartburn can be a symptom of occasional acid reflux or of chronic acid reflux (known as gastroesophageal reflux disease, or GERD). On its own, occasional heartburn is not a serious condition, just as occasional acid reflux isn't a major cause for concern.

Occasional heartburn is very common, affecting more than 60 million Americans at least once a month, and it usually resolves on its own. The vast majority of heartburn cases come about in response to a food or beverage trigger. The most frequent causes of heartburn are spicy foods; citrus foods (including oranges, grapefruit, lemons, limes, and tomatoes); alliums, such as garlic, onions, and shallots; fatty or fried foods; acidic drinks, such as coffee or high-acid juices such as orange, grapefruit, and pineapple; alcohol; chocolate; caffeine; and mint. The first food cure for heartburn is to take note of the food or beverage that triggered your heartburn and eliminate it from your diet. Remaining upright after eating, eating slowly, smoking cessation, losing weight, and eating smaller meals will help as well.[1]

The healing foods for heartburn are the same healing foods used to treat acid reflux. Low-acid foods with a pH value of 5 or higher (the higher the pH number, the lower the acid content) may help reduce stomach acid and prevent further irritation. (Lemon juice, for example, has a pH of 2, while crabmeat has a pH of about 7.)[2] Foods such as oatmeal, bananas, melons, brown rice (which has more fiber than white rice), and whole grain breads made from unprocessed flour are all low in acid. For protein, avoid all fried foods and instead eat lean fish or poultry that's grilled, poached, steamed, or baked, and make sure to remove the skin. Organic tofu and fresh egg whites, with pH values of about 7 and 8, respectively,[3] are good vegetarian sources of low-acid protein.

There is clinical evidence of the efficacy of ginger, fennel, licorice, and chamomile in quelling heartburn. Ginger has long been established as an antinausea and antivomiting remedy, safe even during pregnancy, but it also has anti-inflammatory properties.[4] It can be consumed in many forms, including fresh, pickled, powdered, and as a tea. For heartburn, it's best to skip the pickled ginger.

Fennel has been shown to soothe nausea, ease stomach pain, and act as an anti-inflammatory.[5] With its anise-like flavor and its crunchy texture, fennel is delicious raw or cooked. Like ginger, fennel can also be consumed as a tea, or you can chew dried fennel seeds after a meal to aid digestion and prevent bloating, gas, and general gastrointestinal (GI) irritation.

Licorice has long been used to soothe many GI symptoms. It stimulates the production of gastric mucus, which lends a protective coating to your esophagus, stomach lining, and any existing ulcers, making your digestive tract more resistant to irritating stomach acid.[6] You can add licorice to your diet by chewing on licorice root or drinking licorice root tea. The tea is readily available at health food stores and large supermarkets, or you can steep 1 to 5 grams of dried licorice root in boiling water and drink the tea up to three times a day to soothe the pangs of acid reflux and its number one symptom, heartburn.[7] All this said, proceed with a dose of caution: The active ingredient in licorice, glycyrrhizin, comes with a host of possible side effects, especially at high doses or when used for the long term. Do not eat licorice if you are pregnant or breastfeeding or have heart, liver, or kidney disease, a hormone-sensitive cancer, erectile dysfunction, or diabetes. Licorice also has the potential to interfere with many medications, among them blood pressure medications, MAO inhibitors (a common type of antidepressant), ACE inhibitors and diuretics, insulin, oral contraceptives, warfarin (Coumadin), digoxin, and corticosteroids.[8] A form of licorice from which the glycyrrhizin has been removed, called deglycyrrhizinated licorice, or DGL for short, is available as an herbal supplement and has far fewer potential contraindications than the whole food. In any form, if you plan to include licorice regularly in your self-care routine, it's best to consult a health-care provider.

In contrast, chamomile is considered generally safe, though it should be avoided during pregnancy. An ancient remedy for relieving heartburn, indigestion, ulcers, and general stomach upset, chamomile has been shown to neutralize gastric acidity and help dispel gas and relax intestinal muscles.[9] Chamomile tea is the primary way to include this delightfully floral herb in your diet, and in some people, it has the added benefit of enhancing sleep. Chamomile tea bags are available at most supermarkets, or brew the flowers by steeping for 10 to 15 minutes. Drink one to four cups daily as needed for relief.

A spice to try for treating heartburn is turmeric. Like its cousin ginger, turmeric has long been used in traditional and Ayurvedic medicine to treat a wide range of gastrointestinal complaints. A large systematic review is currently under way to study the effects of turmeric on many digestive disorders, but clinical trials have already shown its ability to reduce the symptoms of dyspepsia and ulcerative colitis, to inhibit intestinal spasms and ulcer formation, and to protect the GI tract through its natural anti-inflammatory properties.[10]

Finally, don't underestimate the power of water to help with heartburn. Water (preferably filtered) flushes stomach acid down where it belongs. Drink up after experiencing symptoms.

See also: Acid Reflux (page 148), Gastritis (page 290), Indigestion (page 345)

hemorrhoids

Also known as piles, hemorrhoids are swollen, inflamed veins located in the lower rectum or anus. They're caused by increased pressure in the anal area, usually due to pregnancy, childbirth, constipation, straining during bowel movements, or, less commonly, chronic diarrhea. Being overweight also causes undue pressure on the anal area and can lead to hemorrhoids. Hemorrhoids, which can be internal or external, are very common and occur in up to half of adults after the age of 50. The most effective ways to prevent hemorrhoids are to maintain a healthy weight, eat a high-fiber diet with adequate fluids to prevent constipation, and to have a bowel movement as soon as possible once the urge arises. Regular exercise also helps, as does taking frequent breaks during periods of prolonged sitting.

To prevent constipation, a top cause of hemorrhoids, drink plenty of fluids and increase your fiber intake. A high-fiber diet was shown to decrease rectal bleeding by 50 percent and relieve hemorrhoid symptoms.[1] Foods high in fiber include fruits (blueberries, chokeberries, strawberries, dates, prunes, apricots, raisins, apples, pears, and grapes); dark, leafy greens (kale, spinach, Brussels sprouts, and broccoli); legumes (lentils, beans, and split peas); whole grains (oatmeal, buckwheat, barley, bulgur, quinoa, and whole grain breads and cereals); and seeds (flaxseeds and chia seeds).

For topical relief, always make sure the anal area is clean and dry after a bowel movement. Adding 1 cup of colloidal oatmeal (oatmeal that has been finely ground so it will dissolve in water) to a warm bath can bring fast relief from itching—soak for 15 to 20 minutes twice a day. If you don't have colloidal oatmeal on hand, finely grind regular oats in a food processor.

For food-based topical agents, a mixture of honey, olive oil, and beeswax has been found to be effective at treating hemorrhoids.[2] Patients applied a mixture consisting of 50 percent honey, 29 percent olive oil, and 21 percent beeswax twice a day, including once before bedtime. The results were remarkable. All patients reported significant pain relief within 1 week and complete resolution of pain within 3 weeks—and a complete cessation of itching after 2 weeks. After

3 weeks, no patients had a relapse of hemorrhoids. All patients experienced a significant reduction in bleeding, and two of the patients whose hemorrhoids were so severe that they'd been scheduled for surgery experienced such improvement within 4 weeks that they no longer required surgery.[3] Honey alone may bring some relief, as it has been shown to have both anti-inflammatory and analgesic properties, and it can speed wound healing.[4]

high blood pressure (hypertension)

Hypertension occurs when the pressure of blood against arterial walls is too great. It is measured by a systolic reading (the pressure as your heart fills with blood) and a diastolic reading (the pressure as your heart relaxes and refills with blood). High blood pressure is a very common condition, affecting nearly 79 million Americans—or one in three adults—every year. It causes no symptoms of its own, but high blood pressure is a major risk factor for a host of deadly conditions: heart attack, stroke, vascular dementia, kidney failure, and more.

The results of the SPRINT (systolic blood pressure intervention trial) study could revolutionize the way we manage blood pressure. The study randomly assigned 9,300 men and women age 50 and over to one of two systolic blood pressure targets: under 140 mmHg (millimeters of mercury) or under 120 mmHg. The study was scheduled to conclude in 2017, but the preliminary results were so striking and of such importance to public health that researchers released news of the results immediately. The study found that people who reached a systolic reading of below 120 reduced their risk of heart attack, stroke, and heart failure by one-third and their risk of death by nearly one-quarter.[1] Another study that's just been released found that those with high blood pressure have a nearly 60 percent greater chance of developing diabetes. Based upon data from 4.1 million adults who were diabetes-free and cardiovascular disease-free at the outset of the study, researchers found that for every 20 mmHg increase in systolic pressure there was a 58 percent greater chance of developing diabetes. For every 10 mmHg increase in systolic pressure there was a 52 percent higher risk.[2]

Clearly there is a great deal at stake, and there are extensive health benefits to be gained by keeping blood pressure at or below the normal range. (Currently, the American Heart Association considers normal blood pressure to be 120/80 or less, but these guidelines may change as a result of the SPRINT study and other developing evidence. Note that blood pressure should not fall below 90/60, a condition known as hypotension.) Fortunately, there's a great deal of evidence that healing foods can effectively and safely lower blood pressure. Let's take a look at the latest research.

Flavonoids, the polyphenolic compounds found widely in plants, are nature's answer to high blood pressure. There are more than 5,000 known flavonoids and more are sure to be discovered, and they include well-known subclasses such as flavanols, flavanones, and anthocyanidins. What's one of the best-known sources of flavanols? Cocoa.

A metastudy involving 856 people examined the effect of cocoa on blood pressure and found that flavanol-rich cocoa products had a significant lowering effect on blood pressure. (Flavanols are the most abundant flavonoids found in foods.) The average reduction in systolic pressure was 2.77 mmHg, and the average reduction in diastolic pressure was 2.20 mmHg.[3] Another study comparing the effects of dark chocolate and white chocolate on blood pressure found even more striking results: Those who consumed 25 g a day of dark chocolate for 8 weeks experienced an average systolic reduction of nearly 6 mmHg and an average diastolic reduction of 6.4 mmHg. Those who ate white chocolate, which contains little to no flavanols, experi-

enced an average drop of only 1.07 mmHg (systolic) and 0.17 mmHg (diastolic). Dark chocolate has a beneficial effect on blood pressure because the flavanols in cocoa beans increase nitric oxide production, which relaxes blood vessels.[4]

Another study combined dietary flavonoids with standard blood pressure medications to evaluate a possible enhanced effect. In this study, the flavonoids consisted of an infusion made from dark chocolate, dehydrated red apple, and green tea. The combination of blood pressure medications and flavonoids resulted in an additional reduction in systolic and diastolic blood pressure of 5 mmHg and 4 mmHg, respectively, compared to controls. Participants also experienced a reduction in C-reactive protein plasma levels, triglyceride levels, and leptin (a hormone that signals satiety) levels.[5] A study focusing on tea alone, which is rich in flavonoids, found a significant correlation between green or black tea consumption and a lowered risk of hypertension.[6] A metastudy on tea and blood pressure found that while tea did not immediately lower blood pressure after intake, long-term tea drinking (12 weeks or more) resulted in a reduction in systolic pressure of 1.8 mmHg and in diastolic pressure of 1.4 mmHg. When researchers looked at green and black tea separately, they found that green tea reduced systolic pressure by 2.1 mmHg and diastolic pressure by 1.7 mmHg, and black tea reduced systolic pressure by 1.4 and diastolic pressure by 1.1 mmHg,[7] suggesting that flavanol-rich green tea is more beneficial for hypertension than black tea.

Coffee has something of a bad reputation when it comes to hypertension and cardiovascular disease, perhaps in part because consuming it does cause a temporary spike in blood pressure. But a study in the *American Journal of Cardiology* sought to determine once and for all whether or not coffee contributes to hypertension. Researchers gathered data from 25 studies published between 2010 and 2015 and found that coffee either had a neutral or beneficial effect on cardiovascular health. They concluded that coffee is safe to drink for those with preexisting hypertension or cardiovascular conditions.[8] Lastly, green coffee beans—beans that have not yet been roasted—deserve special mention. Unroasted coffee beans contain greater amounts of chlorogenic acid, an antioxidant that has blood-pressure-lowering effects. In a study comparing the antihypertensive effects of black coffee to those of green coffee, green coffee significantly reduced systolic and diastolic blood pressure and improved arterial elasticity. (Black coffee also reduced blood pressure, but not by as much as green coffee did.) Interestingly, cortisol levels in the green coffee drinkers fell by 39 percent, but they *increased* by 5 percent in the black coffee drinkers.[9]

Several studies have demonstrated the antihypertensive effect of the flavonoid quercetin. It works because it reduces oxidative stress, improves endothelial function (vasodilation and vasoconstriction), and inhibits a hormone that prompts vasoconstriction. Capers provide the highest concentration of quercetin, with 234 milligrams (mg) of quercetin per 100 grams (g) of raw capers, or 173 g of quercetin per 100 g of canned capers. Apples are also an excellent source of quercetin, as are onions, tea, and cocoa.

Garlic, another potent source of flavonoids, has long been studied as a natural means of lowering blood pressure. The latest research shows that it is most effective at lowering blood pressure in hypertensive individuals, rather than in people with normal blood pressure. Results from 17 studies on garlic were pooled, showing an average 4.4 mmHg reduction in systolic blood pressure and 2.68 mmHg reduction in diastolic blood pressure in hypertensive patients.[10]

One of the best sources of the flavonoid subclass anthocyanidins is blueberries. A study of 48 postmenopausal

eat and drink your way to lower blood pressure

High blood pressure is often treated with medicine, but there are many foods that can help fight the condition, as well.

Foods to Eat

- In general: fresh fruits and vegetables, especially citrus fruits and dark, leafy greens
- Apples
- Avocados
- Bananas
- Beans
- Beet greens
- Blueberries
- Broccoli
- Cantaloupe
- Capers
- Celery and celery seed extract
- Chia seeds and chia flour
- Cocoa products
- Dark chocolate
- Dried apricots
- Dried peaches
- Flaxseeds, flaxseed powder, and flaxseed oil
- Garlic
- Honeydew melon
- Lentils
- Mushrooms
- Nuts: almonds and pistachios especially, but also Brazil nuts, walnuts, cashews, hazelnuts, macadamia nuts, pecans, peanuts, pine nuts, and soy nuts
- Onions
- Prunes
- Red grapes
- Seafood and fish: clams, halibut, cod, tuna, and salmon
- Soybeans
- Spinach
- Sweet potatoes
- Tomato products
- Winter squash
- Yogurt

Beverages to Drink

- Beetroot juice
- Red wine (in moderation)
- Green tea
- Black tea
- Kale juice

Foods and Beverages to Avoid or Reduce

- Alcohol, in excess
- Coffee
- Foods that are high in sodium
- Fried foods
- Licorice and licorice tea
- Processed foods

women found that daily blueberry consumption resulted in lower blood pressure and improved arterial stiffness after 8 weeks. Nitric oxide levels were also greater in the blueberry group.[11]

Celery contains 3-n-butylphthalide (NBP), a compound that has been shown to have antihypertensive and vasorelaxant properties. In a study of celery seed extract with a NBP concentration of 85 percent, patients with mild to moderate hypertension experienced an average systolic drop of 8.2 mmHg and a diastolic drop of 8.5 mmHg after 6 weeks of supplementation. Patients took 150 mg of celery seed extract a day.[12] The beneficial effects of celery on hypertension have been more extensively studied in animal models than in humans, but results are consistently promising,[13] and some have shown a positive effect not only on blood pressure but on cholesterol and lipid profiles, as well.[14]

Another group of foods that has shown promising results for lowering blood pressure is nuts. In a study of 100 overweight or obese women, the group that ate 50 g of almonds a day for 3 months experienced lower blood pressure and lower fasting blood sugar levels than women in the nut-free group. The almond group also lost significantly more weight than the nut-free group: an average of more than 8 pounds, compared to less than 3 pounds for the nut-free group.[15] A metastudy of 21 randomized, controlled trials on nut consumption and blood pressure found that nut consumption leads to a significant reduction in systolic blood pressure in those without type 2 diabetes and that pistachios are particularly effective. This study also revealed that pistachios and mixed nuts are effective at reducing diastolic blood pressure.[16] Data from more than 14,000 individuals found that those who ate tree nuts had lower systolic blood pressure by an average of 3 mmHg than those who did not eat nuts. Tree nut consumption was also associated with a lower body mass index, smaller waist circumference, lower insulin resistance, lower likelihood of overweight/obesity, and higher average HDL (high-density lipoprotein, or "good" cholesterol) levels.[17]

Seeds can play a role in controlling blood pressure, as well. A metastudy on the effect of flaxseeds on blood pressure found that on average, flaxseed consumption lowered systolic blood pressure by 1.7 mmHg and diastolic blood pressure by about 1.5 mmHg. However, consuming whole flaxseeds had a greater effect on diastolic blood pressure, bringing the total decrease to nearly 2 mmHg; the effect was greatest in those who consumed flaxseeds for 12 weeks or more.[18] Another metastudy found significant reductions in both systolic and diastolic blood pressure following flaxseed supplementation.

According to this study, the most effective forms for reducing systolic blood pressure were flaxseed powder and lignan extract, while the best forms for reducing diastolic blood pressure were flaxseed powder or oil.[19] A study on chia supplementation found that chia flour was able to reduce blood pressure for patients taking blood pressure medication as well as for those whose hypertension was untreated. In this study, patients consumed 35 g of chia flour a day for 12 weeks and saw a reduction in both systolic and diastolic readings.[20] Chia flour is available at health foods stores, or you can make your own by pulsing chia seeds in a food processor. Some people substitute chia flour in any recipe that calls for regular flour, while others use part chia flour and part regular or gluten-free flour.

The antihypertensive effect of nitrates is also under investigation. Spinach is one of the greatest dietary sources of nitrates, and one study followed participants who ate a nitrate-rich spinach soup daily for 1 week and a control group that ate a very low-nitrate asparagus soup. Compared to the asparagus group, those in the spinach group experienced a systolic blood pressure reduction of 4.05 mmHg after 7 days, as well as reduced arterial stiffness.[21] A study of healthy women who ate a high-nitrate vegetable diet echoed these

results: The high-nitrate diet significantly reduced systolic blood pressure, from 107 mmHg to 103 mmHg, while no change occurred in those who ate a control diet.[22] Likewise, a study that investigated the role of inorganic nitrate in physical performance found that consuming inorganic nitrate—which is found in abundance in beetroot juice—enhances bloodflow and leads to reductions in both systolic and diastolic blood pressure. The study authors concluded that drinking about 2 cups of beetroot juice a day constitutes an effective, low-cost treatment for those with hypertension and other bloodflow disorders.[23]

If you prefer to go green, try kale juice. One study found that drinking 300 ml of kale juice per day for 6 weeks lowered systolic blood pressure by as much as 5.2 percent and diastolic pressure by as much as 3.7 percent. As in other studies, additional health benefits occurred: Those in the kale juice group also experienced a reduction in body fat percentage and blood glucose levels.[24]

Other minerals that have a direct effect on blood pressure are sodium and potassium. Sodium has long been known to increase blood pressure, so avoid foods that are high in sodium and cut back on adding salt to foods. Processed, prepackaged, and fast foods contain very high levels of sodium, so it's best to eliminate those from your diet.

Potassium, on the other hand, lowers blood pressure. In a longitudinal study of more than 24,000 adults, researchers found that for every 1 mg/kcal intake of potassium, systolic blood pressure decreased by 1.01 mmHg.[25] A metareview of studies on potassium and blood pressure revealed that in hypertensive adults, increased potassium intake reduced systolic blood pressure by 3.49 mmHg and diastolic by nearly 2 mmHg. When the potassium intake was increased to 90 to 120 mmol (millimoles) per day, systolic pressure fell by 7.16 mmHg. This study also found that increased potassium intake resulted in a 24 percent lower risk of stroke.[26] Potassium-rich foods include beans; dark, leafy greens; squash; fish; avocados; and bananas.

Clearly there are a great many foods that have proven roles in managing blood pressure. For an overall antihypertensive dietary pattern, look to the Dietary Approaches to Stop Hypertension (DASH) diet, which was specifically formulated to lower blood pressure. (Visit www.dashdiet.org for more information.)[27]

See also: Alzheimer's Disease (page 160), Anxiety (page 165), Dementia (page 226), Diabetes (page 238), Heart Disease (Cardiovascular Disease) (page 313), High Cholesterol (page 334), Kidney Stones (page 364), Overweight and Obesity (page 396), Stress (page 419), Stroke (page 423)

high cholesterol

For years cholesterol, a fatlike substance found in most body tissues, has been declaimed as one of the most dangerous substances in your diet. But the very latest in emerging research is beginning to repair dietary cholesterol's bad reputation. In fact, the Scientific Report submitted by the 2015 Dietary Guidelines Advisory Committee, which is responsible for updating and creating dietary guidelines every 5 years, plainly states, "Cholesterol is not considered a nutrient of concern for overconsumption."[1] Why? Because there's growing evidence that food sources of cholesterol only account for about 20 percent of blood cholesterol levels. It's when an excess amount of cholesterol accumulates *in your bloodstream* that you run into serious negative health consequences.

Low-density lipoprotein (LDL) justly earned its reputation as the "bad" cholesterol because it delivers cholesterol to artery walls, where it contributes to the formation of plaque, which can clog and stiffen your arteries. On the other hand, high-density lipoprotein, the HDL or "good" cholesterol, sweeps LDL cholesterol away and takes it to your liver, where it is metabolized and then excreted from your body. High levels of LDL and low levels of HDL are significant risk factors for atherosclerosis, heart attack, stroke, and peripheral artery disease. The higher your total cholesterol level, the greater your chances of developing heart disease—the number one killer of American adults—or having a heart attack.

Cholesterol is measured by a blood test, and your total cholesterol score is calculated by the equation HDL + LDL + 20 percent of your triglyceride level. Triglycerides are the most common fats in your body, and levels vary according to age and gender. The latest guidelines for cholesterol show no limit, whereas in the past, a maximum of 300 milligrams (mg) a day was recommended. They did add that individuals should eat as little dietary cholesterol as possible because "foods that are higher in dietary cholesterol, such as fatty meats and high-fat dairy products, are also higher in saturated fats."

High cholesterol, also known as hypercholesterolemia, is influenced by lifestyle and diet, but the latest research confirms that heredity is the number one contributor to high cholesterol. That said, you can make lifestyle and dietary choices that decrease your LDL or "bad" cholesterol and increase your HDL or "good" cholesterol. The two main lifestyle factors that contribute to high cholesterol are being overweight and not engaging in physical activity: Both raise LDL cholesterol and lower HDL cholesterol.

Before turning your attention to the healing foods that improve cholesterol levels, let's take a look at the foods that have a negative impact on your cholesterol levels and cardiovascular health. Eliminate or reduce red meat (beef, pork, and lamb), saturated fats (butter, cheese, cream, lard, poultry with skin, potato chips, and palm oil), trans fats (anything containing a hydrogenated or hydrolyzed vegetable oil), processed foods (including prepared desserts and baked goods), and fast food. Fortunately, there are many delicious foods that naturally lower cholesterol and/or boost HDL cholesterol. For example, a study involving overweight people with high cholesterol compared a moderate-fat diet to a moderate-fat diet that included one Hass avocado a day. Researchers found that the avocado diet had greater lowering effects on LDL, LDL particles, and non-HDL cholesterol. One Hass avocado contains about 13 grams of oleic acid (omega-9) and is a nutrient-dense source of monounsaturated fats.[2] In a study that compared twice-daily servings of a cocoa milk drink to plain milk over a 4-week period, researchers observed an increase in HDL ("good" cholesterol) and fiber intake without producing any weight gain.[3] Speaking of fiber, soluble fiber, which forms a gel when mixed with liquid, has long been established as a clinically effective agent in lowering cholesterol. Examples of soluble fiber include oatmeal, oat bran, psyllium, barley, nuts, seeds, beans, lentils, and many fruits and vegetables, including peas, passion fruit, figs, avocados, apples, nuts, blueberries, Brussels sprouts, greens, asparagus, sweet potatoes, soybeans, oranges, prunes, peaches, flaxseeds, and chia seeds, though there are many more. Recent research has shown that the viscosity of a gel-forming fiber is a better predictor of cholesterol-lowering efficacy than the quantity of fiber consumed. Soluble fiber lowers cholesterol by trapping and eliminating bile. Cholesterol is a component of bile, and when bile leaves your body through a bowel movement, your liver uses stored cholesterol to produce more bile, effectively lowering LDL cholesterol while keeping HDL cholesterol intact.[4]

Plant sterols and stanols are types of phytosterols. They are steroid compounds that have a similar structure to cholesterol; they lower serum cholesterol by inhibiting cholesterol absorption. A daily nonvegetarian diet contains 250 mg of unsaturated phytosterols while a vegetarian diet contains more than 500 mg.[5] Plant sterols have such powerful cholesterol-lowering effects that they're now added to some foods. But they occur naturally in many fruits, grains, legumes, nuts, and seeds. A study of 9,660 adults found that increasing legume consumption lowered triglycerides and increased HDL cholesterol. In this particular study, the legumes consumed were lentils, peas, beans, mung beans, and soy protein. Researchers also found an inverse dose–response effect between legume consumption and the risk of high triglycerides, low HDL, and high LDL, suggesting that the more legumes eaten, the greater the cardiovascular protection.[6] Other legumes include black beans, chickpeas, kidney beans, peanuts, green beans, fava beans, and butter beans. Other studies have found that legumes reduce total cholesterol and LDL cholesterol[7] and that eating legumes three times a week reduces total cholesterol, LDL, and C-reactive protein, a marker of inflammation.[8]

A study of 48 people with elevated LDL cholesterol compared the effects of a cholesterol-lowering diet plus almonds to a cholesterol-lowering diet alone for two periods of 6 weeks. The almond diet decreased non-HDL cholesterol (total cholesterol minus HDL) and LDL cholesterol—and it reduced abdominal fat and leg fat, as well, despite causing no changes in weight. Further, the control diet increased HDL or "good" cholesterol![9] A study of the effect of almonds on patients with coronary artery disease and low HDL found that almonds significantly increased HDL cholesterol. Patients were directed to eat 10 g of skinless almonds every day before breakfast for 12 weeks. At week 6, HDL was 12 to 14 percent higher, and at week 12, it was 14 to 16 percent higher. Patients also experienced an improvement in total cholesterol, triglycerides, LDL cholesterol, and VLDL (very low-density lipoprotein) cholesterol.[10]

Walnuts also have a beneficial effect on cholesterol. Researchers tested a walnut-enriched diet (43 g of walnuts per day) on 40 subjects for 8 weeks, then, after a 2-week washout period, tested a typical Western-style diet for 8 weeks. The walnut diet resulted in a significant decrease in non-HDL cholesterol and apolipoprotein B, the main protein component of LDL and VLDL. Researchers concluded that walnuts lower cholesterol and protect against coronary heart disease.[11]

A study on pistachios and vascular health found exciting results. One group was assigned lifestyle modifications while a second group did lifestyle modifications along with daily consumption of 1.5 ounces of shelled pistachios. At the end of 3 months, there was no change in the lifestyle modification group, but the pistachio group had a significant increase in HDL cholesterol and a significant decrease in LDL cholesterol, total cholesterol, and fasting blood sugar levels. The pistachio group also saw improvements in vascular stiffness and endothelial function.[12]

For years, whole oats have been one of the go-to healing foods for lowering cholesterol—and with good reason. A metastudy examined the role of oats and cardiovascular heart disease risk. Of the 64 studies that assessed lipid markers, 58 percent showed a reduction in total cholesterol and 49 percent showed a reduction in LDL cholesterol. Researchers concluded that long-term intake of oats or oat bran has a beneficial effect upon cholesterol.[13] A metastudy of the effect of whole grains on cholesterol found that compared to controls, whole grains lowered LDL cholesterol, triglycerides, and total cholesterol—and that whole grain oats had the greatest effect on total cholesterol.[14] Yet another metastudy looked specifically at oat beta-glucan, the soluble fiber found in oats that is responsible for many of its cholesterol-lowering properties. Results were consistent: On average, oat consumption is associated with a 5 percent reduction in total cholesterol and a 7 percent reduction in LDL cholesterol levels. Results of this review also showed that eating at least 3 g of oat beta-glucan a day can reduce

LDL levels by 5 to 10 percent in people with normal or high cholesterol.[15] This amount can be found in 40 g of oat bran or about ⅔ cup of raw oatmeal. In another study, adults with high cholesterol participated in a comparison of oatmeal and rice porridge. Group 1 consumed 70 g (3 g of beta-glucan) of oatmeal daily for 4 weeks, then switched to 70 g of rice porridge daily for the next 4 weeks. Group 2 consumed rice porridge first and then oatmeal. Following daily oatmeal consumption, total cholesterol and LDL cholesterol levels were significantly lower than baseline levels and lower than the levels observed with rice consumption. Oat consumption reduced total cholesterol by 5 percent and LDL cholesterol by 10 percent from baseline levels.[16]

Of all plants, one type may reign supreme with regards to cholesterol control: A metastudy of 77 clinical trials found that garlic powder significantly reduced total cholesterol and LDL cholesterol levels, fasting blood glucose, and blood pressure, demonstrating its protective effect against several cardiovascular risk factors.[17] Another metastudy of 39 clinical trials found that garlic was effective at reducing total serum cholesterol by roughly 17 points and LDL cholesterol by about 9 points in individuals with cholesterol levels above 200—provided garlic is used for longer than 2 months. This study also pointed out that an 8 percent reduction in total cholesterol is associated with a 38 percent reduction in risk of coronary events at age 50 and that with few side effects, garlic has a higher safety profile than conventional cholesterol-lowering medications.[18] In patients with mild hypercholesterolemia, aged black garlic was shown to increase HDL cholesterol and decrease levels of apolipoprotein B, the main protein constituent in LDL and VLDL cholesterol.[19]

A hugely significant part of the Mediterranean diet, olive oil has been shown to decrease postprandial blood glucose (blood sugar levels after a meal), LDL cholesterol, and oxidized LDL.[20] Other studies have shown that olive oil improves your lipid profile by increasing HDL cholesterol and reducing LDL cholesterol and triglyceride levels, reducing oxidative stress, and inhibiting human lipoprotein oxidation, making LDL less atherogenic (less likely to form fatty plaques).[21] Omega-3 fatty acids, found in abundance in cold-water fish such as salmon, tuna, halibut, mackerel, herring, and sardines, are also an important part of the Mediterranean diet and are known to reduce triglyceride levels.[22] One study set out to better understand why lean seafood has cardioprotective benefits. Twenty healthy subjects ate a diet in which the main protein source was either seafood or lean beef. The seafood diet, which was rich in omega-3s, reduced fasting and postprandial triglyceride levels. Further, researchers found that the seafood diet prevented the elevated ratio of total cholesterol to HDL cholesterol that was observed after the nonseafood intervention.[23]

Both green and black tea have been extensively studied for their potential cholesterol-lowering effects. A metastudy of 14 clinical trials with 1,136 subjects found that green tea consumption lowered total cholesterol by an average of 7.20 mg/dl and LDL cholesterol by an average of 2.19 mg/dl.[24] A high daily dose (nearly 857 mg) of green tea extract (containing epigallocatechin gallate, or EGCG) has been shown to reduce body mass index, weight, waist circumference, total cholesterol, and LDL cholesterol.[25] Results on studies of black tea have been mixed or inconclusive,[26] but a metastudy of 10 clinical trials with 411 participants found that black tea significantly lowered LDL cholesterol, especially in participants with higher cardiovascular risk.[27] Oolong tea has been shown to decrease weight, subcutaneous fat, total cholesterol, and triglycerides in as little as 6 weeks.[28]

See also: Diabetes (page 238), Gallstones (page 287), Heart Disease (Cardiovascular Disease) (page 313), High Blood Pressure (Hypertension) (page 327), Stroke (page 423)

hives

Hives are a very common itchy skin rash that comes about in reaction to a food, medicine, insect bite or sting, or other irritant. In some cases, hives are triggered by stress. Hives are different from other common skin rashes in a few key ways: (1) These large, red welts can occur on any part of your body; (2) they can "move around," disappearing and reappearing anywhere over short periods of time; and (3) they exhibit a "blanching" effect (they turn white in the center when pressed). Hives are usually not dangerous and most cases resolve on their own within 24 hours, but they can last as long as 6 weeks. In rare cases, hives can become more severe and cause your throat to swell. If you have trouble breathing or swallowing, seek medical attention right away.

To prevent hives, the first step is to identify your trigger and avoid it. Sometimes this is quite obvious, as in hives resulting from penicillin or an insect bite, but sometimes it can take some sleuthing. Food allergens can cause hives, for example, and sometimes it isn't clear which food is triggering an allergic reaction unless you're keeping a food diary or trying an elimination diet. But among the first places to look are common food allergens such as peanuts, tree nuts, soy, wheat, fish, shellfish (shrimp, crab, and lobster), eggs, or dairy. Chronic hives, or hives lasting longer than 6 weeks, are usually the result of a common allergen, or they can be the result of stress. Again, the most effective means of prevention is to avoid the trigger, whether it be pollen, pet dander, a soap or perfume, a food, or too much stress in your life.

Healing foods for hives include foods to eat as well as topical solutions to be applied to your skin to soothe itching. To cut down on the stress that can trigger hives, eat foods rich in B vitamins. B vitamins have been shown to reduce the effects of workplace stress and enhance mood.[1] Good whole foods sources of B vitamins include fish; poultry; meat; dairy products; oat bran; eggs; beans; peas; papayas; oranges; cantaloupe; whole grains; and dark, leafy greens, such as kale, Swiss chard, spinach, and arugula.[2]

For a natural antihistamine, try apples, onions, tea, capers, peppers, blueberries, grapefruit, okra, and red wine. These sources are loaded with the antioxidant quercetin, which has been shown to have an antihistamine[3] and anti-inflammatory effect.[4]

To eat to reduce inflammation, get plenty of omega-3s. The best sources of these essential fatty acids include wild-caught seafood (salmon, mackerel, tuna, herring, sardines, and halibut), walnuts, flaxseeds, flaxseed oil, and pumpkin seeds. Other foods on your anti-inflammatory defense menu include foods that inhibit COX-2, an enzyme that triggers inflammation. That includes any food rich in vitamin C (citrus fruits; papayas; guavas; peppers; mangoes; tomatoes; kiwifruit; cantaloupe; dark, leafy greens; and parsley), turmeric, ginger, pineapple, and green tea.

As for topical preparations, oatmeal has long been used to decrease itching. Modern science reveals that it does so because it has both anti-inflammatory and antihistamine properties. For fast itch relief, add 1 cup of colloidal oatmeal (oatmeal that has been finely ground so it will dissolve in water) to your bath, and soak for 15 to 20 minutes.[5] If you only have whole oats on hand, you can grind them in a food processor. Another natural cure for itching is peppermint oil, which can be applied topically (mixed with coconut oil) or added to bathwater.[6] An oatmeal bath with a few drops of peppermint oil and lavender oil will give you a double dose of itch relief, along with the relaxing benefits of lavender.

See also: Food Allergies (page 278)

hyperhidrosis (excessive sweating)

The International Hyperhidrosis Society estimates that some 3 percent of the population—many millions of people, in other words—experience excessive sweating. Numbers are probably higher because the condition is underreported. Primary focal hyperhidrosis, or excessive sweating that isn't due to a medication or underlying condition, isn't life threatening, but it can have devastating effects on your social, professional, and family life. Many hyperhidrosis sufferers report spending significant time managing or trying to conceal their excessive sweating, and some people avoid social situations and even have trouble maintaining relationships or jobs because of their condition.

Excessive sweating usually occurs in your armpits or on your hands, feet, or face, but it can potentially occur anywhere on your body, including your groin, back, between or under your breasts, and even on your upper lip or nose. There are very few clinical studies to draw upon regarding food remedies for excessive sweating, but one time-honored treatment that has been studied is sage, which has astringent and antihydrotic (tending to reduce sweat secretions) effects.[1] Sage tea has been recommended to treat hyperhidrosis and is high in antioxidants, as well.[2] Sage tea is available in stores, or you may want to add fresh sage leaves to cool or cold water. Fresh or dried sage can be added to many food dishes, as well. Some sources recommend that the best antisweating effects require sage at larger doses, however. Andrew Weil, MD, recommends taking a 1,000 milligram dried sage capsule twice a day. Note: Pregnant women should not take sage because it can cause uterine contractions.[3]

Another treatment to consider is bergamot essential oil. Though evidence is limited, it has been used to treat hyperhidrosis because of its antiseptic and antibacterial properties. Further, with its proven ability to assuage symptoms of stress and anxiety, it may help preclude some of the excessive sweating associated with nervousness and stress.[4]

The American Academy of Dermatology also cites common foods that can trigger or worsen hyperhidrosis. They include foods containing monosodium glutamate (MSG), caffeine (tea, coffee, and chocolate), hot sauces, spices such as curry or cumin, and alcohol.[5] Eliminating or reducing these triggers can help prevent some types of excessive sweating.

It's recommended that people with hyperhidrosis follow an antianxiety or antistress diet, as anxiety and stress are two of the primary causes of excessive sweating. Additionally, you should avoid skipping meals or eating meals or snacks that are high in sugar, as hypoglycemia can cause sweating.

See also: Anxiety (page 165), Hypoglycemia (page 343), Stress (page 419)

hypoglycemia

Hypoglycemia is the state of having an abnormally low blood sugar (glucose) level. Generally, glucose levels should not fall below 70 mg/dl. Most often, hypoglycemia occurs when you're not getting enough calories for your body's needs—you've skipped a meal, gone too long between meals, or are dieting—and eating is the simple, quick solution to bringing glucose levels back up. Low blood sugar also occurs in response to a high-sugar meal in a phenomenon called reactive hypoglycemia. A high-sugar meal causes blood glucose levels to rise quickly, which triggers an overproduction of insulin in order to bring glucose levels back down. Less commonly, some people experience nighttime hypoglycemia, which occurs as blood glucose levels fall during sleep. Alcohol can also cause hypoglycemia, especially on an empty stomach, as can increased physical activity, because your body demands more calories. Hypoglycemia is a particular concern for diabetics. It occurs any time there's too much insulin in your blood and not enough sugar and can result from injecting too much insulin, skipping meals, or overexertion. Diabetics should treat hypoglycemia promptly; untreated diabetic hypoglycemia can result in seizures, loss of consciousness, and in rare cases, death. Further, in people with type 2 diabetes, severe hypoglycemia is one of the strongest predictors of cardiovascular events and all-cause mortality.[1]

The symptoms of hypoglycemia occur because your brain is not getting enough glucose. Mild hypoglycemia can cause headache, hunger, shakiness, confusion, faintness, sweating, nervousness, anxiety, and irritability. As it worsens, hypoglycemia can cause migraine, nausea, and hypothermia; in extreme, prolonged cases, loss of consciousness and even death can occur, though this is very rare.

Unless there is some underlying condition (such as diabetes), hypoglycemia is easily prevented by eating regular meals and avoiding high-sugar foods and beverages. The right kinds of foods and beverages also make an enormous difference. To prevent hypoglycemia, opt for foods that are rich in fiber, plant-based protein, and complex carbohydrates. These foods will leave you feeling full longer, and they're digested more slowly, which means glucose is released into your bloodstream more slowly, precluding the overproduction of insulin that leads to hypoglycemia. If you do find yourself consuming a high-sugar food or beverage, try pairing it with a plant-based protein such as tofu, tempeh, beans, nuts, or a nut butter; these can slow digestion and prevent or reduce the hypoglycemic effect. If you're dieting, try eating smaller, more frequent meals, and plan to lose weight gradually. Ultimately, you'll have more success with keeping the weight off if you lose smaller amounts over a longer period of time.

Cut down on or eliminate sugary desserts, sugary cereals, muffins with frosted or crumble toppings (some of the hearty breakfast-type muffins made with whole grains may be okay, especially if they're paired with a protein), and simple carbohydrates (white bread, white pasta, bagels made with white flour, white rice, biscuits, and rolls), as they're digested quickly and cause a spike in blood sugar levels followed by the inevitable drop. Also avoid processed and refined foods, as they usually contain added sweeteners and artificial flavorings. Eliminate sodas entirely. Sugary, caffeinated soft drinks and energy drinks are notorious for causing a quick rush of energy followed by the hypoglycemic "crash." Some people respond in a hypoglycemic manner to caffeine alone—and the effect is doubled if they're drinking sweetened caffeinated beverages such as cola or coffee with sugar. So in addition to eliminating caffeinated sodas, you can try cutting back on chocolate, tea, and coffee.

If you do find yourself in a hypoglycemic state and need quick relief, some sources will tell you to drink soda, eat jelly beans, or even eat a small amount of plain sugar.[2] And while these means *will* deliver a fast dose of sugar and relieve the symptoms of hypoglycemia (and you should certainly use what you have in an emergency), they will only spark the familiar cycle of precipitous spikes and drops in glucose levels, leaving you back where you started. A far better alternative is to eat a healthier, more complex form of carbohydrate. If you're prone to hypoglycemia, it's a great idea to keep "quick fix" foods on hand—good choices include dried apricots, dried figs, a piece of fresh fruit, ½ cup of fruit juice, 3 teaspoons of honey, or a 6-ounce serving of yogurt. You can also choose a protein and carbohydrate combination, such as crackers and cheese,[3] hummus with carrots, or whole grain toast with peanut butter.

See also: Adrenal Exhaustion/Adrenal Fatigue (page 153), Anxiety (page 165), Diabetes (page 238), Lightheadedness (page 368), Stress (page 419)

indigestion

Indigestion (also called dyspepsia) is a general term that refers to abdominal discomfort. Symptoms can include belching, bloating, heartburn, nausea, abdominal pain, and a feeling of fullness after eating small amounts. Indigestion can arise from overeating, eating spicy or high-fat foods, eating too quickly, eating too much, drinking alcohol, or stress. Indigestion can also occur as a reaction to a medication; aspirin and other NSAIDs (nonsteroidal anti-inflammatory drugs) such as ibuprofen and naproxen are common culprits. Rarely is indigestion a serious problem, and it usually resolves on its own within a few hours. Occasionally, indigestion is a symptom of a more serious gastrointestinal (GI) condition, such as gallstones, gastritis, gastroesophageal reflux disease (GERD), irritable bowel syndrome (IBS), pancreatitis, or ulcers. If indigestion persists for more than a few days or if it's accompanied by blood in your vomit or stool; sudden, severe pain; sudden weight loss; or a loss of appetite, see your doctor for an evaluation.

The primary ways to prevent indigestion are to eat more slowly, not eat past the feeling of satiety, and eliminate foods that cause symptoms. Identifying your indigestion triggers may be easy if you always experience indigestion after eating spicy foods, or it may require keeping a food diary in order to discover dietary patterns or specific foods that prompt indigestion. Chronic indigestion can be an indication of a food allergy or sensitivity, or, in the case of indigestion in response to wheat products, an indication of celiac disease. Among the most common triggers for indigestion are alcohol; caffeinated drinks; spicy foods; acidic foods such as citrus fruits and tomatoes; alliums such as garlic, onions, and shallots; fatty and/or fried foods; chocolate; and mint.

The foods that prompt indigestion can be highly specific from one person to another, but there are some commonalities. A yearlong study of 384 patients who sought treatment for indigestion found that the most frequent triggers were sausage and bolognas, pickles, vinegar, soft drinks, certain grains, tea, salt, pizza, watermelon, red peppers, and macaroni. On the other hand, the foods that most frequently led to a decrease in symptoms were apples, rice, hard candy, bread, caraway seed, dates, honey, yogurt, quince, and walnuts.[1]

When indigestion does strike, in most cases it's best to cease eating and give your digestive system a rest. Any healing foods and beverages consumed to relieve the symptoms of indigestion should be consumed slowly and in small quantities. Ginger has been shown to relieve nausea, queasiness, and even vomiting. It's safe even during pregnancy and has anti-inflammatory properties.[2] It can be consumed in many forms, though for indigestion ginger tea is best, and small amounts of fresh ginger are your next best bet.

Artichoke leaf extract has been shown to relieve the symptoms of indigestion. In a study of 244 people with dyspepsia, an artichoke leaf extract taken twice a day for 6 weeks caused significant improvement in indigestion symptoms as well as overall quality of life scores.[3]

Building on the promising results of ginger and artichoke, researchers devised a ginger and artichoke supplement and tested it on 126 dyspepsia patients for 4 weeks. After only 14 days, only the group receiving the supplement showed improvement in symptoms. This trend continued throughout the study, and by its end, patients in the supplement group showed improvements in nausea, bloating, pain, and satiation.[4]

Fennel has been shown to soothe nausea, ease stomach pain, and act as an anti-inflammatory.[5] Like ginger, fennel can also be consumed as a tea, or you can chew dried fennel seeds after a meal to aid digestion and prevent bloating, gas, and general GI irritation.

Like its cousin ginger, turmeric has long been used in traditional and Ayurvedic medicine to treat a wide range of gastrointestinal complaints. A large systematic review is currently under way to study the effects of turmeric on many digestive disorders, but clinical trials have already shown its ability to reduce the symptoms of dyspepsia and ulcerative colitis, to inhibit intestinal spasms and ulcer formation, and to protect the GI tract through its natural anti-inflammatory properties.[6]

Black cumin (caraway) is another spice that has long been used to treat indigestion and other gastrointestinal problems. You can chew seeds after a meal to settle your stomach.[7]

Probiotics have been shown to relieve bloating.[8] The probiotic known as *Bifidobacterium infantis* is particularly effective and is able to relieve a variety of GI symptoms including indigestion, bloating, flatulence, constipation, and diarrhea.[9] It's found in probiotic yogurts, drinks such as kefir, and some cheeses.

Licorice has long been used to soothe

many GI symptoms. It stimulates the production of gastric mucus, which lends a protective coating to your esophagus, stomach lining, and any existing ulcers, making your digestive tract more resistant to irritating stomach acid.[10] You can add licorice to your diet by chewing on licorice root or drinking licorice root tea. The tea is readily available at health food stores and large supermarkets, or DIYers can steep 1 to 5 grams of dried licorice root in boiling water and drink the tea up to three times a day.[11] All this said, proceed with a dose of caution: The active ingredient in licorice, glycyrrhizin, comes with a host of possible side effects, especially at high doses or when used long term. Do not eat licorice if you are pregnant or breastfeeding or have heart, liver, or kidney disease; a hormone-sensitive cancer; erectile dysfunction; or diabetes. Licorice also has the potential to interfere with many medications, among them blood pressure medications, MAO inhibitors (a common type of antidepressants), ACE inhibitors, diuretics, insulin, oral contraceptives, warfarin (Coumadin),

digoxin, and corticosteroids.[12] A form of licorice from which the glycyrrhizin has been removed, called deglycyrrhizinated licorice (or DGL), is available as an herbal supplement and has far fewer potential contraindications than the whole food. In any form, if you plan to include licorice regularly in your self-care routine, it's best to consult with a health-care provider first.

In contrast, chamomile is considered generally safe, though it should be avoided during pregnancy. An ancient remedy for relieving heartburn, indigestion, ulcers, and general stomach upset, chamomile has been shown to neutralize gastric acidity and help dispel gas and relax intestinal muscles.[13] Chamomile tea is the primary way to include this delightfully floral herb in your diet, and in some people, it has the added benefit of enhancing sleep. Chamomile tea bags are available at most supermarkets, or brew it from scratch by steeping the flowers for 10 to 15 minutes.

See also: Acid Reflux (page 148), Food Allergies (page 278), Irritable Bowel Syndrome (page 360)

infertility

nfertility is defined as the inability to conceive after a year of unprotected sex; some definitions further specify infertility as the inability to conceive after a year of unprotected sex in each of those months with the same partner. Still others specify according to a woman's age: Infertility is the inability of a couple to become pregnant after 1 year of unprotected sex in women under 35 and after 6 months in women 35 and older. There are many causes of infertility and several different types of infertility in both men and women. General risk factors for infertility include female age over 35, male age over 40, tobacco use, drug use, excessive alcohol consumption, exposure to environmental toxins, overweight or obesity, the presence of sexually transmitted infections, and, in women only, being underweight or engaging in strenuous athletic training, both of which can negatively impact ovulation.

There are multiple interventions available to help couples conceive, from relatively simple lifestyle changes to medications to surgical procedures to assisted reproductive technology (ART) methods in which both egg and sperm are manipulated in order to increase your chances of conception. Here, we'll look at nutritional interventions on both ends of the spectrum: foods and dietary patterns that raise your risk of infertility as well as foods and dietary patterns that can best increase your chances of becoming pregnant.

In terms of overall diet, one of the most prevalent causes of infertility will be no surprise: the Western dietary pattern. Research results presented at the 2015 meeting of the American Society for Reproductive Medicine found that a high-fat diet negatively impacts fertility in men and women. A research team from the Harvard T. H. Chan School of Public Health and Massachusetts General Hospital found that men who consumed the highest levels of trans fats had the lowest fertilization rates. In a separate study, researchers examined blood from women undergoing in vitro fertilization (IVF) treatment for the presence of fatty acid chains. They found that elaidic acid, which is found in hydrogenated oils and fried foods, had a negative impact on several measures of ART outcome, including fertilization rate and number of usable blastocysts ("pre-embryos") and embryos.[1] Additional studies have found similar results. To examine the relationship between diet and asthenozoospermia (low sperm motility) risk, researchers examined the diets of 107 men with low sperm motility and 235 age-matched controls. Two overall dietary patterns emerged. The first is the "prudent" pattern, characterized by consumption of dark, leafy greens; yellow vegetables; other vegetables; tomatoes; fish and other seafood; fruits and natural fruit juices; legumes; whole grains; poultry; tea and coffee; low-fat dairy products; and vegetable oils. The second is the familiar Western dietary pattern, which is characterized by consumption of red and processed meats, sugar, soft drinks and sweets, pasta, rice, refined grains, potatoes, French fries, fast foods, high-fat dairy products, hydrogenated fats, mayonnaise and fatty sauces, and snacks. Men with the highest adherence to the prudent pattern had a 54 percent lower risk of asthenozoospermia.[2]

Further, obesity is a significant factor in infertility for both men and women. Obese men are three times as likely as men of normal weight to exhibit a reduction in semen quality—including (but not limited to) decreased

sperm motility, decreased sperm concentration, and DNA damage in sperm.[3] For women, there is evidence indicating that it takes obese women longer to get pregnant because of ovulatory disorders, damage to eggs, and/or negative effects to the endometrium.[4] Obese women also have a significantly higher likelihood of miscarriage.[5] But there is good news on both counts: Weight loss has been shown to improve chances of conception and to restart ovulation in previously anovulatory women.[6]

For both men and women, an overall healthy and varied diet is clearly the best nutritional means to increase the chances of conception and to help maintain a healthy, full-term pregnancy. Now let's look at some specific vitamins and food groups that play special roles in fertility.

In women, consuming animal protein has been shown to increase the risk of ovulatory infertility. But consuming vegetable protein instead of animal protein or carbohydrates was shown to substantially lower the risk of ovulatory infertility. The association was particularly strong in women 32 years old and older. This study also highlighted red meat and chicken as particularly problematic and suggested that replacing them with vegetable protein may reduce the risk of infertility due to anovulation.[7] Vegetable sources of protein include soy products, lentils, dairy products, eggs, beans, quinoa, seeds (pumpkin, sunflower, and flax), nuts, and nut butters.

Trans fats, those industrially produced fats that raise LDL ("bad") cholesterol and lower HDL ("good") cholesterol, have been shown to have an enormous negative impact on healthy ovulation. In one study, consuming trans fats instead of carbohydrates resulted in a 73 percent increased risk of an ovulatory disorder.[8] To avoid trans fats, don't eat anything that includes "partially hydrogenated oils" on the ingredients list. Thankfully, in June of 2015 the FDA gave food companies 3 years to remove partially hydrogenated oils from their products, so you won't have to check labels for much longer.[9]

In women with polycystic ovary syndrome (PCOS), losing weight improves fertility. A study of 60 women with PCOS and a body mass index (BMI) greater than 30 assigned half the women to a calorie-restricted diet while the other half were given no calorie restrictions. At the end of 6 months, the intervention group had lost weight and had significantly improved menstrual regularity.[10]

Vitamin D is recommended for women trying to get pregnant. In one study, women with PCOS experienced increased endometrial thickness and lower serum lipids while receiving vitamin D. A high vitamin D intake may also be protective against endometriosis.[11] One of the best sources of vitamin D is exposure to sunlight, but it can also be found in fatty fish such as salmon, tuna, and mackerel, and cod liver oil contains 340 percent of the recommended daily value of vitamin D for people age 4 and over. Other food sources of vitamin D include fortified milk, beef liver, mushrooms, cheese, and egg yolks.[12]

A recent meta-analysis of studies on the relationship between caffeine and coffee consumption and pregnancy loss concluded that both were associated with an elevated risk of pregnancy loss. The results also suggested that risk of pregnancy loss rose by 19 percent for every increase in caffeine intake of 150 milligrams (mg) a day and by 8 percent for every increase in coffee intake of 2 cups per day.[13] At amounts over 500 mg per day, caffeine has been associated with a 9.5-month increase in the time it takes to get pregnant.[14]

For men, eating a diet rich in carbohydrates, fruits and vegetables, fiber, folate, and lycopene is associated with improved semen quality. Eating a diet that's lower in proteins and fats also improves semen quality.[15] Lycopene is a powerful antioxidant found in tomatoes and tomato products, watermelon, and pink grapefruit. Folate is a B vitamin found in food sources such as avocados; asparagus; beans; broccoli; Brussels sprouts; citrus fruits and juices; dark, leafy greens; eggs; grains; seafood; and spinach.[16]

Oxidative stress has a significant negative impact upon sperm. A metareview of studies that examined antioxidant therapy to reduce oxidative stress in sperm found overwhelmingly positive results. There was also strong evidence of improved sperm motility.[17] To boost your antioxidant intake, eat any fresh, colorful fruits and vegetables. Other sources of antioxidants include beans, dark chocolate, tea, coffee, and wine. Don't overdo it with the wine, however, as overconsumption of alcohol has been linked to decreased sperm count, decreased sperm motility, and lower semen volume.[18]

There is some evidence that ginger can act as an aphrodisiac by increasing testosterone—not to mention sperm count, viability, and motility, suggesting that it may play a beneficial role in fertility as well.[19] And maca, an herbaceous plant native to Peru that has quickly gained a reputation as a superfood, has been shown to improve sperm concentration and motility in men ages 20 to 40 after 12 weeks of treatment. In this study, men ingested 1.75 g of maca powder per day.[20] Maca is also available as an extract, a tea, and in capsule form.

See also: Decreased Libido (page 224); Erection Problems, Erectile Dysfunction (page 263)

influenza

The flu, one of the most common and most dreaded infectious illnesses, is a respiratory infection caused by the influenza virus. The flu primarily affects your nose, throat, and lungs, but it also causes a high fever, muscle aches, fatigue, headache, cough, and chills. There are several different strains of influenza viruses, and they mutate often. Most people recover within 2 weeks, but influenza has the potential to be deadly. Infants and young children, the elderly, those with preexisting illnesses, and people with a compromised immune system are most at risk.

Dietary interventions to prevent the flu include any foods that can boost your immune system. The powerful antioxidants known as flavonoids, found in abundance in fruits and vegetables, possess anti-inflammatory and immune-boosting properties.[1] Among the best sources of flavonoids are apples, arugula, aronia berries (chokeberries), beans, blueberries, capers, chocolate, coriander, cranberries, currants, dock, elderberries, fennel, grapefruit, hot peppers, juniper berries, kale, kumquats, lovage, onions, oregano, parsley, plums, radicchio, radishes, raspberries (black), red cabbage, red wine, and serviceberries.[2] Some of the best vitamins and minerals for immune system support include vitamin A, vitamin B_2, vitamin B_6, vitamin C, vitamin D, vitamin E, folate, iron, selenium, and zinc. Eating a well-balanced diet consisting of plenty of fresh fruits and vegetables, whole grains, lean proteins, and adequate fluid intake will provide most if not all of these vitamins and minerals. The exception is vitamin D, which can be found in dairy products, eggs, fish and fish oil, fortified orange juice,[3] and mushrooms, but sun exposure is the best source. Food sources for zinc include oysters, wheat germ, chicken, crab, beans, oatmeal, yogurt, pumpkin seeds, and pine nuts. Food sources for the rest of the immune-supporting nutrients include almonds; bananas; barley; beans; berries of any variety; Brazil nuts; cantaloupe; carrots; chickpeas; citrus fruits; dark, leafy greens; garlic; hazelnuts; lean poultry; mackerel; papayas; peppers of any variety; quinoa; salmon; squash; sweet potatoes;

tuna; and yogurt. Probiotics have also been shown to help prevent the flu.[4] Probiotics work by blocking the replication of the flu virus. Food sources include yogurt, kefir, miso soup, sauerkraut, tempeh, and kombucha, a type of fermented black tea.

If the flu does strike, you may not feel like eating, but continue to eat small amounts of immune-boosting, antioxidant-rich foods as you're able to. It's equally important to stay hydrated, as eating less than normal and the high fever that sometimes accompanies the flu are both dehydrating. Drink as much water, 100 percent fruit juices (or fruit juices diluted with water), or herbal tea as you can. (Don't forget the kombucha!)

Add honey, which has antiviral properties, to regular tea. One study found that honey, and manuka honey in particular, significantly inhibits influenza virus replication.[5] One study even found that one of our tastiest beverages has anti-influenza effects: cocoa. Researchers compared two groups: Both groups were vaccinated against influenza, but one group drank cocoa for 3 weeks before and after vaccination. The cocoa group had higher, more elevated levels of natural killer cell activity. Researchers concluded that drinking cocoa activates your natural immunity and enhances the effect of the flu vaccination, providing stronger protection against the flu.[6]

insect/spider bites and stings

Most insect bites and stings result in a set of mild reactions that will resolve on their own in a few days. Symptoms vary depending on what type of insect caused the bite or sting. Bites from mosquitoes, fleas, chiggers, and mites itch and can cause redness and minor swelling. Bites from ants or spiders usually cause more pain than itching, as do stings from bees, wasps, yellow jackets, hornets, and scorpions. Any bite can cause localized swelling and redness.

Common bites or stings can be cared for at home through simple measures we'll describe below. There are certain cases, however, that require medical attention, usually for one of three reasons: (1) the person is allergic to the venom, such as may be the case with a bee sting allergy; (2) the person has been bitten by a poisonous pest, such as a black widow or brown recluse spider; or (3) the person falls ill after the bite, as in the case of the West Nile virus or Rocky Mountain spotted fever. (See "When to Seek Medical Attention for Insect Bites and Stings" for more information.)

For at-home treatment of minor bites and stings, first clean the wound and remove the stinger, if it's lodged in your skin. Apply ice to reduce swelling and pain. Then, to beat the itch of a bite or sting, make a paste of oatmeal mixed with a little water and apply it directly to the bite. Oatmeal has both anti-inflammatory and antihistamine properties. If you have extensive bites, add 1 cup of colloidal oatmeal (oatmeal that has been finely ground so it will dissolve in water) to your bath and soak for 15 to 20 minutes.[1] If you only have whole oats on hand, you can grind them in a food processor. Another natural cure for itching is peppermint oil, which can be applied topically (mix it with coconut oil to apply it easily) or added to bathwater.[2] (If you don't have peppermint oil on hand, try rubbing mint toothpaste directly onto the bite.) Lavender oil can also be applied topically to stop itching and treat insect bites.[3] An oatmeal bath with a few drops of peppermint oil or lavender oil

when to seek medical attention for insect bites and stings

Follow the advice here and you'll never have to wonder whether you should see a doctor or head to the ER after you've been bitten or stung.

Seek Emergency Medical Attention If . . .

- You have trouble breathing or feel as if your throat is swelling.
- You have difficulty swallowing.
- Your lips, tongue, or face swells.
- You begin vomiting.
- You experience chest pain.
- You experience excessive sweating.
- An infant or child has been stung by a scorpion.
- You've been bitten by a black widow or brown recluse spider. (Some people experience mild reactions to black widow or brown recluse bites and care for the wound at home. But as the venom of these two spiders is poisonous, it's better to be safe than sorry.)
- The bitten area swells excessively or becomes discolored (other than redness).
- You develop a very high fever or a fever accompanied by a spotty rash.

Follow Up with Your Doctor If . . .

- Pain and swelling worsen over the 48 hours following the bite or sting.
- You develop a red, donut-shaped rash after a tick bite, which could be a sign of Lyme disease.
- You develop flulike symptoms after a bite.

will give you a double dose of itch relief.

To relieve pain and swelling, apply a bit of honey, which has been shown to have antibacterial, anti-inflammatory, and analgesic properties. Honey can also speed wound healing.[4]

healing foods

Though there were few human clinical trials to support their use, there is strong anecdotal evidence for using the following healing foods in the treatment of common insect bites and stings.

- **BASIL:** Apply crushed basil or basil oil directly to your skin to relieve itching; basil plants also help repel mosquitoes.

- **LEMON OR LIME JUICE:** Apply the juice directly to your skin for itch relief; lemon and lime juice also have antibacterial properties.

- **MILK AND WATER:** Mix in equal parts and dab onto your skin for itch and pain relief.

- **USED TEA BAGS:** Apply to your skin to draw out fluid; the tannins in tea are astringent and can reduce swelling and inflammation.

- **APPLE CIDER VINEGAR:** This works as an anti-inflammatory and antibacterial; dab it onto bites or, for allover relief, add 1 cup of apple cider vinegar to a bath and soak in it.

insomnia

Insomnia is the inability to fall asleep or to remain asleep through the night. (Some people experience both kinds.) Insomnia is often a temporary problem that arises in response to stress, anxiety, the use of alcohol, the use of stimulants, illness or pain, hormonal changes, or environmental factors (such as noise, an overheated room, jet lag, or light pollution). Insomnia caused by factors such as these is called acute insomnia, and it usually resolves without treatment.

But an alarming number of Americans are now plagued with chronic insomnia, which is insomnia that occurs 3 nights a week (or more) for a month or longer. Its effects go well beyond the daytime sleepiness, irritability, inability to focus or concentrate, and general tiredness that accompany even one night of insomnia. The most recent research confirms that chronic insomnia is a far more serious condition than we once thought, resulting in negative health consequences such as obesity, long-term cognitive impairment, accelerated aging, higher incidence of chronic pain, and weakened immunity. Chronic insomnia also increases your risk of cardiovascular disease, depression and anxiety, type 2 diabetes, cancer, stroke, and even death.[1]

So what specific foods can help in your effort to sleep well and live well? Ginseng improves sleep by reducing total wake time and increasing sleep duration. It also has an antianxiety effect.[2] The lingzhi (or reishi) mushroom contains natural sleep-promoting agents.[3] Tart cherry juice increases melatonin, resulting in significant increases in time in bed, total sleep time, and sleep efficiency ratio (the amount of time spent sleeping versus the total amount of time in bed).[4] Walnuts can help improve sleep because of their natural melatonin, serotonin, and polyphenol content.[5] Kiwifruit has been found to improve overall sleep quality, decrease waking time after sleep onset, and decrease the amount of time it takes to fall asleep. It can also increase total sleep time and sleep efficiency. In this particular study, people ate two kiwis 1 hour before bedtime for their sleep-promoting effects.[6]

The National Sleep Foundation recommends eating a prebedtime snack containing protein and carbohydrates, such as cheese and crackers or peanut butter on toast. Why? Because proteins are the building blocks of tryptophan, the amino acid that can induce sleepiness, and carbohydrates increase the bioavailability of tryptophan.[7] Other great protein and carb combos include yogurt and kiwis, lean turkey and brown rice, whole grain cereal and low-fat milk, or whole oats with bananas.

A deficiency of B vitamins and minerals also seems to disrupt sleep, most likely because these nutrients contribute to the secretion of melatonin and are necessary for the synthesis of serotonin. Vitamin B_3 (niacin) increased REM (rapid eye movement) sleep in people with normal sleep patterns and improved the sleep efficacy in those with moderate to severe insomnia.[8]

Food sources of niacin include tuna, salmon, chicken, turkey, cremini mushrooms, brown rice, lamb, beef, asparagus, and tomatoes. Magnesium supplementation in those who are deficient has also been shown to enhance sleep quality. Magnesium promotes melatonin secretion and has a relaxing effect. So eat sesame seeds; sunflower seeds; almonds; oats; dark, leafy greens; avocados; and bananas. Tryptophan is also needed by your body to produce serotonin, which can induce feelings of calmness and drowsiness.[9] To increase your tryptophan intake, eat lean turkey, seaweed, spinach, soy protein, sesame seeds, crab, lobster, mozzarella cheese, bananas, and egg whites.

As there was older evidence showing that eating a meal with a high glycemic index before bed could help people fall

healthy insight

Looking for an unconventional means to put insomnia to rest? A recent study found that Japanese sake yeast increased delta sleep power during the first cycle of slow-wave sleep (or the quality of deep sleep) by 110 percent and also decreased next-day fatigue and sleepiness. In this study, participants took a supplement containing 500 milligrams of sake yeast 1 hour before bedtime. It also increased human growth hormone as measured in morning urine by 137 percent,[10] which is associated with increased energy and enhanced cognitive function.

asleep faster,[11] researchers more recently examined the role of rice, bread, and noodles in sleep quality among 1,848 adults. They found that indeed, a high glycemic index was associated with better sleep—but only when it came to rice, which contains high levels of melatonin. Bread had no relationship with sleep quality, and noodle intake actually promoted poor sleep.[12]

Finally, putting it all together, a recent study found that those who slept best were those who ate the widest variety of foods. Those who had the least variety in their diets either slept less than 5 hours a night *or* greater than 9 hours a night, neither of which meets the ideal of 7 to 8 hours of sleep per night for adults.[13] Once again, we see the benefits of an overall healthy dietary pattern.

See also: Anxiety (page 165), Colds (page 214), Depression (page 232), Diabetes (page 238), Heart Disease (Cardiovascular Disease) (page 313), High Blood Pressure (Hypertension) (page 327), Overweight and Obesity (page 396), Stress (page 419), Stroke (page 423)

irritable bowel syndrome

I rritable bowel syndrome (IBS), once referred to as spastic colon and not to be confused with inflammatory bowel disease, is a group of abdominal symptoms that occur concurrently. It is the most common gastrointestinal condition and can affect anyone at any age. The primary symptoms include abdominal pain or discomfort, changes in bowel habits (constipation, diarrhea, or both, and these may change over time), and a change in the appearance of stools (most often, mucus in the stool). Other symptoms that may appear include bloating, the sensation of incomplete bowel movements, and urgency (the need to move your bowels right away). One of the vexing characteristics of IBS is its mutability: Symptoms can flare up or diminish or disappear over time, and bowel habits can range from diarrhea to constipation. The causes of IBS are not entirely understood, but some people have a genetic predisposition toward the condition, some sufferers report that specific foods cause or exacerbate symptoms, and stress seems to play a role in triggering IBS and in exacerbating subsequent flare-ups. (Interestingly, chronic stress experienced before the age of 18 has been shown to be associated with an increased prevalence of IBS.)[1] An intestinal infection seems to predispose some people to IBS, as well.

One challenge to creating an anti-IBS diet is that in addition to divergent symptoms—your diet will look quite different depending on whether you're suffering from constipation or diarrhea, for instance—different foods have different effects on IBS sufferers. You should thus be aware of your unique food triggers that cause flare-ups or worsen symptoms, and you should eliminate those from your diet. That said, there are general guidelines that will work for most people with IBS.

One of the latest overall dietary plans to treat IBS is called the low FODMAP diet. Developed by a research team in Australia, where roughly one in seven adults suffers from IBS, FODMAP is an acronym for fermentable oligosaccharides, disaccharides, monosaccharides, and polyols. In brief, FODMAPs are short-chain carbohydrates that are poorly absorbed in your small intestine and are thus quickly fermented by bacteria in your gut. The fermentation process naturally produces gas, which can lead to bloating and stomach distension. And because these carbohydrates are poorly absorbed, they can lead to irritation in many people's guts, resulting in the familiar "intestinal distress" symptoms of diarrhea and/or constipation. Many IBS sufferers have found great relief by avoiding high FODMAP foods. In a metastudy of 22 clinical trials, IBS sufferers who followed the low FODMAP diet experienced a significant reduction in symptom severity scores overall, including abdominal pain and bloating. Quality of life scores improved significantly, as well.[2]

The full list of high FODMAP foods is too long to list here,[3] but in brief, they include:

- Foods high in fructose (apples, cherries, mangoes, peaches, pears, watermelon, asparagus, artichokes, sugar snap peas, honey, fruit juices, and any processed food made with high-fructose corn syrup)
- Lactose (milk, yogurt, soft cheeses, butter, and ice cream)
- Oligosaccharides (peaches, persimmons, watermelon, artichokes, asparagus, beans, beetroot, Brussels sprouts, cabbage, chicory, fennel, garlic, leeks, shallots, okra, onions, peas, wheat, rye, barley, pistachios, lentils, chickpeas, soy products, chicory drinks, and the common food additive inulin)
- Sugar alcohols known as polyols (such as sorbitol and xylitol, including foods like apricots, avocados, blackberries, cherries, lychees, nectarines, plums, prunes, cauliflower, mushrooms, snow peas, and any food containing an artificial sweetener)[4]
- Onions, garlic, and wheat products (avoid entirely, if possible)

The full list of foods to avoid according to the FODMAP diet is extensive, but the good news is that in most cases, this diet is a temporary measure you should follow for 6 to 8 weeks, or until your IBS symptoms subside. If you have IBS you may, under the guidance of your doctor, wish to follow the FODMAP diet for extended periods of time.

Research is still emerging, but one of the most exciting developments in healing foods for IBS concerns the management of IBS through probiotics. Studies have shown that up to 20 percent of IBS cases are preceded by an intestinal infection, and a meta-analysis study showed that small intestinal bacterial overgrowth (SIBO) was present in up to 54 percent of IBS cases. There is also some evidence that IBS is a condition of low-grade inflammation.[5] Probiotics that modulate the intestinal flora and

help for irritable bowel syndrome: foods to calm your gut (and your mind)

There are plenty of old wives' tales about how to treat an upset stomach or abdominal discomfort. These foods are recommended specifically for IBS symptoms.

Foods to Eat to Treat Constipation

- Apricots
- Beans (but proceed with caution; they're notorious for causing gas)
- Blueberries
- Dates
- Dark, leafy greens: kale, spinach, Swiss chard, arugula, collard greens, and lettuces
- Lentils
- Prunes
- Raisins

Foods to Eat to Treat Diarrhea

- Probiotics: yogurt and kefir
- Liquids to keep you hydrated: water, herbal tea, and diluted fruit juices

Foods to Eat to Treat Stress

- Probiotic foods such as yogurt, kefir, sauerkraut, miso, natto, kimchi, and tempeh
- Foods containing omega-3s: wild-caught fish such as salmon, mackerel, herring, and sardines; walnuts; and flaxseeds
- Avocados
- Bananas
- Brown rice
- Cantaloupe
- Holy basil
- Lean chicken or turkey (skin removed)
- Papayas
- Seaweed
- Tofu
- Whole grains

Foods to Avoid for IBS

- Any of your unique food triggers—keep a food diary if you're unsure of yours
- Caffeine
- Fried foods
- Spicy foods

exert effects upon the gut–brain axis are indicated for all of these factors. In a metastudy of 1,793 IBS patients, researchers found that compared to a placebo, probiotic users experienced a reduction in abdominal pain severity, bloating, and flatulence.[6] In a study of 274 constipation-predominant IBS patients, those who consumed a fermented yogurt containing *Bifidobacterium animalis* experienced improvements in quality of life scores, bloating, and an increase in stool frequency in those with fewer than three bowel movements per week. *Bifidobacterium* strains produced IBS symptom relief in additional studies, either alone or in combination with other probiotic strains.[7]

One natural remedy that shouldn't be overlooked is peppermint oil. Not all IBS sufferers benefit from it, but some do. In a metareview of four studies that compared peppermint oil to placebos, 65 percent of IBS patients had persistent symptoms while only 26 percent of those who used peppermint oil did.[8] Now a new form of peppermint oil designed for sustained release in the small intestine has been investigated for the treatment of IBS. Seventy-two IBS patients were randomized either to the peppermint oil treatment or a placebo. After 4 weeks, peppermint oil was associated with a 40 percent reduction in total IBS symptom score (an index of common IBS symptoms), while there was only a 24.3 percent improvement in the placebo group. Patients in the peppermint group also experienced greater improvement in multiple individual gastrointestinal symptoms as well as in "severe or unbearable" symptoms, compared to a placebo.[9]

An anti-IBS diet should also address stress. Stress triggers a whole-body response in everyone, and one of the most common responses is an increase in bowel movements. As people with IBS have especially sensitive gastrointestinal tracts, foods that exert a calming effect on your mind and body are smart choices to best prepare to deal with stressful events and to lower stress level overall. For a full list, see Anxiety (page 165) and Stress (page 419). When choosing any of these stress-relieving foods, make sure to cross-reference them with any of your personal IBS food triggers and/or with the low FODMAP diet, if you're following it.

See also: Constipation (page 218), Diarrhea (page 245), Flatulence (page 276), Food Allergies (page 278), Indigestion (page 345)

kidney stones

Kidney stones form when crystalline substances such as calcium, oxalate, or uric acid accumulate in urine and stick together. Kidney stones can make their way from your kidneys into your ureters and on into your bladder, where they are passed out of your body through your urine. Some kidney stones are so small that they're excreted undetected, but if they become large the condition can be terribly painful. Symptoms include pain in your side, back, groin, and/or lower abdomen, which can fluctuate and be quite severe; painful urination; discolored urine; the presence of blood in your urine; nausea and vomiting; a frequent need to urinate; low urine output; and fever. It's best to see your doctor if you suspect a kidney stone, especially if this is your first attack.

There are several key healing foods that can help prevent kidney stones—and at the top of the list is not a food, but a beverage. Many kidney stones form when urine isn't sufficiently diluted, allowing minerals and salts to stick together—in other words, when you're dehydrated. So drink plenty of water: The goal is to produce 2 liters or more of urine per day.[1] (Many sources recommend a daily urine output of 2.5 liters, especially if you suffer from recurrent kidney stones.) There is also evidence that increasing citrates (citric acid) can prevent kidney stone formation by (1) binding with urinary calcium and (2) binding calcium oxalate crystals and preventing crystal growth. Easy ways to get more citric acid into your diet are to drink more fruit juices (orange, lemon, lime, and melon) and to add fruit juices such as lemon or lime to water. Juices to be *avoided*, on the other hand, are tomato juice, because of its high sodium content, and grapefruit and cranberry juice, because of their oxalate content.[2] Potassium citrate also raises the pH of urine and plays a role in the prevention of kidney stones.[3] Good food sources include bananas, prunes, prune juice, orange juice, tomatoes, raisins, artichokes, lima beans, acorn squash, spinach, sunflower seeds, almonds, and molasses.[4]

Oxalates have been implicated in the creation of calcium oxalate kidney stones, but the evidence is mixed, and because oxalates are prevalent in so many healthy foods, many health-care professionals only recommend a low-oxalate diet if you have hyperoxaluria, a condition in which you produce too much oxalate and there is too much oxalate in your urine. Though generally uncommon, hyperoxaluria is found in about 20 percent of people with kidney stones. If your doctor determines that oxalates are contributing to your kidney stones, eliminate or greatly reduce spinach, rhubarb, beets, strawberries, chocolate, nuts and nut butters, and black tea. Otherwise, the National Kidney Foundation recommends eating oxalate-rich foods along with calcium-rich foods, as oxalate and calcium bind together in your stomach and intestines before your kidneys are involved, thus decreasing the chances of kidney stone formation.[5] Another thing to keep in mind concerning oxalates is vitamin C:

sneaky ways to lower your sodium intake

Eating less sodium isn't just about putting away the saltshaker. You can count on processed and fast foods to be loaded with excess sodium, so the next step should be obvious: Use fresh food products whenever possible. Fruits, vegetables, and proteins in their natural state have no added sodium.

Next, examine labels with a beady eye. Foods that look healthy at first glance—or even foods that specifically claim to be healthy or all natural—can contain high amounts of sodium. For example, canned soups, broths, canned vegetables, crackers, pretzels, frozen foods (including veggie burgers and protein patties!), prepared sauces, breads and other baked goods, and fortified cereals can contain more sodium than you'd think. One of the most surprising sources of sodium is cottage cheese. One cup of 1% cottage cheese contains an eye-popping 918 milligrams (mg) of sodium—nearly half of the recommended daily allowance. (And remember that 2,300 mg is the *upper* limit.) If you do use canned vegetables and beans, rinse them before cooking with or eating them; you can drain away as much as 35 percent of the sodium.

Instead of salting dishes during food preparation, try cutting back or even eliminating salt and letting people salt their meals according to individual taste. If you can't break the salt habit entirely, try cutting added salt in half and adding pizzazz to dishes by using black pepper, herbs, or spices. When they're in season, chopped fresh herbs are a delicious addition to many dishes; use dried herbs throughout the year.

At superdosages, vitamin C increases urine oxalate concentrations. But vitamin B_6 has the opposite effect, and studies have shown that vitamin B_6 intake is linked to a lower prevalence of kidney stones. Foods high in vitamin B_6 include avocados, bananas, halibut, mangoes, oatmeal, soybeans, and fortified cereals.[6]

Likewise, many people are told to cut their calcium intake in order to prevent kidney stones. But actually, quite the opposite is true. There is substantial evidence demonstrating that a diet high in calcium is associated with a lower risk of kidney stones, for the very reason mentioned above: Calcium binds to oxalate in your gut, thereby reducing oxalate absorption.[7] People who form calcium oxalate stones should make sure that they're getting sufficient calcium, not only to prevent kidney stones but also to maintain bone density.[8] The National Institutes of Health (NIH) recommends that men and women ages 19 to 70 get at least 1,000 milligrams (mg) of calcium per day; those 71 and older should get 1,200 mg. Food sources of calcium include milk, yogurt, cheese, soy milk, tofu, salmon, kale, turnip greens, bok choy, and cabbage. One surprising source of calcium is canned sardines: Three ounces give you 33 percent of the recommended daily allowance of calcium.[9]

High intakes of sodium and protein—especially animal protein—are generally accepted as nutritional risk factors for kidney stones. Sodium increases the amount of calcium your kidneys must filter, and it increases the amount of calcium in your urine. It is also strongly associated with other renal disorders, such as chronic kidney disease. In a study of more than 3,900 patients, a higher sodium and potassium intake was linked to a faster progression of chronic kidney disease. Sodium intake was particularly distressing: On average, participants in this study consumed 3,700 mg of sodium per day,[10] which far exceeds the USDA's recommendation to limit sodium intake to 2,300 mg or less per day. Many medical professionals think this limit is also too high; an intake of no more than 1,500 mg of sodium per day is recommended by proponents of the DASH (Dietary Approaches to Stop Hypertension) diet, as well as by the American Heart Association.

Limiting animal protein can also help. Uric acid is produced when your body metabolizes animal protein, and it shows up in large quantities in your urine. Animal protein also lowers the pH of urine, and these two conditions—supersaturation with uric acid plus low pH—are prime factors for uric acid stones. A study published in the *Journal* of Renal Nutrition concluded that high-protein diets cause an increased risk of kidney stones, hypertension due to increased sodium, and glomerular hyperfiltration, which can result in excessive protein in the urine and may contribute to chronic kidney disease.[11] Those who have risk factors for kidney stones and those who have suffered from them before should adopt a diet that is low in animal protein (including dairy and eggs). Instead, consider safer, plant-based protein sources such as legumes (lentils, peas, and beans), quinoa, buckwheat, spirulina, chia seeds, and soy products.

lightheadedness

Lightheadedness is the feeling that you're going to faint, or the kind of swimmy-headed or "floaty" feeling that can occur intermittently. Unlike dizziness (or vertigo), you don't feel as if the room is moving or spinning, and in most cases lightheadedness improves or goes away once you lie down. Brief episodes of lightheadedness are usually not serious and occur when your brain doesn't get enough blood. The most common causes are getting up too quickly (this occurs especially in older people and during pregnancy), a sudden change in blood pressure, dehydration, hyperventilation, hypoglycemia, or feeling anxious or stressed. Lightheadedness can also accompany an illness such as a cold or flu, especially when fever is present, and it can result from the use of alcohol, illicit drugs, or certain prescription medications. If lightheadedness doesn't resolve on its own or is accompanied by additional symptoms, such as fatigue or heart arrhythmia, or if you experience multiple fainting spells, see a medical professional for an evaluation.

As one of the most common causes of lightheadedness is dehydration, make sure you're taking in adequate hydration every day. The best beverages are filtered water and herbal teas. Fruit juices are fine in moderation, but be careful of getting too much sugar. Caffeine and alcohol actually have dehydrating effects, so if you're feeling lightheaded, you'll want to reduce or eliminate caffeinated and alcoholic beverages and rely on water and/or herbal teas until you feel better. Of course, hydration comes from food sources as well. Some of the foods with the highest water content are celery, apples, cucumbers, blueberries, peaches, mangoes, water chestnuts, fennel, grapes, bell peppers, watermelon, strawberries, broths, and broth-based soups. If dehydration is severe, consider some of the low-sugar energy drinks that are on the market; they can restore your electrolyte balance. Or try making your own with the World Health Organization's recipe: Stir 6 teaspoons of sugar and $\frac{1}{2}$ teaspoon of salt into 5 cups of water. You can flavor this drink with a squeeze or lemon, lime, or orange, or drop in some sliced cucumber for a refreshing taste.

Lightheadedness can just as easily

come from being in a hypoglycemic state—meaning that your blood sugar has dropped temporarily. If you're skipping meals or eating meals that are high in sugar, you'll inevitably experience a drop in blood sugar, which can leave you feeling lightheaded, shaky, and irritable. Eating meals that are high in protein can prevent lightheadedness and can treat it if it occurs. Opt for lean proteins such as seafood, lean poultry, eggs, organic soy products, and nut butters. They'll keep you feeling full longer and will keep your blood sugar stable. If you need a quick fix to boost your blood sugar level, eat a handful of dried apricots. They're full of concentrated carbs, which can give you a fast boost when you need it most, and they're far healthier than sources of simple sugars such as candies, white breads, or desserts.

To improve circulation over the long haul, eat cold-water fish such as salmon, mackerel, herring, sardines, and tuna. Studies have shown that omega-3s can improve blood circulation and stabilize arterial pressure,[1] and with their high protein content, they'll prevent hypoglycemia, as well. For vegetarian sources of omega-3s, eat flaxseeds, flaxseed oil, and nuts. If your blood pressure is chronically low and your health-care provider okays it, try licorice or licorice tea for raising blood pressure. The active component in licorice, glycyrrhizin, is known to elevate blood pressure. But it comes with a list of potential unwanted side effects and has caused cases of hypertension, headache, low potassium, edema, and platelet deficiency,[2] especially when taken in excessive amounts or with extended use, so seek guidance before trying this healing food.

See also: Anxiety (page 165), Hypoglycemia (page 343), Stress (page 419)

lupus

Lupus is a chronic inflammatory autoimmune disorder that occurs when your immune system malfunctions and attacks your own tissues and organs. The exact cause of lupus is unknown, but many scientists believe it's caused by a combination of environmental, genetic, and hormonal factors. The most commonly cited environmental factors are ultraviolet light (which is present in sunlight), infections, and exposure to silica dust. Lupus runs in families, and even if there is no family history of lupus, it's more likely to develop when family members have other autoimmune disorders. Lupus also occurs more frequently in women, and symptoms tend to be worse during pregnancy or just before a woman's menstrual period, when estrogen levels are high. There are four main types of lupus and several subtypes, but the most common type (and the type we'll be addressing here) is known as systemic lupus erythematosus (SLE). Though no two cases of lupus are exactly alike, the most common symptoms are joint pain and swelling; fatigue; chest pain; shortness of breath; a red, butterfly-shaped facial rash; dry eyes; hair loss; edema; and headaches. Many people with lupus develop photosensitivity; skin lesions can appear and/or worsen after exposure to sunlight. Lupus comes in "waves," or alternating periods of flare-ups and remission. There is no cure for lupus and severe cases are life threatening, but with proper rest, medical care, and management of symptoms during flares, the vast majority of lupus sufferers can expect to live a normal life span and engage in normal activities.

Good nutrition is an integral part of lupus management, so let's take a look at the latest recommendations and research findings. There is no single diet plan for everyone with lupus, but as it is a disease affecting multiple organs and causing widespread inflammation, lupus sufferers benefit greatly from eating patterns that provide whole-body nutrition and that emphasize antioxidant-rich foods such as colorful fruits and vegetables, beans, dark chocolate, tea, coffee, and wine. Further, considering their elevated risk of atherosclerosis, metabolic syndrome, and diabetes, lupus patients can benefit from following any of the well-known heart-healthy diet plans, such as the Mediterranean diet, the DASH diet, or the Nordic diet (also predominantly plant-based and containing oily fish; shellfish; foraged foods like mushrooms; fruits; berries; wild meat; and whole grains). Any dietary pattern that emphasizes fresh, whole foods; fruits and vegetables; complex carbs; lean proteins; and healthy fats is recommended.

In contrast, steer clear of the typical Western dietary pattern, which is heavy on processed and refined foods, fast food, fried foods, and sugary drinks and desserts. Though evidence is somewhat mixed, the Lupus Foundation of America also advises people with lupus to avoid alfalfa, as it has the potential to trigger flares or other lupuslike effects such as muscle pain, fatigue, and kidney problems. Further, if you're taking corticosteroids, limit your salt and fat intake, as corticosteroids can elevate blood pressure, cholesterol, and lipids. (There is some evidence that vitamin A, found in fish and fish oils, sweet potatoes, spinach, carrots, cantaloupe, sweet peppers, mangoes, black-eyed peas, apricots, broccoli, eggs, and fortified milk and cereal, can reverse the damaging immunosuppressive effects of corticosteroids.)[1] Finally, alcohol can interfere with the efficacy of some medications, such as anticoagulation medicines.[2] Check with your doctor to make sure, but in most cases moderate alcohol consumption is fine for people with lupus. With this framework of healthy foods in place, we can turn our attention to specific foods and nutrients that can help prevent and manage disease activity.

Omega-3 fatty acids provide multiple benefits for people with lupus. These polyunsaturated fatty acids have anti-inflammatory and antiautoimmune effects, and they lower triglycerides. Omega-3s provide further benefits for lupus sufferers because they can suppress macrophage activity, reduce protein in your urine, and protect your kidneys against the effect of free radicals. Flaxseed oil alone has been shown to reduce protein in urine, preserve kidney function, and inhibit platelet activating factor, which is commonly elevated in lupus patients.[3] A study comparing 114 lupus patients with 122 healthy controls found that higher levels of DHA (docosahexaenoic acid) and EPA (eicosapentaenoic acid), both long-chain omega-3 fatty acids, decreased disease activity and reduced atherosclerotic plaques. Conversely, higher levels of omega-6s, which are found primarily in vegetable oils, had the opposite effect; in this study, higher carbohydrate intake was associated with higher omega-6 levels.[4] Another study compared fish oil supplementation with an olive oil placebo in patients with lupus;

results were recorded at baseline and after 6 months of treatment. Those receiving fish oil experienced a reduction in biomarkers of inflammation and an improvement in scores of their energy and emotional well-being.[5] Omega-3s are found in flaxseeds and flaxseed oil, canola oil, olive oil, nuts, fish oil, and fish such as salmon, herring, sardines, and tuna.

Another nutrient that has been the subject of extensive study in relation to lupus is vitamin D, which has multiple immunomodulating effects. Vitamin D deficiency is common in the general population and even more so in those with lupus. In a study of 177 lupus patients, 82 percent had low vitamin D, and this deficiency was associated with elevated disease activity as well as elevated markers of antibodies that attack double-stranded DNA. Low vitamin D has also been associated with carotid artery plaque in lupus patients.[6] A study examining the effects of vitamin D randomized 267 lupus patients to receive either a placebo or 2,000 international units (IU) a day of vitamin D for 12 months. At the start of the study, 69 percent of the patients had suboptimal levels of vitamin D, and 39 percent were vitamin D deficient (having serum levels of less than 10 ng/ml). Lower levels of vitamin D correlated with significantly higher disease activity (as

opposed to periods of dormancy). After 12 months of treatment, there was significant improvement in disease activity scores and C4 (a protein that protects against infection) levels, as well as a significant reduction in markers of inflammation and autoantibodies.[7] Low vitamin D levels are also associated with decreased bone mineral density,[8] which is further exacerbated by extended use of corticosteroids.

One reason people with lupus tend to have abnormally low levels of vitamin D is that lupus can cause photosensitivity, an unusual sensitivity to sunlight. Sunlight can cause a rash in photosensitive lupus sufferers, or it can trigger full-blown flares that bring joint pain, fatigue, weakness, and fever. About two-thirds of lupus patients have photosensitivity, and as our main source of vitamin D is sun exposure, lupus sufferers are especially at risk for vitamin D deficiency. Researchers have also pointed out that those with darker pigmentation have a harder time getting sufficient vitamin D from sun exposure—and that African-Americans and Hispanics are disproportionately affected by lupus and tend to have more severe cases.[9] The extended use of steroids can also play a part in the lower levels of vitamin D in lupus patients, as can hypoparathyroidism.[10] Vitamin D can be found in foods such as dairy products, eggs, fish, fish oil, fortified orange juice, and mushrooms, but with so many deleterious effects resulting from vitamin D deficiency for lupus sufferers and so many health benefits to gain, those with lupus should consider a supplement, as well.

As lupus sufferers are already at heightened risk for osteoporosis and decreased bone mineral density due to vitamin D deficiency, the use of corticosteroids, early menopause due to exposure to cytotoxic agents, and disease activity generally, adequate calcium intake is extremely important. One study found that women with lupus are five times more likely to suffer fractures than healthy women of the same age.[11] Calcium-rich foods include dairy products, tofu, sardines, shrimp, collards, broccoli, broccoli rabe, kale, soybeans, bok choy, okra, white beans, black-eyed peas, dried figs, oranges, fortified orange juice, fortified cereals, and milk substitutes such as almond milk, soy milk, and rice milk.

Vitamin C is recommended, as it has been shown to lower the risk of lupus-related inflammatory activity and inhibit the release of inflammatory mediators. Vitamin C also plays a vital role in heart health and has been shown to improve vasodilation in lupus patients with heart disease.[12] Vitamin C can be found in citrus fruits and their juices, papayas, tomatoes, broccoli, kiwifruit, strawberries, red peppers, Brussels sprouts, cauliflower, cantaloupe, guavas, parsley, and acerola cherries (West Indian cherries).

Finally, one food in particular deserves special mention when it comes to lupus, and that's turmeric. Multiple studies have demonstrated the healing effects of this aromatic spice, which is known for its powerful anti-inflammatory abilities. Patients with lupus nephritis, an inflammation of the kidney caused by lupus, received turmeric supplements with each meal for 3 months, while a control group received a placebo. Volunteers were assessed at baseline and again after 1, 2, and 3 months. Those in the turmeric group had significantly less protein in their urine at each assessment. By the end of the study period, systolic blood pressure and the presence of blood in the urine had also significantly decreased.[13] Curcumin is the active ingredient in turmeric, and it's been shown to inhibit autoimmune diseases by regulating inflammatory cytokines.[14] It's also been shown to inhibit the binding of lupus autoantibodies to their respective antigens by up to 52 percent.[15]

See also: Arthritis and Joint Pain (page 171), Dry Eyes (page 250), Fatigue (page 266)

macular degeneration

Macular degeneration is often referred to as age-related macular degeneration, or AMD, as it mostly occurs in adults over the age of 50. It's the leading cause of blindness in people who are 65 and older. AMD affects central vision, resulting in blurry or dark spots directly ahead. Over time, the distorted spots grow larger, further obscuring vision and making everyday tasks such as reading or driving impossible. Risk factors for AMD include age, race (Caucasians are more likely to develop the condition), family history of AMD, smoking, and a sedentary lifestyle.

There are two types of macular degeneration, dry (nonneovascular) and wet (neovascular). Dry AMD is the much more common type, affecting some 85 to 90 percent of AMD sufferers. Currently there is no known cure for either type of AMD, so interventions focus on prevention and on slowing the disease once it is diagnosed. AMD can be detected during a routine eye exam even before there is any discernible loss of vision.

Lifestyle factors such as not smoking, getting sufficient exercise, and eating a healthy diet that emphasizes dark, leafy greens; fruits; and seafood can help prevent AMD. If AMD does occur, these same factors can help slow the progression of the disease and preserve vision. Let's look specifically at the nutritional interventions that can support eye health.

A major clinical trial sponsored by the National Eye Institute called the Age-Related Eye Disease Study (AREDS) found that high levels of antioxidants and zinc can reduce the risk of AMD and its associated vision loss by as much as 25 percent. This study followed 3,640 individuals ages 55 to 80 for more than 6 years. The levels of supplementation were as follows: vitamin C, 500 milligrams (mg); vitamin E, 400 international units (IU); beta-carotene, 15 mg; zinc, 80 mg in the form of zinc oxide. (Additionally, participants received 2 mg of copper as cupric oxide in order to prevent copper deficiency anemia, which can be caused by high levels of zinc.)[1] Some companies have created eye vitamin formulations based upon the results of this landmark study. Board-certified ophthalmologist Elizabeth Brown, MD, notes that since the publication of the first AREDS study,

"it's become the standard of care for ophthalmologists to recommend a diet rich in antioxidants to their patients with macular degeneration. Because it can be difficult to consume the quantities outlined in the study, we also recommend supplements with the AREDS formula of vitamins. An antioxidant-rich diet is the first line of defense we have in a [fight against this] potentially devastating disease." Dr. Brown also recommends that anyone with a family history of AMD should "make a conscious, daily effort to consume a diet rich in antioxidants."

Five years after the first AREDS study, the National Eye Institute launched AREDS2, a 5-year study that would examine whether the original AREDS recommendations could be improved by adding omega-3 fatty acids; the plant-derived carotenoids lutein and zeaxanthin; removing beta-carotene; and/or reducing zinc, which was found to produce gastrointestinal side effects in some people. The study also examined how different combinations of these supplements could help. The results were released in 2013, and the main findings were that omega-3 fatty acids have no additional effect on the original AREDS formulation, but that lutein and zeaxanthin are a safe alternative to beta-carotene, which was found to increase the risk of lung cancer in smokers.[2] Recent data confirms the efficacy of lutein, zeaxanthin, and other carotenoids on vision health. Carotenoids are the yellow, orange, and red pigments synthesized by plants, and they have strong antioxidant effects. The results of an AMD study that followed more than 102,000 people for more than 20 years found about a 40 percent risk reduction for advanced AMD in men and women who consumed the highest levels of lutein and zeaxanthin and a 25 to 35 percent lower risk in those who consumed the highest levels of other carotenoids (beta-cryptoxanthin, alpha-carotene, and beta-carotene).[3]

Finally, a Korean study has found that the toxic heavy metals mercury and cadmium are associated with late-stage age-related macular degeneration and that lead is associated with both

> **BONUS TIP:** Though peer-reviewed research is quite limited in this area, there is some evidence that certain foods play a role in helping to detoxify your body of the effects of heavy metals such as mercury, cadmium, and lead. These foods include coriander/cilantro, garlic, green tea, onions, and turmeric,[4] among many others (such as chlorella, milk thistle, and cloves) that are commonly cited by naturopaths and other complementary medicine practitioners.

early- and late-stage age-related macular degeneration (see Bonus Tip on page 375). On the other hand, manganese and zinc were found to have a protective effect against late-stage age-related macular degeneration.[5]

So, from *all* of these results, what can we conclude are the best whole foods to help prevent AMD? Here are some of the best food sources to support eye health.

Antioxidants are found in abundance in fresh fruits and vegetables and also in tea, coffee, red wine, and cocoa. Sources of antioxidants include pineapple, berries, tomatoes, red grapes, red cabbage, kale, spinach, arugula, onions, apples, broccoli, soybeans, apricots, beets, cantaloupe, carrots, mangoes, oranges, winter squash, yellow and orange peppers, green tea, dark chocolate, and papayas. For zinc, eat oysters, wheat germ, chicken, crab, beans, oatmeal, yogurt, sunflower seeds, pumpkin seeds, and pine nuts. For food sources of lutein and zeaxanthin (both are types of carotenoids), eat einkorn (an ancient wheat), durum wheat (used to make pasta), yellow corn, cantaloupe, carrots, orange and yellow peppers, oranges, salmon and other fish, kale, spinach, turnip greens, collards, parsley, watercress, fresh basil, and eggs. Some of the best sources of manganese are black tea, blueberries, wheat bran, spinach, amaranth leaves, fresh basil, hearts of palm, mollusks, and the ground spices ginger, saffron, cardamom, and cinnamon.[6]

memory loss (short term)

All of us experience a decline in memory as we age; occasionally forgetting words or names is quite common and not a matter of urgent concern. People often wonder about the line between normal forgetfulness and the kind of memory loss that necessitates a trip to the doctor. One reliable determining factor is the degree to which memory loss is impacting your daily life. Does it amount to an occasional irritation—for example, occasionally misplacing your glasses or car keys or having difficulty recalling a word—or is it preventing you from living a full and productive life? If it's the latter, you should follow up with your health-care provider. The entries on Alzheimer's Disease (page 160) and Dementia (page 226) address more serious forms of memory loss. Here, we'll look at nutritional interventions that can help with routine lapses in short-term memory.

For nutritional interventions to preserve memory and prevent cognitive decline, the first word to remember is *flavonoids.* Flavonoids are compounds found in abundance in fruits, vegetables, and tea, and they have powerful antioxidant and anti-inflammatory properties. Some researchers believe that age-related memory loss occurs because of free radical damage to neurons—and flavonoids have been found to scavenge free radicals and exert powerful anti-inflammatory effects. In a study of 2,574 middle-aged men and women, a higher flavonoid intake was shown to help preserve verbal memory. More specifically, a higher intake of the flavonoid subclasses cate-chins, theaflavins, flavonols, and hydroxybenzoic acids was positively associated with language and verbal memory and especially with episodic memory,[1] which is the ability to recall autobiographical events.

One of the best food sources of flavonoids is berries, and numerous studies have found that berries can improve cognition. In a long-term study that examined data from more than 16,000 participants in the Nurses' Health Study, researchers found that a greater intake of strawberries and blueberries resulted in slower rates of cognitive decline—a delay in cognitive aging of up to 2.5 years, in fact.[2] Berries are particularly rich in a class of flavonoid called anthocyanins, which can cross the blood-brain barrier and directly affect the hippocampus, a brain region associated with learning and memory.[3]

Getting more flavonoids can even be as simple as quenching your thirst. In a study of men ages 30 to 65, the group that consumed flavonoid-rich orange juice performed significantly better on tests of executive function and psycho-motor speed compared to the group who drank a calorie-matched placebo.[4] The protective effect extends to older populations, as well: A study that examined the effect of high-flavanone orange juice in volunteers with an average age of 67 found a significant benefit to global cognitive function.[5] A study on adults with mild cognitive impairment found that drinking Concord grape juice improved their performance on memory tests; fMRI scans also showed greater activation in the anterior and posterior regions of the right hemisphere of the brains in the grape juice group.[6] Resveratrol, a phytochemical found in grape juice and red wine, and pterostilbene, a phytochemical found in grapes, blue-berries, and their juices, have both been shown to protect against cogni-tive loss on a cellular level by activat-ing signaling pathways that protect your brain against oxidative stress and inflammation.[7]

B vitamins have also been shown to have a beneficial effect on memory. A study that followed patients 70 years old and older for 2 years found that those who consumed a supplement containing vitamin B_6, vitamin B_{12}, and folic acid experienced a much slower rate of brain atrophy than those who consumed a placebo. These B vita-mins lowered homocysteine, an amino acid and by-product of protein metabo-lism that, at elevated levels, is a known risk factor for brain atrophy, cognitive decline, and dementia.[8] A more recent study on vitamin B sup-plementation and cognitive decline found that vitamin B treatment slowed brain atrophy rate by 40 percent—but only in those who had a high baseline of omega-3 fatty acids.[9] Foods that are good sources of B vitamins are listed in "Best Foods and Beverages for Short-Term Memory Protection" on the opposite page.

Studies have shown that a higher intake of polyunsaturated fatty acids (PUFAs), as well as a higher ratio of PUFAs to saturated fats, reduces your risk of memory impairment, and a higher intake of omega-3 PUFAs is linked to a lower risk of cognitive decline, including decline caused by Alzheimer's. Conversely, a higher intake of carbohydrates, simple sugars in par-ticular, is associated with lower cogni-tive function.[10] Seafood is a natural

best foods and beverages for short-term memory protection

If you're eating a plant-based diet, chances are you already eat a number of foods that protect against short-term memory loss.

Foods to Eat

- Foods rich in B vitamins: fruits; vegetables; whole grains; lean poultry; fish; dark, leafy greens; papayas; cantaloupe; oranges; eggs; and low-fat dairy (milk and yogurt)
- Omega-3-rich foods: salmon, mackerel, herring, tuna, cod, halibut, sardines, trout, walnuts, walnut oil, flaxseeds, and flaxseed oil
- Apples
- Apricots
- Beans: fava, black, pinto, kidney, and great northern
- Berries: blueberries, goji berries, mulberries, strawberries, blackberries, and acai berries
- Celery
- Coconut
- Dark, leafy greens: broccoli, kale, spinach, and lettuces
- Dark chocolate
- Extra-virgin olive oil
- Fruit juices, in moderation, especially orange juice, Concord grape juice, and blueberry juice
- Garlic
- Grapes
- Onions
- Parsley
- Pomegranates
- Red wine (in moderation)
- Seafood
- Soy products: tofu, tempeh, soybeans, soy milk, and miso
- Tea: green, black, and oolong
- Tomatoes
- Turmeric
- Vanilla

Foods to Avoid or Limit

- Fast foods
- Fried foods
- Processed foods
- Simple sugars: syrup, candies, refined carbohydrates, and soft drinks
- Sugary desserts
- Trans fats, including margarine and anything with partially hydrogenated oils

source of omega-3 PUFAs, so get more in your diet; see "Best Foods and Beverages for Short-Term Memory Protection" on page 379 for a full list of omega-3-rich foods. Examples of simple sugars to avoid are candies, cakes, syrups, and soft drinks. Fruit juices also fall into the category of simple sugars, so consume them in moderation.

An herbal supplement that always receives a great deal of attention when it comes to memory improvement is ginkgo biloba. Also known as the maidenhair tree, ginkgo is a rich source of flavonoids and is one of the most popular natural remedies for protecting memory. But clinical studies have found mixed results. A meta-analysis based on data from 2,576 people found that ginkgo biloba had no discernible effect on memory, executive function, or attention in healthy people.[11] However, in people who *already* have some signs of memory loss or dementia, ginkgo biloba extract at 240 milligrams a day appears to be helpful.[12]

Maintaining a healthy body mass index (BMI) is also crucial in protecting memory. Studies have found that obe-sity in middle age is independently associated with later cognitive impairments and that it causes more rapid cognitive decline.[13] The effect of BMI upon memory can even be seen in children. An Australian study found that 14-year-olds who ate a Western diet (characterized by a high intake of fast food, fried food, processed foods, and soft drinks) experienced diminished cognitive decline just 3 years later. Not surprisingly, this study also found positive associations between increased fruit and dark, leafy green consumption and improved cognitive performance.[14] A recent study confirms the benefits of an overall healthy diet to protect memory and overall cognition: Both the Mediterranean diet with increased olive oil consumption *and* the Mediterranean diet plus increased soy isoflavone consumption were found to improve memory. The Mediterranean dietary patterns improved global cognition, as well.[15]

See also: Alzheimer's Disease (page 160), Dementia (page 226), Depression (page 232), Insomnia (page 357), Overweight and Obesity (page 396)

menopause

Menopause is a normal biological process and not a disease or illness, but it does come with an increased risk of certain illnesses, as well as unwanted symptoms of its own. The absence of menstrual periods for 12 consecutive months, menopause is preceded by perimenopause, the transitional span of time that can last for several years. During the time leading up to full menopause, many women experience hot flashes, night sweats, irregular periods, changes in menstrual flow, vaginal dryness, insomnia, mood swings, thinning hair, dry skin, decreased libido, weight gain, and loss of breast fullness. Some women experience an increased susceptibility to bladder infections and urinary incontinence. After menopause, women are more susceptible to osteoporosis and heart disease. Changes in estrogen levels are linked to both of these conditions.

Menopause is inevitable, but many of its symptoms can be prevented, and in some women it may be possible to delay menopause through lifestyle changes, as well. Let's look at the research on healing foods for menopause.

To prevent osteoporosis, which affects about one out of every three postmenopausal women, eat foods that are rich in calcium, protein, and vitamin D. (Weight-bearing exercise, not smoking, and reducing alcohol consumption also help.)[1] Good food choices for bone health include low-fat dairy products, such as skim milk and yogurt; dark, leafy greens; lean, skinless poultry; seafood and fish; and nuts and nut butters. According to preliminary results, soy isoflavones can also help protect menopausal women against osteoporosis. Researchers gave 200 women in early menopause a daily supplement with soy protein or soy protein plus 66 milligrams (mg) of isoflavones for 6 months. The women in the isoflavone group showed significantly lower levels of the protein βCTX (a marker for bone loss), suggesting that their rate of bone loss was slower. The 66 mg of soy isoflavones is equivalent to a traditional Asian diet, whereas the typical Western diet contains only 2 to 16 mg of isoflavones.[2] Soy isoflavones are found in soybeans, tofu, miso, tempeh, and soy milk. Soy isoflavones have also been shown to alleviate hot flashes and can potentially reduce heart disease by lowering LDL cholesterol and improving endothelial function.[3] Speaking of hot flashes—perhaps the most well-known symptom of perimenopause and menopause—a new study has found a clinical and epidemiological relationship between the common menopause symptoms of hot flashes, poor sleep quality, and irritability. Researchers found that a combination of tryptophan, resveratrol, glycine, and vitamin E can improve these symptoms.[4] Tryptophan is found in turkey, cheese, and nuts. Resveratrol is found in red wine, grapes, peanuts, dark-colored berries, and cocoa. Glycine is an amino acid found in meat, fish, dairy products, and protein-rich vegetables. Vitamin E is found in almonds, hazelnuts, peanuts, sunflower seeds, spinach, and wheat germ. A higher adherence to the Mediterranean diet and a higher consumption of fruit can further help reduce hot flashes and night sweats. Conversely, diets that are high in fat or sugar are associated with an increased incidence of hot flashes and night sweats. This data was based on a study of 6,040 menopausal women who were followed for 9 years.[5] Folic acid has been shown to be effective in reducing the severity, duration, and frequency of hot flashes.[6] Folic acid, also known as vitamin B_9, is the synthetic form of folate and is found in supple-

ments and fortified foods. Folate is the natural form of vitamin B_9. Food sources of folate include avocados; asparagus; beans; broccoli; Brussels sprouts; citrus fruits and juices; dark, leafy greens; eggs; grains; seafood; and spinach.[7]

Next to hot flashes, weight gain is one of the most common menopause-related complaints, and menopause-related fat tends to gather in your abdomen. While weight gain is in part due to changes in hormones and is influenced by genetics, as well, exercise and an overall healthy dietary pattern can keep the weight off. A study of 535 premenopausal women ages 44 to 50 assigned one group to a diet of 1,300 calories per day and exercise sufficient to burn 1,000 to 1,500 calories per week. A control group was given no specific instructions. After 4.5 years, 55 percent of the intervention group was at or below their baseline weight, compared to 26 percent for controls.[8] Losing weight also reduces night sweats and hot flashes.[9]

To prevent or treat dry skin, another common menopause symptom, drink plenty of water and herbal tea and eat probiotic-rich foods. One clinical trial examined the effect of *Lactobacillus plantarum* on women ages 41 to 59 who had dry skin and wrinkles. Sixty-one volunteers received a daily probiotic for 12 weeks, and 49 served as controls. At week 12, volunteers in the probiotic group experienced a significant increase in skin water content in their faces and hands and less transepidermal water loss. What's more, the probiotic group experienced a significant reduction in wrinkle depth, better skin gloss, and a 21.8 percent improvement in skin elasticity by week 12.[10] Probiotics are found in yogurt, kefir, sauerkraut, kimchi, miso soup, sour pickles, kombucha tea, and some soft cheeses, such as Gouda and Swiss. For topical treatment of dry skin, try virgin coconut oil,[11] avocado oil, or grape seed oil.[12] Other topical treatments that can be found in your kitchen pantry include olive oil, almond oil, and flaxseed oil.

Finally, red clover extract just may qualify as a superfood for the treatment of menopause symptoms. Postmenopausal women were assigned to take either an 80 mg supplement of red clover extract or a placebo for 90 days. The women in the experimental group reported better moisture, texture, and overall condition of their skin; an improvement in scalp hair; and improvements to mood, libido, sleep, and tiredness.[13]

See also: Anxiety (page 165), Decreased Libido (page 224), Depression (page 232), Dry Skin (page 254), Hair Loss (page 304), Insomnia (page 357), Osteoporosis (page 392), Overweight and Obesity (page 396), Stress (page 419)

menstrual cramps (dysmenorrhea)

Menstrual cramps are the painful cramping sensations in your lower abdomen (and sometimes in your back) that occur just before and/or during your menstrual period. Dysmenorrhea is the most common gynecological complaint regardless of age and nationality.[1] Cramps are caused by high levels of prostaglandins, chemicals that are released as the lining of your uterus breaks down each month. Prostaglandins trigger muscle contractions, and they also promote inflammation. Oral contraceptives prevent ovulation and thus reduce the amount of prostaglandins your uterus produces, which is why women on birth control pills experience less menstrual pain. Menstrual cramp pain can range from mild to severe, and stress has been found to worsen symptoms. Women with a family history of dysmenorrhea are more prone to the condition, and a high intake of caffeine has been shown to exacerbate symptoms.[2] Most menstrual cramps are not a serious medical condition and can be treated with an over-the-counter pain reliever and/or heating pad. In some cases, cramps can be a sign of endometriosis, pelvic inflammatory disease, fibroid tumors of the uterus or ovaries, or other, less common conditions that require medical treatment. See your doctor if your menstrual cramps are severe, if they begin suddenly, or if they're accompanied by a fever or an unusual vaginal discharge.

If you dread your monthly cycle, there's good news for you, as the latest research reveals a host of effective, natural food cures for the pain of dysmenorrhea. For example, a recent study found that dill was as effective as mefenamic acid in reducing the pain of menstrual cramps.[3] Mefenamic acid is an NSAID (nonsteroidal anti-inflammatory drug) prescribed for menstrual pain, but it is not commonly used because of harmful side effects. Ginger was also found to be just as effective as mefenamic acid in reducing menstrual cramp pain—and this was in women with moderate to severe dysmenorrhea.[4] A study that compared ginger to a placebo found that ginger was superior to the placebo in relieving both the intensity and the duration of menstrual cramps.[5]

Wheat germ has also been found to relieve the pain of menstrual cramps. Compared to a placebo group, wheat germ was also effective in relieving fatigue, headache, and mood swings. Researchers attribute its pain-relieving capabilities to its anti-inflammatory effects.[6]

Another study compared the effects of fenugreek seed powder to a placebo and found that the fenugreek group experienced significantly less pain and that other menstrual symptoms, including headache, fatigue, nausea, vomiting, and fainting, decreased in the fenugreek group, as well.[7]

A study comparing the effects of cinnamon, ibuprofen, and a placebo found that both cinnamon and ibuprofen reduced the severity and duration of menstrual cramp pain, though the effects of ibuprofen were superior.[8] A different study found that cinnamon was superior to a placebo in relieving pain—and that it had the added benefit of decreasing menstrual bleeding and relieving nausea and vomiting.[9] With these results as well as ibuprofen's side effects in mind, cinnamon emerges as the preferred treatment for many women. Try drinking cinnamon tea as needed to relieve cramps. Simply boil a cinnamon stick in a cup of water for 10 minutes, then add a bag of caffeine-free tea, such as chamomile (see next column), and steep for a minute or two longer. If desired, add honey for taste.

If you enjoy hot beverages, skip the coffee (caffeine can exacerbate menstrual cramping) and opt for chamomile tea, which can reduce menstrual pain and relieve associated tension. In one study, women drank 2 cups of chamomile tea per day, beginning 1 week prior to menstruation and continuing for the first 5 days of their periods. After just 1 month of using chamomile tea, they had significantly less pain, anxiety, and distress than a placebo group.

Vitamin B_1 has been shown to reduce the pain severity and intensity of menstrual cramps.[10] Vitamin B_1, or thiamin, is found in abundance in whole grains and fortified cereals. It's also in rice, black beans, pork, trout, mussels, tuna, seeds, yogurt,[11] wheat germ, lentils, and green peas.[12] Similarly, omega-3 fatty acids can help relieve menstrual cramp pain. In one study, women with primary dysmenorrhea experienced a significant reduction in pain intensity after 3 months of treatment with omega-3 fatty acids and required fewer "rescue" doses of ibuprofen than a control group.[13] Food sources of omega-3s include flaxseeds, flaxseed oil, walnuts, sardines, salmon, mackerel, herring, shrimp, soybeans, and tofu.

See also: PMS (Premenstrual Syndrome) (page 404)

motion sickness

Motion sickness is a temporary but very uncomfortable condition characterized by nausea and vomiting, dizziness, cold sweats, and fatigue. It most often occurs when traveling by boat, car, airplane, or train, but it can also occur after being on an amusement park ride or even seeing a movie that features a lot of camera movement. The cause is a miscommunication between what your eye perceives, what your inner ear senses, and what your brain interprets. The result is that awful set of symptoms, but the good news is that the condition passes quickly once the stimulus stops.

If you're prone to motion sickness and can't avoid travel, there are medications designed to prevent motion sickness or to deal with the symptoms. But the side effects of many of these are drowsiness and sluggishness.

The most effective food remedy for motion sickness, ginger, targets the accompanying nausea: Ginger's role in treating motion sickness generally has been mixed. An older study that was conducted on navy cadets found that ginger powder was effective in preventing vomiting and cold sweats, and subjects reported less nausea and vertigo, as well.[1] But a study conducted 5 years later on volunteers in whom motion sickness was induced by timed head movements in a rotating chair did not find any efficacy of ginger for motion sickness.[2] An even more recent study

also looked at the effects of ginger on motion sickness induced in a lab. In this study, volunteers with a history of motion sickness consumed a 1,000-calorie meal and then sat in a drum that rotated until the subject experienced nausea. Those who were treated with ginger before the experiment began experienced less severe nausea, and the time it took for them to feel nauseated was longer than for those who did not receive ginger. They also experienced a shorter recovery time after the drum ceased

BONUS TIP: Grapefruit juice has been shown to increase the bioavailability of the motion sickness drug scopolamine, so if your doctor prescribes that drug for you, consider taking it with some grapefruit juice—in addition to crackers.[3]

spinning. This study was conducted with ginger capsules, and interestingly, a dose of 1,000 milligrams (mg) was effective but those who took a dose of 2,000 mg experienced no benefit.[4] But part of the difference in results could be due to the different ways individuals experience motion sickness.

A study released in 2015 observed that "the polysymptomatic nature of motion sickness, high interindividual variability, and the extensive brain regions involved may preclude a single, decisive treatment."[5] This means that ginger will work for some people, but not for others. Bottom line? There's strong clinical evidence in support of ginger's effectiveness at treating nausea and vomiting, so it's worth a shot. For best results, eat ginger or drink ginger tea about an hour before you travel. If you find your stomach just won't tolerate anything, try ginger aromatherapy.

A review of five studies with a total of 328 respondents found that inhaling ginger essential oil vapor reduced the incidence and severity of nausea and vomiting and decreased the need for antiemetics (medications that reduce vomiting).[6]

If you're prone to motion sickness, do not eat a large meal before traveling, and avoid spicy, greasy, or high-fat foods. Also avoid alcohol. While there is also some evidence that vitamin C taken in pill form can suppress symptoms of seasickness, presumably because it regulates histamine,[7] avoid citrus foods and juices (the acid is hard to digest). Pack bland foods that are convenient for travel, such as crackers or pretzels, and munch on these a little at a time to help settle your stomach.

See also: Nausea (page 390), Vertigo (page 446)

muscle cramps

Muscle cramps—the sudden, painful contraction of muscles—are extremely common, and you become more likely to experience them as you age. Pregnancy, being dehydrated, general fatigue, overexertion (especially of a particular muscle or muscle group), and certain illnesses such as hypothyroidism, liver disease, and nerve injury can also predispose you to cramps. Alcoholism and obesity increase your risk of developing muscle cramps, and they are a fairly common side effect of several medications.

One of the main dietary ways to prevent muscle cramps is to stay properly hydrated. Many exercise experts recommend drinking 7 to 10 ounces of fluid every 10 to 20 minutes while you exercise to stay hydrated. Some people turn to sports drinks, especially during and after long workouts, but water works fine. To stay hydrated at any point, water, coconut water, herbal teas, and occasional fruit juices are all great choices. If you're worried about the sugar content in fruit juice, dilute it with water, or just flavor your water with fresh lemon, lime, or orange juice.

Muscle cramps are one of the primary symptoms of magnesium deficiency.[1] To get more magnesium in your diet, eat pumpkin seeds, sesame seeds, sunflower seeds, almonds, Brazil nuts, cashews, pine nuts, spinach, Swiss chard, soybeans, black beans, navy beans, quinoa, and brown rice. Low calcium may play a role in the spontaneous leg cramps that are common during pregnancy and that occur more often as you age, especially at night. The other two minerals that are commonly associated with cramps—especially the painful nighttime leg cramping known as a charley horse—are potassium and calcium.[2] To boost your calcium, eat dairy products; dark, leafy greens; nuts; salmon; almonds; tofu; black-eyed peas; green peas; baked beans; and oranges; and drink soy milk.[3] High-potassium foods include sweet potatoes; tomato products; beet greens; beans; yogurt; clams; halibut; soybeans; tuna; winter squash; cod; bananas; spinach; dried peaches; dried apricots; prunes; cantaloupe; milk; honeydew melon; lentils; and orange, carrot, and prune juice.[4]

There is also some evidence that vitamin E can help. In a study of dialysis patients experiencing muscle cramps, a vitamin E supplement of 400 international units (IU) a day for 12 weeks decreased cramps by 68.3 percent.[5] Food sources of vitamin E include almonds, hazelnuts, peanuts, sunflower seeds, spinach, and wheat germ.

But for muscle cramps, we may have saved the best for last: Believe it or not, one of the most effective treatments is pickle juice. Ten brave male athletes participated in a study that required them to become slightly dehydrated and then endure electrically induced cramps. The first set of cramps lasted about 2.5 minutes on average. But on the second round, volunteers were given 2.5 ounces of either deionized water or pickle juice to drink when the cramps began. Those who drank pickle juice enjoyed relief from cramping within about 85 seconds, whereas the men who drank water continued to cramp.[6] Pickle juice has become such a relied-upon means for preventing and stopping cramps that up to 25 percent of athletic trainers routinely recommend pickle juice to treat cramping. There does not appear to be any risk of reaching dangerous levels of sodium or potassium after drinking pickle juice, and it does not inhibit short-term rehydration.[7]

See also: Thyroid Disease (page 429)

nausea

Nausea is one of those conditions that hardly needs an explanation—it's impossible to forget that miserable sensation of queasiness that usually results in vomiting. Nausea has dozens of potential causes: Everything from pregnancy to food poisoning or a food sensitivity, from anxiety to motion sickness to chemotherapy can cause nausea, and it's a hallmark of many gastrointestinal disorders. When you're feeling nauseated, food and drink may be the very last thing you want to think about. And while it's true that often the best cure for nausea is vomiting, followed by resting your digestive system, there are food and beverage remedies that can calm a queasy stomach.

The most well-researched food cure for nausea is ginger. Ginger has been used for thousands of years as a natural remedy for nausea, and it's so safe that it can be used during pregnancy to relieve nausea and vomiting.[1] It has also been used to treat the nausea associated with surgery, postoperative nausea and vomiting, and chemotherapy.[2] One study examined the effect of oral ginger on chemotherapy patients suffering from nausea and vomiting. (All patients received standard antiemetic, or vomit-reducing, drugs.) Compared to the control group, the patients who ate ginger experienced a significant reduction in nausea and fewer episodes of vomiting.[3] A study of 576 chemotherapy patients found that ginger significantly reduced acute nausea severity compared to a placebo.[4] If your stomach just won't tolerate anything, try ginger aromatherapy. A review of five studies with a total of 328 respondents found that inhaling ginger essential oil vapor reduced the incidence and severity of nausea and vomiting and decreased the need for antiemetics.[5]

Whenever there is vomiting, dehydration is a concern, so try to keep hydrated with water, clear broths, gin-

> BONUS TIP: Though the scientific evidence is mixed, there is substantial anecdotal evidence to support the use of mint and lemon, either taken orally or used as aromatherapy, to soothe a queasy stomach. Try mint tea or tea flavored with lemon, or add mint leaves or fresh lemon juice to water or any tea.

ger tea, or diluted juices. Once you feel that you can eat solid foods, avoid spicy, fried, and fatty foods. Eat very small amounts, and stick to bland foods such as crackers, dry toast, bananas, applesauce, plain oatmeal, or farina. Some sources also recommend nuts or peanut butter for protein, if you're not allergic.

See also: Acid Reflux (page 148), Irritable Bowel Syndrome (page 360), Motion Sickness (page 386)

osteoporosis

Osteoporosis is a very common chronic condition in which bones become weak, porous, and brittle. The International Osteoporosis Foundation estimates that globally, one in three women and one in five men are at risk for an osteoporotic fracture; indeed, such fractures occur approximately every 3 seconds.[1] Hip fractures have the most serious consequences. Some people never regain complete mobility even after recovery, and about one in five hip fracture patients over age 50 die within a year of their fracture as a result of medical complications. Vertebral fractures have also been linked with increased mortality in older people.[2] Postmenopausal women are most at risk for developing osteoporosis, and the risk increases with age, but other risk factors include a family history of osteoporosis, a body mass index of less than 19, having rheumatoid arthritis, lack of exercise, taking glucocorticoids for 3 months or longer, insufficient intake of vitamin D and/or calcium, overconsumption of alcohol, and smoking. Smoking doubles your risk of developing osteoporosis.

Prevention is the most effective means of avoiding this irreversible disease and its potentially devastating consequences, and the earlier one attends to bone health, the better. Some researchers have even argued that osteoporosis can be thought of as a pediatric disease, as well, because there is a clear relationship between the bone density obtained in adolescence and the development of osteoporosis later.[3] Certainly it's well known that peak bone mass is achieved by early adulthood and that calcium absorption drastically diminishes as we age, so it's wise to get an adequate intake of calcium, vitamin D, and protein from childhood on. For women, bone mass tends to stay steady from about the age of 30 until menopause, whereupon most women go through rapid bone mass loss for a few years, which then slows but continues throughout the rest of their lives.[4] Next, we'll discuss what to eat to preserve as much bone mass as possible, but the other crucial means of maintaining bone density is to get at least half an hour per day of weight-bearing exercise.

To best support bone health, eat a varied diet that's rich in fresh fruits and vegetables (especially citrus fruits and dark, leafy greens), lean sources of protein, low-fat dairy products, nuts, and legumes, and make your primary source of fat olive oil—in other words, the Mediterranean diet or some similar dietary pattern. One study examined the effect of the Mediterranean diet on bone density in two groups of women, one premenopausal and one postmenopausal. In both groups of women, consumption of fruits and vegetables was found to have a beneficial effect on bone mineral density. In postmenopausal women, nuts were also positively associated with bone mineral density. Both outcomes suggest that a varied diet based on Mediterranean dietary patterns is beneficial to the prevention of osteoporosis.[5]

Another dietary pattern that has achieved notoriety for its role in osteoporosis prevention is the Scarborough Fair diet. The Scarborough Fair Study gained wide attention in 2013, when the protocol and the study design were described. Researchers hoped to demonstrate in humans the bone resorbing–inhibiting properties of specific foods; these properties had previously only been shown in animal models. In this 3-month study, 150 postmenopausal women were randomly assigned to three groups: The intervention group consisted of 50 women each in two study arms (group A and group B), while 50 women served as controls (group C). Both groups A and B increased their fruit and vegetable consumption to nine or more servings a day, but group B ate fruits and vegetables specifically cho-

sen for their bone resorbing–inhibiting properties. This latter meal plan was called the Scarborough Fair Diet.[6] The results were published in 2015. Significantly less urinary calcium loss was seen in both groups A and B, but the most significant finding of the study was a decrease in bone turnover markers in group B's osteopenic women. Osteopenia is bone density that is lower than normal but that has not yet progressed to osteoporosis. Thus the Scarborough Fair Diet was shown to exert an antiresorption effect in women with increased bone loss. So, what are the Scarborough Fair Diet fruits and vegetables? Here they are, in terms of servings per day.

HERBS: One serving of garlic, parsley, rosemary, sage, and thyme

PRUNES: One serving

ORANGES OR OTHER CITRUS FRUITS: One serving

ADDITIONAL FRUITS: One serving, *not including* banana or apple

GREEN, LEAFY VEGETABLES: One serving of Chinese cabbage, bok choy, arugula, lettuce, etc.

OTHER VEGETABLES: Two or three servings (or more) of onions, broccoli, tomatoes, mushrooms, cucumbers, leeks, and green beans, plus one or two servings of self-selected vegetables[7]

Further demonstrating the need for a varied diet, a recent study demonstrated the synergistic interaction of calcium, vitamin D, protein, and inorganic phosphate in reducing bone resorption (where bone loses calcium), increasing bone formation, and attenuating age-related bone loss. Bone composition and structural integrity are dependent upon calcium, protein, and phosphate. All of these nutrients require adequate vitamin D to function properly, and dairy products are a rich source of all four of these nutrients.[11] Vitamin D insufficiency is widespread, and some studies have noted that it is particularly insufficient in postmenopausal women with osteoporosis. In a recent survey of more than 200 postmenopausal women with osteoporosis, dietary vitamin D intake was an average of 167 international units (IU) per day, which is well below both the established target of 400 IU per day and the more recent, higher guideline recommended for postmenopausal women of 800 to 1,300 IU per

kale, spinach, and lettuces are all great choices.

■ Yellow and orange vegetables. A study of nearly 24,000 men showed that dietary total vegetables, green vegetables, and yellow-orange vegetables, as well as total and specific carotenoids, including alpha-carotene, beta-carotene, lutein, and zeaxanthin, were significantly inversely associated with hip fractures. Beta-carotene had the most protective effect: Compared to the men who ate the least beta-carotene, the men with the highest consumption had a 37 percent decreased risk of hip fracture.[9] Carotenoids are found in yellow, orange, and red vegetables and in dark, leafy greens. Foods that are high in beta-carotene include pumpkin, sweet potatoes, carrots, winter squash, cantaloupe, spinach, kale, collards, and turnip greens.

■ Olive oil. This monounsaturated fat is rich in phenolic compounds and boasts a host of health benefits, including that it prevents the loss of bone mass.[10]

■ Oolong tea and green tea, both of which have antiosteoporotic properties.

■ Herbs, specifically parsley, sage, thyme, rosemary, and garlic.

day. Dietary vitamin D intake was even lower for participants who were 75 and older, at an average of 120 IU per day.[12] Though there are food sources of vitamin D (see "Feed Your Bones: Recommendations for Osteoporosis Prevention and Management through Nutrition") and it can be absorbed through exposure to sunlight, in this particular population, supplementation is recommended. Vitamin D plus calcium supplementation has been found to be more effective in preventing fractures than vitamin D supplementation alone in both men and women.[13]

Postmenopausal women who regularly drink oolong tea had greater bone density than non-tea-drinkers.[14] Research has also demonstrated the osteoporosis-preventing effects of green tea polyphenols, which can suppress inflammation, inhibit oxidative stress, increase bone mass, and suppress bone resorption.[15]

overweight and obesity

Overweight and obesity have become major global public health concerns. The small Polynesian island kingdom of Tonga currently holds the dubious distinction of being the most overweight country in the world, with an estimated 86.1 percent of its adult citizens considered overweight (i.e., with a BMI of over 25). BMI is the acronym for body mass index, which is the ratio of a person's height and weight. For adults, a BMI between 18.5 and 24.9 is considered healthy.[1] A BMI of 25 and over is considered overweight, and a BMI of 30 is considered obese. According to worldwide rates of overweight and obesity, the United States is in 27th place out of 188 countries, with an estimated 66.3 percent of the adult populace overweight. (If one reconfigures the statistics to search only for obesity, the United States moves up to 19th place, with 32.8 percent of adults considered obese.)[2] Recent statistics from the World Health Organization indicate that as of 2014, 11 percent of men and 15 percent of women worldwide were obese, meaning that more than half a billion adults across the globe are considered obese.[3]

The complications of overweight and obesity are well known but are worth reviewing, if only in brief. People who are overweight are at greater risk for a host of illnesses and health conditions, including but not limited to: cardiovascular disease, diabetes, metabolic disorders, dementia, hypertension, sleep disorders, asthma, stroke, gallbladder disease, certain types of cancer (including breast, endometrial, gallbladder, prostate, and colon cancer), gastrointestinal disorders, high cholesterol, infertility, kidney stones, depression, arthritis, osteoporosis, and premature death. There is even evidence that overweight people have a greater susceptibility to pain.[4]

You may not have been aware that obesity is related to Alzheimer's disease (AD), but studies have shown that carrying extra pounds at midlife increases your chances of developing Alzheimer's. A study published in *Molecular Psychiatry* found that midlife adiposity also predicts an earlier onset of Alzheimer's. Every unit of increase in BMI at age 50 and above predicts an earlier onset of 6.7 months.[5] In fact, there's such a strong link between obesity and Alzheimer's that AD has been called "type 3 diabetes." What's the connection? Science doesn't yet have all the answers, but brain imaging has shown that obese people have smaller brain volumes, which increases their risk of AD.[6] Some theories suggest that AD is linked with obesity-induced insulin resistance and/or impaired insulin signaling, which results in decreased glucose metabolism, a symptom of Alzheimer's.[7] Whatever the exact relationship is, the results are undisputed: Obesity is an established risk factor for AD.

The worldwide epidemic of overweight and obesity constitutes a true public health concern with devastating physical, mental, emotional, social, and economic repercussions. This is true on a global as well as an individual scale. Many of the recommendations for how to prevent weight gain and lose extra weight are well known, but like the health consequences of overweight and

the nonnegotiables

When it comes to overweight and obesity, the food you eat and the level of exercise you maintain are key to regaining your good health, so follow these guidelines.

- ■ Limit consumption of foods and beverages that are high in saturated fats and sugars. More specifically, limit red meat, fried foods, desserts, pastries, sodas, and sugary baked goods. With these nonnegotiable basics in place, we can add on tips for faster weight loss and consider some individual foods and food groups that play special roles in weight loss.

- ■ Eliminate all processed foods and trans fats, which means eliminating all fast foods. If you can't eliminate

fast foods entirely, cut back as much as you can, and opt for the healthiest menu items.

- ■ Increase your consumption of fruits, legumes, nuts, seeds, vegetables, and whole grains.

- ■ Engage in regular physical activity. Adults should aim for a minimum of 150 minutes of moderate aerobic activity per week.

- ■ Consume alcohol in moderation: one serving per night for women, two servings per night for men.

obesity, they are worth reviewing in brief. We'll begin with general guidelines and then move into some specific healing-foods methods that will help you eat and drink your way to a healthy weight. But always keep in mind the number one overarching guideline for losing weight: The most successful weight-loss program combines eating fewer calories with burning more calories.

If you're looking for an overall dietary pattern that supports whole-body health as well as weight loss, the Mediterranean diet is recommended. Researchers assigned 5,801 volunteers to one of three diets: the Mediterranean diet supplemented with extra-virgin olive oil, the Mediterranean diet supplemented with nuts, or a low-fat diet. They followed the volunteers for 4.8 years, and they found some surprising results: The people who ate a low-fat diet did not show improvement in weight, but both groups who ate the Mediterranean diet showed significant decreases in central (abdominal) obesity.[8]

The New Nordic diet has also showed positive results for weight loss. Danish researchers assigned 147 adults with central obesity and an average BMI of 30.2 to either the New Nordic diet or an average Danish diet for 26 weeks. By the end of the study, those on the Nordic diet lost an average of 10.4 pounds, com-pared to only 3.3 pounds for those in the control group. Those who followed the New Nordic diet also experienced greater reductions in both systolic and diastolic blood pressure. So what did each group eat? The New Nordic diet is comprised of the following 15 foods and food groups, most of which should be local and organically grown: "fruit and vegetables (especially berries, cabbages, root vegetables, and legumes), potatoes, fresh herbs, plants and mushrooms gathered from the wild, nuts, whole grains, meats from livestock and game, fish and shellfish, and seaweed." The regular Danish diet was characterized by "refined grains including pasta and rice, meat, dairy and cheese, sugary products, convenience foods, and, to a lesser extent, low-fiber vegetables and imported fruit."[9]

There is evidence that the plant phenolic compounds known as lignans can slow weight gain. Lignans are found in abundance in flax and sesame seeds and also in whole grains, nuts, fruits, vegetables, coffee, tea, and wine. Researchers examined urine samples from more than 48,000 women and found that those with the highest urinary excretion of lignans had the lowest baseline BMIs. These women also gained an average of 0.6 pound less per year over a 10-year follow-up period compared with the women who had the lowest levels of lignans. Higher lignan excretion generally suggested a higher intake of coffee, fruits, red wine, vegetables, and whole grains.[10]

A 3-year study of overall dietary habits and weight loss found that for men, decreasing sugar intake had the biggest impact on weight loss. Compared to no change in their sugar intake, decreasing sugar more than doubled their likelihood of weight loss. In women, it was vegetables and whole grains that had the biggest impact on weight loss: Eating fewer vegetables decreased women's likelihood of weight loss by 56 percent, and compared to women who ate whole grains regularly, researchers observed a 92 percent increase in the risk of weight gain in the women who ate fewer whole grains.[11] Another study revealed some useful data on weight loss: Participants who lost the most weight and had the greatest change in BMI over 3 months consumed the highest amounts of fruits, low-fat dairy products, and high-fiber foods and the least amounts of fatty meats, non-whole-grain cereals, overall fat, and overall calories.[12] Another study compared the effects of a low-fat diet to a low-carbohydrate diet on weight loss and incidence of atherosclerotic cardiovascular disease (ASCVD). Based upon data from 17 trials that lasted anywhere from 8 to 24 months and followed a total of 1,797 patients, the low-carb diet won. While *both* diets resulted in weight loss and a reduction in ASCVD risk, the low-carb diet on average resulted in an additional 4 pounds of weight loss and a greater reduction in ASCVD risk.[13] Echoing these results, a study in the *Lancet* found that low-carbohydrate diets are significantly more effective for long-term weight loss than low-fat diets.[14]

A large study of 133,468 adults examined the effect of fruit and vegetable intake on change in weight from the years 1986 through 2010; assessments were taken every 4 years. After adjusting for smoking, physical activity, and other aspects of diet, researchers found that increased intake of several individual fruits led to less weight gain over time; these included blueberries, prunes, apples, pears, strawberries, raisins, grapes, and grapefruit. Increased intakes of many individual foods and vegetables were also inversely associated with weight change; these included tofu/soy; peppers; carrots; cauliflower; and cruciferous and dark, leafy greens. On the other hand, increased intake of starchy vegetables, including corn, peas, and potatoes, was associated with weight gain.[15]

Researchers are also looking into the role that the gut microbiome plays in overweight and obesity—and how probiotics and prebiotics can help with weight loss. There is evidence that being overweight creates chronic low-grade inflammation throughout your body, as do diets that are high in meats, fat, and sugar. But probiotics and prebiotics are able to attenuate some of this inflammation and thus slow the progression of metabolic diseases such as obesity and type 2 diabetes.[16] In a study of 75 overweight and obese volunteers, those who ate a low-calorie diet with a probiotic yogurt for 8 weeks experienced greater

real-life tricks for faster weight loss

■ **EAT HOT PEPPERS BEFORE A MEAL.** Meta-analysis findings have shown that eating capsaicinoids, the naturally occurring chemicals that give hot peppers their kick, reduces energy intake by an average of 74 calories per meal. At least 2 milligrams (mg) of capsaicinoids are necessary for this calorie-curbing effect. Researchers think these fiery chemicals inspire a preference for carbohydrate-rich foods rather than high-fat foods.[18] Capsaicins are found in chile peppers (hot chiles, red chiles, and green chiles), cayenne peppers, jalapeño peppers, and habanero peppers, among others, and the amount each contains depends on the growing conditions of the plant. Concentrations can range from 2.5 mg/g to 60 mg/g or more.[19] Generally, the hotter the pepper, the higher the capsaicin content.

■ **EAT MORE CUMIN.** In one study, 88 overweight or obese women were randomly assigned to two groups. The experimental group ate yogurt with 3 grams of cumin powder at two meals every day for 3 months. The control group ate the same amount of yogurt, but without the cumin powder. The results? The group who ate cumin powder experienced a significant reduction in weight, BMI, waist circumference, and percentage of fat mass. The bonus? Their total cholesterol, triglycerides, and LDL cholesterol numbers fell, and their HDL cholesterol levels rose.[20]

■ **EAT MORE SAFFRON.** An 8-week study on mildly obese women examined the effects of saffron supplementation (176.5 mg a day) on snacking behaviors and weight loss. Snacking decreased by 55 percent in the saffron group but only 26 percent in the placebo group. The saffron group also lost about 2 more pounds on average than the placebo group.[21]

■ **EAT MORE CALORIES EARLY.** Researchers studied two groups who ate

reduction in BMI, fat percentage, and leptin levels than those who ate a low-calorie diet with regular yogurt or those who just added a probiotic yogurt to their diets. Markers of inflammation fell, as well.[17] More specifically, the pre-biotic alpha-galacto-oligosaccharide, which is derived from legumes, was found to reduce appetite, food intake, and inflammation in 88 overweight adults. In this study, participants drank a tea that was supplemented with 8, 12,

the same Mediterranean-style diet for 3 months, but in different calorie distributions. The first group ate 70 percent of their calories over breakfast, a morning snack, and lunch, and they ate the remaining 30 percent over an afternoon snack and dinner. The second group ate 55 percent of their calories over breakfast, morning snack, and lunch, and they ate the remaining 45 percent over afternoon snack and dinner. The first group had greater reductions in weight, waist circumference, and fat mass, and greater improvements in insulin sensitivity.[22] In another 20-week study, findings showed that eating the largest meal earlier in the day resulted in more weight loss and a higher rate of weight loss compared to those who ate their main meal later, and this result was independent of 24-hour calorie intake.[23]

■ EAT HALF AN AVOCADO WITH LUNCH. A study of overweight individuals found that adding half a Hass avocado to a normal lunch increased satisfaction by 23 percent and decreased the desire to eat by 28 percent compared to a control meal without avocado. Though the avocado added about 112 calories, the effect of satiety lasted up to 5 hours, discouraging between-meal snacking.[24]

■ PUT YOUR HEALTHIEST FOODS IN THE SPOTLIGHT. In a study of 300 adults, researchers found that normal-weight individuals were more likely than obese individuals to have fresh fruit prominently displayed on their kitchen counters and less likely to have soda and baked goods in sight. Women who kept soft drinks on their counters or in other highly visible locations in the kitchen weighed up to 26 pounds more than those who did not. Keeping cereal on the counter was associated with an additional 20 pounds in women, and candy on the counter was associated with an additional 17 pounds in men.[25]

or 18 grams of the prebiotic, and the higher the dose, the greater the effects.[26] Several studies have found that probiotics, especially of the *Lactobacillus* and *Bifidobacterium* strains, exert multiple beneficial effects in people with metabolic syndrome: They promote weight loss and the reduction of visceral adiposity (abdominal fat), improve glucose tolerance, and modulate low-grade inflammation of the intestines.[27] In one study, subjects with a BMI of 24.2 to 30.7 were assigned to drink a fermented milk drink containing *Lactobacillus gasseri* or a fermented milk drink without *L. gasseri* every day for 12 weeks. In the probiotic group, abdominal fat and subcutaneous fat decreased by an average of 4.6 percent. Body weight, BMI, and waist and hip circumference also decreased significantly, while those who did not receive the probiotic experienced no significant reductions in any of these parameters.[28] A more recent study on *L. gasseri* found that obese adults who added *L. gasseri* to their diets lost an average of more than 8 percent of abdominal fat over 12 weeks of supplementation. A dose as low as 10 colony-forming units per day can achieve these effects, but constant consumption may be needed to maintain them.[29] *L. gasseri* can be found in certain yogurts (make

sure it says "live active cultures"), tempeh, kimchi, kefir, sauerkraut, lassi, miso soup, and natto.

Green tea and black tea have also been thoroughly researched for their potential role in weight loss, though results are sometimes conflicting.[30] In a review of 12 human studies on tea consumption and body weight, however, 10 confirmed that drinking green tea or consuming its active ingredient, epigallocatechin gallate (EGCG), could reduce weight and body fat. Additional studies have demonstrated green tea's positive effects on waist circumference and fat oxidation, as well as habitual tea consumption's ability to prevent or alleviate metabolic disease.[31] A high daily dose (nearly 857 milligrams) of green tea extract (EGCG) has been shown to reduce BMI, weight, waist circumference, total cholesterol, and LDL cholesterol.[32] Oolong tea has been shown to decrease weight, subcutaneous fat, total cholesterol, and triglycerides in as little as 6 weeks.[33] The South American tea known as yerba maté has been shown to promote feelings of satiety, delay gastric emptying, and modulate and potentially even inhibit the production of fat cells.[34]

Clearly there are many benefits to drinking tea, and now there's a new tea in town that looks like it can super-charge your weight-loss efforts. Kenya's purple tea, 25 years in the making and developed as a medicinal tea that's high in anthocyanins, became available in the United States in 2012. Purple tea has powerful antioxidant ability and is lower in caffeine than green or black tea. As it's still so new, most clinical studies have been performed on animals. But those results have shown that purple tea can inhibit weight gain and prevent abdominal and liver fat accumulations. In a small study done on 10 mildly obese individuals, drinking purple tea daily for 4 weeks resulted in a reduction in BMI, weight, body fat mass, abdominal fat, body fat ratio (measuring the percentage of fat compared to your total weight), waist size, hip size, and abdominal and right upper arm fat thickness.[35]

pms (premenstrual syndrome)

Premenstrual syndrome (PMS) is a very common condition that affects nearly half of girls and women of reproductive age.[1] The symptoms are numerous and can range greatly in severity with each menstrual cycle. As the name implies, PMS occurs just before the onset of your monthly period, usually 7 to 10 days before, and it subsides once menstrual flow begins. The symptoms are emotional and physical, and the most common are abdominal cramping (dysmenorrhea), acne breakouts, anxiety, backache, bloating, swollen or tender breasts, changes in appetite and/or food cravings, depression, fatigue, gastrointestinal complaints such as constipation or diarrhea, headache, irritability, mood swings, sleep disturbances, and trouble with memory or concentration. Natural changes in hormones during your menstrual cycle seem to be responsible for PMS, but neurochemical changes could play a part, as well. Over-the-counter pain relievers can be used for achiness and cramping, but lifestyle changes, including exercise and dietary changes, may have the greatest impact on relieving PMS symptoms.

Fennel has been shown to have an analgesic, anti-inflammatory, and anti-spasmodic effect. It's able to inhibit uterine contractions (so it alleviates painful cramping) and shorten period duration by facilitating the discharge of blood in a shorter time. It's also been shown to relieve fatigue and lethargy associated with PMS. Fennel's root, leaves, and fruit can be used, and it's available as an essential oil and a tea, as well.[2]

In a study comparing the effects of cinnamon, ibuprofen, and a placebo on dysmenorrhea pain, ibuprofen and cinnamon were both effective at relieving pain. Cinnamon was most effective 8 hours after ingestion. For those who cannot tolerate the side effects of ibuprofen, cinnamon is a low-cost, effective remedy with no side effects.[3] Boil a cinnamon stick in a cup of water for 10 minutes, then steep a bag of caffeine-free tea, such as chamomile (see below), in the water for 1 to 2 minutes. Add honey to taste, if desired. Drink as needed.

Chamomile is another time-honored natural treatment for PMS, prized for its anti-inflammatory, antispasmodic, and antianxiety effects. In clinical trials, chamomile has proven effective in reducing anxiety, menstrual pain, depression, and anger.[4] In one study, women who drank chamomile tea twice a day 1 week prior to menstruation and for the first 5 days of their periods experienced less pain, anxiety, and distress than a placebo group, and this was with just 1 month of tea drinking.

In a study comparing college students who took a vitamin B_1 supplement over two cycles to a placebo group, the vitamin B_1 group experienced a significant improvement in many PMS symptoms, including anxiety, depression, fatigue, poor concentration, sleep disturbances, and tension. Overall, vitamin B_1 reduced mean mental (35 percent) and physical (21 percent) symptoms significantly.[5] Vitamin B_1 has also been shown to reduce the pain severity and intensity of menstrual cramps.[6] Vitamin B_1, or thiamin, is found in abundance in whole grains and fortified cereals. It's also in rice, black beans, pork, trout, mussels, tuna, seeds, yogurt,[7] wheat germ, lentils, and green peas.[8] Another study found that dietary intake of thiamin (vitamin B_1) and riboflavin (vitamin B_2) was associated with a 35 percent lower risk of developing PMS. This is especially notable because the effect was present with food sources only—a B-complex vitamin supplement had no effect on risk of PMS. Study authors noted that the effective level for both was considerably above current recommendations. The recommended daily allowance (RDA) for thiamin is 1.1 milligrams (mg), but women consuming about 1.9 mg daily had a 25 percent lower risk of PMS than did those consuming 1.2 mg daily. This level of intake can be achieved by consuming two or three servings a day of thiamin-rich foods, such as fortified cereals, legumes, and nuts. The RDA for riboflavin is also 1.1 mg, but women consuming about 2.5 mg daily had a 35 percent lower risk of PMS than did those consuming 1.4 mg per day. This level of intake can be achieved with one or two servings of fortified cereal a day or six or seven servings of riboflavin-rich foods such as milk, soy milk, spinach, and red meats.[9] Additional food sources of riboflavin include cheddar cheese, eggs, almonds, salmon, halibut, chicken, broccoli, asparagus, and whole wheat bread.[10]

Wheat germ extract has been shown to reduce a variety of PMS symptoms. One study followed 100 women with a diagnosis of PMS for two consecutive cycles; one group received 400 mg of wheat germ extract, and the second group received a placebo. Wheat germ significantly reduced physical symptoms (by 63. 6 percent), psychological symptoms (by 66.3 percent), and the women's general PMS symptoms (by 65.0. percent). What's more, physical symptoms only decreased in the wheat germ group. The greatest reductions occurred in the following symptoms: fatigue, irritability, heart palpitations, tension, breast tenderness, headache, sleep problems, increased appetite, acne, mood swings, food cravings, wish to be alone, depression, forgetfulness, anxiety, poor concentration, crying, and swelling.[11]

Certain mineral deficiencies have been shown to exacerbate premenstrual symptoms, especially deficiencies of calcium, iron, and magnesium. One study followed 93 women for 3 months and monitored their calcium, sodium, iron, and magnesium levels. Researchers found that 83 percent of the participants had below-normal levels of calcium, and 14 percent had insufficient levels of magnesium; there was a correlation between low levels of calcium and magnesium and the common PMS symptoms of anxiety, irritability, depression, constipation, and nausea. Restoring proper calcium and magnesium levels can have a positive effect on PMS symptoms.[12] Calcium-rich foods include dairy products (milk, yogurt, and cheese); dark, leafy greens; nuts; salmon; soy milk; almonds; tofu; black-eyed peas; green peas; baked beans; and oranges.[13] Food sources of magnesium include almonds, spinach, cashews, peanuts, soy milk, black beans, soybeans, avocados, oatmeal, yogurt, salmon, halibut, brown rice, and chicken breast.[14]

Another study found that women who had the highest levels of iron intake had a 31 percent lower risk of PMS. But there's a fascinating caveat: The lower risk was associated only with nonheme iron; heme iron was unrelated to PMS risk.[15] (Heme iron comes from animal sources, whereas nonheme iron comes from plants and fortified foods.) Good food sources of nonheme iron include fortified whole grain cereals, white beans, dark chocolate, lentils, spinach, tofu, kidney beans, chickpeas, tomatoes, and cashews.[16]

See also: Anxiety (page 165), Depression (page 232), Fatigue (page 266), Headaches/ Migraines (page 309), Insomnia (page 357), Memory Loss (Short Term) (page 377), Menstrual Cramps (Dysmenorrhea) (page 384), Stress (page 419)

pneumonia

Pneumonia is a bacterial, fungal, or viral infection of the lungs in which the air sacs, known as alveoli, become inflamed and filled with fluid. Symptoms include fever, productive cough (a cough that produces phlegm, which can be dark yellow, green, or tinged with blood), chest pain, rapid breathing, breathing difficulties, tachycardia (rapid heart rate), chills, and fatigue. In some cases nausea, vomiting, or diarrhea can occur, as can mental confusion, especially in older adults. Err on the side of caution when it comes to pneumonia, as it can worsen quickly and does have the potential to be lethal. If you suspect you have pneumonia, seek immediate medical treatment if you have a preexisting condition such as HIV/AIDS, asthma, cardiovascular disease, pulmonary disease, diabetes, or any other condition that would impair your ability to fight off an infection. The elderly and children should also receive medical treatment for pneumonia. There is a one-time vaccine for pneumococcal pneumonia, and yearly influenza vaccinations can help prevent pneumonia that results from certain types of flu.

To help prevent pneumonia, make sure you're getting enough sleep and enough exercise; both support immune function, and exercise promotes deep breathing and prevents fluid buildup. Though there is no consensus on a definitive "immune system diet," some of the best vitamins and minerals for immune system support include vitamin A, vitamin B_2, vitamin B_6, vitamin C, vitamin D, vitamin E, folate, iron, selenium, and zinc. Zinc has been studied specifically in connection with pneumonia; it's been found to play a role in protecting against pneumonia as well as shortening the duration of pneumonia in children,[1] and normal zinc levels in an elderly population resulted in a lower incidence of pneumonia and a shorter duration of pneumonia if they did develop the condition.[2] A well-balanced diet consisting of plenty of fresh fruits and vegetables, whole grains, and lean proteins, plus adequate fluid intake, will provide most if not all of these vitamins and minerals. The exception is vitamin D, which can be found in dairy products, eggs, fish and fish oil, fortified orange juice,[3] and mushrooms but sun exposure is the best source. Food sources for zinc include oysters, wheat germ, chicken, crab, beans, oatmeal, yogurt, pumpkin seeds, and pine nuts. Food sources for the rest of the immune-supporting nutrients include almonds; bananas; barley; beans; berries of any variety; Brazil nuts; cantaloupe; carrots; chickpeas; citrus fruits; dark, leafy greens; garlic (a natural antibacterial); hazelnuts; lean poultry; mackerel; papayas; peppers of any variety; quinoa; salmon; squash; sweet potatoes; tuna; and yogurt.

There is also growing evidence that probiotics can help prevent pneumonia. A study of 150 patients found that probiotic supplementation (in this case, with *Lactobacillus casei*) helped prevent ventilator-associated pneumonia. The study also found a trend for fewer resistant bacteria in the probiotic group.[4] The common *Lactobacillus* strain of probiotics has been shown to be effective in fighting *Klebsiella* pneumonia.[5] Another study compared the effects of an 8-day regimen of thrice-daily probiotics given to critically ill infants to those of a placebo. Those who received probiotics—in this case consisting of two strains of *Lactobacillus* (*L. casei* and *L. acidophilus*), *Bacillus subtilis*, and *Enterococcus faecalis*—were far less likely to develop pneumonia: 18 percent versus 36 percent, in the placebo group.[6] Yet another study found

that the probiotic *Streptococcus salivarius* was effective at preventing *S. pneumoniae* from binding to the epithelial lining of the nasopharynx (where the nasal passage connects to the throat). Left unchecked, *Streptococcus* can colonize the nasopharynx and result in pneumonia.[7] Probiotics can also help treat pneumonia. If your doctor prescribes antibiotics, probiotics can protect healthy gut flora and help prevent yeast infections and antibiotic-associated diarrhea. Food sources of probiotics include yogurt, kefir, sauerkraut, kimchi, miso soup, sour pickles, kombucha tea, and some soft cheeses, such as Gouda or Swiss.

The same healthy diet described on page 407 can help you recover from pneumonia. Avoid any foods containing trans fats or saturated fats, such as processed, prepackaged, and fast foods. Your body needs fresh fruits and vegetables that are rich in antioxidants for recovery. You may also want to eliminate or reduce dairy consumption, as dairy is inflammatory and promotes mucus production. Staying hydrated is also essential. Fluids are necessary to help thin and loosen mucus and to replace fluids lost through fever and coughing. To help calm a dry cough and soothe a throat that's sore from coughing, try honey, licorice, eucalyptus, or ginger. Ginger tea sweetened with honey may be your best bet, as ginger has anti-inflammatory effects, and the honey and warm liquid will help soothe your throat and reduce cough. Eucalyptus and licorice tea are also available, but use caution when consuming licorice, as too much can elevate your blood pressure, and don't use any licorice product if you're nursing or breastfeeding.

The other main component of food remedies for pneumonia is any food that has an anti-inflammatory effect. The best foods to reduce inflammation are antioxidants, found in abundance in fresh fruits and vegetables (pineapple; berries; dark, leafy greens; mushrooms; tomatoes; and olive oil are especially good), and any food with omega-3s, including salmon, mackerel, herring, flaxseeds, and walnuts. Ginger and turmeric are also excellent foods to fight inflammation.

See also: Bronchitis (page 186), Colds (page 214), Coughs (page 220)

psoriasis

Psoriasis is a chronic, autoimmune skin disease that causes skin cells to build up rapidly on the surface of your skin, resulting in redness, scaling, itchiness, dry skin, and pain. These patches of red, raised, scaly skin are known as psoriasis lesions. They can appear anywhere on your body, though they most often show up on your scalp, knees, and elbows. The causes of psoriasis aren't entirely clear, but the latest research points to a genetic predisposition combined with an environmental trigger.

Many people have observed that certain foods exacerbate their psoriasis. Determining your food triggers is partly a matter of paying attention to your diet and outbreaks, but one place to start may be with gluten. Psoriasis patients have a higher prevalence of other autoimmune conditions, including celiac disease; some studies suggest that having psoriasis roughly doubles your chances of being diagnosed with celiac disease.[1] A number of studies have also noted that these conditions share common genetic and inflammatory pathways,[2] and they both involve inflammatory immune responses. One study found that 42 percent of psoriasis in patients with celiac disease could be attributed to the underlying celiac disease,[3] suggesting that treatment of celiac disease would treat psoriasis in these patients. A small study showed that seven out of eight psoriasis patients experienced great improvement in skin lesions after adopting a gluten-free diet for 6 months.[4] Another study compared the effects of a gluten-free diet in 30 psoriasis patients who had antibodies to gliadin (AGA), an indicator of celiac disease, with six psoriasis patients who were AGA-negative. After 3 months on a gluten-free diet, all of the AGA-positive patients showed a highly significant decrease in their Psoriasis Area and Severity Index (PASI) scores, whereas the AGA-negative patients showed no improvement. In those who improved, 82 percent also exhibited lower AGA values.[5] Overall, research suggests that for those with psoriasis *and* celiac disease, following a gluten-free diet can improve psoriasis symptoms. (Going "g-free" does not appear to ease psoriasis symptoms in psoriasis patients without celiac disease.)

Many studies have noted a connection between overweight and obesity, and psoriasis. Psoriasis sufferers have an increased risk of cardiovascular disease, and obesity—which promotes a chronic inflammatory state—plays a key role in linking these two comorbidities. Further, weight loss has been shown to decrease psoriasis severity and enhance response to treatment.[6] Sixty obese patients with psoriasis were divided into two weight-loss groups: one that ate 800 to 1,000 calories a day for 8 weeks, followed by 8 weeks of normal food intake that reached 1,200 calories a day, and a second group that was advised to eat normal, healthy foods. At the outset of the study, PASI scores were an average of 5.4. After 16 weeks, those in the weight-loss group lost an average of nearly 35 pounds, compared to just under 1 pound on average for the control group. The intervention group also experienced an average change of −2.3 in their PASI scores, as opposed to just −0.3 in the control group, and the intervention group reported significantly greater improvement in their skin-related quality of life. Researchers also noted that the greatest reduction in

PASI scores occurred during the first half of the study, when the greatest weight loss occurred. PASI scores leveled out after 8 weeks, when subjects returned to their normal diets.[7] Further, body weight and BMI influence the response to treatment, with higher BMIs making some psoriasis drug therapies less effective.[8] So not only do overweight and obesity and psoriasis appear to be linked medically, overweight and obesity, this study suggests, further complicate treatment for psoriasis.

As for specific foods and nutrients that can help psoriasis sufferers, researchers have studied nutritional interventions such as omega-3 fatty acids, vitamin B_{12}, and selenium. Clinical trials have delivered mixed results on each of these, but omega-3s seem to be the most promising. A recent metareview of the effect of fish oil on psoriasis evaluated results from 15 trials. Twelve trials showed clinical improvement in psoriasis and three showed no improvement.[9] The efficacy of omega-3 fatty acids could be due to their anti-inflammatory effects, leading some to hypothesize that an overall anti-inflammatory diet could help treat psoriasis. The National Psoriasis Foundation notes that many sufferers do see an improvement in their symptoms by following an anti-inflammatory diet, and so they recommend avoiding fatty red meats, dairy products, processed foods, refined sugars, and "nightshade" vegetables such as peppers, potatoes, and tomatoes. On the other hand, foods with an anti-inflammatory effect include omega-3-rich cold-water fish such as albacore tuna, mackerel, salmon, herring, and lake trout; flaxseeds; olive oil; pumpkin seeds; walnuts; and colorful, fresh fruits and vegetables.[10] Other foods that are known to exert an anti-inflammatory effect include turmeric (combine it with black pepper to increase its effect); ginger; pineapple; papayas; mangoes; capers; apples; citrus fruits and their juices; dark, leafy greens (arugula, kale, spinach, Swiss chard, etc.); aronia berries (chokeberries); blueberries; cilantro; mushrooms; sweet potatoes; coffee; tea; and dark chocolate.

Finally, though clinical trials have not demonstrated their efficacy, some people report an improvement in psoriasis symptoms after using home remedies such as topically applied tea tree oil, oatmeal baths (which have been shown to relieve itching), a topical solution made of apple cider vinegar and water, or aloe vera gel. Psoriasis sufferers should take care to keep their skin moisturized through adequate fluid intake as well as topical creams.

See also: Dry Skin (page 254), Eczema (page 259), Food Allergies (page 278), Overweight and Obesity (page 396)

shingles

Shingles is an infection caused by the varicella-zoster virus and is also known as herpes zoster or zoster. Varicella-zoster is the same virus responsible for chicken pox. The condition is most common in people over 50, but anyone who has had chicken pox or received a chicken pox vaccine can develop shingles—indeed, nearly one out of three Americans will develop shingles at some point in their lives.[1] A vaccine is recommended for anyone 60 and older.

Shingles is characterized by a painful rash that develops on one side of your body. Usually it occurs on your torso, but it can appear on your face, as well. (A rash that develops near your eye should be treated as soon as possible to prevent permanent damage to that eye.) Shingles can also cause fever, headache, nausea, fatigue, and sensitivity to light. The standard treatment is a course of antivirals that, while they do not cure the condition, can lessen its duration and decrease the severity of your symptoms. Topical creams can cut down on the itching and help to dry up blisters.

Healing foods interventions for shingles are first of all about prevention. The higher incidence of shingles that occurs as we age is thought to be the result of a decline in cell-mediated immunity. Increasing health problems as we grow older and social-environmental changes, such as stressful life events, also play a part in triggering the activation of varicella-zoster.[2] It's also well known that any factor that weakens your immune system, such as HIV infection, diabetes, cancer, or taking immunosuppressive drugs, leaves you more susceptible to shingles. And, not surprisingly, poor nutrition has also been linked to the incidence of shingles as well as its most common complication, postherpetic neuralgia (nerve pain due to damage from the varicella-zoster virus).[3] Without proper nutrition your immune system simply isn't able to function at optimal levels.

Though there is no definitive "immune system diet," eating a well-balanced diet consisting of plenty of fresh fruits and vegetables, whole grains, lean proteins, and adequate fluid intake will provide most of the vitamins and minerals your immune system needs. The exception is vitamin D, which your body synthesizes from sun exposure, but it can also be found in dairy products, eggs, fish, fish oil, fortified orange juice,[4] and mushrooms. Some of the most important nutrients for immune system support—antioxidants—are found in fresh fruits and vegetables, which are high in these anti-inflammatory and immune-boosting flavonoids.[5] Among the best sources of flavonoids are apples, aronia berries (chokeberries), beans, blueberries, capers, chocolate, coriander, cranberries, currants, dock, elderberries, fennel, garlic, grapefruit, hot peppers, juniper berries, kumquats, lovage, onions, oregano, parsley, plums, radicchio, radishes, raspberries, red cabbage, and red wine.[6] Any dark, leafy green is a great source of antioxidants, including arugula, broccoli, chicory, collard greens, kale, lettuces, mustard greens, spinach, and watercress. Also add any brightly colored fruits and vegetables to your list of immune-supporting foods: apricots, beets, cantaloupe, carrots, lemons, limes, mangoes, oranges, peppers of any type, tomatoes, and winter squash. These foods are excellent sources of immune-supporting vitamins A and C. Another essential mineral for immune support is zinc. Food sources of zinc include oysters, wheat germ, chicken, crab, beans, oatmeal, yogurt, pumpkin seeds, and pine nuts.

If you do come down with shingles, continue with an antioxidant-rich diet to support immune- and whole-body health so the outbreak will pass as quickly as possible. You may want to try licorice root extract—it's available as a tea but licorice root can be chewed, as well—as it's been found to have some antiviral activity against varicella-zoster.[7] Do not consume licorice, however, if you have high blood pressure or if you are pregnant or breastfeeding. For pain control, there is some evidence that topical capsaicin, a cream made from the heat compound found in hot chile peppers, can provide pain relief for shingles. But because capsaicin causes a burning sensation, it may not be tolerated well by everyone, and you may want to take an analgesic before using the cream.[8] A more pleasant home remedy may be turmeric paste, which you can make by combining ground turmeric with water and coconut oil. Curcumin, the active ingredient in turmeric, has been shown to be effective in inhibiting the herpes simplex virus.[9] You can also try drinking turmeric tea—sweeten it with local honey for an extra dose of a natural antiviral. With turmeric's known antioxidant and anti-inflammatory properties, it's a great idea to add it to your diet.

sinusitis

The most basic definition of sinusitis is inflamed sinuses. Sinusitis is most often the result of a cold, a sinus infection, or allergies, but it can also be caused by nasal polyps or a structural abnormality such as a deviated septum. Whatever the cause, sinusitis causes swelling of the tissue lining your sinuses, which results in congestion, nasal discharge, sinus pain and pressure, cough, and loss of your sense of smell. Sinusitis can also lead to halitosis, sore throat, and sleep difficulties or fatigue, and fever is associated with sinusitis caused by infection.

Antibiotics are the conventional treatment for sinusitis caused by bacterial infection, but many health-care providers now caution against the overuse of antibiotics and the possibility of creating antibiotic-resistant strains of bacteria. Corticosteroids in the form of nasal sprays, oral medications, or injection are used for severe cases of sinusitis. And though there are no foods that can outright cure a sinus infection, there are plenty of nutritional interventions and nonmedication remedies that can help your body heal more quickly and that can bring you quick relief from some of the symptoms of sinusitis. To keep your immune system strong and to fight off a sinus infection more quickly, load your diet with antioxidants (especially vitamins A and C), vitamin D, and zinc. To do this, eat apples, aronia berries (chokeberries), beans, blueberries, capers, chocolate, coriander, cranberries, currants, dock, elderberries, fennel, grapefruit, hot peppers, juniper berries, kumquats, lovage, onions, oregano, parsley, plums, radicchio, radishes, raspberries, red cabbage, and red wine.[1] Dark, leafy greens (arugula, broccoli, chicory, collard greens, kale, lettuces, mustard greens, spinach, and watercress) are also great sources of antioxidants, as are brightly colored fruits and vegetables such as apricots, beets, cantaloupe, carrots, lemons, limes, mangoes, oranges, peppers of any type, tomatoes, and winter squash. To get vitamin D, spend a little time in the sun, and eat dairy products, eggs, fish, fish oil, fortified orange juice, and mushrooms. Food sources of zinc include oysters, wheat germ, chicken, crab, beans, oatmeal, yogurt, sunflower seeds, pumpkin seeds, and pine nuts. For further antibacterial benefits, add garlic and ginger.

The other foods you'll want to concentrate on are any foods that can relieve inflammation. The classics here are omega-3s, which are found in cold-water fish (salmon, herring, mackerel, tuna, trout, and sardines); walnuts; flaxseeds; flaxseed oil; and olive oil. Other excellent natural anti-inflammatory foods are turmeric, which has been used for thousands of years to reduce inflammation;[2] ginger, which has anti-inflammatory, antioxidant, and anti-allergy effects;[3] and pineapple, because of its high bromelain content. Bromelain has specifically been linked to the treatment of sinusitis and has a high absorption rate in the body.[4]

To open up swollen sinuses and promote nasal discharge, spicy foods are a guaranteed natural remedy. Try hot peppers, horseradish, spicy mustard, and hot sauces with all-natural ingredients. Hot teas and hot soups can also promote nasal discharge, and certain teas can provide extra benefits. For example, green tea is loaded with antioxidants and has anti-inflammatory properties, as well. Licorice root tea has anti-inflammatory and antiviral effects and has been shown to prevent inflammation of the nasal mucous membranes.[5] Honey has been shown to reduce inflammation of mucous membranes, and it has an antioxidant effect.[6]

Finally, try a simple saline solution. The American Academy of Otolaryngology—Head and Neck Surgery recommends this recipe for saline solution: Combine 1 quart (4 cups) of boiled or distilled water, 1 teaspoon of baking soda, and 1 teaspoon of non-iodized salt.[7] Use this solution in a neti pot or a bulb syringe. (Both are available at most any corner drugstore.) To use a neti pot, start by preparing the warm saline solution. After adding it to the pot, lean over your sink, tilt your head sideways so your face is horizontal, and insert the spout into your upper nostril. Allow the solution to drain into the nostril, then tilt your head so that the solution drains into the sink. Repeat with the remaining nostril. Nasal irrigation can be used as needed to clear nasal passages of mucus, sweep out infection, and soothe irritated membranes. To use a bulb syringe, squeeze the air out of the bulb, place the tip of the bulb into a nostril, then release the bulb to let the air back into the bulb. Remove from your nostril and squeeze the mucus out of the bulb and onto a tissue. Repeat with your remaining nostril. A metastudy found that nasal symptoms—defined as congestion, itching, sneezing, and discharge—decreased by an average of nearly 28 percent as a result of nasal irrigation and that overall quality of life rose by nearly 28 percent, as well.[8]

See also: Allergic Rhinitis (Hay Fever) (page 156), Colds (page 214), Coughs (page 220), Halitosis (page 307), Sore Throat (page 417)

sore throat

Pain and inflammation in your throat can arise from any number of factors, including the common cold, allergies, laryngitis (inflammation of the larynx), tonsillitis (inflammation of the tonsils), GERD (gastroesophageal reflux disease), smoking, exposure to pollutants, strep throat, or the presence of tumors. By far the most common cause of a sore throat is viral pharyngitis (inflammation of the pharynx). Mild, short-term sore throats can be treated at home, and most go away within a week. But if the pain is severe, sudden, and/or accompanied by a fever, you should be evaluated by your doctor. A severe sore throat accompanied by a fever, enlarged lymph nodes, and patchy white spots on your tonsils is most likely strep throat, and antibiotics are required to treat it.

Many of the best healing "foods" for sore throat are actually beverages. Gargling with warm salt water, just like your grandmother recommended, still works like a charm. The warmth soothes your throat and eases the pain, and the salt draws out fluid, which decreases swelling (and pain). Gargling can be done as needed to treat pain and discomfort. The warm water also helps any nasal mucus to thin and drain.

Any warm liquid, from soup to broth to tea, will ease the pain of a sore throat. Sage tea is one of the best options, as it's high in antioxidants and has long been used as a home remedy to treat inflammation of the mouth and throat.[1] Licorice root tea is another good choice, as it has anti-inflammatory and antiviral effects, and it has been shown to prevent inflammation of the nasal mucous membranes.[2] Don't ingest any licorice product if you have hypertension or are pregnant or breastfeeding, however. Licorice also interacts with various medications, including warfarin (Coumadin), so familiarize yourself with the full list of possible side effects and interactions before drinking licorice root tea. An option with no reported side effects is marshmallow root.[3] It's available as a tea, an extract, and a capsule, but your best bet for sore throat relief is the tea, which will bring the benefits of a soothing warm liquid, as well. There's also some evidence that marshmallow root tea relieves a cough.[4] If you like to sweeten your tea, bypass sugar and go for antioxidant-rich honey, which has been shown to reduce inflammation of mucous membranes.[5]

There is also some evidence that probiotics can help prevent and treat sore throat. The oral probiotic *Streptococcus salivarius* was found to be effective in reducing the number of sore throat episodes in adults with recurrent streptococcal pharyngitis (strep throat). Study participants took this probiotic for 90 days and experienced an 80 percent reduction in streptococcal pharyngeal infection and a 60 percent reduction in reported strep during the 6-month follow-up period.[6] An older study also confirmed the efficacy of *S. salivarius* in fighting strep.[7] This particular probiotic is available as a supplement, lozenge, or gum, but considering the power of common probiotics to prevent and treat the common cold—and considering that colds are among the most common causes of sore throat—adding probiotics to your diet is advisable. Food sources of probiotics include yogurt, kefir, sauerkraut, kimchi, miso soup, sour pickles, kombucha tea, and some soft cheeses, such as Gouda and Swiss. For additional specific foods that help prevent and treat colds, see Colds on page 214.

stress

Stress hardly needs an introduction—most of us are probably all too well acquainted with experiences of tension, anxiety, and psychological distress. The causes of stress are endless and can range from simple daily nuisances like running late to the moderate stressors of giving a presentation to life-altering events such as losing a loved one. Stress triggers an incredibly complex set of concurrent responses that involve your entire body. Your brain triggers the release of adrenaline and norepinephrine from your adrenal glands. These hormones flood your system and in turn trigger a host of physical symptoms: heart rate increases, respiration increases, pupils dilate, blood vessels constrict, and muscles tighten.

These *temporary* states of high arousal can be beneficial when we need increased focus and extra strength to deal with a perceived threat or to deal with events that require high performance and attention to detail. But your body and mind can be badly harmed when stress becomes unrelenting or *chronic*. We're simply not built to remain in a long-term state of hyperarousal.

Chronic stress has been linked to anxiety disorders and depression,[1] insomnia, fatigue, substance abuse problems, hypertension, gastrointestinal problems, weight changes, cognitive impairment, accelerated aging, elevated risk of cardiovascular disease, and even increased all-cause morbidity. Stress can also cause compromised immunity, increased risk of infection, and slower wound healing.[2] A meta-analysis of studies on workplace stress and stroke risk that examined data from 138,782 people found that people with high-stress jobs had a 22 percent higher risk of stroke of any type and a 58 percent higher risk of ischemic stroke than people with low-stress jobs. (Ischemic strokes occur as a result of an obstructed blood vessel that supplies blood to the brain.) The risk was especially pronounced in women: Women with high-stress jobs had a 33 percent greater risk of stroke than women with low-stress jobs.[3] Chronic stress has long been associated with coronary heart disease,[4] and a recent study based on evidence from more than 600,000 people found that work stressors such as long working hours and job strain are associated with an elevated risk of coronary heart disease and stroke.[5] And in a study on social stressors and mortality, researchers found that frequent worries or demands from a partner or children were associated with an elevated mortality risk of anywhere from 50 to 100 percent! The study was based upon 9,875 adults between the ages of 36 and 52. Frequent arguing was associated with two to three times increased mortality risk. The study also found that men and the unemployed were more vulnerable to the deleterious effects of stressful social relations.[6] Early-life adversity and posttraumatic stress disorder have even been linked to negative effects on sleeping and to poorer diet quality all around, including a higher consumption of trans fats.[7]

Fortunately there are many effective ways to lower stress, including therapy, meditation, exercise, spending time with loved ones (including pets), diaphragmatic breathing practices, aromatherapy, massage, taking a vacation (or even just a day off), listening to relaxing music, journaling, and laughing. It's also vitally important to get proper sleep and to eat a healthy diet. Let's take a look at what the latest research advises on nutritional support for stress management.

A study of 281 young adults found that their mood was better on days they ate more fruits and vegetables. Further, fruit and vegetable consumption predicted positive mood for the next day, as well. Researchers suggest you eat seven or eight daily servings of fruits and vegetables for positive mood.[8] But never fear, you can have your treats, too: Dark and milk chocolate were shown to decrease perceived stress in students who were given 40 grams of chocolate per day. The effect was stronger in women than in men.[9]

Probiotics have been shown to improve symptoms of both anxiety and

healthy insight

Now for the results of a study you may not want to hear. Researchers have found that dishwashing—performed mindfully—is an effective stress buster. The experimental group was asked to be "fully aware" that they were washing dishes by focusing on the warmth of the water, the smell of the dish soap, and so on. Compared to a control group, the mindful dishwashers experienced a 27 percent reduction in nervousness and reported greater mental inspiration. Researchers believe their findings can apply to any mundane task performed mindfully.[10]

depression. In one study, volunteers consumed the probiotics *Lactobacillus helveticus* and *Bifidobacterium longum* in combination for 30 days, and even in people with lower cortisol levels, mood was improved.[11] There is increasing evidence that gut microbiota communicate with and influence your central nervous system and that probiotics can modulate gut microbiota such that mood and anxiety disorders can be treated and even prevented.[12] In one study, subjects were assigned to consume a probiotic yogurt plus a placebo capsule, a conventional yogurt plus a probiotic capsule, or a conventional yogurt and a placebo capsule. After 6 weeks, a significant improvement in general health and in scores measuring anxiety and depression occurred in the group that took the probiotic yogurt and the one that took probiotic capsules. Those who ate the probiotic yogurt had the most improvement.[13] And in a study that found that fermented foods have a beneficial effect on social anxiety, researchers speculated that fermented foods may have an antianxiety effect above and beyond probiotic supplements because of the presence of peptides and other chemicals that affect the brain.[14] Fermented whole foods include yogurt, kimchi, tempeh, kefir, soy milk, sauerkraut, sour cream, natto, some soft cheeses, pickles, miso soup, and dark chocolate.

The medicinal plant known as *Ocimum sanctum,* or holy basil, is effective at reducing anxiety and stress. In one study, 35 adults took 500 milligram (mg) capsules of holy basil twice a day for 60 days. By the end of the trial, subjects experienced less anxiety and less depression and had significant reductions in stress index scores: At baseline the average stress score was about 96, but by day 60 it had fallen to about 68.[15]

There is evidence that the neurological peptide called carnosine can enhance cortisol metabolism. In animal studies it was shown to suppress stress, and in human studies it improved behavior, cognition, and well-being.[16] Food sources of carnosine include beef, chicken, fish, milk, eggs, and cheese. It is also available as a supplement.

The B vitamins have long been studied for their ability to regulate mood; vitamin B supplementation has been shown to be effective at improving mood by helping your body deal with stress.[17] Sixty workers experiencing occupational stress who were given a daily vitamin B complex supplement for 12 weeks experienced significantly lower personal strain and a reduction in confusion and depressed/dejected mood.[18] A deficiency in vitamin B_{12} has been linked to increased psychological distress,[19] and low concentrations of vitamin B_6 (which is depleted by chronic stress) and iron have been observed in people suffering from panic attacks. Moreover, vitamin B_6

and iron play key roles in the production of serotonin and dopamine, and studies have shown that low serotonin is partially responsible for panic attacks.[20] To get more vitamin B_6 into your diet, eat avocados, bananas, brown rice, chicken breast, fish, potatoes,[21] molasses, pistachios, and turkey breast.[22] Vitamin B_{12} is only found in animal products—with the exception of nori and sea lettuce. Some of the best food sources are clams, mussels, and mackerel, but it's also found in crab, beef, salmon, turkey, chicken, eggs, and dairy products.[23] Iron is also found in animal products such as beef and pork, but it can also be found in fortified whole grain cereals, white beans, dark chocolate, lentils, spinach, tofu, kidney beans, chickpeas, tomatoes, and cashews.[24]

Vitamin C has been shown to reduce anxiety, and with its powerful antioxidant properties, it may play a key role in reversing the free radical damage caused by chronic stress.[25] Your brain and your adrenal glands are your organs with the highest concentrations of vitamin C, and a lack of it may impair your ability to deal with stress.[26] To increase your vitamin C intake, eat fresh citrus fruits such as oranges, grapefruits, lemons, and limes. Other sources are kiwifruit, strawberries, tomatoes, acerola cherries (West Indian cherries), red peppers, broccoli, papayas, Brussels sprouts, cauliflower, cantaloupe, guavas, and parsley.

Magnesium has a well-deserved reputation as a natural stress buster. It's known to have a relaxing effect, and it promotes melatonin secretion, which can help with a good night's sleep. Symptoms of magnesium deficiency include agitation and anxiety, not to mention insomnia, hyperventilation, and irritability, which are all symptoms of anxiety, as well.[27] To add calming magnesium to your diet, eat sesame seeds; sunflower seeds; almonds; cashews; walnuts; oats; dark, leafy greens; seaweed; tofu; whole grains; avocados; and bananas.

Zinc is a cofactor in adrenaline and neurotransmitter synthesis, and a deficiency will influence cognitive functioning and may impair your ability to deal with stress.[28] To boost your zinc intake, eat oysters, beef, wheat germ, fortified cereals, pumpkin seeds, or sesame seeds.

Both stress and depression are known to trigger inflammatory cytokine production. But higher levels of omega-3s as well as lower ratios of omega-6s to omega-3s are both associated with lower proinflammatory cytokine production. To protect against the negative health consequences of stress, increase your omega-3 fatty acid consumption with foods like fish, fish oil, flax oil and flaxseeds, walnuts, and walnut oil.[29]

See also: Anxiety (page 165), Depression (page 232), Heart Disease (Cardiovascular Disease) (page 313), Insomnia (page 357), Stroke (page 423)

stroke

Astroke occurs when bloodflow to your brain is blocked, resulting in cell death. Though nearly 800,000 people in the United States experience a stroke every year,[1] quick medical intervention dramatically increases your chances of survival and of avoiding permanent disability. (Of that 800,000, only about 130,000 strokes result in death.)[2] The most common signs and symptoms of stroke appear suddenly: numbness or weakness, often on one side of the body; severe headache; confusion; trouble seeing in one or both eyes; dizziness, which may result in a loss of balance and coordination; and confusion, which may result in difficulty in speaking or understanding speech. Transient ischemic attacks (TIA), often referred to as mini strokes, are caused by a transient (temporary) clot and exhibit the same symptoms as strokes, but most last less than 5 minutes. Though most TIAs cause no lasting brain damage, they are serious warning signs of increased risk of stroke; about one-third of people who experience a TIA go on to have a stroke within a year.[3]

Risk factors for stroke include overweight and obesity, high cholesterol, high blood pressure, heart disease, tobacco use, overconsumption of alcohol, sedentary lifestyle, poor diet, and age. Chronic stress combined with any of these risk factors substantially increases your risk, as well. Of all of these, age is the only unavoidable risk factor, but on the other hand, a healthy diet and sufficient exercise (at least 150 minutes a week) will prevent or mitigate the other risk factors.

Healing foods for stroke are all about *prevention*. To eat to avoid stroke, adhere to the general guidelines for healthy living as seen in the entries on Heart Disease (page 313) and High Blood Pressure (page 327), as you want to eat to keep your cardiovascular system healthy. Dietary recommendations for a healthy cardiovascular system are essentially the same as those for stroke prevention. High blood pressure is the biggest contributor to your risk of stroke, so choose foods that reduce blood pressure. Epidemiological studies have revealed that diets that are low in sodium and high in fruits and vegetables lower your risk of stroke.[4] (See High Blood Pressure on page 327 for specific recommendations.) An overall dietary pattern that significantly reduces your risk of stroke will follow the Mediterranean diet or a similar heart-healthy diet, such as the DASH diet, MIND diet, Nordic diet, or traditional Japanese diet. Adherence to the Mediterranean diet is associated with a lower risk of heart attack, heart failure, and ischemic stroke.[5] Emphasize fresh fruits and vegetables, especially citrus fruits and dark, leafy greens. Data from the Nurses' Health Study based on 14 years of follow-up showed that increased intake of flavonoids, primarily from citrus fruits, was associated with a reduced risk of ischemic stroke.[6] Get your protein from omega-3-rich seafood; plant-based proteins, such as soy products, nuts, and nut butters; and occasional lean poultry. Eliminate or drastically reduce your consumption of red and processed meats, both of which have been linked to a significantly increased risk of stroke—especially ischemic stroke.[7] Eliminate all trans fats—anything that contains hydrogenated vegetable oils. Watch out for hidden sources of trans fats, such as commercially prepared baked goods or fast foods. Eat whole grains, legumes, nuts, and seeds; avoid refined carbohydrates. Drink alcohol in moderation. Red wine may be the best form of alcohol for cardiovascular health, as it's rich in resveratrol and anthocyanins.

Many studies have demonstrated that a high-sodium diet increases your risk of stroke,[8] so eat less than 2,300 milligrams (mg) of sodium a day—though 1,500 mg or less of sodium lowers blood pressure even more and is recommended for those with hypertension.[9] Limit consumption of sugary beverages and sweets to five or fewer a week. Overall, eat foods that are high in fiber and low in cholesterol and saturated fats. Avoid foods that are processed and/or that have artificial ingredients.

With these general recommendations in mind, let's look at some of the specific foods that can help protect against stroke. A high consumption of dietary flavonols has been shown to decrease your risk of stroke. A metareview of eight studies, with 5,228 stroke cases among 280,174 participants, showed a significant association between the highest flavonol intake and a reduced risk for stroke, especially among men. Further, an increase in flavonol intake of 20 mg a day was associated with a 14 percent decrease in the risk for developing stroke.[10] Flavonols belong to the large group of compounds called flavonoids, and they're found in abundance in fruits, vegetables, red wine, cocoa products, and tea. Other food sources include apples, apricots, beans, berries, broccoli, capers, cherries, chives, cranberries, dark chocolate, grapes, kale, leeks, lettuces, onions, pears, and tomatoes.

Higher fiber consumption has also been shown to have a significant impact on decreasing your risk of stroke. A metareview of six studies on a total of 314,864 subjects and 8,920 stroke cases were assessed for fiber consumption. For every 10 grams a day of increased dietary fiber intake, stroke risk fell by 12 percent.[11] Good sources of fiber include fruits (blueberries, chokeberries, dates, prunes, apricots, figs, raisins, apples, oranges, peaches, passion fruit, pears, and grapes); dark, leafy greens (arugula, kale, spinach, Brussels sprouts, lettuces, and broccoli); legumes (lentils, beans, chickpeas, and split peas); flaxseeds and chia seeds; and whole grains (oatmeal, barley, bulgur, quinoa, and whole grain breads and cereals).

As high cholesterol is a known risk factor for stroke, eat foods that have been shown to lower total serum cholesterol and LDL cholesterol. Good examples include avocados, foods with fiber (see above), garlic, legumes, nuts (especially almonds, pistachios, and walnuts), oats and oat bran, olive oil, and green tea.[12] And while we're speaking of tea, both black and green tea have been shown to be protective against stroke generally. A study of nearly 195,000 individuals showed that drinking 3 or more cups of tea a day, green or black, was associated with a 21 percent lower risk of stroke than for those who drank only 1 cup per day.[13]

Research studies have demonstrated a link between potassium intake and stroke. Researchers followed more than 90,000 women ages 50 to 79 (at the outset of the study) for an average of 11 years. The highest intake of potassium was associated with a lower incidence of stroke and total mortality. The protective effect was strongest in those who were not hypertensive.[14] In a metastudy that examined data from 10 studies with a total of 8,695 stroke cases and 268,276 participants, researchers observed a significant inverse association between potassium intake and risk of stroke. For every 1,000 mg per day increase in potassium intake, the risk of stroke decreased by 11 percent.[15] Potassium-rich foods include sweet potatoes (694 mg potassium), tomato paste (664 mg per $\frac{1}{4}$ cup), beet greens (665 mg per $\frac{1}{2}$ cup), white beans (595 mg per $\frac{1}{2}$ cup), yogurt (579 mg per 8-ounce container), clams (534 mg per 3-ounce serving), halibut (490 mg per 3-ounce serving), soybeans (485 mg per $\frac{1}{2}$ cup), winter squash (448 mg per $\frac{1}{2}$ cup), bananas (422 mg for one medium banana), and spinach (419 mg per $\frac{1}{2}$ cup). Other excellent sources of potassium include tuna, cod, dried peaches, dried apricots, prunes, cantaloupe, milk, honeydew melon, lentils, and orange, carrot, and prune juice.[16]

If you do have a stroke or experience a TIA, as you recover it's more important than ever to make lifestyle and dietary changes that lower your blood pressure and cholesterol and help you maintain a healthy BMI: Recurrent strokes make up about one out of four of the nearly 800,000 strokes Americans experience each year.[17] Follow all of the recommendations stipulated as previously mentioned, as well as any specific instructions on diet, medications, and exercise from your doctor. And if chronic stress is a part of your life,

make changes to lower your stress level. A meta-analysis of studies on workplace stress and stroke risk that examined data from 138,782 people found that those with high-stress jobs had a 22 percent higher risk of stroke of any type and a 58 percent greater risk of ischemic stroke than people with low-stress jobs. The risk was especially pronounced in women: Women with high-stress jobs had a 33 percent greater risk of stroke than women with low-stress jobs.[18]

See also: Heart Disease (Cardiovascular Disease) (page 313), High Blood Pressure (Hypertension) (page 327), High Cholesterol (page 334), Stress (page 419)

sunburn

Sunburn is caused by overexposure to UV radiation. Overexposure usually happens when you stay out in the sun too long, but tanning beds can also cause sunburn. Its symptoms are reddened skin and pain, and more severe cases can cause blisters and flulike symptoms. People with lighter skin are more susceptible to sunburn, as are young children and adults over 65. While sunburn subsides on its own and rarely requires professional treatment, the Skin Cancer Foundation warns that a single blistering sunburn in childhood more than *doubles* a person's chances of later developing melanoma.[1]

Most of the time we think of treating sunburn only after the damage is done, but there are actually healing foods that have built-in sun protection. Carotenoids are a class of phytochemicals that have photoprotective effects. Beta-carotene and lycopene, the pigments found in carrots and tomatoes, respectively, are usually the dominating carotenoids in human blood and tissues. There is evidence that they protect your skin against sunburn by increasing your basal defense against UV damage.[2] Clinical trials have shown that beta-carotene supplementation decreases the intensity of sunburn and protects against suppression of the immune system caused by sunburn.[3] In vitro data also suggest that the carotenoid lutein has some photoprotective benefit.[4] Sources of beta-carotene include yellow and orange fruits, such as mangoes and papayas; orange root vegetables, such as carrots and yams; and dark, leafy greens, such as spinach and kale. Lycopene is found in tomatoes, grapefruit, watermelon, gac fruit, and guavas. Lutein is found in dark, leafy greens, especially kale and spinach, but also watercress, dandelion greens, turnip greens, Swiss chard, and collards.

The polyphenols in green tea have been shown to be photoprotective in both animal and human models. Topical application of epigallocatechin gallate (EGCG), the main catechin in green tea, resulted in the inhibition of UVB-induced sunburn, oxidative stress, and infiltration of inflammatory leukocytes, and by drinking green tea you benefit from its antioxidant and anti-inflammatory effects, as well.[5]

Finally, there is evidence that omega-3 fatty acids provide systemic photoprotection by protecting your skin against acute UV radiation–induced inflammation. Clinical trials have shown that omega-3 supplementation reduces UV ray sensitivity. One study examined the topical application of PUFA-rich sardine oil and found that it reduced sunburn by 24.5 percent compared to controls.[6] Omega-3 fatty acids are found in cold-water fish such as salmon, mackerel, herring, sardines, tuna, and cod, and in walnuts, flaxseeds, and their oils.

thyroid disease

Your thyroid is a small, butterfly-shaped endocrine gland located at the base of your neck. It produces thyroid hormone, which controls your body's metabolic processes, body temperature, and tissue growth. How fast and how efficiently you burn energy is controlled by your thyroid gland.

The three main thyroid disorders are hyperthyroidism, which results from an overactive thyroid that produces too much thyroid hormone; hypothyroidism, which results from an underactive thyroid that produces insufficient thyroid hormone; and thyroid cancer. For reasons that are unclear, thyroid disorders are three times more likely to occur in women than in men. Many people suffer from a confusing set of symptoms that may seem unrelated; that cover a range of physical, mental, and emotional complaints; and/or that are mistaken for other conditions—so it's no wonder that thyroid problems often go missed or misdiagnosed.

Signs of hypothyroidism, or underactive thyroid, can include constipation, depression, dry skin, fatigue, muscle aches or weakness, hoarseness, thinning hair, impaired memory, increased sensitivity to cold, high cholesterol, puffy face (puffiness can also occur in the hands or feet), periods that are heavier than normal, irregular periods, and weight gain.

Signs of hyperthyroidism, or overactive thyroid, can include anxiety, increased appetite, an increase in bowel movements, difficulty sleeping, fatigue, rapid heartbeat, palpitations, high blood pressure, sweating, shaking, thinning hair, hair loss, goiter (an enlarged, visibly swollen thyroid gland), itchy or clammy skin, unexplained weight loss, and breast development in men. In addition, one of the telltale signs of hyperthyroidism is protruding eyeballs, a phenomenon known as exophthalmos. Eyes can also become dry, red, and swollen, and disturbances to vision can occur.

Signs and symptoms of thyroid cancer can include goiter, swollen lymph nodes, neck pain, hoarseness, trouble swallowing, trouble breathing, or a persistent cough not due to cold. Though the vast majority of lumps or nodules on the thyroid are benign, it's important to see your doctor right away if you experience any of these symptoms.

The most important nutrient for thyroid function is iodine, as it's required for the synthesis of thyroid hormones. Iodine is present in salt, dairy products, seafood, green sea vegetables, yogurt, and eggs. Too little iodine results in hypothyroidism; too much results in hyperthyroidism. The safe upper limit of iodine for adults is about 1.1 milligrams (mg) per day. To put that into perspective, $\frac{1}{4}$ teaspoon of iodized salt contains 0.071 mg of iodine, and 3 ounces of cod contains about 0.1 mg. Seaweed is the best food source of iodine, but be sure to double-check nutritional values, as the iodine content can vary widely— anywhere from 0.016 mg per gram of seaweed to a whopping 1.9 mg of iodine per gram, which exceeds the recommended daily value.[1]

Selenium is second only to iodine for its importance in healthy thyroid function. Selenium is also crucial for thyroid hormone synthesis, and a deficiency in selenium worsens iodine deficiency. Deficiencies of these nutrients result in hypothyroidism. Selenium-rich foods include mushrooms, garlic, onions, eggs, beef liver, shellfish, wheat germ, sunflower seeds, and sesame seeds.[2]

The amino acid tyrosine is essential for healthy thyroid function. Most people get enough in their diets, but some sources recommend additional tyrosine (also known as L-tyrosine) to ensure proper thyroid function.[3] Food sources that are high in tyrosine include seaweed, soy products, cottage cheese, salmon, poultry, eggs, shrimp, and mustard greens.[4] Do not take a tyrosine supplement if you have high blood pressure, and if you're on thyroid medication already, check with your doctor before increasing your tyrosine intake.

Goitrogenic foods play a major role in thyroid disease. Goitrogens are any substances that interfere with thyroid hormone synthesis by inhibiting iodine uptake and the activity of thyroid peroxidase (an enzyme critical to thyroid function).[5] Various drugs and chemicals are goitrogens, and there are quite a few foods that are goitrogenic. Examples include bamboo shoots, cassava, pine nuts, peanuts, strawberries, pears, peaches, sweet potatoes, millet, and soy products, as well as cruciferous vegetables in the *Brassica* family such as Brussels sprouts, cauliflower, bok choy, broccoli, kohlrabi, cabbage, collard greens, mustard greens, kale, rutabaga, radishes, and turnips. For people with healthy thyroid function, goitrogenic foods don't pose a problem. But if thyroid function is compromised, these foods can further interfere with thyroid hormone production, resulting in the enlargement of the thyroid gland (goiter). Cooking these foods attenuates the goitrogenic effect, so people with compromised thyroid function can still enjoy goitrogenic foods in moderation. Fermentation, on the other hand, increases goitrogenic activity, so you may want to avoid fermented foods.

The other option is to add foods to your diet that counteract the goitrogenic effect. One study on goitrogenesis was conducted in Pakistan, as the South Asian population has a high prevalence of thyroid disorders due to iodine deficiency and goitrogen use. Data from 2,335 people was collected, and nearly 29 percent had a palpable goiter. But researchers noted that goiter was less common among those who consumed daily milk, daily ghee (clarified butter), chiles, turmeric, and other spices. Turmeric was associated specifically with reduced goitrogenesis. Researchers concluded that those consuming a diet high in goitrogens should incorporate turmeric, spices, iodized salt, and green chiles into their diets and recipes to reduce their risk of goiter development.[6]

To protect against any sort of thyroid disease, there may be some benefit to following a vegan diet. In a study based on data from nearly 66,000 people, vegan, lacto-ovo (vegetarian plus dairy and eggs), and pescatarian (vegetarian plus seafood) diets were associated with lower risk of *hyper*thyroidism compared with omnivorous diets. A vegan diet, which excludes all animal products, was associated with 52 percent lower odds of hyperthyroidism compared with omnivorous diets. Lacto-ovo vegetarian and pescatarian diets were associated with intermediate protection.[7] A different study based on the same data, however, found that vegan diets tended to be protective against *hypo*thyroidism, though the association was not great enough to be statistically significant, and a lacto-ovo vegetarian diet was associated with an increased risk of hypothyroidism.[8]

tinnitus

Tinnitus is the experience of ringing or buzzing in your ears. (The word comes from the Latin word *tinnire,* which means "to ring.") It's one of the most common complaints in the United States, affecting about one in five people. It can come and go, or it can be a constant, high-pitched whine. Tinnitus can be caused by trauma to the ear, excessive noise exposure, the normal aging process, cancer drugs, aspirin, an ear infection, or even excess wax in the ear. It often accompanies hearing loss, and it has been linked with hypertension and diabetes. (And in fact, having both hypertension and diabetes constitutes an independent risk factor for tinnitus.)[1] Tinnitus is also one of the defining symptoms of Ménière's disease, an inner ear disorder involving episodes of vertigo and progressive hearing loss.

Though there is no foolproof cure for tinnitus, there are many treatment and symptom management options. White noise machines can distract from the ringing and help you fall asleep—special pillows with built-in speakers are available. Small masking devices worn in your ears can provide continuous white noise that can distract you from tinnitus symptoms. Tinnitus retraining therapy exposes the tinnitus sufferer to constant low levels of background noise or music in an attempt to habituate the person to tinnitus noise and is usually accompanied by counseling. Some people have been helped by cognitive-behavioral therapy, acupuncture, hypnosis, relaxation techniques, meditation, and pursuing activities that distract them from their tinnitus symptoms. Research on nerve stimulation and transcranial magnetic stimulation for tinnitus relief is ongoing, but early results are promising. For many people, a combination of interventions works best.

There is a connection between tinnitus and diet, so some people can find relief by changing what they eat. If tinnitus is a result of Ménière's disease, lower your sodium intake. Excess sodium promotes fluid retention, and fluid in your ears worsens tinnitus. Even if you don't have a formal diagnosis of Ménière's, lowering your salt intake is advisable: You may experience symptom relief, and a high sodium intake is also associated with hypertension, which itself can cause tinnitus. For specific recommendations on how to lower your sodium intake, see High Blood Pressure (page 327).

Research has shown that the prevalence of hearing impairment and tinnitus is more common in people with type 2 diabetes, and these problems develop at an earlier age than in those without diabetes.[2] There is also an association between tinnitus and hypertension, atherosclerosis, and other blood vessel disorders. The links between tinnitus and cardiovascular conditions and diabetes suggest that an overall healthy diet could be essential to preventing tinnitus and possibly alleviating symptoms. The American Tinnitus Association recommends a health-conscious diet that can reduce high blood pressure and weight, increase bloodflow, and enhance energy levels and emotional well-being—all of which can bring tinnitus relief.[3] An overall healthy dietary pattern such as the Mediterranean diet provides an excellent road map for eating habits that can support tinnitus symptom relief as well as whole-body health.

Researchers have looked for specific food triggers that can cause tinnitus, such as caffeine, alcohol, dairy, sugar, and wheat, but results have been inconclusive and, at times, contradictory. In the past, caffeine consumption was implicated in the development of tinnitus, but more recent research has found no connection. In a trial that examined the effect of caffeine abstinence on 66 tinnitus sufferers, researchers found that not only did the cessation of caffeine have no effect on tinnitus, caffeine withdrawal symptoms actually added to the burden of tinnitus.[4] And in fact, a large, multiyear study of more than 65,000 women found that greater caffeine intake was associated with a lower risk of tinnitus. Regardless of age, women who consumed 450 to 599 milligrams (mg) of caffeine per day had a 15 percent lower risk of tinnitus than women who consumed less than 150 mg per day of caffeine, or the amount of caffeine in one 8-ounce cup of coffee. In this study, caffeine consumption was based upon intake from any source, including coffee, tea, chocolate, and sodas.[5]

Excitotoxins (compounds known to overstimulate neuron receptors) may play a role in worsening some tinnitus symptoms,[6] and glutamate excitotoxicity is directly related to tinnitus that occurs after injury to the ear.[7] The two main dietary sources of excitotoxins are glutamate and aspartame. Though research in this area is scant, there are established links between aspartame and tinnitus in some sufferers,[8] and glutamate antagonists have been prescribed for tinnitus sufferers.[9] Thus, eliminating these two excitotoxins from your diet is worth a try. The main source of dietary glutamate is monosodium glutamate, or MSG. Remember that MSG can show up on labels in many different forms, including anything with the word "glutamate," "glutamic," or "hydrolyzed." MSG also occurs naturally in foods such as tomatoes, seaweed, some cheeses, and plant proteins. Aspartame is a different story in that it is purely artificial. It's most often found in diet soft drinks, but it can show up in candies, chewing gum, syrups, jellies, low-fat yogurts, and breath mints.

Many people wonder about natural or alternative treatments for tinnitus, but clinical evidence is limited. One of the most studied treatments is ginkgo biloba, but the research results were mixed at best, and a 2013 metareview concluded that ginkgo biloba was not effective at treating patients with a primary complaint of tinnitus.[10] Korean red ginseng, though not as thoroughly researched as ginkgo biloba, has been found to be effective in managing tinni-

tus and improving quality of life. In one study, 59 tinnitus sufferers took 3,000 mg of Korean red ginseng every day for 4 weeks. They reported significant improvement according to the Tinnitus Handicap Inventory, as well as improved mental and emotional health scores, according to a survey.[11]

Overall, given the lack of consistency and conclusive evidence on healing foods for tinnitus, it seems that the best recommendation is to adopt an overall healthy diet that ameliorates many of the cardiovascular risk factors associated with tinnitus and with worsening tinnitus symptoms. Stress management is also essential, as stress is both a cause and a result of tinnitus. Following the Mediterranean diet, getting adequate exercise, and reducing stress are some of the best interventions both to prevent and to treat tinnitus.

See also: Anxiety (page 165), Diabetes (page 238), Heart Disease (Cardiovascular Disease) (page 313), High Blood Pressure (Hypertension) (page 327), Stress (page 419), Vertigo (page 446)

tooth decay

Tooth decay is a very common—and very preventable—condition. Proper dental hygiene is the primary means of avoiding a host of dental conditions, including tooth decay, cavities, periodontal disease, gingivitis, halitosis, and yes, the inevitable toothaches that come with many of these conditions. The American Dental Association recommends, at a minimum, flossing and brushing twice a day. For optimal oral health, you should brush after every meal and avoid sugary drinks and foods, which eat away at tooth enamel and lead to cavities and other problems. Mouthwashes also protect against plaque and freshen breath.

To eat for strong teeth and to prevent tooth decay, make sure you're getting enough calcium and vitamin D. Teeth are specialized bones, after all, and you want to build strong teeth from the inside out. A study of 1,162 women found that compared to the group of women who had the lowest level of calcium intake, women with the highest calcium intake had the lowest prevalence of periodontal disease.[1] Want another reason to like calcium? Researchers found that people who added milk to their tea experienced less tooth staining than those who drink their tea straight up. The credit goes to casein, which makes up 80 percent of the protein content in cow's milk.[2] To increase your calcium and vitamin D intake, eat dairy products; seafood; dark, leafy greens; eggs; fortified juices; fortified soy milk; or fortified nut milks.

But calcium isn't the only mineral that's involved in dental health—it turns out copper also plays a significant role in protecting teeth from undue wear. Fifty patients with severe tooth wear were compared to 20 age-, sex- and BMI-matched healthy controls and assessed on a number of nutrient levels. The results may surprise you. The patients with tooth wear all had reduced lumbar spine bone mineral density compared to controls, and they all had significantly lower copper content in their tooth enamel.[3] More research is needed to determine the connection between tooth wear, reduced bone mineral density, and copper, but healthy sources of copper, which cannot be made by your body and must be ingested, include soy products, seeds, avocados, and dark chocolate.

In a healthy, varied diet, most people will get enough copper, as well as the rest of the vitamins and minerals they need to support periodontal health—and there's substantial evidence that an *overall* healthy diet is one of the best defenses against tooth decay. Researchers recruited 27 patients who, with a BMI over 25 and with impaired glucose tolerance, were at high risk for periodontal disease. After 8 weeks of eating a high-fiber, low-fat diet, all subjects experienced improvement in periodontal disease markers, including probing depth, clinical attachment loss, and bleeding on probing. Body weight and overall health improved, as well.[4] A study on oral hygiene, food intake, and risk of dental caries followed 935 women and found that consuming milk, fruits, and vegetables 4 or more days a week protected against dental caries. Consuming chocolate and soft drinks increased the risk of cavities, but the women who cleaned their teeth after eating sweets and chocolates and had no gingivitis were at less risk of dental caries than other women.[5] A healthy diet also lends protection to tooth roots, which is good news for anyone who's

healthy insight

If you need any additional motivation to avoid tooth decay, consider the results of a study published in the *Journal of Prosthodontics*: There is a clear and proven association between the loss of teeth and a host of serious illnesses, including obesity, cardiovascular disease, rheumatoid arthritis, dementia, pulmonary diseases, certain cancers (lung, bladder, esophageal, and head and neck among them), and even death. The exact relationship between tooth loss and these illnesses is complex and far beyond the scope of this book, but the study's conclusions are straightforward: People with missing or no teeth are at an increased risk for obesity, chronic obstructive pulmonary disease (COPD), head and neck cancer, the loss of cognitive function, and mortality. And edentulism, or the complete loss of teeth, is so strongly associated with cardiovascular disease that it is an independent predictor of death from cardiovascular disease.[6]

ever had a root canal. A study of 533 men ages 47 through 90 examined the association between root caries and dietary habits. Diets were scored according to adherence to the Dietary Approaches to Stop Hypertension (DASH) guidelines, which assessed diet according to 10 food groups: fruits, vegetables, total dairy, low-fat dairy, meat, total grains, high-fiber grains, legumes, fats, and sweets. After controlling for age, number of teeth at risk for root caries, time at risk of root caries, calculus (plaque on teeth), use of dentures, history of dental cleanings and x-rays, BMI, and smoking, researchers found that the men with the highest adherence to the DASH diet had a 30 percent lower indication of root caries risk. Risk was lower with greater vegetable and total grain intake and higher with greater consumption of sweetened carbonated beverages.[7]

It's clear that sugar causes tooth decay, but if you want a less harmful sweetener, choose honey. Researchers exposed extracted, cavity-free molars to solutions of honey, glucose, and fructose and measured the effects of these substances upon demineralization depth. For least damage, the clear winner was honey, which caused far fewer cavities than glucose and fructose. (The most harmful, by the way, was glucose.)[8]

Honey, which has natural antibacterial properties, has also been shown to actually inhibit the growth of bacteria that lead to dental caries.[9]

The other dietary component frequently implicated in tooth decay is acid: Foods and beverages that are highly acidic cause erosion and abrasion of enamel. Progression of erosion occurs more swiftly in older adults than in younger adults, in people who use a hard-bristle toothbrush, and in those who consume four or more acidic foods or beverages per day. Some of the most erosive foods and beverages include sports and energy drinks; sodas; carrot juice; multiple fruits and their juices, including apple, orange, grapefruit, pineapple, kiwi, and apricot; alcoholic beverages; flavored mineral water; kombucha; and rose hip tea. See "Reducing Acid Damage," page 438, for more pointers on how to cut down on enamel damage from acid.

Finally, you may want to consider the age-old Indian custom of oil pulling. Oil pulling is simply the practice of swishing an edible oil—such as sunflower, sesame, olive, or coconut oil—in your mouth for 10 to 15 minutes. It works by "pulling" bacteria and other disease-promoting microorganisms from your mouth, and it should be followed up with normal brushing. Oil

reducing acid damage

Rather than eliminating all acidic foods from your diet if you are prone to cavities and enamel erosion, you can just reduce your intake. Everyone would benefit from a few simple steps that reduce the time acid is in contact with teeth.[10]

1. Try not to consume highly acidic foods or beverages before bed.
2. Avoid sipping, swishing, or holding acidic beverages in your mouth. Use a straw to reduce acid exposure.
3. Choose juices that are fortified with calcium, which cuts down on the acid content. Finish meals with dairy products, which counteract acid.
4. If you're prone to acid reflux or gastroesophageal reflux disease (GERD), avoid reflux-causing foods and beverages such as wine, citrus fruits and their juices, vinegar, fatty or fried foods, tomatoes, peppermint, coffee, black tea, carbonated drinks, and chocolate.
5. Chew sugar-free gum after meals to stimulate salivation and reduce reflux.
6. If vomiting occurs, don't brush your teeth immediately afterward. Instead, rinse with water, milk, or a solution of baking soda (1 teaspoon) and water (1 cup).
7. Be aware of acidic medications, such as cold and flu medications in liquid form.[11]

pulling has been shown to reduce the presence of *Streptococcus mutans*,[12] the main cause of tooth decay and dental plaque,[13] and many people experience a teeth-whitening effect, as well. Oil pulling is an excellent option for those who want to maintain oral health without using the harsh chemicals found in conventional mouthwash.

See also: Alzheimer's Disease (page 160), Dementia (page 226), Dry Mouth (page 252), Heart Disease (Cardiovascular Disease) (page 313), Gingivitis (page 293), Halitosis (page 307), Overweight and Obesity (page 396)

ulcers (peptic)

Peptic ulcers are painful, open lesions on the surface of your upper gastrointestinal tract, including your esophagus, stomach, or small intestine. The term *peptic ulcers* is sometimes used interchangeably with *gastric ulcers,* or simply *stomach ulcers.* Symptoms include a gnawing or burning sensation in your abdomen, especially after eating; bloating; heartburn; nausea; vomiting; and loss of appetite. In severe cases, blood may be present in the stool or vomit, pain can be extreme, and weight loss may occur. Peptic ulcers can heal and recur, resulting in pain that flares up for a few days or weeks and then subsides.

For many years, stress was thought to be the primary cause of stomach ulcers, but more recent research has revealed that a common bacteria known as *Helicobacter pylori* is responsible for approximately 60 percent of cases (and up to 90 percent of duodenal ulcers). Long-term use of NSAIDs such as ibuprofen and aspirin can cause ulcers as well, as can glucocorticoids. Stress, while it may not be the cause of peptic ulcers (the matter is still under investigation), is a complicating factor. Stress is known to increase the production of stomach acid, and *H. pylori* thrive in an acidic environment.[1]

As for healing foods for peptic ulcers, avoid caffeine, at least when ulcers are active. Caffeine can't cause peptic ulcers, but it does stimulate the production of stomach acid, which will aggra-vate existing ulcers. Avoid the overconsumption of alcohol generally. Ulcers are more common in people with cirrhosis, which is associated with heavy drinking.[2] You may want to avoid soft drinks, as well, as they increase acid production and promote gas and gastric distension.[3]

For many years, traditional medicine has used herbal and dietary remedies to heal peptic ulcers, and clinical trials have demonstrated the efficacy of various fruits, herbs, and vegetables. Some target the bacteria directly, while others have protective properties. For example, barberry is a shrub with extremely tart, acidic, edible berries. The active component of its fruit, berberine, has been shown to be effective in inhibiting the growth of *H. pylori.* With its antioxidant activity, barberry fruit has shown a protective effect against small intestinal injury.[4] Grape skins and grape seeds have likewise shown anti–*H. pylori* effects. Grape seed extract shows higher gastroprotective and antioxidant properties than vitamins C and E, and the seed showed wound-healing properties. Resveratrol, a polyphenolic compound in red grapes, suppresses *H. pylori* and, at low doses, demonstrates ulcer-healing activity.[5] Probiotics of the species *Lactobacillus* have shown in vitro and in vivo success against *H. pylori*. *Lactobacillus* also has anti-inflammatory properties and shows immune-stimulating activity. It can be found in many probiotic yogurts and also in kimchi, sauerkraut, miso, and tempeh.[6] Broccoli sprouts have been shown to be effective against *H. pylori*, too. Broccoli's high content of sulforaphane is thought to have an antibiotic effect against *H. pylori,* and it's been shown to make inactive the *H. pylori*

urease (an enzyme by-product), as well.[7] Mulberry leaves have shown protective activity against peptic ulcers and *H. pylori* and are high in antioxidants.[8] Indian gooseberries, which are available online and in some Asian markets, are rich in antioxidants and have been shown to heal gastric ulcers.

If you prefer to take your remedies as beverages, two juices can be of use in healing gastric ulcers. In in vitro studies, cranberry juice has been shown to inhibit the growth of *H. pylori* and exhibit antiadhesion activity against *H. pylori.* It has also been shown to be effective in human studies, though regular consumption may be required to sustain the effect.[9] Quince juice similarly exhibited strong anti–*H. pylori* activity. Quince juice, peel, pulp, and seeds all have strong antioxidant activity, and the phenolic compounds from its fruit show gastroprotective properties.[10] An extract made from the peel of

healthy insight

Smoking increases your chances of developing ulcers and slows their healing. Smoking increases the production of pepsin, a protein-metabolizing enzyme that can harm your stomach lining. It also decreases bloodflow to your stomach lining, reduces protective mucus secretion, and decreases the production of acid-neutralizing sodium bicarbonate.[11]

pomegranates exhibits anti–*H. pylori* activity and decreases gastric acidity. The tannins from the fruit have been shown to prevent gastric ulcer, increase nitric oxide level, stimulate the secretion of adherent and free mucus, and exhibit antioxidant activity in gastric mucosa.[12]

While apple peels are effective at combating *H. pylori*,[13] apples in general have strong antioxidant capabilities and have been shown to reduce gastric endothelial cell injury. Other foods, such as pumpkin, have shown protective activity against ulcers by increasing mucosal thickness and by increasing alkaline phosphate enzymes in stomach tissue. Pumpkin seeds protected against ulcers by reducing gastric secretions and the acidity of gastric juices.[14] Though studies have only been conducted on animal models and in vitro, arugula is such a healthy food that we're including it in this list. Arugula, also known as rocket, has been shown to reduce gastric acid secretion and acidity and to help prevent ulcer formation as well as treat existing ulcers.[15] Curcumin, the active ingredient in turmeric, has been shown to reduce peptic ulcers and aid in their healing.[16] Perhaps counterintuitively, capsaicin, the compound that lends spiciness to chile peppers, cayenne peppers, and other hot peppers, is a healing food for peptic ulcers. Capsaicin does not stimulate but rather inhibits acid secretion, and it stimulates alkali, mucus secretions, and gastric mucosal bloodflow, which help in preventing and healing ulcers.[17] Capsaicin, by altering the acid balance in your stomach, creates an inhospitable environment for *H. pylori.* Be careful with this one, though: Peppers and spicy foods create irritation in the gastric mucosa in some people.[18]

vaginitis

Though sometimes used interchangeably (and erroneously) with the term *vaginal infection*, vaginitis is a general term that refers to any inflammation of the mucous membranes lining the vagina. Symptoms include abnormal vaginal discharge, a burning sensation, redness, inflammation, discomfort during urination, and itching. A foul odor can occur, especially in the case of infection. Any change in the natural vaginal flora can cause vaginitis, and these changes can be brought on by sexual intercourse; hormonal fluctuations (such as declining estrogen in aging women, which is the cause of atrophic vaginitis, a condition in which the vaginal walls thin and shrink); douching; or the use of antibiotics, spermicides, or any product containing potential irritants, such as perfumes, scented lotions, scented tampons, vaginal contraceptives, or even fabric softeners and detergents. Infection is also a primary cause of vaginitis. Vaginitis symptoms can be exacerbated by wearing tight clothing, which, especially if it's made of synthetic fibers, doesn't "breathe."

Cases of vaginitis, especially if accompanied by an abnormal discharge and/or a foul odor, should be evaluated by your doctor to determine the cause of the inflammation. Treatment depends on the causative agent and could include over-the-counter antifungal medications, oral or topical antifungals, oral or topical antibiotics, or estrogen creams. A sitz bath (soaking only the buttocks and hips in warm water) or oatmeal bath (a soothing bath prepared with colloidal oatmeal and warm water) can help relieve symptoms.

There is some evidence that probiotics can help treat bacterial vaginosis, a form of vaginitis, and prevent its recurrence. The normal vaginal microbiota is dominated by lactobacilli, especially *Lactobacillus crispatus, Lactobacillus jensenii, Lactobacillus iners*, and *Lactobacillus gasseri*, which together defend against pathogens. Compared with normal women, women with bacterial vaginosis more commonly have certain types of vaginal microbiotas, including *Gardnerella vaginalis, Mycoplasma hominis, Prevotella, Streptococcus, Mobiluncus*, and *Bacteroides* species in higher numbers, while lactobacilli are found less frequently and in lower numbers. Evidence suggests that the absence of lactobacilli is associated with the development of bacterial vaginosis—and that probiotics can restore vaginal flora and prevent relapses of bacterial vaginosis. *Lactobacillus rhamnosus, L. acidophilus,* and *L. delbrueckii* have all shown efficacy in protecting against microbial infection. Probiotics for vaginitis can be taken orally through supplements or in probiotic-rich foods such as yogurt, kefir, sauerkraut, kimchi, miso soup, sour pickles, kombucha tea, and some soft cheeses. Additionally, plain yogurt with live cultures may be administered vaginally for relief.[1]

To help prevent infection of any type, eat a diet that's high in antioxidants—any fresh, brightly colored fruit or vegetable will provide antioxidants. Just a few examples include berries, tomatoes, red grapes, red cabbage, kale, spinach, arugula, onions, apples, broccoli, soybeans, apricots, beets, cantaloupe, carrots, mangoes, oranges, winter squash, yellow and orange peppers, tea, dark chocolate, red wine, and papayas. Pineapple will provide extra inflammation relief due to its bromelain content,[2] as will turmeric, due to its main compound curcumin, a powerful anti-inflammatory that can inhibit the activity of enzymes responsible for inflammation and pain[3] in much the same way that nonsteroidal anti-inflammatory drugs (NSAIDs) do. Ginger also acts against inflammation in a manner similar to NSAIDs, and it modulates biochemical pathways that are activated in chronic inflammation.[4] Garlic has antibacterial, antiviral, and antifungal properties, and the allicin in garlic reduces inflammation.[5] To keep your immune system strong, keep up with the antioxidants, and increase your zinc intake. Zinc plays a key role in immune function by helping to produce antibodies and ensure proper lymphocyte functioning.[6] To boost your zinc intake, eat oysters, shellfish, crab, shrimp, lima beans, pinto beans, miso, green beans, pumpkin, or sunflower seeds.

See also: Fungal Infections, General (Yeast Infections, Candidiasis) (page 281)

varicose veins

Varicose veins are unsightly, bulging veins that have become enlarged due to a weakening of the vessel wall. Varicose veins are usually harmless, but they can cause discomfort or aching pain, itching, leg cramps, swelling, and a feeling of heaviness in your legs. They almost always occur in the legs and the feet, and they're quite common, affecting up to 60 percent of people. Women are more susceptible to varicose veins than men, as are people who sit or stand for prolonged periods of time and those who don't get enough exercise. Pregnancy and being overweight also increase your chances of developing varicose veins because of the excess pressure these conditions put on your legs and circulatory system. Other factors that raise your risk of varicose veins are smoking or repeated heavy lifting that puts undue strain on your legs.

To prevent varicose veins, maintain a healthy BMI (body mass index) and exercise. Avoid prolonged sitting, and don't cross your legs while seated. Wear clothing that doesn't constrict blood-flow, especially in your waist, groin, or legs. Some practitioners also warn against wearing high heels.[1] Elevating your legs while seated also helps.

As for dietary interventions, eating a high-fiber, low-salt diet can help prevent varicose veins. Cruciferous vegetables such as kale, spinach, lettuces, arugula, and chard are great sources of fiber, as are whole grains such as oatmeal, buckwheat, barley, bulgur, quinoa; whole grain breads and cereals; beans; flaxseeds; and chia seeds. Fruits, especially prunes, apricots, apples, raisins, blueberries, strawberries, dates, apples, pears, and grapes are also good sources of fiber. To reduce sodium, eliminate processed and fast foods, which are loaded with excess sodium. Read food labels and avoid high-sodium products. Even foods that claim to be healthy or all natural (such as canned soups, broths, canned vegetables, crackers, pretzels, frozen foods including veggie burgers and protein patties, premade sauces, breads and other baked goods, and fortified cereals) can contain high amounts of sodium. One of the most surprising sources of sodium is cottage cheese. One cup of 1% cottage cheese contains an eye-popping 918 milligrams of sodium. If you do use canned vegetables and beans, rinse them before cooking with or eating them; you can drain away as much as 35 percent of the sodium. You can also try cutting added salt in half and swapping in black pepper, herbs, or spices.

There are a few specific healing foods that can play a part in preventing varicose veins. *Centella asiatica*, also known as Indian pennywort or gotu kola, has been shown to strengthen connective tissue of the vascular wall and improve venous insufficiency.[2] There is some evidence that the anthocyanins found in berries have antiangiogenic properties that could discourage the unwanted growth of blood vessels that can lead to varicose veins. Based upon in vitro tests of berry extracts—including wild blueberry, bilberry, cranberry, elderberry, raspberry, and strawberry—there is some evidence that the anthocyanins in berries have antiangiogenic properties that

could discourage the unwanted growth of blood vessels that can lead to varicose veins.[3] The flavonoid rutin, found in abundance in buckwheat and also in apples, amaranth leaves, asparagus, elderflower tea, figs, and rooibos tea, is associated with improving vascular function and swelling in the legs.[4] Studies have shown that pycnogenol, a natural plant extract from French maritime pine bark, improves the appearance, discomfort, and swelling of pregnancy-related varicose veins and spider veins.[5] Pycnogenol has also been shown to improve vascular tone and elasticity[6] and is used in the treatment of chronic venous insufficiency and other vascular disorders such as deep vein thrombosis, postthrombotic syndrome, long-haul air-travel-related leg edema, venous ulcers, and acute hemorrhoids.[7]

See also: Hemorrhoids (page 325), High Blood Pressure (Hypertension) (page 327)

vertigo

Vertigo, or dizziness, is related to but different from lightheadedness. With the latter, you feel like you're going to faint or pass out, and in most cases lightheadedness improves or goes away once you lie down. Vertigo brings the sensation of spinning, whirling, tilting, or other forms of movement that throw off your balance, and it can cause nausea and vomiting. It can be a very distressing condition even if it lasts for only a short time, as it brings a serious risk of falling and makes normal activities such as walking, reading, or driving impossible.

Vertigo has many possible causes, including hypoglycemia (though this is more often associated with lightheadedness), metabolic disorders, hypertension, anxiety or panic attacks, dehydration, head injury, migraine headaches, motion sickness, excessive consumption of alcohol, Ménière's disease, multiple sclerosis, and injury to or disorders of the inner ear, where your seat of balance is located. Less commonly, vertigo can be the result of a brain tumor or a growth of any type behind your eardrum. If vertigo begins suddenly, it could be a sign of a stroke or transient ischemic attack, and you should seek immediate medical attention.

Healing foods recommendations for vertigo depend entirely on the underlying cause of the condition, so refer to the entries on individual conditions that may be causing the condition (see "See also" on the next page). Generally speaking, however, make sure you're staying properly hydrated—8 to 10 glasses of water a day is optimal, but herbal teas and (occasionally) fruit juice are fine for hydration, as well. Eating at regular intervals will preclude hypoglycemia and any concomitant dizziness; high-protein foods that keep blood glucose stable help, too. Avoid eating foods that are high in sugar, as they will cause spikes in blood glucose followed by dips that can trigger dizziness. If you suffer from migraines, know your food triggers and avoid them. Common dietary migraine triggers include MSG (monosodium glutamate), sulfites (found in beer, wine, and processed foods, including meats, fish, fruits, and vegetables preserved with sulfites), caffeine, chocolate, aged cheeses, fermented foods, potato chips, nuts, and tomato products. Diets that are high in sodium are thought to change the delicate composition of inner ear fluid,[1] so reducing sodium intake could prevent some cases of vertigo.

A study of benign paroxysmal positional vertigo (BPPV), a disorder of the inner ear and the most common cause of vertigo in adults, found a significant relationship between BPPV, excessive carbohydrate intake, and insufficient fiber intake. Researchers noted that their results correlate with dyslipidemia (high "bad" cholesterol) and hypertriglyceridemia (elevated triglycerides) status, underscoring the need to reduce your intake of fats and carbohydrates and increase fiber intake to stabilize triglycerides and thus minimize harmful effects on your inner ear.[2] Foods that are high in fiber include fruits (blueberries, dates, prunes, apricots, raisins, apples, pears, and grapes); dark, leafy greens (kale, spinach, arugula, Brussels sprouts, and broccoli); legumes (lentils, beans, and split peas); and whole grains (oatmeal, barley, bulgur, quinoa, and whole grain breads and cereals).

Lastly, as there is also a known association between stress and vertigo,[3] taking measures to reduce stress may help prevent vertigo or lessen the severity of symptoms.

See also: Anxiety (page 165), Diabetes (page 238), Earache (page 257), Headaches/Migraines (page 309), High Blood Pressure (Hypertension) (page 327), Lightheadedness (page 368), Motion Sickness (page 386), Stress (page 419), Stroke (page 423)

warts (common)

Warts are small, rough skin growths caused by the human papillomavirus (HPV). Warts usually disappear without treatment but they can take many months to go away, and recurrence is common. Warts can appear anywhere on your body, but they most often appear on fingers or hands. This type of wart is relatively harmless but quite contagious, and many people have them removed because they're unsightly. Other types include plantar warts, which appear on the soles of the feet; flat warts, which are pinhead-size warts that usually occur in children and adolescents; and genital warts, a highly contagious sexually transmitted disease that causes warts on the genitals, anus, and cervix. Genital warts should be monitored by a health-care professional. The HPV vaccine Gardasil protects against two types of HPV that cause genital warts.

For natural, food-based ways to treat common warts, try applying garlic or garlic extract directly to the wart. In a study of 50 patients with recurrent common warts, topical garlic extract resulted in a complete resolution in 96 percent of patients, and the warts did not recur.[1] Another study of garlic extract found the same results. Garlic is thought to be effective because of its natural antiviral properties.[2] If you'd rather not use garlic extract, you can simply apply a bit of olive oil or tea tree oil directly to the wart and then tape a slice of fresh garlic in place. This method should be used nightly for up to 3 weeks; the wart will blacken as it begins to die.[3] There is also some evidence that banana peels can be used to treat warts, though this method may be particularly effective for plantar warts.[4] The easiest way to use the banana peel treatment is to cut a small piece of banana peel and tape it in place overnight, repeating until the wart disappears.

Zinc has also been shown to be effective at curing warts. Oral zinc or topical, in the form of zinc oxide or zinc sulfate, has been shown to clear warts completely.[5] Zinc also has an immune-boosting effect, which can help fight off HPV as well as other viruses. To boost your zinc intake, eat oysters, beef, wheat germ, fortified cereals, pumpkin seeds, or sesame seeds.

Finally, to continue boosting your immune system, eat a high level of antioxidants. Dark, leafy greens, such as arugula, broccoli, chicory, collard greens, kale, lettuces, mustard greens, spinach, and watercress, and brightly colored fruits and vegetables, such as apricots, beets, berries, cantaloupe, carrots, mangoes, oranges, tomatoes, winter squash, and yellow and orange peppers, are excellent sources of immune-supporting vitamins A and C. There is also evidence that tea's polyphenolic compounds can protect against many health conditions and infections, including genital warts.[6]

wounds

In its broadest sense, a wound is any type of damage that breaks the skin barrier; wounds may or may not damage underlying tissue. Superficial wounds can be cared for at home, but more serious wounds require medical attention.

Initial wound care involves cleaning and disinfecting the wound and controlling bleeding. Call your doctor if a minor wound shows signs of infection, such as thick pus, pus with a foul odor, an increase in swelling or drainage, or fever, or if a wound just isn't healing. In addition to basic care, you can speed healing from the inside out by getting proper nutrition to support wound healing. Malnutrition slows wound healing and makes you more susceptible to infection, and malnutrition alone is a risk factor for pressure ulcer (bedsore) development.[1] As your body will begin to divert energy to grow new tissue, it's more essential than ever to eat a well-balanced diet to promote healing, support your immune system so as to ward off infection, and keep inflammation in check. Generally, eat a varied diet rich in antioxidants, which will speed healing and ward off infection; up to three servings of protein a day to help repair damaged tissue, form new connective tissue, and build collagen;

fats and fatty acids for cell membrane support; and complex carbohydrates to support your body's greater energy demands. Beyond these general guidelines, a few nutrients deserve a special mention.

Zinc helps your body synthesize protein, build collagen, and stop bleeding, and it plays a key role in immune function by helping to produce antibodies and ensure proper lymphocyte functioning.[2] As 20 percent of your body's zinc stores are found in your skin, people with large wounds face significant zinc loss; zinc deficiency is common in people with burn wounds and with chronic leg ulcers. Even without significant loss of zinc through your skin, your body needs higher levels of zinc in order to recover from wounds.[3] A deficiency in zinc is known to prolong wound healing.[4] To boost your zinc intake, eat oysters, beef, wheat germ, fortified cereals, pumpkin seeds, or sesame seeds.

To reduce inflammation—both at the wound site and throughout your body on a cellular level as your body responds to the stress of being wounded—increase your intake of omega-3 fatty acids and decrease your intake of omega-6s. Omega-6s can promote inflammation, while omega-3s regulate and reduce inflammation.[5] There is also evidence that omega-3s can reduce wound infection rates and decrease the length of hospital stays. A metastudy that examined data from more than 1,500 patients found that those who received omega-3 supplementation after surgery had a significant reduction in infection, less inflammation, and reduced hospital stays, both in the intensive care unit (ICU) and overall.[6] There is evidence that arginine combined with omega-3s has an even greater effect on reducing infection, wound healing complications, and hospital stays.[7] The amino acid arginine plays a key role in collagen synthesis,[8] increases bloodflow, and stimulates the release of growth hormone and of insulin-like growth factor. Arginine is produced by your body and is found in protein, but additional arginine is recommended after suffering a wound.[9] Food sources of omega-3s include salmon, mackerel, herring, cod, halibut, sardines, anchovies, trout, walnuts, walnut oil, flaxseeds, and flaxseed oil. Healthy sources of arginine include soy protein (including tofu), crab, shrimp,

lobster, crayfish, mollusks, spinach, seaweed, orange roughy, and watercress.[10] Cut back on food sources of omega-6s while a wound is healing. Examples include corn oil, safflower oil, soybean oil, palm oil, cottonseed oil, hempseeds, and hempseed oil.

Glutamine is another amino acid that plays a key role in wound healing. Like arginine, glutamine is produced in sufficient quantities by your body, but during wound healing your body requires greater amounts. Glutamine is a precursor to glutathione, an antioxidant necessary for the stabilization of cell membranes and transporting amino acids across membranes; and it is a cofactor for enzymatic reactions, meaning it is essential to cell repair.[11] Some of the best food sources of glutamine include beef, poultry, milk, yogurt, ricotta cheese, cottage cheese, raw spinach, raw parsley, and cabbage.[12]

And speaking of yogurt, emerging evidence demonstrates the role of prebiotics and probiotics in wound healing. Their main source of efficacy lies in their ability to stimulate growth of helpful bacteria in your gut, which helps to ward off infection, alleviate inflammatory responses, and even prevent and treat chronic wounds.[13] There is also evidence that consuming probiotics after an injury can shorten the time it takes for a wound to heal.[14] If antibiotics are prescribed, which is not unusual when a wound is healing, prebiotics and probiotics protect your intestinal microbiota and support efficient wound healing.[15]

The antioxidants vitamin A and vitamin C are also important for wound healing. Like zinc, vitamin C levels decrease at the site of a wound, and extra vitamin C is required for proper healing. Vitamin C is instrumental in the formation of collagen, and its antioxidant capabilities can reduce the free radical damage caused by inflammation.[16] Low vitamin C levels are known to impair wound healing.[17] Vitamin A is crucial for the functioning of your immune system; those with a vitamin A deficiency have a much greater susceptibility to infection[18] and experience slower wound healing. Vitamin A is required for epithelial formation and cellular differentiation.[19] Vitamin A can also reverse the damaging immunosuppressive effects of corticosteroids that slow wound healing.[20] Healthy sources of vitamin A include fish and fish oils, papayas, sweet potatoes, spinach, carrots, cantaloupe, sweet peppers, mangoes, black-eyed peas, apricots, broccoli, eggs, and fortified milk and cereal. Vitamin C is found in abundance in citrus fruits, yellow bell peppers, papayas, black currants, guavas, kale, acerola cherries (West Indian cherries), chile

peppers, potatoes, and parsley. In terms of vitamin A and C content, papaya is a superfood for wound healing: One large papaya contains 148 percent of your recommended daily intake of vitamin A and 792 percent of your vitamin C!

There are also several foods that can be used topically to speed wound healing and decrease the likelihood of infection. Papaya has been used for centuries for wound healing—and now that we know about its super levels of vitamins A and C, it's clear why. In one clinical trial, 64 patients were divided into two groups, one receiving a papaya wound dressing and the other a hydrogen peroxide dressing. The time required to induce wound granulation (a phase of wound healing in which new connective tissue and vasculature grow) was 6.2 days in the peroxide group but only 2.5 days in the papaya group. Hospital duration was an average of 19.2 days for the peroxide group but just under 13 for the papaya group. What's more, only about 3 percent of the papaya group required additional wound debridement (removal of dead tissue from the site), whereas 56 percent of the peroxide group did.[21] In addition to speeding healing, papaya extract has also been shown to prevent infection.[22]

Since antiquity honey has been used to aid in wound healing, and now there is extensive scientific evidence that explains how it works. On a practical level, honey is an ideal wound dressing because it moisturizes injured tissue, fights infection, soothes inflammation, and keeps gauze from sticking to wounds. But on a cellular level, honey has been found to promote the growth of new blood vessels, connective tissue, and the epidermis, and it stimulates the production of white blood cells as well as phagocytes.[23]

Another traditional topical aid for wound healing is banana pulp and peel. Bananas contain multiple antioxidants and phenolic compounds and are rich in vitamin A. Banana pulp or banana peel applied directly to a wound has been shown to speed healing.[24]

Grape seed extract has antioxidant and anti-inflammatory properties and can speed wound healing when applied topically. It also stimulates vascular endothelial growth factor, which results in restoring oxygen supply to tissue.[25]

Turmeric applied directly to a wound can stop bleeding, accelerate wound healing, and lighten scars.[26] It also has anti-inflammatory and antimicrobial properties and plays a role in muscle regeneration after serious injury.[27]

Though human studies are limited, there is also some evidence that green tea extract applied to a wound can aid healing and prevent scarring.[28]

Finally, it is important to remain sufficiently hydrated during wound healing. Especially in the case of large wounds, fluid loss can be substantial, so drink plenty of water. Epithelial cells require moisture to migrate from the borders of a wound and close it up, and improving fluid intake has been shown to increase tissue oxygenation, which is required for wound healing.[29] Fruit juices are also recommended for the short term because of their high vitamin C content. The catechins in green tea are known to have powerful antioxidant and anti-inflammatory properties, so green tea is a good choice during wound healing, as well.

See also: Bruises (page 188), Burns (page 189)

wrinkles

Wrinkles are an inevitable consequence of normal aging—but there are lifestyle factors under our control that can delay, prevent, and possibly even reverse some wrinkling. Factors that accelerate the aging process include exposure to pollutants or environmental toxins, chronic stress, insomnia, use of tobacco products, use of illegal drugs, overconsumption of alcohol, overexposure to UV rays, and poor nutrition. Heredity also plays a part in wrinkling. Any of these factors can lead to earlier wrinkling, as well as to deeper wrinkles.

As for poor nutrition, it works both ways: Not getting enough of the nutrients your body needs to support skin health *and* consuming too many unhealthy foods and beverages can both promote wrinkling. The typical Western diet, with its emphasis on fast foods, processed foods, refined foods, sugar, and foods with artificial colors and other additives, has been shown to accelerate the aging process—both on a cellular level and on the visible epidermal layer. Sugar in particular has been shown to accelerate sagging skin and loss of elasticity, as it promotes cross-linking of collagen fibers.[1]

The basis of any nutritional anti-wrinkle regimen is all about antioxidants. Antioxidants scavenge your body of those free radicals that come from the highly inflammatory Western diet, from UV exposure, from cigarette smoke, from environmental pollutants, and even from exercise and perfectly normal metabolic processes like breathing. Basically, anything that taxes your body will produce free radicals. It's impossible to avoid free radicals entirely, and despite their current reputation, they're not inherently evil. What you want to avoid is having too many free radicals circulating about and causing oxidative stress, or put another way, you want to have a proper balance between antioxidants and free radicals. It's when free radicals get out of hand that they cause cell damage and accelerate the aging process. Any antioxidant will help inhibit the oxidative damage caused by free radicals, but with regard to aging skin, the antioxidants to focus on are vitamins, polyphenols, and flavonoids, which reduce the breakdown of collagen by removing free radicals from tissue.

454

First, let's look at the antioxidants vitamin C and vitamin E. Vitamin C, also known as ascorbic acid, benefits your skin by stabilizing collagen[2] and stimulating collagen synthesis.[3] Vitamin C is a common ingredient in many antiaging and skin-care creams because of its free-radical-scavenging ability. A study of a vitamin C moisturizing cream found that it was extremely effective at promoting collagen synthesis in a wide range of ages. The study was conducted on 60 women, ages 20 to 75, along with age-matched controls.[4] To increase your vitamin C intake, eat citrus fruits, yellow bell peppers, papayas, black currants, guavas, acerola cherries (West Indian cherries), gac fruit, kale, chile peppers, potatoes, and parsley. Vitamin E can control inflammation associated with ultraviolet (UV) exposure, inhibit the oxidative degradation of lipids (damage caused by free radicals), and improve excessive pigmentation in the skin (age spots).[5] Vitamin C and vitamin E work synergistically, so try to eat foods that contain both at the same time. Food sources of vitamin E include almonds, hazelnuts, peanuts, sunflower seeds, spinach, and wheat germ.

In a recent antiaging study—one notable for its focus on men—subjects used a supplement consisting of marine protein, vitamin C, grape seed extract, tomato extract, and zinc for 180 days.

All subjects who completed the study experienced improvement in skin redness, hydration, radiance, and "overall appearance," which included a reduction in fine lines and increased smoothness of skin.[6] The amount of each ingredient in the supplement was modest enough. Specifically, the amounts were: marine protein (105 mg), vitamin C (27 mg), grape seed extract (13.75 mg), zinc (2 mg), and tomato extract (14.38 mg). You can easily obtain the same results through eating whole foods (see specific recommendations, below). Similarly, a recent study that followed 160 postmenopausal women for 14 weeks found that a liquid supplement containing soy isoflavones, lycopene, vitamin C, vitamin E, and omega-3 fish oil resulted in significant improvement in depth of "crow's-feet" wrinkles and increased deposits of new collagen fibers.[7] To get marine protein and omega-3s into your diet, eat wild-caught salmon, which is high in essential omega-3 fatty acids. Omega-3s have been shown to play a direct role in protecting your skin from UV rays that can accelerate the aging of skin, and linoleic acid, an omega-6, is associated with a lower incidence of dry and thinning skin.[9] Instead of grape seed extract, you can eat whole grapes with their seeds. Grape seeds, though bitter, are entirely edible, and the sweetness of the grape flesh will help this medicine go down. If you absolutely can't stand the seeds, grape flesh does contain some vitamin C and other powerful antioxidants, or have a glass of red wine to get the benefits of the antioxidant resveratrol. Zinc, which plays a role in reducing oxidative stress, has been shown to fight wrinkles and hyperpigmentation (age spots).[9] Add zinc to your diet—and get that marine protein simultaneously—by eating oysters. For vegetarian sources of zinc, eat wheat germ, fortified cereals, pumpkin seeds, or sesame seeds. To get lycopene, eat tomatoes. Tomatoes are chock-full of lycopene, which helps protect your skin against sun damage and prevents the breakdown of collagen. Lycopene is also present in tomato products, such as

sauces and salsa, and in watermelon and grapefruit. The soy isoflavone glycitein has been shown to promote collagen production, prevent the breakdown of elastin, and decrease β-galactosidase, which is associated with aging skin cells.[11] The best sources of soy isoflavones are organic, non-GMO (genetically modified organism) soybeans and soy products. Boiled soybeans have 47 milligrams (mg) of isoflavones per $\frac{1}{2}$ cup, and miso has 59 mg per $\frac{1}{2}$ cup. Other sources of isoflavones are tofu and tempeh.[12]

Avocados may prevent wrinkles by lending UV protection to your skin, and they are a good source of both vitamin C and vitamin E. They're also an excellent source of monounsaturated fats, and a study of more than 700 women found that total dietary fat was associated with more skin elasticity and that a higher intake of green and yellow vegetables was associated with fewer wrinkles.[13]

You may associate argan oil with hair-care products, but it's used in many skin-care products, as well—and it's also edible. In a study of 60 postmenopausal women, the consumption of 25 milliliters a day of argan oil led to improved skin elasticity. Don't feel like eating your argan oil? Not to worry: The topical application of argan oil worked just as well.[14]

> BONUS TIP: An extract of gac fruit has been shown to be an effective antiwrinkle ingredient. Gac extract has higher antioxidant activity than vitamins C and E, and a clinical trial of gac extract cream showed increased skin hydration, increased smoothness, and decreased roughness.[10] Gac fruit has 70 times the lycopene found in tomatoes. Gac fruit is still hard to find in the United States; you're more likely to see it as an ingredient in a supplement than in its whole form at your local health food store. Gac oil supplements are also available, as is gac fruit juice. It can be ordered in whole or dried form online, and some enterprising health enthusiasts are growing it.

One clinical trial examined the effect of *Lactobacillus plantarum* on women ages 41 to 59 with dry skin and wrinkles. Sixty-one volunteers received a daily probiotic for 12 weeks, and 49 served as controls. At week 12, there was a significant increase in skin water content in the faces and hands of the probiotic group, as well as less trans-epidermal water loss. What's more, the probiotic group experienced a significant reduction in wrinkle depth, better skin gloss, and a 21.7 percent improvement in skin elasticity by week 12.[15] *L. plantarum* has also been shown to have antiaging effects on skin damaged by sun exposure.[16]

Women who consumed a green tea beverage totaling 1,402 total catechins daily for 12 weeks experienced increased skin elasticity, density, and hydration and less roughness and scaly skin.[17] Green tea is an abundant source of polyphenols, which protect against UV-accelerated skin aging and confer antiwrinkle, anti-inflammation, and antioxidant effects.[18]

Red ginseng may be effective in fighting wrinkles. In a study of 82 women, an intervention group took 3 grams a day of red ginseng extract for 24 weeks. Compared to controls, who took a placebo, the intervention group had decreased facial wrinkles, increased type I procollagen synthesis (related to skin rejuvenation), and an increase in fibrillin-1 fiber length (related to skin elasticity).[19]

See also: Dry Skin (page 254), Insomnia (page 357), Stress (page 419), Sunburn (page 427)

Extraordinary People, Extraordinary Healing

Lia Huber, 45

Even with a busy life as a mom, an entrepreneur, a small business owner, a writer, and a professional recipe developer, Lia Huber makes time for preparing and eating fresh, locally grown whole foods and sustainably sourced proteins. Her conversion from processed foods to fresh, whole foods brought her joy and a brand new career path—and it also saved her life.

A self-proclaimed "fat phobic" in her twenties, Lia did what a lot of us did in the days of the low-fat diet craze: She ate very little fat, but she included low-nutrient foods such as pretzels or processed desserts like SnackWell's cookies in her diet. She also hated vegetables, avoiding them entirely except for potatoes, cucumbers, and raw carrots. "I had no concept of what eating well meant," she said. "I was just doing the low-fat hack." And despite her efforts, she was still 20 pounds overweight and had very little energy. "I was always on a diet and always failing," she said. "I was never comfortable in my body."

It was only so long before her body began to complain. Besides the extra weight, Lia began to experience deep body aches and joint pain, as well as weakness so severe that at times she couldn't unscrew the cap on a tube of toothpaste. A rash appeared on her face and she was constantly exhausted. "I started to panic," she said. "I worried that if I felt this bad in my twenties, I wouldn't be able to get out of bed by the time I was 60."

For years she went from specialist to specialist seeking answers, but no one could come up with a diagnosis. "They'd shoot me up with injections, give me pills, or think I was making it up," Lia said. "There was such shame that I just tried to grin and bear it, yet I was miserable and scared." She also still felt awful. Eventually, a rheumatologist diagnosed her with lupus. A year later, Lia was diagnosed with a rare and deadly type of precancer, and she had a hysterectomy at the age of 27. She remembers thinking, "No way. I'm not even 30—something is really wrong here."

Serendipitously, Lia was just getting into food and travel writing, and to try and understand what was happening and how she could feel better, she asked for assignments that were focused on nutrition. "I wanted to talk to the experts," she said. "I wanted to know what I should be eating and why my diet wasn't working and why I felt like I was dying."

What she heard over and over from nutrition experts was to eat lots of fresh vegetables, whole grains, and healthy fats. This last bit of advice was so counter to the way Lia had eaten for years that she knew she'd have to retrain herself entirely. She resolved to give herself a year to learn the fundamentals of healthy eating and how to make meals she loved.

By that time she was living in California, which offered an abundance of farmers' markets. "Freshly grown vegetables made all the difference in the world," she said. "Lettuces from the famers' market or grown in my backyard were nothing like the iceberg lettuce from a salad bar. Tomatoes right off the vine literally brought tears to my eyes. Learning about seasonable vegetables was a huge shift for me. I started to love healthy foods." Shortly thereafter she went to a new doctor, who diagnosed her with fibromyalgia instead of lupus, and she went off her lupus medications.

And then, "without even trying or paying attention," Lia lost the weight she'd struggled years to lose. Within 6 months, the 20 pounds were gone. The rash on her face cleared up, her aches and pains disappeared, and her energy returned. "I was like a new person," she said. "I finally felt amazing in my body." Her experience with healing foods led Lia to her life's work. "The Nourish Evolution program gives people a framework for seeing where they are on the journey and what they need to do to make the lasting shift to whole foods," she said. "It gives them meal planning ideas and recipes they can use in their own kitchens."

These days, Lia's fibromyalgia is "almost nonexistent." She experiences a flare-up once a year or less, and her energy level is high. Those 20 pounds never returned. "What I cultivated over the course of that year of learning was a lifelong eating practice," she said. "I found a way to eat that I loved, that healed my body, and that brought joy back to my life."

Lisa Rae Rosenberg

At first, Lisa Rae Rosenberg was skeptical of the extremes of a raw vegan diet—no cooked food, no dairy, no meat—and not so thrilled by the prospect of giving up glazed doughnuts and chicken-fried steak. But in a last-ditch attempt to curb her rising cholesterol, she stifled her doubts and resolved to try it for 7 days. "After that week, I felt so much better that I decided to add another week, and after about a month, I felt like I had superpowers," she says. She dropped 20 pounds, and her total cholesterol plunged 60 points in 8 months. "People started telling me I looked radiant instead of telling me how tired I looked," she says. "My skin is clearer and my eyes are brighter." The changes—and all of the questions from friends—inspired Lisa to start MyRawBlog.com, a chronicle of recipes and tips illustrating how anyone can adopt the diet. "I wanted to show people it's not hard, and you can do this," she says. "You can feel better."

Maria Gordon

Maria Gordon was 23 when she was diagnosed with type 2 diabetes and told she needed daily medication. In 2013, after 3 years of dependence on the drugs, she started to feel trapped. "I talked to my doctor about maybe getting off them, and he told me he wasn't sure I could completely," she says. Maria took this sobering news as a message that she had to do something—fast. She started by nixing her go-to vices, like frozen TV dinners, chips, and cookies, in exchange for whole wheat bread, tofu, and almond milk. She slowly increased her intake of fruits and vegetables until they made up about 80 percent of her diet. At the same time, she scaled back her meat consumption and started cooking her own meals, taking walks, and drinking more water. Each change was small, but the combined effects—and Maria's dogged dedication—paid off in a jaw-dropping way: In just over a year, she lost more than 100 pounds and reversed her diabetes so effectively that she now needs no drugs at all. But those two massive changes weren't even the most gratifying part: the rebirth of her self-confidence. "I was in the background for most of my life, being overweight and then being sick," she says. "But I'm not afraid anymore to get out there and be noticed."

Samantha Yeager

Samantha Yaeger didn't think much about the rash that first showed up on her stomach 2 years ago. She assumed it was just irritation, a pesky memento of a recent tropical vacation. But when it started to spread and then covered her body from chest to ankles, she needed a diagnosis. Five months later, she got it: lichen planus, an autoimmune condition that has no cure but would likely clear up on its own in, oh, a couple of years. "I just couldn't accept that—I had to look for my own solution," she says. She found one randomly, on a trip to Costco: the book *Clean Gut*, by Alejandro Junger, MD. He promises big improvements for irritated skin if readers take on a monthlong cleanse that eliminates dairy, gluten, added sugars, soy, coffee, or certain other food groups. It was extreme—but then again, so was the maddening itch. A few days into the cleanse, changes started. "The itching was subsiding, the bumps were less inflamed, and I became less irritable," she says. Samantha continued to avoid gluten, dairy, and added sugars after that month was behind her, and the symptoms stayed away. A year after the itching ended, she has lost 55 pounds and shaved 10 points from her body mass index (BMI). Emboldened by her transformation, she has decided to study to become a registered holistic nutritionist. "I have a new passion for healing that food awakened in me," she says. "I've gone from stumbling through life to being excited by it."

Aaron and Jen

Before he had even turned 40, Aaron was 40 pounds overweight with a kid, a busy career, and little motivation to eat well or exercise. That all changed when his wife, Jen, was diagnosed with a chronic condition that caused doctors to prescribe her everything from anxiety drugs to steroid injections. Frustrated, Jen saw a naturopath, who told her to stop eating packaged foods, dairy, gluten, soy, and refined sugar. Within 3 months, Jen's daily migraines became monthly and her list of medications dropped from 10 to zero. Aaron was so stunned that he began, slowly, to eat more whole foods, too. "I lost 50 pounds, my acne cleared up, and my depression symptoms improved," he says.

Today, eating clean is a family affair. Case in point: Their fast-food-loving son was recently spotted making a spinach salad, unprompted.

Andrea Boje

Andrea Boje had her doctors stumped. For years she had battled headaches, achy joints, and severe seasonal allergies, only to be told to "eat better" and exercise. Then, in 2004, she saw a nutritionist who told her she was allergic to gluten and dairy. "It was dramatic how much my body responded to not eating them," she says. "The headaches went away, the joint pain went away, the allergies went away." Eight months later, without exercising or even consciously trying, Andrea had lost 50 pounds. She began to teach herself how to cook without gluten and dairy, and before long she had decided to leave her job in publishing to pursue one as a chef, studying at the Natural Gourmet Institute, where she honed traditional French techniques along with modern nutritional know-how. After graduation, Andrea launched her private chef service, Holistic Chef (theholisticchef.com), for others with food allergies and sensitivities. Today she has a thriving business and a new perspective on life without gluten and dairy. "Being healthy is about eating as many unprocessed foods as possible. Eating real food—things you make at home and from scratch," she says.

Endnotes

PART 1: FOODS

BEANS AND LEGUMES

1   http://www.sciencedirect.com/science
    /article/pii/S0308814613004561.
2   http://www.ncbi.nlm.nih.gov/pmc/articles
    /PMC4555112/.
3   http://www.ncbi.nlm.nih.gov
    /pubmed/23046862/.
4   http://www.cmaj.ca/content
    /early/2014/04/07/cmaj.131727.
5   http://www.ncbi.nlm.nih.gov
    /pubmed/25442631.
6   http://journals.cambridge.org/action
    /displayAbstract?fromPage=online
    &aid=9887385&fileId=S0007114515001725.
7   K. Beck et al., "Gold Kiwifruit Consumed with
    an Iron-Fortified Breakfast Cereal Meal
    Improves Iron Status in Women with Low
    Iron Stores: A 16-Week Randomized
    Controlled Trial," *British Journal of
    Nutrition*, 5, no. 1 (2011): 101–9, http://
    www.ncbi.nlm.nih.gov/pubmed/20727238.
8   http://www.nature.com/ejcn/journal/v69/n5
    /full/ejcn2014228a.html.
9   http://nutritiondata.self.com/facts
    /vegetables-and-vegetable-products
    /2333/2.
10 http://nutritiondata.self.com/facts
    /legumes-and-legume-products/4349/2.
11 http://www.ncbi.nlm.nih.gov/pmc/articles
    /PMC4461985/.
12 http://www.ncbi.nlm.nih.gov
    /pubmed/25423740.
13 http://www.ncbi.nlm.nih.gov/pmc/articles
    /PMC3522559/.
14 http://www.ncbi.nlm.nih.gov
    /pubmed/26572874.
15 http://www.ncbi.nlm.nih.gov
    /pubmed/25871313.
16 http://www.ncbi.nlm.nih.gov
    /pubmed/23514011.
17 http://www.ncbi.nlm.nih.gov
    /pubmed/22916816.
18 http://nutritiondata.self.com/facts
    /legumes-and-legume-products/4354/2.
19 http://www.ncbi.nlm.nih.gov
    /pubmed/22916818.
20 http://www.ncbi.nlm.nih.gov
    /pubmed/20807459.
21 http://www.ncbi.nlm.nih.gov
    /pubmed/22916813.
22 Ibid.
23 http://www.ncbi.nlm.nih.gov
    /pubmed/21792822.
24 http://journals.plos.org/plosone
    /article?id=10.1371/journal.pone.0099325.
25 http://www.ncbi.nlm.nih.gov/pmc
    /articles/PMC3071778/.
26 http://www.ncbi.nlm.nih.gov
    /pubmed/22916816.

BEVERAGES

1   http://circ.ahajournals.org/content
    /early/2015/11/10/CIRCULATION
    AHA.115.017341.abstract.
2   http://onlinelibrary.wiley.com/doi/10.1002
    /scin.2015.188007017/abstract.
3   http://care.diabetesjournals.org
    /content/37/2/569.full.
4   http://www.tandfonline.com/doi
    /full/10.3109/15622975.2013.795243.
5   http://onlinelibrary.wiley.com/doi/10.1002
    /scin.2015.188007017/abstract.
6   http://jnci.oxfordjournals.org/content/107/2
    /dju421.long; http://onlinelibrary.wiley.com
    /doi/10.1002/scin.2015.188007017/abstract.
7   http://jnci.oxfordjournals.org/content
    /early/2011/05/17/jnci.djr151.abstract.
8   http://circ.ahajournals.org
    /content/129/6/643.long.

9   http://www.ncbi.nlm.nih.gov
    /pubmed/25041334.

10 http://www.ncbi.nlm.nih.gov
    /pubmed/25062326.

11 http://russiapedia.rt.com/of-russian
    -origin/kefir/.

12 http://www.ncbi.nlm.nih.gov/pmc/articles
    /PMC3833126/.

13 http://www.ncbi.nlm.nih.gov
    /pubmed/26298752.

14 http://www.ncbi.nlm.nih.gov
    /pubmed/26655888.

15 http://www.ams.ac.ir/AIM
    /NEWPUB/15/18/12/0011.pdf.

16 http://www.ncbi.nlm.nih.gov
    /pubmed/23498346.

17 http://www.ncbi.nlm.nih.gov
    /pubmed/24774066.

18 http://www.ncbi.nlm.nih.gov
    /pubmed/24898224.

19 http://www.ncbi.nlm.nih.gov
    /pubmed/22648714.

20 http://www.ncbi.nlm.nih.gov
    /pubmed/24915350; http://www.ncbi.nlm
    .nih.gov/pubmed/23448443; http://
    www.ncbi.nlm.nih.gov/pmc/articles
    /PMC2855614/.

21 http://www.ncbi.nlm.nih.gov
    /pubmed/26024546.

22 http://anp.sagepub.com/content/49/4/334
    .long#T2.

23 http://www.ncbi.nlm.nih.gov
    /pubmed/24331002.

24 http://www.ncbi.nlm.nih.gov
    /pubmed/24522468.

25 http://stroke.ahajournals.org
    /content/40/5/1786.long.

26 http://journals.plos.org/plosone
    /article?id=10.1371/journal.pone.0096013;
    http://www.cpmedical.net/newsletter
    /green-tea-reduces-risk-of-dementia.

27 http://www.ncbi.nlm.nih.gov
    /pubmed/22202078.

28 http://www.ncbi.nlm.nih.gov
    /pubmed/26092629.

29 http://www.ncbi.nlm.nih.gov/pubmed/?term
    =brain+food+for+alzheimer-free+aging+focus.

30 http://www.ctcpjournal.com/article/S1744
    -3881(13)00091-1/fulltext.

31 R. J. Green et al., "Common Tea Formulations
    Modulate in Vitro Digestive Recovery of
    Green Tea Catechins," *Molecular Nutrition &
    Food Research* 51, no. 9 (2007): 1152–62,
    http://www.ncbi.nlm.nih.gov/
    pubmed/17688297.

32 http://www.ncbi.nlm.nih.gov/pmc
    /articles/PMC3942920/; http://www.ncbi
    .nlm.nih.gov/pubmed/24172305; http://
    www.ncbi.nlm.nih.gov/pmc/articles
    /PMC4322420/.

33 http://www.ncbi.nlm.nih.gov/pmc/articles
    /PMC3459493/.

34 http://www.ncbi.nlm.nih.gov/pmc
    /articles/PMC4207053/.

35 http://www.ncbi.nlm.nih.gov
    /pubmed/21736786/.

36 http://www.ncbi.nlm.nih.gov/pmc/articles
    /PMC3553795/.

37 http://www.sciencedirect.com/science
    /article/pii/S0195666315002287.

38 http://www.ncbi.nlm.nih.gov
    /pubmed/21084879.

39 http://www.ncbi.nlm.nih.gov/pmc/articles
    /PMC4504608/.

40 http://www.who.int/features/qa/66/en/.

41 http://www.cdc.gov/alcohol/faqs.htm.

42 http://www.biomedcentral.com/1741
    -7015/11/192.

43 http://www.ncbi.nlm.nih.gov/pmc
    /articles/PMC3347010/.

44 http://www.ncbi.nlm.nih.gov
    /pubmed/21614415/.

45 http://www.ncbi.nlm.nih.gov/pmc
    /articles/PMC3407993/.

46 http://www.ncbi.nlm.nih.gov/pmc
    /articles/PMC4334149/.

47 http://www.hindawi.com/journals
    /omcl/2014/681318/.

48 http://www.ncbi.nlm.nih.gov
    /pubmed/25617534.

DAIRY PRODUCTS

1   http://health.gov/dietaryguidelines
    /2015-BINDER/meeting7/docs/DGAC
    -Meeting-7-SC-1.pdf.

2   http://ajcn.nutrition.org/content
    /early/2015/05/27/ajcn.115.111062.abstract.

3   J. E. Kim et al., "Effects of Egg Consumption
    on Carotenoid Absorption from
    Co-consumed, Raw Vegetables," *American
    Journal of Clinical Nutrition* 102, no. 1
    (2015): 75–83, http://ajcn.nutrition.org
    /content/early/2015/05/27/ajcn.115
    .111062.abstract.

4   http://ajcn.nutrition.org/content/101/5
    /1088.abstract.

5   http://www.ncbi.nlm.nih.gov
    /pubmed/23880191.

6   http://www.ncbi.nlm.nih.gov
    /pubmed/24079288/.

7   http://www.ncbi.nlm.nih.gov
    /pubmed/26258087.

8   http://www.hsph.harvard.edu
    /nutritionsource/healthy-eating-plate
    -vs-usda-myplate/.

9   J. L. Rosenblum et al., "Calcium and Vitamin D
    Supplementation Is Associated with Decreased
    Abdominal Visceral Adipose Tissue in
    Overweight and Obese Adults," *The
    American Journal of Clinical Nutrition* 95,

no. 1 (2012): 101–8, http://www
.ncbi.nlm.nih.gov/pubmed/?term
=Calcium+and+vitamin+D+supplementation
+is+associated+with+decreased
+abdominal+visceral+adipose+tissue+in
+overweight+and+obese+adults.

10 http://www.ers.usda.gov/data-products
/dairy-data.aspx.

11 http://www.ncbi.nlm.nih.gov/pmc/articles
/PMC3759377/.

12 https://www.jstage.jst.go.jp/article/jnsv/61
/Supplement/61_S139/_pdf.

13 http://www.ncbi.nlm.nih.gov
/pubmed/25740747.

14 http://www.ncbi.nlm.nih.gov
/pubmed/26511614.

FRUITS

1 http://www.ncbi.nlm.nih.gov/pmc/articles
/PMC3183591/; http://www.ncbi.nlm.nih
.gov/pmc/articles/PMC4488768/#B6
-nutrients-07-03959.

2 http://www.ncbi.nlm.nih.gov/pmc/articles
/PMC442131/; http://www.ncbi.nlm.nih.gov
/pmc/articles/PMC3183591/.

3 http://www.ncbi.nlm.nih.gov
/pubmed/20681654/.

4 http://www.ncbi.nlm.nih.gov
/pubmed/23511050.

5 http://www.ncbi.nlm.nih.gov/pmc/articles
/PMC4258571/.

6 http://www.ncbi.nlm.nih.gov/pmc/articles
/PMC4000498/.

7 http://www.ncbi.nlm.nih.gov/pmc/articles
/PMC4541379/.

8 http://www.ncbi.nlm.nih.gov/pmc/articles
/PMC3183591/.

9 Ibid.

10 http://www.ncbi.nlm.nih.gov/pmc/articles
/PMC4579562/.

11 http://www.ncbi.nlm.nih.gov/pmc/articles
/PMC4377870/; http://www.ncbi.nlm.nih
.gov/pmc/articles/PMC3183591/.

12 C. M. Adams et al., "Identification and Small
Molecule Inhibition of an ATF4-Dependent
Pathway to Age-Related Skeletal Muscle
Weakness and Atrophy," *Journal of Biological
Chemistry* (2015): 290: 25497–511.

13 http://www.ncbi.nlm.nih.gov
/pubmed/20170359.

14 http://www.ncbi.nlm.nih.gov
/pubmed/23941506.

15 http://www.ncbi.nlm.nih.gov
/pubmed/20170359; http://www.ncbi
.nlm.nih.gov/pubmed/26561060.

16 http://www.ncbi.nlm.nih.gov/pmc/articles
/PMC4276299/.

17 http://www.ncbi.nlm.nih.gov
/pubmed/24433076.

18 http://www.ncbi.nlm.nih.gov
/pubmed/25973889.

15 http://aboutyogurt.com/index.asp
?bid=29.

16 http://www.nejm.org/doi/full/10.1056
/NEJMoa1014296.

17 http://ajcn.nutrition.org/content/99/5
/1263S.long#ref-31.

18 http://www.ncbi.nlm.nih.gov
/pubmed/26340330.

19 Ibid.

20 http://www.ncbi.nlm.nih.gov/pmc/articles
/PMC4502710/.

21 http://www.ncbi.nlm.nih.gov/pmc/articles
/PMC4662178/.

22 http://www.sciencedirect.com/science
/article/pii/S095816691400175X.

19 http://www.ncbi.nlm.nih.gov
/pubmed/21863241.

20 http://www.ncbi.nlm.nih.gov/pmc/articles
/PMC3397218/.

21 http://ndb.nal.usda.gov/ndb/foods
/show/2157?manu=&fgcd=.

22 http://www.ncbi.nlm.nih.gov/pmc/articles
/PMC4222592/.

23 http://www.ncbi.nlm.nih.gov/pmc/articles
/PMC3545982/.

24 http://www.ncbi.nlm.nih.gov/pmc/articles
/PMC3664913/.

25 http://cancerres.aacrjournals.org
/content/75/12/2478.abstract.

26 http://www.ncbi.nlm.nih.gov/pmc/articles
/PMC3664913/.

27 http://www.ncbi.nlm.nih.gov/pmc/articles
/PMC3762447/.

28 L. S. McAnulty et al., "Effect of Blueberry
Ingestion on Natural Killer Cell Counts, Oxidative Stress, and Inflammation Prior To and
After 2.5 h of Running," *Applied Physiology,
Nutrition, and Metabolism* 36, no. 6 (2011):
976–84, http://www.ncbi.nlm.nih.gov
/pubmed/?term=Effect+of+blueberry
+ingestion+on+natural+killer
+cell+counts%2C+oxidative
+stress%2C+and+inflammation
+prior+to+and+after+2.5+h+of+running.

29 http://www.researchgate.net/profile/Sarah
_Johnson39/publication/270910487_Daily_
Blueberry_Consumption_Improves
_Blood_Pressure_and_Arterial_Stiffness
_in_Postmenopausal_Women_with
_Pre-_and_Stage_1-Hypertension_A
_Randomized_Double-Blind_Placebo
-Controlled_Clinical_Trial/
links/54eba8f60cf2082851be543f.pdf

30 http://www.ncbi.nlm.nih.gov/pmc/articles
/PMC4346840/; http://www.ncbi.nlm.nih
.gov/pubmed/23387969.

31 http://www.ncbi.nlm.nih.gov
/pubmed/23507228/.

32 http://www.nrcresearchpress.com/doi
    /abs/10.1139/apnm-2014-0247
    #.Vkx57HhNxxp.
33 http://nutritiondata.self.com/facts
    /fruits-and-fruit-juices/1807/2.
34 http://www.ncbi.nlm.nih.gov
    /pubmed/23727631.
35 R. Terkeltaub, "Are Cherries Now Ripe for
    Use as a Complementary Therapeutic in
    Gout? Appraisal of the State of Evidence,"
    Evidence-Based Medicine 18, no. 6
    (December 2013): 230–31. http://www.ncbi
    .nlm.nih.gov/pubmed/23023818.
36 http://www.ncbi.nlm.nih.gov
    / pubmed/23023818.
37 http://www.ncbi.nlm.nih.gov/pmc/articles
    /PMC4326390/.
38 K. S. Kuehl, "Cherry Juice Targets
    Antioxidant Potential and Pain Relief,"
    Medicine and Science in Sports and Exercise
    59 (2012): 86–93.
39 http://www.ncbi.nlm.nih.gov
    /pubmed/25983669.
40 http://www.mdpi.com/1420
    -3049/19/2/2629/htm.
41 http://www.ncbi.nlm.nih.gov
    /pubmed/23254473.
42 http://www.ncbi.nlm.nih.gov
    /pubmed/26016866.
43 http://www.ncbi.nlm.nih.gov/pmc/articles
    /PMC3360888/.
44 http://ajcn.nutrition.org/content/101/3/506
    .abstract.
45 http://www.researchgate.net/
    publication/263927188_Impact_of_Orange
    _Juice_Consumption_on_Bone_Health_of
    _the_U.S._Population_in_the_National
    _Health_and_Nutrition
    _Examination_Survey_20032006.
46 http://www.ncbi.nlm.nih.gov/pmc/articles
    /PMC3743276/.
47 http://www.researchgate.net
    /publication/261345432_Underutilized
    _citrus_fruits.
48 http://www.hindawi.com/journals
    /jnme/2014/912684/.
49 http://www.ncbi.nlm.nih.gov
    /pubmed/26471075.
50 http://cnr.sagepub.com/content/23/1/54
    .long; http://www.jurology.com/article/
    S0022-5347(14)04646-1/pdf; http://www
    .ncbi.nlm.nih.gov/pubmed/24499122; http://
    www.ncbi.nlm.nih.gov/pmc/articles
    /PMC3853585/.
51 http://www.ncbi.nlm.nih.gov
    /pubmed/26378019; http://www.ncbi.nlm
    .nih.gov/pubmed/22388548; http://www
    .ncbi.nlm.nih.gov/pubmed/21922132; http://
    www.ncbi.nlm.nih.gov/pubmed/21994123;
    http://www.ncbi.nlm.nih.gov
    /pubmed/17182824; http://www.ncbi
    .nlm.nih.gov/pubmed/16968064.
52 http://www.ncbi.nlm.nih.gov
    /pubmed/15107065; http://www.ncbi.nlm
    .nih.gov/pubmed/21906930.
53 http://www.ncbi.nlm.nih.gov/pmc/articles
    /PMC3878739/.
54 http://www.ncbi.nlm.nih.gov/pmc/articles
    /PMC3612419/.
55 http://onlinelibrary.wiley.com/doi/10.1111
    /j.1745-4514.2009.00296.x/abstract.
56 http://www.ncbi.nlm.nih.gov
    /pubmed/23098877.
57 http://www.ncbi.nlm.nih.gov
    /pubmed/25214106.
58 http://onlinelibrary.wiley.com/doi/10.1111
    /ijfs.12721/abstract.
59 http://www.ncbi.nlm.nih.gov
    /pubmed/26454905.
60 http://www.spandidos-publications
    .com/10.3892/ijo.26.4.881; http://www.ncbi
    .nlm.nih.gov/pubmed/26252798.
61 http://www.ncbi.nlm.nih.gov/
    pubmed/25649746; http://www.ncbi.nlm
    .nih.gov/pubmed/23020228.
62 http://onlinelibrary.wiley.com/doi/10.1111
    /ijfs.12721/abstract.
63 http://www.ncbi.nlm.nih.gov
    /pubmed/24841279.
64 http://www.ncbi.nlm.nih.gov/pmc/articles
    /PMC3916869/.
65 http://www.ncbi.nlm.nih.gov
    /pubmed/21548775/.
66 http://www.ncbi.nlm.nih.gov
    /pubmed/22468945/.
67 http://www.ncbi.nlm.nih.gov/pmc/articles
    /PMC3916869/.
68 http://www.bmj.com/content/347/bmj.f5001.
69 http://www.ncbi.nlm.nih.gov
    /pubmed/24007424.
70 Ibid.
71 http://ndb.nal.usda.gov/ndb/foods
    /show/2305?manu=&fgcd=; https://ods.od
    .nih.gov/factsheets/VitaminC-Consumer/.
72 http://www.ncbi.nlm.nih.gov
    /pubmed/25526570.
73 http://www.ncbi.nlm.nih.gov/pmc/articles
    /PMC4091614/.
74 http://www.ncbi.nlm.nih.gov
    /pubmed/26436036.
75 http://www.karger.com/Article/FullText
    /357477.
76 http://www.ncbi.nlm.nih.gov
    /pubmed/23212988.
77 http://www.ncbi.nlm.nih.gov
    /pubmed/26518672.
78 http://www.ncbi.nlm.nih.gov
    /pubmed/26518672.
79 http://www.ncbi.nlm.nih.gov
    /pubmed/23137025.
80 http://www.ncbi.nlm.nih.gov
    /pubmed/23930843.
81 http://www.ncbi.nlm.nih.gov
    /pubmed/11052704.

82 http://www.ncbi.nlm.nih.gov/pmc/articles/PMC3400101/.
83 http://www.ncbi.nlm.nih.gov/pubmed/22342388; http://www.ncbi.nlm.nih.gov/pubmed/25999265; http://www.ncbi.nlm.nih.gov/pubmed/26091382.
84 http://www.ncbi.nlm.nih.gov/pmc/articles/PMC4153032/.
85 http://onlinelibrary.wiley.com/doi/10.1002/biof.1199/full.
86 http://www.ncbi.nlm.nih.gov/pmc/articles/PMC4007340/; http://www.ncbi.nlm.nih.gov/pmc/articles/PMC4477247/.
87 http://www.ncbi.nlm.nih.gov/pmc/articles/PMC4477247/.
88 http://www.ncbi.nlm.nih.gov/pubmed/23684435.
89 http://ajcn.nutrition.org/content/early/2013/11/20/ajcn.113.069641.
90 http://www.ncbi.nlm.nih.gov/pubmed/24706588.
91 S. U. Mertens-Talcott et al., "Ellagic Acid Potentiates the Effect of Quercetin on p21wafl/cipl, p53, and MAP-Kinases without Affecting Intracellular Generation of Reactive Oxygen Species in Vitro," *Journal of Nutrition* 135, no. 3 (2005): 609–14, http://www.ncbi.nlm.nih.gov/pubmed/15735102.
92 http://www.ncbi.nlm.nih.gov/pubmed/23982695.
93 http://www.ncbi.nlm.nih.gov/pmc/articles/PMC4192974/.
94 http://www.ncbi.nlm.nih.gov/pmc/articles/PMC4192974/.
95 http://www.ncbi.nlm.nih.gov/pubmed/26357900; http://www.ncbi.nlm.nih.gov/pubmed/26392037.
96 http://onlinelibrary.wiley.com/doi/10.1002/ana.23594abstract;jsessionid=183E2BD28E03F88801DEF90A9840A4AA.f02t02
97 http://pubs.acs.org/doi/abs/10.1021/jf405455n.
98 http://www.sciencedirect.com/science/article/pii/S0955286313002490.
99 http://www.ncbi.nlm.nih.gov/pubmed/24334868.
100 http://www.ncbi.nlm.nih.gov/pubmed/25156566.
101 http://www.ncbi.nlm.nih.gov/pubmed/22331646.
102 http://www.ncbi.nlm.nih.gov/pmc/articles/PMC4406031/.
103 http://www.nutritionjrnl.com/article/S0899-9007(14)00502-4/abstract.
104 http://www.sciencedaily.com/releases/2008/06/080630165707.htm.
105 http://www.ncbi.nlm.nih.gov/pubmed/21195829.
106 http://www.ncbi.nlm.nih.gov/pmc/articles/PMC4616444/.
107 http://pubs.acs.org/doi/full/10.1021/jf400964r.
108 http://ajh.oxfordjournals.org/content/27/7/899.
109 http://www.ncbi.nlm.nih.gov/pubmed/23615650.

HERBS AND SPICES

1 http://www.ncbi.nlm.nih.gov/pubmed/26688969.
2 http://www.notulaebotanicae.ro/index.php/nbha/article/view/3534.
3 http://www.ncbi.nlm.nih.gov/pubmed/23523869; http://www.notulaebotanicae.ro/index.php/nbha/article/view/3534; http://www.ncbi.nlm.nih.gov/pmc/articles/PMC4280134/; http://www.ncbi.nlm.nih.gov/pubmed/26455352.
4 http://www.ncbi.nlm.nih.gov/pubmed/23682780.
5 http://www.ncbi.nlm.nih.gov/pubmed/24266685.
6 http://www.ncbi.nlm.nih.gov/pmc/articles/PMC3185238/
7 http://www.ncbi.nlm.nih.gov/pubmed/26571987.
8 http://www.ncbi.nlm.nih.gov/pubmed/23625885.
9 http://www.ncbi.nlm.nih.gov/pubmed/26146123.
10 http://www.ncbi.nlm.nih.gov/pubmed/20839630.
11 http://www.ncbi.nlm.nih.gov/pubmed/25915608; http://www.ncbi.nlm.nih.gov/pubmed/24377461; http://www.ncbi.nlm.nih.gov/pubmed/20887269.
12 http://www.ncbi.nlm.nih.gov/pubmed/24050578.
13 http://www.ncbi.nlm.nih.gov/pubmed/19019643.
14 http://www.ncbi.nlm.nih.gov/pubmed/23122099.
15 http://www.phytojournal.com/vol2Issue6/Issue_feb_2014/32.1.pdf.
16 http://www.ncbi.nlm.nih.gov/pubmed/25148954.
17 http://journals.plos.org/plosone/article?id=10.1371/journal.pone.0099086.
18 http://www.ncbi.nlm.nih.gov/pubmed/26109513.
19 http://www.ncbi.nlm.nih.gov/pubmed/25019675.
20 http://www.ncbi.nlm.nih.gov/pubmed/25776008.
21 http://www.ncbi.nlm.nih.gov/pmc/articles/PMC3955423/.

22 http://www.ncbi.nlm.nih.gov/pubmed
    /25914334.
23 http://www.ncbi.nlm.nih.gov/pubmed
    /26436036.
24 http://www.ncbi.nlm.nih.gov/pubmed
    /24102093/.
25 http://www.ncbi.nlm.nih.gov/pmc/articles
    /PMC4103721/; http://www.ncbi.nlm.nih.
    gov/pmc/articles/PMC3874089/; http://www
    .ncbi.nlm.nih.gov/pubmed/25386977.
26 S. Gautam, K. Platel, and K. Srinivasan,
    "Higher Bioaccessibility of Iron and Zinc
    from Food Grains in the Presence of Garlic
    and Onion," *Journal of Agricultural and
    Food Chemistry* 58, no. 15 (2010): 8426–29,
    http://pubs.acs.org/doi/abs/10.1021
    /jf100716t.
27 http://www.ncbi.nlm.nih.gov
    /pubmed/26551789.
28 http://www.ncbi.nlm.nih.gov
    /pubmed/23583806.
29 http://www.researchgate.net/publication
    /233379240_Role_of_garlic_(Allium
    _sativum)_in_various_diseases_An
    _overview.
30 http://www.ncbi.nlm.nih.gov/pmc/articles
    /PMC4550798/.
31 http://www.sciencedirect.com/science
    /article/pii/S0944711315000264.
32 http://www.ncbi.nlm.nih.gov
    /pubmed/25411831.
33 http://www.ncbi.nlm.nih.gov
    /pubmed/26693740.
34 http://www.ncbi.nlm.nih.gov
    /pubmed/23590705.
35 http://www.ncbi.nlm.nih.gov
    /pubmed/23991965.
36 http://www.ncbi.nlm.nih.gov
    /pubmed/25414888; http://www.ncbi.nlm
    .nih.gov/pubmed/24218997; http://www.
    ncbi.nlm.nih.gov/pubmed/26414587; http://
    www.ncbi.nlm.nih.gov/pubmed/24820858.
37 http://www.ncbi.nlm.nih.gov/pmc/articles
    /PMC4461790/.
38 http://www.ncbi.nlm.nih.gov/pmc/articles
    /PMC4436156/.
39 http://www.ncbi.nlm.nih.gov
    /pubmed/25300574.
40 http://www.ncbi.nlm.nih.gov
    /pubmed/24282290; http://www.ncbi.nlm
    .nih.gov/pmc/articles/PMC3847409/;
    http://www.ncbi.nlm.nih.gov/
    pubmed/26621832; http://www.ncbi
    .nlm.nih.gov/pubmed/25838819; http://
    www.ncbi.nlm.nih.gov/pubmed
    /25961833.
41 http://www.ncbi.nlm.nih.gov/pmc/articles
    /PMC4277626/.
42 http://www.ncbi.nlm.nih.gov
    /pubmed/24559810.
43 http://www.ncbi.nlm.nih.gov
    /pubmed/25298352.
44 http://koreascience.or.kr/search/articlepdf
    _ocean.jsp?url=http://ocean.kisti.re.kr
    /downfile/volume/skg/GROSBR/2013
    /v37n1/GROSBR_2013_v37n1_8.pdf&admNo
    =GROSB_2013_v37n1_8.
45 http://www.ncbi.nlm.nih.gov/pmc/articles
    /PMC3659550/.
46 http://www.ncbi.nlm.nih.gov/pmc/articles
    /PMC3629193/.
47 http://www.ncbi.nlm.nih.gov
    /pubmed/23301896.
48 Ibid.
49 http://www.ncbi.nlm.nih.gov
    /pubmed/26579460.
50 http://www.ncbi.nlm.nih.gov/pmc/articles
    /PMC3123991; M. N. Asl and H. Hosseinzadeh,
    "Review of Pharmacological Effects of
    Glycyrrhiza sp. and Its Bioactive Compounds,"
    Phytotherapy Research 22 (2008): 709–24.
51 http://www.liebertpub.com/dcontent/files
    /samplechapters/Sample_ClinicalNatural
    MedicineHandbook.pdf.
52 http://www.ncbi.nlm.nih.gov/pmc/articles
    /PMC3123991/.
53 http://www.hindawi.com/journals
    /bmri/2014/872139/.
54 http://www.ncbi.nlm.nih.gov/pmc/articles
    /PMC4629407/.
55 http://jn.nutrition.org/content/133/5/1286
    .abstract.
56 http://www.ncbi.nlm.nih.gov
    /pubmed/25763467.
57 http://www.ncbi.nlm.nih.gov
    /pubmed/25230257.
58 http://www.ncbi.nlm.nih.gov
    /pubmed/25194985.
59 http://www.ncbi.nlm.nih.gov
    /pubmed/24737278.
60 http://www.ncbi.nlm.nih.gov
    /pubmed/26481920.
61 http://www.ncbi.nlm.nih.gov
    /pubmed/25038680.
62 https://www.researchgate.net
    /publication/261065967_Parsley_a_review
    _of_ethnopharmacology_phytochemistry
    _and_biological_activities.
63 http://www.ncbi.nlm.nih.gov
    /pubmed/25019465.
64 http://www.ncbi.nlm.nih.gov
    /pubmed/26483970.
65 http://www.ncbi.nlm.nih.gov
    /pubmed/26596707.
66 http://www.ncbi.nlm.nih.gov
    /pubmed/22944717.
67 http://www.ncbi.nlm.nih.gov
    /pubmed/26170168.
68 http://www.ncbi.nlm.nih.gov
    /pubmed/26092628.
69 http://www.ncbi.nlm.nih.gov
    /pubmed/26114303.
70 University of Arkansas, Food Safety
    Consortium, "To Block the Carcinogens, Add

a Touch Of Rosemary When Grilling Meats," *Science Daily,* May 24, 2008, http://www.sciencedaily.com/releases /2008/05/080521184129.htm.

71 http://online.liebertpub.com/doi/ abs/10.1089/jmf.2011.0005.

72 http://www.hindawi.com/journals /ecam/2012/564927/.

73 http://www.ncbi.nlm.nih.gov /pubmed/21955093/.

74 http://www.ncbi.nlm.nih.gov /pubmed/24615943.

75 http://www.ncbi.nlm.nih.gov /pubmed/26114303.

76 http://www.ncbi.nlm.nih.gov /pubmed/24802524.

77 http://www.ncbi.nlm.nih.gov/pmc /articles/PMC2769154/.

78 http://www.ncbi.nlm.nih.gov /pubmed/24050577.

79 http://www.ncbi.nlm.nih.gov /pubmed/24836739.

80 http://www.ncbi.nlm.nih.gov /pubmed/25379783.

81 http://www.ncbi.nlm.nih.gov /pubmed/25749238.

82 http://www.ncbi.nlm.nih.gov /pubmed/26481920.

83 http://www.ncbi.nlm.nih.gov /pubmed/9619120.

84 http://www.mdpi.com/1420-3049/20/5/9183 /htm; http://www.ncbi.nlm.nih.gov/pmc /articles/PMC3942920/; https://www .researchgate.net/publication/230658704 _Multitargeting_by_turmeric_the_golden _spice_From_kitchen_to_clinic.

85 http://www.ncbi.nlm.nih.gov /pubmed/26308760; http://www.mdpi .com/1420-3049/20/5/9183/htm; http://www .ncbi.nlm.nih.gov/pmc/articles /PMC3942920/.

86 http://www.clinicalnutritionjournal.com /article/S0261-5614%2815%2900002-3 /abstract.

87 http://www.ncbi.nlm.nih.gov /pubmed/23438873

88 http://www.ncbi.nlm.nih.gov /pubmed/24445038

89 http://www.ncbi.nlm.nih.gov /pubmed/22407780

90 http://www.ncbi.nlm.nih.gov /pubmed/26652155.

91 http://www.ncbi.nlm.nih.gov /pubmed/25200875.

92 http://www.ncbi.nlm.nih.gov /pubmed/26610378.

NUTS

1 http://www.ncbi.nlm.nih.gov /pubmed/26148924.

2 http://www.ncbi.nlm.nih.gov /pubmed/25138064.

3 http://www.ncbi.nlm.nih.gov /pubmed/26148914.

4 G. Mandalari et al., "In Vitro Evaluation of the Pre-Biotic Properties of Almond Skins (*Amygdalus communis L.*)," *FEMS Microbiology Letters* 304, no. 2 (2010): 116–22, http://www.ncbi.nlm.nih.gov /pubmed/20146750.

5 http://www.ncbi.nlm.nih.gov /pubmed/25670361.

6 https://ods.od.nih.gov/factsheets/Selenium -HealthProfessional/.

7 http://www.ncbi.nlm.nih.gov /pubmed/25395121.

8 http://www.ncbi.nlm.nih.gov/pmc /articles/PMC3693158/.

9 S. Akhtar et al., "Physicochemical Characteristics, Functional Properties, and Nutritional Benefits of Peanut Oil: A Review" *Critical Reviews in Food Science and Nutrition* 54, no. 12 (2014): 1562–75.

10 P.A. van den Brandt and L. J. Schouten, "Relationship of Tree Nut, Peanut and Peanut Butter Intake with Total and Cause-Specific Mortality: A Cohort Study and Meta-Analysis," *International Journal of Epidemiology*, 44, no. 3 (2015): 1038–49.

11 H. N. Luuet al., "Prospective Evaluation of the Association of Nut/Peanut Consumption With Total and Cause-Specific Mortality" *JAMA Internal Medicine* 175, no. 5 (2015): 755–66.

12 R. R. Bansode et al., "Bioavailability and Hypolipidemic Effects of Peanut Skin Polyphenols," *Journal of Medicinal Food* 18, no. 3 (March 2015): 265-272.

13 http://www.ncbi.nlm.nih.gov /pubmed/25305221.

14 http://www.ncbi.nlm.nih.gov /pubmed/26450069.

15 http://jn.nutrition.org/content/141/1/56.long.

16 http://www.ncbi.nlm.nih.gov/pubmed /24279287; http://www.ncbi.nlm.nih.gov /pubmed/22691487.

17 http://www.ncbi.nlm.nih.gov /pubmed/21924598.

18 http://www.ncbi.nlm.nih.gov /pubmed/26148925.

19 http://www.ncbi.nlm.nih.gov /pubmed/22458696.

20 http://www.ncbi.nlm.nih.gov /pubmed/24377454.

21 http://www.ncbi.nlm.nih.gov /pubmed/25396407.

22 http://www.ncbi.nlm.nih.gov /pubmed/25809855.

23 http://www.ncbi.nlm.nih.gov /pubmed/25125505.

24 http://www.ncbi.nlm.nih .gov/pubmed/25466114; http://www.ncbi .nlm.nih.gov/pubmed/22187094.

25 http://jn.nutrition.org/content/144/4/547S .long.

26 http://www.ncbi.nlm.nih.gov /pubmed/22349682.

27 http://www.ncbi.nlm.nih.gov /pubmed/23756586.

28 http://www.sciencedirect.com/science /article/pii/S0026049513003879.

29 http://www.ncbi.nlm.nih.gov /pubmed/25336096.

OILS

1 http://ajcn.nutrition.org/content/102/2/479 .long.

2 S. R. Goltz et al., "Meal Triacylglycerol Profile Modulates Postprandial Absorption of Carotenoids in Humans," *Molecular Nutrition & Food Research*, 56, no. 6 (2012): 866–77, http://www.ncbi.nlm.nih.gov/ pubmed/22707262.

3 http://www.ncbi .nlm.nih.gov/pmc /articles/PMC4568762/.

4 http://www.ncbi.nlm.nih.gov /pubmed/26040366.

5 http://www.biomedcentral.com/1741 -7015/12/78.

6 http://www.ncbi.nlm.nih.gov /pubmed/26450601.

7 http://www.ncbi.nlm.nih.gov /pubmed/26092624.

8 http://www.ncbi.nlm.nih.gov /pubmed/26565552.

9 http://www.ncbi.nlm.nih.gov /pubmed/25172701.

10 http://ajcn.nutrition.org/content/100 /Supplement_1/443S.long.

11 http://www.ncbi.nlm.nih.gov/pmc/articles /PMC4409715/#CR14

12 http://www.ncbi.nlm.nih.gov /pubmed/26543357.

13 http://www.ncbi.nlm.nih.gov /pubmed/21088453.

14 http://www.ncbi.nlm.nih.gov /pubmed/25688177; http://www.ncbi.nlm .nih.gov/pmc/articles/PMC3775252/.

15 http://www.ncbi.nlm.nih.gov /pubmed/20095133; http://www.ncbi .nlm.nih.gov/pmc/articles/PMC4365303/.

16 http://www.ncbi.nlm.nih.gov/pmc/articles /PMC4365303/.

17 http://www.ncbi.nlm.nih.gov /pubmed/20095133.

18 http://ar.iiarjournals.org/content/35/1/97 .long.

19 http://www.researchgate.net/publication /265475789_Virgin_Coconut_Oil_and_Its _Potential_Cardioprotective_Effects.

20 http://www.aulamedica.es/nh/pdf /9642.pdf.

21 http://www.ncbi.nlm.nih.gov/pmc/articles /PMC4176590/.

22 http://msphere.asm.org/documents /mSphere.00020-15.pdf.

SEAFOOD AND FISH

1 https://ods.od.nih.gov/factsheets /Zinc-HealthProfessional/.

2 http://oceana.org/sites/default/files/MBA _SeafoodWatch_NationalGuide_0.pdf.

3 http://www.aacijournal.com/content /11/1/30.

4 https://ods.od.nih.gov/factsheets/Zinc -HealthProfessional/.

5 http://ndb.nal.usda.gov/ndb/nutrients /report/nutrientsfrm?max=25&offset=0 &totCount=0&nutrient1=309& nutrient2=&nutrient3=&subset=0& fg=15&sort=c&measureby=m.

6 http://www.ncbi.nlm.nih.gov /pubmed/24148607/.

7 http://www.ncbi.nlm.nih.gov /pubmed/25624228.

8 http://www.seafoodhealthfacts.org /seafood-nutrition/healthcare-professionals /omega-3-content-frequently-consumed -seafood-products.

9 http://oceana.org/sites/default/files/MBA _SeafoodWatch_NationalGuide_0.pdf.

10 http://www.ncbi.nlm.nih.gov /pubmed/24694001.

11 G. I. Smith et al., "Omega-3 Polyunsaturated Fatty Acids Augment the Muscle Protein Anabolic Response to Hyperinsulinaemia- Hyperaminoacidaemia in Healthy Young and Middle-Aged Men and Women," *Clinical Science (Lond)* 121, no. 6 (2011): 267–78, http://www.ncbi.nlm.nih.gov /pubmed/?term=Omega-3+polyunsaturated +fatty+acids+augment+the+muscle+protein +anabolic+response+to+hyperinsulinaemia -hyperaminoacidaemia+in+healthy +young+and+middle-aged+men +and+women.

12 http://www.ncbi.nlm.nih.gov
    /pubmed/25720716.
13 http://www.ncbi.nlm.nih.gov
    /pubmed/26260547.
14 http://www.ncbi.nlm.nih.gov
    /pubmed/25446949.
15 http://www.ncbi.nlm.nih.gov
    /pubmed/26420180.
16 http://www.ncbi.nlm.nih.gov
    /pubmed/25720716.
17 http://www.ncbi.nlm.nih.gov
    /pubmed/23571649.
18 http://www.ncbi.nlm.nih.gov
    /pubmed/25514035.
19 http://www.ncbi.nlm.nih.gov
    /pubmed/26463349.
20 http://www.seafoodwatch.org/seafood
    -recommendations/groups/sardine.
21 http://www.ncbi.nlm.nih.gov
    /pubmed/22221769.
22 A. J. Adler and B. J. Holub, "Effect of Garlic
    and Fish-Oil Supplementation on Serum
    Lipid and Lipoprotein Concentrations in
    Hypercholesterolemic Men," *American*

Journal of Clinical Nutrition 65, no. 2 (1997):
445–50, http://www.ncbi.nlm.nih.gov
/pubmed/9022529.
23 http://www.ncbi.nlm.nih.gov
    /pubmed/26260547.
24 https://www.researchgate.net/publication
    /266204598_Chew_on_this_Sardines
    _are_still_a_healthy_choice_against
    _SUDEP.
25 http://oceana.org/sites/default/files
    /MBA_SeafoodWatch_NationalGuide
    _0.pdf.
26 http://www.ncbi.nlm.nih.gov
    /pubmed/25962922.
27 https://www.jstage.jst.go.jp/article
    /jtm/21/5/21_5_215/_article.
28 http://www.ncbi.nlm.nih.gov
    /pubmed/26635922.
29 http://www.ncbi.nlm.nih.gov
    /pubmed/25149823.
30 http://www.ncbi.nlm.nih.gov
    /pubmed/25752887; http://www.ncbi.nlm
    .nih.gov/pubmed/26325092.

SEEDS

1   http://www.ncbi.nlm.nih.gov
    /pubmed/24811150.
2   http://www.ncbi.nlm.nih.gov
    /pubmed/25403867.
3   http://www.ncbi.nlm.nih.gov/pmc/articles
    /PMC4237475/.
4   http://www.ncbi.nlm.nih.gov
    /pubmed/22361189.
5   http://www.ncbi.nlm.nih.gov
    /pubmed/23354422.
6   http://www.ncbi.nlm.nih.gov
    /pubmed/26232691.
7   http://www.ncbi.nlm.nih.gov
    /pubmed/24434020.
8   http://www.ncbi.nlm.nih.gov
    /pubmed/24463788.
9   http://jn.nutrition.org/content/145
    /4/758.full.

10 http://www.ncbi.nlm.nih.gov/pmc/articles
    /PMC4032845/.
11 http://www.ncbi.nlm.nih.gov
    /pubmed/24864154.
12 http://www.ncbi.nlm.nih.gov
    /pubmed/23506532; http://www.ncbi.nlm
    .nih.gov/pubmed/24564589.
13 http://www.ncbi.nlm.nih.gov
    /pubmed/25871017.
14 http://www.ncbi.nlm.nih.gov
    /pubmed/21827664.
15 http://www.ncbi.nlm.nih.gov
    /pubmed/23933354.
16 http://www.ncbi.nlm.nih.gov
    /pubmed/22995032.
17 http://www.ncbi.nlm.nih.gov/pmc/articles
    /PMC4045277/.

SWEETS

1   http://www.ncbi.nlm.nih.gov/pmc/articles
    /PMC4596528/.
2   http://onlinelibrary.wiley.com/doi/10.1002
    /ieam.1594/full.
3   http://www.njmonline.nl/getpdf
    .php?id=1269.
4   http://onlinelibrary.wiley.com/doi/10.1002
    /mnfr.201300277/abstract.
5   http://www.ncbi.nlm.nih.gov
    /pubmed/24582922.
6   C. S. Kwok et al., "Habitual Chocolate
    Consumption and Risk of Cardiovascular

Disease Among Healthy Men and
Women," *Heart* (2015): 1–9, doi:10
.1136/heartjnl-2014
-307050.
7   http://www.fasebj.org/content/28/3/1464
    .abstract.
8   http://www.njmonline.nl/getpdf
    .php?id=1269.
9   http://ajcn.nutrition.org/content
    /early/2014/12/16/ajcn.114.092189.
10 http://www.ncbi.nlm.nih.gov
    /pubmed/26456559.

11 http://www.ncbi.nlm.nih.gov/pmc/articles/PMC3583289/

12 http://www.ncbi.nlm.nih.gov/pmc/articles/PMC3758027/.

13 http://www.ncbi.nlm.nih.gov/pubmed/22866051; http://onlinelibrary.wiley.com/doi/10.1111/j.1365-2621.2004.tb15509.x/abstract.

14 http://www.ncbi.nlm.nih.gov/pmc/articles/PMC3743976/.

15 http://www.ncbi.nlm.nih.gov/pmc/articles/PMC3758027/.

16 http://www.ncbi.nlm.nih.gov/pmc/articles/PMC4158441/; http://www.ncbi.nlm.nih.gov/pmc/articles/PMC3758027/.

17 http://www.ctcpjournal.com/article/S1744-3881(13)00091-1/fulltext; http://www.ncbi.nlm.nih.gov/pubmed/19916918.

18 http://www.hindawi.com/journals/ecam/2011/295494/.

19 http://www.ncbi.nlm.nih.gov/pmc/articles/PMC4020454/.

20 http://www.ncbi.nlm.nih.gov/pubmed/25193590.

21 http://www.ncbi.nlm.nih.gov/pubmed/26453201.

22 http://www.ncbi.nlm.nih.gov/pubmed/24305429.

23 http://www.ncbi.nlm.nih.gov/pubmed/23256446/.

24 http://www.ncbi.nlm.nih.gov/pubmed/24605717.

25 http://www.ncbi.nlm.nih.gov/pubmed/26171198.

26 http://www.ncbi.nlm.nih.gov/pubmed/26613081.

VEGETABLES

1 http://www.ncbi.nlm.nih.gov/pubmed/26310198.

2 Ibid.

3 Ibid.

4 http://www.ncbi.nlm.nih.gov/pubmed/22746542.

5 http://www.ncbi.nlm.nih.gov/pubmed/15353023.

6 http://www.ncbi.nlm.nih.gov/pmc/articles/PMC4627240/.

7 http://www.ncbi.nlm.nih.gov/pubmed/23923586.

8 Ibid.

9 http://www.ncbi.nlm.nih.gov/pmc/articles/PMC4477242/.

10 http://www.ncbi.nlm.nih.gov/pubmed/26463825.

11 http://www.ncbi.nlm.nih.gov/pmc/articles/PMC3869575/.

12 http://www.arjournals.org/index.php/ijpm/article/view/1598/817.

13 http://www.ncbi.nlm.nih.gov/pubmed/20951824.

14 http://www.ncbi.nlm.nih.gov/pubmed/23640589.

15 http://ajpregu.physiology.org/content/305/12/R1441.long.

16 http://circheartfailure.ahajournals.org/content/8/5/914.abstract?sid=c7972c37-593e-4ce1-a7d2-a895bcce2e67.

17 http://www.ncbi.nlm.nih.gov/pubmed/22709704.

18 E R. Bertone-Johnson et al., "Calcium and Vitamin D Intake and Risk of Incident Premenstrual Syndrome," *Archives of Internal Medicine* 165, no. 11 (2005): 1246–52, http://www.ncbi.nlm.nih.gov/pubmed/15956003.

19 http://www.ncbi.nlm.nih.gov/pubmed/26400430; http://www.ncbi.nlm.nih.gov/pubmed/26165427.

20 http://www.ncbi.nlm.nih.gov/pubmed/25225771.

21 http://www.ncbi.nlm.nih.gov/pubmed/21160094.

22 Ibid.

23 Ibid.

24 http://www.ncbi.nlm.nih.gov/pubmed/24287881.

25 http://www.ncbi.nlm.nih.gov/pmc/articles/PMC4570035/.

26 http://www.ncbi.nlm.nih.gov/pubmed/25774338.

27 http://www.ncbi.nlm.nih.gov/pmc/articles/PMC4637098/.

28 http://eds.b.ebscohost.com/eds/detail/detail?sid=eca9d0e8-5540-4a2e-806e-1cc924c40322%40sessionmgr113&vid=0&hid=112&bdata=JnNpdGU9ZWRzLWxpdmU%3d#AN=ejs36147078&db=edo.

29 http://www.ncbi.nlm.nih.gov/pmc/articles/PMC4063312/.

30 http://online.liebertpub.com/doi/abs/10.1089/jmf.2012.2563?src=recsys.

31 http://archopht.jamanetwork.com/article.aspx?articleid=268224.

32 http://nutritiondata.self.com/facts/vegetables-and-vegetable-products/2383/2.

33 http://www.researchgate.net/publication/260149876_Dietary_carrot_consumption_and_the_risk_of_prostate_cancer.

34 http://www.ncbi.nlm.nih.gov/pmc/articles/PMC4203935/; http://www.ncbi.nlm.nih.gov/pubmed/22815230; http://www.ncbi.nlm.nih.gov/pubmed/25684522.

35 http://www.ncbi.nlm.nih.gov/pubmed/26610885.

36 http://www.ncbi.nlm.nih.gov/pubmed/26148912.

37 http://www.ncbi.nlm.nih.gov/pmc/articles/PMC2874783/.

38 http://www.idosi.org/gjp/9(1)15/20.pdf.

39 http://www.biomedcentral.com/1471-2407/14/591.

40 http://www.ncbi.nlm.nih.gov/pmc/articles/PMC4137549/.

41 http://www.ncbi.nlm.nih.gov/pubmed/22010973.

42 http://www.johcd.org/pdf/May_August_2014/04_An%20in-Vivo%20Evaluation.pdf.

43 http://www.ncbi.nlm.nih.gov/pubmed/22447109.

44 http://www.ncbi.nlm.nih.gov/pubmed/22010973.

45 http://www.ncbi.nlm.nih.gov/pmc/articles/PMC4525133/.

46 http://www.ncbi.nlm.nih.gov/pubmed/25085020.

47 http://www.ncbi.nlm.nih.gov/pubmed/22393831/.

48 http://www.ncbi.nlm.nih.gov/pmc/articles/PMC4049200/.

49 http://www.ars.usda.gov/News/docs.htm?docid=23199; http://www2.ca.uky.edu/agc/pubs/FCS3/FCS3567/FCS3567.pdf.

50 https://www.nlm.nih.gov/medlineplus/magazine/issues/winter11/articles/winter11pg12.html.

51 http://ndb.nal.usda.gov/ndb/nutrients/report/nutrientsfrm?max=25&offset=0&totCount=0&nutrient1=301&nutrient2=&nutrient3=&subset=0&fg=11&sort=c&measureby=m.

52 http://www.ncbi.nlm.nih.gov/pmc/articles/PMC4603065/.

53 http://www.ncbi.nlm.nih.gov/pmc/articles/PMC4049200/.

54 http://www.ncbi.nlm.nih.gov/pubmed/25085257; http://www.ncbi.nlm.nih.gov/pubmed/24877989; http://www.ncbi.nlm.nih.gov/pubmed/26629253; http://www2.ca.uky.edu/agc/pubs/FCS3/FCS3567/FCS3567.pdf.

55 http://www.ncbi.nlm.nih.gov/pmc/articles/PMC3575935/.

56 http://www.ncbi.nlm.nih.gov/pubmed/23294925.

57 http://www.ncbi.nlm.nih.gov/pmc/articles/PMC3831537/.

58 http://www.ncbi.nlm.nih.gov/pmc/articles/PMC4225228/.

59 http://www.ncbi.nlm.nih.gov/pmc/articles/PMC3891790/.

60 http://www.ncbi.nlm.nih.gov/pubmed/24950293.

61 http://www.ncbi.nlm.nih.gov/pmc/articles/PMC4320875/.

62 http://www.sciencedirect.com/science/article/pii/S1756464612000746.

63 http://www.mdpi.com/1420-3049/20/10/19489/htm.

64 http://www.ncbi.nlm.nih.gov/pubmed/23557365.

65 http://www.ncbi.nlm.nih.gov/pubmed/24056209/.

66 http://www.ncbi.nlm.nih.gov/pmc/articles/PMC4056650/.

67 http://www.fasebj.org/cgi/content/meeting_abstract/27/1_Meeting Abstracts/643.15.

68 http://www.ncbi.nlm.nih.gov/pubmed/24915405.

69 http://www.ncbi.nlm.nih.gov/pubmed/26148912; http://www.ncbi.nlm.nih.gov/pubmed/24820444.

70 http://www.ncbi.nlm.nih.gov/pubmed/26473159.

71 http://www.ncbi.nlm.nih.gov/pubmed/24612081.

72 http://www.ncbi.nlm.nih.gov/pubmed/26385226.

73 http://www.ncbi.nlm.nih.gov/pubmed/17519926.

74 http://pubs.acs.org/doi/pdfplus/10.1021/np300898z.

75 Ibid.

76 http://www.ncbi.nlm.nih.gov/pubmed/21852280/.

77 http://www.ncbi.nlm.nih.gov/pubmed/25675368; http://www.ncbi.nlm.nih.gov/pmc/articles/PMC4422461/; http://www.ncbi.nlm.nih.gov/pubmed/26630428.

78 http://www.nutrition-and-you.com/chili-peppers.html.

79 http://www.ncbi.nlm.nih.gov/pubmed/25603234; http://www.ncbi.nlm.nih.gov/pubmed/25675368.

80 http://www.ncbi.nlm.nih.gov/pubmed/26630428.

81 http://www.ncbi.nlm.nih.gov/pubmed/26171907.

82 http://www.ncbi.nlm.nih.gov/pubmed/26617603; http://www.mdpi.com/1420-3049/19/4/5434/htm; http://www.ncbi.nlm.nih.gov/pubmed/23853433.

83 https://www.researchgate.net/publication/272187657_Biological_Activities_of_Red_Pepper_Capsicum_annuum_and_Its_Pungent_Principle_Capsaicin_A_Review.

84 http://www.nature.com/ijo/journal/vaop/naam/abs/ijo2015253a.html.

85 http://www.ncbi.nlm.nih.gov/pmc/articles/PMC4525189/.

86 http://www.ncbi.nlm.nih.gov/pubmed/25568828.

87 http://pubs.acs.org/doi/abs/10.1021/jf0109017.

88 http://www.ncbi.nlm.nih.gov/pmc/articles
/PMC3529556/; http://www.ncbi.nlm.nih
.gov/pubmed/25152445.

89 http://www.ncbi.nlm.nih.gov/pmc/articles
/PMC3715682/.

90 http://www.ncbi.nlm.nih.gov
/pubmed/22173777/.

91 http://www.ncbi.nlm.nih.gov/pmc/articles
/PMC3715682/.

92 http://www.ncbi.nlm.nih.gov/pmc/articles
/PMC4069315/.

93 M. R. Hilimire et al., "Fermented Foods,
Neuroticism, and Social Anxiety: An
Interaction Model" *Psychiatry Research* 228
(2015): 203–8.

94 http://www.phycologia.org/doi
/full/10.2216/15-77.1.

95 http://www.ncbi.nlm.nih.gov/pmc/articles
/PMC4557030/.

96 http://www.ncbi.nlm.nih.gov/pmc/articles
/PMC4178489/.

97 http://www.ncbi.nlm.nih.gov/pmc/articles
/PMC4557030/.

98 http://www.ncbi.nlm.nih.gov
/pubmed/26433766.

99 http://www.phycologia.org/doi
/full/10.2216/15-77.1.

100 http://online.liebertpub.com/doi
/abs/10.1089/jmf.2012.2468?src=recsys.

101 https://www.researchgate.net/publication
/275260109_Weight_loss_and_reductions
_in_body_mass_index_abdominal-girth
and-depth_after_a_12_week_dietary
_intervention_of_soya_beans_edamame.

102 http://www.ncbi.nlm.nih.gov
/pubmed/25995282.

103 http://apjcn.nhri.org.tw/server
/APJCN/22/2/222.pdf.

104 http://www.ncbi.nlm.nih.gov
/pubmed/26006245.

105 http://www.ncbi.nlm.nih.gov
/pubmed/24629984.

106 http://www.ncbi.nlm.nih.gov
/pubmed/23745032.

107 http://www.ncbi.nlm.nih.gov
/pubmed/26509161.

108 S. Veda and K. Srinivasan, "Influence of
Dietary Spices—Black Pepper, Red Pepper
and Ginger on the Uptake of ß-carotene by
Rat Intestines," *Journal of Functional Foods
1, no.* 4 (2009): 394–98, http://www
.sciencedirect.com/science/article/pii
/S1756464609000656.

109 http://www.ncbi.nlm.nih.gov/pmc/articles
/PMC4293869/.

110 http://www.ncbi.nlm.nih.gov
/pubmed/21861722.

WHOLE GRAINS

1 http://www.ncbi.nlm.nih.gov
/pubmed/25075608.

2 http://www.ncbi.nlm.nih.gov/pmc/articles
/PMC3958897/.

3 http://www.ncbi.nlm.nih.gov
/pubmed/26386056.

4 http://www.ncbi.nlm.nih.gov
/pubmed/24039967.

5 http://www.ncbi.nlm.nih.gov
/pubmed/23577719.

6 http://pubs.acs.org/doi/abs/10.1021
/acs.jafc.5b02498?journalCode
=jafcau.

7 http://pubs.acs.org/doi/abs/10.1021
/acs.jafc.5b02498?journalCode=jafcau;
http://www.ncbi.nlm.nih.gov/
pubmed/25076146.

8 http://pubs.acs.org/doi/abs/10.1021/acs
.jafc.5b02498?journalCode=jafcau.

9 http://www.ncbi.nlm.nih.gov/pubmed
/22962927; http://www.ncbi.nlm.nih.gov
/pubmed/23905830.

10 http://www.ncbi.nlm.nih.gov
/pubmed/26471595.

11 http://www.ncbi.nlm.nih.gov
/pubmed/19941618.

12 http://www.ncbi.nlm.nih.gov
/pubmed/23422921.

13 http://www.ijdvl.com/article.asp?issn=0378
-6323;year=2012;volume=78;issue=2;spage
=142;epage=145;aulast=Pazyar#ft7.

14 http://www.ncbi.nlm.nih.gov
/pubmed/23561127.

15 http://www.ncbi.nlm.nih.gov
/pubmed/24024772.

16 http://www.ncbi.nlm.nih.gov
/pubmed/26273900.

17 http://www.ncbi.nlm.nih.gov
/pubmed/25863614; http://www.ncbi
.nlm.nih.gov/pubmed/25053071.

18 http://www.ncbi.nlm.nih.gov
/pubmed/24344670.

19 http://www.ncbi.nlm.nih.gov
/pubmed/23537598.

20 http://www.nulifemarket.com/media
/files/AwikaRooneySorghumPhyto
chemicalsAndTheirPotentialImpact
OnHum.pdf.

21 http://www.ncbi.nlm.nih.gov
/pubmed/25092385.

22 http://www.ncbi.nlm.nih.gov
/pubmed/24158434/.

23 http://www.ncbi.nlm.nih.gov
/pubmed/26062574.

24 http://www.ncbi.nlm.nih.gov/pmc/articles
/PMC4659141/.

ACID REFLUX

1. http://www.fda.gov/Food/Foodborne IllnessContaminants/CausesOfIllness BadBugBook/ucm122561.htm.
2. http://foodscience.caes.uga.edu/extension /documents/FDAapproximatepHoffoodslacf -phs.pdf.
3. http://www.ncbi.nlm.nih.gov/books /NBK92775/.
4. http://www.ncbi.nlm.nih.gov/pmc/articles /PMC4137549/.
5. http://www.ncbi.nlm.nih.gov /pmc/articles/PMC3123991/#B17;

   M. N. Asl and H. Hosseinzadeh, "Review of Pharmacological Effects of *Glycyrrhiza* sp. and Its Bioactive Compounds," *Phytotherapy Research* 22 (2008): 709–24.
6. http://umm.edu/health/medical/altmed /herb/licorice.
7. Ibid.
8. https://umm.edu/health/medical/altmed /herb/german-chamomile.
9. http://www.ncbi.nlm.nih.gov/pmc/articles /PMC2995283/.

ACNE

1. http://www.ncbi.nlm.nih.gov/pmc/articles /PMC4106357/#B12.
2. H. H. Kwon et al., "Clinical and Histological Effect of a Low Glycemic Load Diet in Treatment of Acne Vulgaris in Korean Patients: A Randomized, Controlled Trial," *Acta Dermato Venereologica* 92, no. 3 (2012): 241–46.
3. http://www.ncbi.nlm.nih.gov/pmc/articles /PMC3780801/.
4. http://www.ncbi.nlm.nih.gov/pmc/articles /PMC4507494/.
5. http://www.ncbi.nlm.nih.gov/pubmed /11349462; http://www.ncbi.nlm.nih.gov /pubmed/19943837.

6. http://www.prevention.com/beauty/ 25-best-foods-for-your-skin?slide=6.
7. I. F. Benzie and S. W. Choi, "Antioxidants in Food: Content, Measurement, Significance, Action, Cautions, Caveats, and Research Needs," *Advances in Food and Nutrition Research* 71 (2014): 1–53, doi:10.1016/B978-0-12-800270 -4.00001-8.
8. http://www.prevention.com/beauty /25-best-foods-for-your-skin?slide=16.
9. http://www.ncbi.nlm.nih.gov/pubmed /26061422; http://www.ncbi.nlm.nih.gov /pubmed/23886975.

ADRENAL EXHAUSTION/ADRENAL FATIGUE

1. Tricia Pingel, NMD, *Total Health Turnaround: The All-Natural Plan to Reverse Adrenal Fatigue, Lose Weight, and Feel Better Fast* (Emmaus, PA: Rodale, 2014).

ALLERGIC RHINITIS (HAY FEVER)

1. Z. A. Asha'ari et al., "Ingestion of Honey Improves the Symptoms of Allergic Rhinitis: Evidence from a Randomized Placebo-Controlled Trial in the East Coast of Peninsular Malaysia," *Annals of Saudi Medicine* 33, no. 5 (Sep–Oct 2013): 469–75.
2. http://www.ncbi.nlm.nih.gov/pmc/articles /PMC4264806/#b8-0601107.
3. http://www.ncbi.nlm.nih.gov /pubmed/23333628.
4. http://www.dissertationtopic.net /doc/2158274; http://www.ncbi.nlm .nih.gov/pubmed/23333628.

5. http://www.ncbi.nlm.nih.gov /pubmed/23281076.
6. http://www.ncbi.nlm.nih.gov /pubmed/16870019.
7. http://www.ncbi.nlm.nih.gov/pmc/articles /PMC3925289/.
8. http://www.ncbi.nlm.nih.gov /pubmed/21395878.
9. http://www.ncbi.nlm.nih.gov/pmc/articles /PMC3904042/.
10. http://www.nature.com/ejcn/journal/v67 /n2/full/ejcn2012197a.html.
11. http://www.ncbi.nlm.nih.gov /pubmed/26045910.

12 http://umm.edu/health/medical/altmed /herb/licorice.

ALZHEIMER'S DISEASE

1   http://www.ncbi.nlm.nih.gov/pmc/articles /PMC3824191/.
2   http://www.ncbi.nlm.nih.gov/pubmed/?term =brain+food+for+alzheimer-free+aging.
3   http://www.ncbi.nlm.nih.gov/pmc/articles /PMC4583585/.
4   http://www.ncbi.nlm.nih.gov/pmc/articles /PMC4005962/.
5   http://www.ncbi.nlm.nih.gov/pmc/articles /PMC3024594/; http://www.ncbi.nlm.nih.gov /pubmed/20182044; http://www.ncbi.nlm. nih.gov/pubmed/21539488; http://www.ncbi .nlm.nih.gov/pubmed/25681666; http://www .ncbi.nlm.nih.gov/pubmed/26086182; http:// www.ncbi.nlm.nih.gov/pubmed/25770254.
6   http://www.ncbi.nlm.nih.gov /pubmed/26342761; http://www.ncbi.nlm .nih.gov/pubmed/25862980.
7   http://www.nature.com/mp/journal/vaop /ncurrent/full/mp2015129a.html.
8   http://www.ncbi.nlm.nih.gov /pubmed/26086182.
9   http://www.ncbi.nlm.nih.gov /pubmed/25681666.
10 http://www.ncbi.nlm.nih.gov /pubmed/26092624.
11 http://www.ncbi.nlm.nih.gov /pubmed/24890399.

13 http://www.ncbi.nlm.nih.gov/pmc/articles /PMC3544658/.

12 http://www.ncbi.nlm.nih.gov /pubmed/25418871.
13 http://www.sciencedirect.com/science /article/pii/S0304394010000546.
14 http://www.ncbi.nlm.nih.gov/pmc/articles /PMC4537710/; http://www.ncbi.nlm.nih .gov/pubmed/26301243.
15 http://www.ncbi.nlm.nih.gov /pubmed/26501267.
16 http://www.sciencedirect.com/science /article/pii/S0197018615300322; http:// www.ncbi.nlm.nih.gov/pmc/articles /PMC4495334/.
17 http://lpi.oregonstate.edu/mic/vitamins /vitamin-B12.
18 http://www.neurobiologyofaging.org/article /S0197-4580(14)00348-0/fulltext.
19 http://www.ncbi.nlm.nih.gov /pubmed/25997382.
20 http://www.ncbi.nlm.nih.gov /pubmed/25043908.
21 http://www.ncbi.nlm.nih.gov /pubmed/26214150.
22 http://www.ncbi.nlm.nih.gov/pmc/articles /PMC4340060/.
23 http://www.ncbi.nlm.nih.gov /pubmed/23810791.

ANXIETY

1   http://www.ncbi.nlm.nih.gov /pubmed/26061411.
2   http://www.ncbi.nlm.nih.gov /pubmed/23295173.
3   http://www.ncbi.nlm.nih.gov/pmc/articles /PMC3355196/.
4   http://www.ncbi.nlm.nih.gov/pmc/articles /PMC4118660/.
5   http://www.ncbi.nlm.nih.gov/pmc/articles /PMC4480845/.
6   http://www.ncbi.nlm.nih.gov/pmc/articles /PMC3560823/.
7   http://www.ncbi.nlm.nih.gov /pubmed/22894890; http://www.ncbi.nlm .nih.gov/pmc/articles/PMC3600416/.
8   http://www.sciencealert.com/taking -probiotics-could-make-you-less-stressed -and-boost-your-memory.
9   http://www.ncbi.nlm.nih.gov /pubmed/25470391.
10 http://www.ncbi.nlm.nih.gov/pubmed /?term=fermented+foods+neuroticism.
11 http://www.hindawi.com/journals /ecam/2013/681304/.

12 http://ncp.sagepub.com/content/26/4/409 .abstract.
13 http://www.ncbi.nlm.nih.gov /pubmed/24717118.
14 http://www.ncbi.nlm.nih.gov/pmc/articles /PMC3191260/.
15 http://www.ncbi.nlm.nih.gov /pubmed/25550171.
16 http://www.ncbi.nlm.nih.gov /pubmed/25776839.
17 http://www.ncbi.nlm.nih.gov /pubmed/9619120.
18 http://www.ncbi.nlm.nih.gov /pubmed/26353411.
19 http://www.ncbi.nlm.nih.gov/pmc/articles /PMC4290459/#CR16.
20 http://www.ncbi.nlm.nih.gov/pmc/articles /PMC2748268/.
21 http://www.lib.okayama-u.ac.jp/www/acta /pdf/67_2_99.pdf.
22 https://umm.edu/health/medical/altmed /supplement/magnesium.

ARTHRITIS AND JOINT PAIN

1   http://www.hsph.harvard.edu
     /nutritionsource/omega-3-fats/.
2   http://ucsdnews.ucsd.edu/pressrelease/why
     _omega_3_oils_help_at_the_cellular_level/.
3   http://www.ncbi.nlm.nih.gov
     /pubmed/25770254; http://www.ncbi.nlm
     .nih.gov/pmc/articles/PMC1315308/; http://
     www.ncbi.nlm.nih.gov/pubmed/23983046.
4   http://www.arthritis-research.com
     /content/12/2/208#B14.
5   http://www.ncbi.nlm.nih.gov/pmc/articles
     /PMC3400101/#bibr78-1759720X11436238.
6   http://www.arthritis-research.com
     /content/12/2/208#B14.
7   http://www.womenshealthmag.com
     /nutrition/green-tea-antioxidant-content.

8   http://www.oarsijournal.com/article/S1063
     -4584(14)01276-X/fulltext.
9   http://www.ncbi.nlm.nih.gov/pmc/articles
     /PMC4230973/.
10   http://www.ncbi.nlm.nih.gov
     /pubmed/24672232.
11   http://www.equinenutriceuticals.com/pdf
     /RA-Study-BCM-95.pdf.
12   http://www.ncbi.nlm.nih.gov
     /pubmed/9619120.
13   http://www.ncbi.nlm.nih.gov
     /pubmed/25675368.
14   http://www.ncbi.nlm.nih.gov/pmc/articles
     /PMC3344210/.
15   http://www.ncbi.nlm.nih.gov
     /pubmed/23727631.

ASTHMA

1   http://www.ncbi.nlm.nih.gov/pmc/articles
     /PMC3725497/.
2   http://www.ars.usda.gov/SP2UserFiles
     /Place/80400525/Data/Flav/Flav_R03-1.pdf.
3   http://www.atsjournals.org/doi/full
     /10.1164/ajrccm.164.10.2104061
     #.VvKDU3hNxxo
4   http://www.ncbi.nlm.nih.gov/pmc/articles
     /PMC3763034/.
5   http://www.atsjournals.org/doi/full/10.1164
     /ajrccm.164.10.2104061#.VdhhK3hNxxo.
6   https://ods.od.nih.gov/factsheets/Selenium
     -HealthProfessional/.
7   http://www.nature.com/nri/journal/v15/n5
     /full/nri3830.html.

8   R. Varraso, "Nutrition and Asthma,"
     Current Allergy Asthma Reports 12 (2012):
     201–210.
9   http://www.ncbi.nlm.nih.gov/pmc
     /articles/PMC3604064/; http://www
     .ncbi.nlm.nih.gov/pmc/articles
     /PMC3930933/.
10   http://www.ncbi.nlm.nih.gov
     /pubmed/25620368.
11   R. Barros et al., "Adherence to the
     Mediterranean Diet and Fresh Fruit
     Intake Are Associated with Improved
     Asthma Control," *Allergy* 63, no. 7 (2008):
     917–23.

ATTENTION DEFICIT HYPERACTIVITY DISORDER (ADHD)

1   http://www.cdc.gov/ncbddd/adhd/features
     /key-findings-adhd72013.html.
2   http://pediatrics.aappublications.org
     /content/129/2/330.long.
3   http://www.ncbi.nlm.nih.gov/pmc/articles
     /PMC4011050/.
4   http://www.ncbi.nlm.nih.gov
     /pubmed/20631199/.
5   http://www.ncbi.nlm.nih.gov/pmc/articles
     /PMC3184556/.
6   http://www.nature.com/npp/journal/v40
     /n10/full/npp201573a.html.
7   http://www.ncbi.nlm.nih.gov
     /pubmed/24214970.
8   http://www.childpsych.theclinics.com
     /article/S1056-4993(14)00034-0/abstract.
9   http://www.clinicaltherapeutics.com
     /article/S0149-2918(15)00226-X/fulltext;
     J. T. Nigg, K. Lewis, T. Edinger, and M. Falk,
     "Meta-Analysis of Attention-Deficit/
     Hyperactivity Disorder or Attention-Deficit/

     Hyperactivity Disorder Symptoms,
     Restriction Diet, and Synthetic Food Color
     Additives," *Journal of the American
     Academy Child & Adolescent Psychiatry*
     51 (2012): 86–97.
10   http://www.ncbi.nlm.nih.gov
     /pubmed/25599186.
11   https://www.mja.com.au/journal/2013
     /198/11/salicylate-elimination-diets
     -children-food-restriction-supported
     -evidence; http://www.akademiai.com/doi
     /pdf/10.1556/AAlim.2014.0017.
12   http://www.ncbi.nlm.nih.gov/pmc/articles
     /PMC4322780/.
13   http://www.ncbi.nlm.nih.gov/pmc/articles
     /PMC4321798/.
14   http://www.ncbi.nlm.nih.gov/pmc/articles
     /PMC3441937/
15   O. Oner et al., "Effects of Zinc and Ferritin
     Levels on Parent and Teacher Reported
     Symptom Scores in Attention Deficit

Hyperactivity Disorder," *Child Psychiatry & Human Development* 41 (2010): 441–47, doi:10.1007/s10578-010-0178-1; http://www.ncbi.nlm.nih.gov/pubmed/20453262/; http://www.ncbi.nlm.nih.gov/pubmed/23082739; http://www.ncbi.nlm.nih.gov/pubmed/25364604.

16 http://www.researchgate.net/profile/Samuele_Cortese/publication/5792824

_Effects_of_iron_supplementation_on_attention_deficit_hyperactivity_disorder_in_children/links/0912f50807c56c36c9000000.pdf.

17 http://www.childpsych.theclinics.com/article/S1056-4993(14)00034-0/abstract.

18 http://www.ncbi.nlm.nih.gov/pubmed/24576365.

BACK PAIN

1 http://onlinelibrary.wiley.com/doi/10.1111/obr.12067/abstract;jsessionid=A8096ED9DA9AF753C4117A99729A6349.f02t02.

2 http://www.chiromt.com/content/21/1/15.

3 http://www.ncbi.nlm.nih.gov/pubmed/23511683.

4 http://www.ncbi.nlm.nih.gov/pmc/articles/PMC4190421/.

5 http://nutritiondata.self.com/foods-000102000000000000000.html.

6 http://www.practicalpainmanagement.com/treatments/complementary

/anti-inflammatory-diet-pain-patients?page=0,1.

7 K. S. Kuehl, "Cherry Juice Targets Antioxidant Potential and Pain Relief," *Medicine and Science in Sports and Exercise* 59 (2012): 86–93.

8 http://www.ncbi.nlm.nih.gov/pmc/articles/PMC3344210/.

9 Ibid.

10 http://commons.pacificu.edu/pa/493/.

11 https://ods.od.nih.gov/factsheets/VitaminB12-HealthProfessional/.

BLADDER INFECTIONS/URINARY TRACT INFECTIONS

1 http://www.ncbi.nlm.nih.gov/pubmed/24310806.

2 http://cnr.sagepub.com/content/23/1/54.long.

3 http://www.ncbi.nlm.nih.gov/pubmed/24499122; http://www.jurology.com/article/S0022-5347(14)04646-1/pdf.

4 http://www.ncbi.nlm.nih.gov/pubmed/25882919.

5 http://www.ncbi.nlm.nih.gov/pmc/articles/PMC3853585/.

6 Chisholm, Annie H. "Probiotics in preventing recurrent urinary tract infections in women: a literature review." *Urologic Nursing* 35 (2015): 18–21.

7 http://www.ncbi.nlm.nih.gov/pubmed/25051393.

8 http://www.ncbi.nlm.nih.gov/pubmed/24316093; http://www.andjrnl.org/article/S2212-2672(15)00371-8/abstract.

BRONCHITIS

1 http://www.pdrhealth.com/diseases/acute-bronchitis-in-adults/treatment.

2 http://umm.edu/health/medical-reference-guide/complementary-and-alternative-medicine-guide/condition/bronchitis.

3 http://www.ncbi.nlm.nih.gov/pmc/articles/PMC3249897/.

4 http://www.ncbi.nlm.nih.gov/pubmed/23583806.

5 http://www.ncbi.nlm.nih.gov/pubmed/25230520.

6 http://www.hindawi.com/journals/grp/2015/142979/#B12.

7 http://www.hindawi.com/journals/mi/2014/805841/.

8 http://www.ncbi.nlm.nih.gov/pmc/articles/PMC3942920/.

9 http://www.ncbi.nlm.nih.gov/pmc/articles/PMC3842692/.

10 http://scialert.net/fulltext/?doi=jbs.2014.1.19.

11 http://www.ncbi.nlm.nih.gov/pubmed/25924532.

12 https://www.thieme-connect.com/products/ejournals/abstract/10.1055/s-0031-1296656.

13 http://www.ncbi.nlm.nih.gov/pubmed/25823507.

14 http://www.ncbi.nlm.nih.gov/pmc/articles/PMC2957147/.

15 http://www.nutritionandmetabolism.com/content/9/1/61.

16 http://www.mdpi.com/1420-3049/20/2/3479/htm.

BRUISES

1 https://www.nlm.nih.gov/medlineplus /druginfo/natural/983.html.
2 https://www.nlm.nih.gov/medlineplus/ency /article/002407.htm.

3 http://www.altmedrev.com /publications/5/2/144.pdf.
4 Ibid.

BURNS

1 N. S. Barbosa and A. N. Kalaaji, "CAM Use in Dermatology. Is There a Potential Role for Honey, Green Tea, and Vitamin C?" *Complementary Therapies in Clinical Practice* 20, no. 1 (2014): 11–15.
2 http://www.ncbi.nlm.nih.gov /pubmed/20649832.
3 http://onlinelibrary.wiley.com/doi/10.1002 /14651858.CD005083.pub4/abstract.
4 http://www.ncbi.nlm.nih.gov /pubmed/26061489.

5 http://www.ncbi.nlm.nih.gov/pmc/articles /PMC3188210/.
6 http://www.ncbi.nlm.nih.gov /pubmed/21991225.
7 http://www.ncbi.nlm.nih.gov/pmc/articles /PMC3188105/.
8 http://www.ncbi.nlm.nih.gov /pubmed/26518672.
9 http://www.ncbi.nlm.nih.gov /pubmed/25306088.

BURSITIS

1 http://www.ncbi.nlm.nih.gov/pmc/articles /PMC3575932/.
2 http://www.ncbi.nlm.nih.gov/pmc/articles /PMC2835915/.
3 http://www.ncbi.nlm.nih.gov /pubmed/26490535.
4 http://www.ars.usda.gov/SP2UserFiles /Place/80400525/Data/Flav /Flav_R03.pdf.

5 http://www.altmedrev.com /publications/14/2/141.pdf.
6 http://www.ncbi.nlm.nih.gov /pubmed/22407780
7 http://www.ncbi.nlm.nih.gov /pubmed/16117603

CANCER

1 http://www.cancer.org/research /acsresearchupdates/more/10-must -know-2015-global-cancer-facts.
2 http://www.who.int/mediacentre/factsheets /fs297/en/.
3 Ibid.
4 http://www.cancer.gov/about-cancer/causes -prevention/risk; http://www.who.int /cancer/prevention/en/.
5 http://www.aicr.org/reduce-your-cancer -risk/weight/reduce_weight_cancer_link .html.
6 http://www.aicr.org/cancer-research -update/2015/10_28/cru_Bacon -Processed-Meats-a-Cause-of-Cancer -Your-FAQs.html.
7 Ibid.; http://www.thelancet.com/journals /lanonc/article/PIIS1470-2045(15)00444-1 /abstract.
8 http://onlinelibrary.wiley.com/doi/10.1002 /cncr.29543/abstract.
9 http://www.ncbi.nlm.nih.gov /pubmed/26192392.
10 http://www.ncbi.nlm.nih.gov /pubmed/26148912.

11 http://www.ncbi.nlm.nih.gov /pubmed/25575572.
12 http://www.ncbi.nlm.nih.gov /pubmed/24366437.
13 http://www.ncbi.nlm.nih.gov /pubmed/26148912.
14 http://www.ncbi.nlm.nih.gov /pubmed/26416794.
15 http://www.aicr.org/foods-that-fight -cancer/legumes.html#research.
16 http://www.sciencedirect.com/science /article/pii/S0308814613004561.
17 http://www.ncbi.nlm.nih.gov/pmc/articles /PMC3522559/.
18 http://www.ncbi.nlm.nih.gov /pubmed/23514011.
19 http://www.aicr.org/foods-that -fight-cancer/foodsthatfightcancer _berries.html.
20 http://pubs.acs.org/doi/abs/10.1021 /jf4044056.
21 http://www.ncbi.nlm.nih.gov /pubmed/25781639.
22 http://www.ncbi.nlm.nih.gov /pubmed/25781639.

23 http://jcp.bmj.com/content/early/2014/07/23/jclinpath-2013-202075.

24 http://www.ncbi.nlm.nih.gov/pubmed/25150116.

25 http://www.ncbi.nlm.nih.gov/pubmed/25781639.

26 http://www.ncbi.nlm.nih.gov/pubmed/26476633.

27 http://www.ncbi.nlm.nih.gov/pmc/articles/PMC4258571/.

28 http://www.ncbi.nlm.nih.gov/pubmed/25329001.

29 http://www.ncbi.nlm.nih.gov/pmc/articles/PMC4346840/.

30 http://www.ncbi.nlm.nih.gov/pubmed/26396333.

31 http://www.ncbi.nlm.nih.gov/pubmed/25781639.

32 http://www.ncbi.nlm.nih.gov/pubmed/24519559.

33 http://www.ncbi.nlm.nih.gov/pmc/articles/PMC4203935/; http://www.ncbi.nlm.nih.gov/pubmed/22815230; http://www.ncbi.nlm.nih.gov/pubmed/25684522.

34 http://www.ncbi.nlm.nih.gov/pubmed/26148912.

35 http://www.ncbi.nlm.nih.gov/pubmed/22455656.

36 http://www.ncbi.nlm.nih.gov/pmc/articles/PMC4616874/.

37 http://www.ncbi.nlm.nih.gov/pubmed/23593085.

38 http://www.ncbi.nlm.nih.gov/pubmed/24932663.

39 F. Gaascht, M. Dicato, and M. Deiderich, "Coffee Provides a Natural Multitarget Pharmacopeia Against the Hallmarks of Cancer," *Genes & Nutrition* 10, no. 6 (2015): 51.

40 Ibid.

41 http://jnci.oxfordjournals.org/content/early/2011/05/17/jnci.djr151.abstract.

42 http://www.ncbi.nlm.nih.gov/pubmed/25691730.

43 http://www.ncbi.nlm.nih.gov/pubmed/24037930.

44 F. Song, A. A. Quereshi, J. Han, "Increased Caffeine Intake Is Associated with Reduced Risk of Basal Cell Carcinoma of the Skin," *Cancer Research*, 72 (2012): 3282.

45 L. M. Ferrucci et al., "Tea, Coffee, and Caffeine and Early-Onset Basal Cell Carcinoma in a Case–Control Study," *European Journal of Cancer Prevention* 23 (2014): 296–302.

46 http://www.ncbi.nlm.nih.gov/pubmed/26298460.

47 http://www.ncbi.nlm.nih.gov/pubmed/25774338.

48 http://www.impactjournals.com/oncotarget/index.php?journal=oncotarget&page=article&op=view&path%5B%5D=4542&path%5B%5D=12753.

49 http://www.ncbi.nlm.nih.gov/pmc/articles/PMC4336706/.

50 http://www.ncbi.nlm.nih.gov/pubmed/24444040/; http://www.ncbi.nlm.nih.gov/pubmed/25740748.

51 http://www.ncbi.nlm.nih.gov/pubmed/22391648.

52 http://www.ncbi.nlm.nih.gov/pubmed/22877795.

53 http://www.ncbi.nlm.nih.gov/pubmed/23859034.

54 http://www.ncbi.nlm.nih.gov/pmc/articles/PMC2901397/.

55 http://www.ncbi.nlm.nih.gov/pubmed/22328735/.

56 http://www.ncbi.nlm.nih.gov/pmc/articles/PMC4603065/.

57 http://www.ncbi.nlm.nih.gov/pmc/articles/PMC3257702/.

58 Ibid.

59 http://www.ncbi.nlm.nih.gov/pmc/articles/PMC4517353/.

60 http://www.ncbi.nlm.nih.gov/pmc/articles/PMC4152533/.

61 http://www.aicr.org/foods-that-fight-cancer/flaxseed.html#research.

62 http://www.ncbi.nlm.nih.gov/pubmed/26298460.

63 http://www.ncbi.nlm.nih.gov/pubmed/26148912.

64 http://jeb.biologists.org/content/218/1/59.long#sec-11.

65 http://www.nature.com/bjc/journal/v112/n7/full/bjc201525a.html.

66 http://ije.oxfordjournals.org/content/37/5/1018/T4.expansion.html.

67 http://www.ncbi.nlm.nih.gov/pubmed/24615943; http://www.ncbi.nlm.nih.gov/pubmed/20449663.

68 http://www.ncbi.nlm.nih.gov/pubmed/23523869.

69 http://www.ncbi.nlm.nih.gov/pubmed/25379783.

70 http://www.hindawi.com/journals/ecam/2012/564927/.

71 http://www.ncbi.nlm.nih.gov/pubmed/18462866/.

72 http://www.ncbi.nlm.nih.gov/pubmed/12680238/.

73 http://www.ncbi.nlm.nih.gov/pmc/articles/PMC4589652/.

74 http://www.ncbi.nlm.nih.gov/pubmed/26192392.

75 http://www.ncbi.nlm.nih.gov/pmc/articles/PMC4589652/.

76 http://www.ncbi.nlm.nih.gov/pubmed/25594891

77 http://www.ncbi.nlm.nih.gov
/pubmed/9619120.

78 http://www.ncbi.nlm.nih.gov
/pubmed/25052987.

79 http://www.mdpi.com/1420-3049/19/2/2497
/htm.

80 http://www.ncbi.nlm.nih.gov
/pubmed/25052987.

81 http://www.cancerepidemiology.net/article
/S1877-7821(15)00070-3/fulltext.

82 Ibid.

83 http://www.mdpi.com/1420-3049/19/2/2497
/htm.

84 http://www.researchgate.net
/publication/271892533_The_role_of_edible
_mushrooms_in_health_Evaluation_of_the
_evidence.

85 http://www.spandidos-publications.com
/or/34/2/547.

86 http://www.ncbi.nlm.nih.gov
/pubmed/26183374.

87 I. Casari, M. Falasca, "Diet and Pancreatic
Cancer Prevention," *Cancers* 7 (2015):
2309–17.

88 http://www.ncbi.nlm.nih.gov
/pubmed/25833976; http://www.ncbi.nlm
.nih.gov/pubmed/26313936.

89 http://www.ncbi.nlm.nih.gov
/pubmed/24841279.

90 http://www.ncbi.nlm.nih.gov
/pubmed/26365989.

91 http://www.ncbi.nlm.nih.gov
/pubmed/26457243.

92 http://www.ncbi.nlm.nih.gov/pmc/articles
/PMC4152533/.

93 http://www.ncbi.nlm.nih.gov
/pubmed/26227583.

94 http://www.ncbi.nlm.nih.gov
/pubmed/25739930.

95 http://www.ncbi.nlm.nih.gov
/pubmed/26298460.

96 http://www.ncbi.nlm.nih.gov
/pubmed/26148912.

97 http://www.ncbi.nlm.nih.gov
/pubmed/24841279.

98 http://www.ncbi.nlm.nih.gov/pmc/articles
/PMC4477247/.

99 http://www.apocpcontrol.org/page
/apjcp_issues_view.php?sid=Entrez:
PubMed&id=pmid:26320438&
key=2015.16.14.5697.

100 http://www.ncbi.nlm.nih.gov/pmc/articles
/PMC4477247/.

101 http://www.ncbi.nlm.nih.gov
/pubmed/25216701.

102 http://www.ncbi.nlm.nih.gov/pmc/articles
/PMC3944519/.

103 http://www.ncbi.nlm.nih.gov
/pubmed/23613993.

104 http://www.ncbi.nlm.nih.gov/pmc/articles
/PMC4446612/.

105 http://www.hindawi.com/journals
/jo/2010/214186/.

106 http://www.ncbi.nlm.nih.gov
/pubmed/25842380.

107 http://www.ncbi.nlm.nih.gov/pmc/articles
/PMC4472533/.

108 http://ajcn.nutrition.org/content/early
/2013/10/30/ajcn.113.059352.full.pdf+html.

109 http://www.ncbi.nlm.nih.gov
/pubmed/24851879.

110 http://www.ncbi.nlm.nih.gov
/pubmed/26148912.

111 http://www.ncbi.nlm.nih.gov
/pubmed/25575572.

112 http://www.ncbi.nlm.nih.gov
/pubmed/25915188.

COLD SORES

1 http://www.ncbi.nlm.nih.gov/pmc/articles
/PMC3283972/.

2 http://www.ncbi.nlm.nih.gov
/pubmed/22390834.

3 http://www.ncbi.nlm.nih.gov
/pubmed/26031763.

4 http://www.ncbi.nlm.nih.gov
/pubmed/25860226.

COLDS

1 http://www.cmaj.ca/content
/early/2014/01/27/cmaj.121442.full.pdf+html.

2 http://bmcfampract.biomedcentral.com
/articles/10.1186/s12875-015-0237-6

3 USDA Nutrient Database zinc rich foods.
www.ndb.nal.usda.gov

4 http://nutritiondata.self.com/foods
-012124000000000000000-w
.html?maxCount=57.

5 http://www.aafp.org/afp/2013/1215/od3
.html.

6 http://www.hindawi.com/journals
/ijmicro/2015/376387/#B8.

7 http://www.ncbi.nlm.nih.gov
/pubmed/25866155.

8 http://www.ncbi.nlm.nih.gov
/pubmed/23643542.

9 http://www.ncbi.nlm.nih.gov
/pubmed/23123794.

10 http://www.cochrane.org/CD006206/ARI
_garlic-common-cold.

11 http://quranmed.com/10111.fulltext.

12 http://www.cmaj.ca/content/early/2014
    /01/27/cmaj.121442.full.pdf+html.
13 http://pediatrics.aappublications.org/content
    /early/2014/03/11/peds.2013-0652.abstract?sid
    =49de3457-2a51-4ef9-8a82-28c600abbad6.
14 http://www.ncbi.nlm.nih.gov/pmc/articles
    /PMC4054664/.

15 http://www.ncbi.nlm.nih.gov
    /pubmed/23840373; http://www
    .ncbi.nlm.nih.gov/pmc/articles
    /PMC3543548/.
16 http://www.ncbi.nlm.nih.gov/pmc/articles
    /PMC3459493/.

CONSTIPATION

1 http://www.ncbi.nlm.nih.gov
   /pubmed/23326148.
2 http://www.ncbi.nlm.nih.gov/pmc/articles
   /PMC4415962/.
3 http://www.nutritionix.com
   /search/item/513fceb875b8d
   bbc21003547.
4 All data on fiber come from the USDA
   Nutrient Database on fiber content.
   www.ndb.nal.usda.gov
5 All data on fiber come from the USDA

   Nutrient Database on fiber content.
   www.ndb.nal.usda.gov
6 http://www.ncbi.nlm.nih.gov
   /pubmed/25099542.
7 http://www.wageningenacademic.com/doi
   /abs/10.3920/BM2014.0113?url_ver=Z39.88
   -2003&rfr_id=ori:rid:crossref.org&rfr
   _dat=cr_pub%3dpubmed.
8 http://www.turkjgastroenterol.org/eng
   /makale/4463/281/Full-Text.

COUGHS

1 http://www.ncbi.nlm.nih.gov/pmc/articles
   /PMC3758027/.
2 http://www.ncbi.nlm.nih.gov
   /pubmed/18056558.
3 http://www.ncbi.nlm.nih.gov/pmc/articles
   /PMC4264806/.
4 http://www.ncbi.nlm.nih.gov/pmc/articles
   /PMC4264806/#b8-0601107.
5 http://www.coughjournal.com
   /content/9/1/27.

6 http://www.nature.com/articles/pcrj201372.
7 http://www.hindawi.com/journals
   /isrn/2014/976264/#B5.
8 http://www.ncbi.nlm.nih.gov/pmc/articles
   /PMC3842692/.
9 http://www.hindawi.com/journals
   /isrn/2014/976264/#B5.
10 http://www.ncbi.nlm.nih.gov/pmc/articles
   /PMC4369959/.

DANDRUFF

1 http://journals.plos.org
   /plospathogens/article?id=10.1371
   /journal.ppat.1002701
   #ppat.1002701-Schwartz1.
2 http://www.ncbi.nlm.nih.gov
   /pubmed/25219371.
3 http://www.ncbi.nlm.nih.gov
   /pubmed/21710859.
4 http://www.ncbi.nlm.nih.gov
   /pubmed/24117781.

5 http://lpi.oregonstate.edu/mic
   /micronutrients-health/skin-health/nutrient
   -index/essential-fatty-acids.
6 N. S. Al-Waili, "Therapeutic and Prophylactic
   Effects of Crude Honey on Chronic
   Seborrheic Dermatitis and Dandruff,"
   European Journal of Medical Research 6
   (2001): 306–8.
7 http://www.ncbi.nlm.nih.gov
   /pubmed/24305429.

DECREASED LIBIDO

1 http://www.ncbi.nlm.nih.gov/pubmed
   /21597089; http://www.ncbi.nlm.nih.gov
   /pubmed/23318529; http://www.ncbi.nlm
   .nih.gov/pubmed/22403029; http://www
   .ncbi.nlm.nih.gov/pubmed/24754044.
2 http://www.ncbi.nlm.nih.gov
   /pubmed/17673936; http://www.ncbi
   .nlm.nih.gov/pubmed/18401349.
3 http://www.ncbi.nlm.nih.gov/pmc/articles
   /PMC4199300/

4 http://nutritiondata.self.com/foods
   -000089000000000000000000.html.
5 http://www.ncbi.nlm.nih.gov
   /pubmed/24362474.
6 http://www.ncbi.nlm.nih.gov/pmc/articles
   /PMC3649098/.
7 http://www.ncbi.nlm.nih.gov
   /pubmed/21671089.
8 http://www.ncbi.nlm.nih.gov
   /pubmed/25475395.

9 http://www.ncbi.nlm.nih.gov/pmc/articles
   /PMC4411442/.
10 http://www.ncbi.nlm.nih.gov/pmc/articles
   /PMC4082836/.
11 http://www.ncbi.nlm.nih.gov/pmc/articles
   /PMC4377061/.

DEMENTIA

1 http://www.hindawi.com/journals
   /bmri/2014/908915/.
2 http://www.ncbi.nlm.nih.gov/pmc/articles
   /PMC3880612/.
3 http://www.ncbi.nlm.nih.gov/pmc/articles
   /PMC4228955/.
4 http://www.ncbi.nlm.nih.gov
   /pubmed/26230648.
5 http://www.ncbi.nlm.nih.gov
   /pubmed/21877951.
6 http://www.ncbi.nlm.nih.gov
   /pubmed/25961184.
7 http://www.ncbi.nlm.nih.gov
   /pubmed/25961184.
8 http://advances.nutrition.org
   /content/6/2/154.long.
9 http://www.alzheimersanddementia.com
   /article/S1552-5260(15)02701-6/fulltext.
10 http://www.ncbi.nlm.nih.gov/pmc/articles
   /PMC3824191/.

DEPRESSION

1 http://www.who.int/mental
   _health/management/depression
   /who_paper_depression_wfmh
   _2012.pdf.
2 http://www.ncbi.nlm.nih.gov
   /pubmed/26359904.
3 http://www.biomedcentral.com/1741
   -7015/11/3.
4 http://www.nature.com
   /aps/journal/v32/n1/full
   /aps2010184a.html.
5 http://circ.ahajournals.org
   /content/118/17/1768.long.
6 http://www.ncbi.nlm.nih.gov/pmc/articles
   /PMC4573281/.
7 http://www.ncbi.nlm.nih.gov
   /pubmed/23332529.
8 http://www.ncbi.nlm.nih.gov
   /pubmed/23295173.
9 http://www.ncbi.nlm.nih.gov/pmc/articles
   /PMC4563885/.
10 http://www.ncbi.nlm.nih.gov/pmc/articles
   /PMC4454450/.
11 http://www.ncbi.nlm.nih.gov
   /pubmed/26208984.
12 http://www.ncbi.nlm.nih.gov/pmc/articles
   /PMC4013121/.
13 http://biomedicine.cmu.edu.tw/doc
   /issue_3/2012-6-5.pdf.

12 http://www.hindawi.com/journals
   /ogi/2011/949302/.
13 http://www.ncbi.nlm.nih.gov/pmc/articles
   /PMC4161099/.
14 https://ods.od.nih.gov/factsheets/Folate
   -HealthProfessional/.

11 http://www.ncbi.nlm.nih.gov/pmc/articles
   /PMC3824191/.
12 http://www.ncbi.nlm.nih.gov
   /pubmed/26086182.
13 http://www.ncbi.nlm.nih.gov
   /pubmed/26325006.
14 http://lpi.oregonstate.edu/mic/dietary
   -factors/phytochemicals/flavonoids.
15 http://www.nature.com/neuro/journal/v17
   /n12/full/nn.3850.html.
16 http://ajcn.nutrition.org/content/101/3/538
   .full.
17 http://onlinelibrary.wiley.com/doi/10.1002
   /ana.23594/abstract;jsessionid
   =183E2BD28E03F88801DEF90
   A9840A4AA.f02t02.
18 http://www.ncbi.nlm.nih.gov/pmc/articles
   /PMC4353806/.
19 http://www.ncbi.nlm.nih.gov
   /pubmed/26366714.

14 http://www.ncbi.nlm.nih.gov
   /pubmed/26333890.
15 http://www.ncbi.nlm.nih.gov/pmc/articles
   /PMC4013121/.
16 http://www.ncbi.nlm.nih.gov
   /pubmed/22500660.
17 http://www.ncbi.nlm.nih.gov
   /pubmed/25733470; http://www.ncbi
   .nlm.nih.gov/pubmed/23636546;
   http://www.ncbi.nlm.nih.gov
   /pubmed/26397113.
18 http://www.ncbi.nlm.nih.gov
   /pubmed/26141257.
19 http://www.ncbi.nlm.nih.gov
   /pubmed/24423304.
20 http://www.ncbi.nlm.nih.gov
   /pubmed/24632894.
21 http://www.ncbi.nlm.nih.gov/pmc/articles
   /PMC3856388/.
22 http://link.springer.com/article/10.1007
   /s12011-013-9723-7.
23 http://www.ncbi.nlm.nih.gov
   /pubmed/21798601.
24 http://www.ncbi.nlm.nih.gov
   /pubmed/23453038.
25 http://www.ncbi.nlm.nih.gov
   /pubmed/19828710.
26 http://www.ncbi.nlm.nih.gov/pmc/articles
   /PMC3355196/#R23.

27 http://www.sciencedirect.com/science
/article/pii/S0195666315002287.
28 http://www.ncbi.nlm.nih.gov/pmc/articles
/PMC3984246/.

29 http://www.ncbi.nlm.nih.gov
/pubmed/22190027/; http://www.ncbi.nlm
.nih.gov/pubmed/22716932.

DIABETES

1 http://www.hsph.harvard.edu
/nutritionsource/preventing-diabetes-full
-story/#ref53.
2 http://www.who.int/mediacentre/factsheets
/fs312/en/.
3 http://www.who.int/features/factfiles
/diabetes/en/.
4 http://www.ncbi.nlm.nih.gov
/pubmed/22649266.
5 http://circ.ahajournals.org/content/131
/Suppl_1/A20.short.
6 http://www.ncbi.nlm.nih.gov/pmc/articles
/PMC3658901/.
7 http://jn.nutrition.org/content/143/9/1474
.long?utm_source=hs_email&utm_medium
=email&utm_content=11473588&_hsenc
=p2ANqtz-_h-f4ghFnYnnV5yFSAYQ4uC
_gtIlRQb0g0Dz2F6QDymd7no0ydmOzRwnh
aOO2I4MXKa6NDWQXV8b-OLVZC
_F3F5lwd8A&_hsmi=11473588#T5.
8 http://jn.nutrition.org/content/144/2/202
.full?sid=3e44c2bb-e2d7-4ec4-891e-
d615ec308daa.
9 J. L. Rios et al., "Natural Products for the
Treatment of Type 2 Diabetes Mellitus,"
Planta Medica 81 (2015): 975–94.
10 http://pubs.acs.org/doi/abs/10.1021/acs
.jafc.5b00776.
11 https://www.thieme-connect.com/products
/ejournals/abstract/10.1055/s-0035-1546131.
12 http://www.ncbi.nlm.nih.gov
/pubmed/26002927.
13 http://www.ncbi.nlm.nih.gov/pmc/articles
/PMC3898757/.
14 J. L. Rios et al., "Natural Products for the
Treatment of Type 2 Diabetes Mellitus,"
Planta Medica 81 (2015): 975–94.

15 http://www.ncbi.nlm.nih.gov/pmc/articles
/PMC4344557/.
16 http://www.ncbi.nlm.nih.gov/pmc/articles
/PMC3980034/.
17 http://www.jbc.org/content/early/2015
/09/02/jbc.M115.672097.long.
18 http://www.nutritionj.com/content/13/1/102.
19 http://www.ncbi.nlm.nih.gov
/pubmed/26436069.
20 http://www.ncbi.nlm.nih.gov/pmc/articles
/PMC3857752/.
21 http://www.ncbi.nlm.nih.gov/pmc/articles
/PMC3476912/.
22 http://www.ncbi.nlm.nih.gov
/pubmed/25745485.
23 http://www.nutritionj.com/content/13/1/102.
24 http://www.ncbi.nlm.nih.gov/pmc/articles
/PMC4609100/.
25 http://www.ncbi.nlm.nih.gov/pmc/articles
/PMC4296439/#ref57.
26 http://www.krepublishers.com/02
-Journals/S-EM/EM-03-0-000-09-Web
/EM-03-1-000-2009-Abst-PDF/EM-03-1
-005-09-098-Kochhar-A/EM-03-1-005-09
-098-Kochhar-A-Tt.pdf.
27 http://www.ncbi.nlm.nih.gov/pmc/articles
/PMC3695574/.
28 http://www.ncbi.nlm.nih.gov
/pubmed/24490949.
29 http://www.ncbi.nlm.nih.gov
/pubmed/24559810.
30 http://www.ncbi.nlm.nih.gov
/pubmed/19177188.
31 http://www.ncbi.nlm.nih.gov
/pubmed/24050577.
32 http://www.ncbi.nlm.nih.gov/pmc/articles
/PMC4310066/.

DIARRHEA

1 http://www.who.int/selection_medicines
/committees/expert/20/EML_2015
_FINAL_amended_JUN2015.pdf
?ua=1.
2 http://rehydrate.org/solutions/homemade
.htm#recipe.
3 S.F. Salfi and K. Holt, "The Role of Probiotics
in Diarrheal Management," *Holistic
Nursing Practice* 26, no. 3 (May–June 2012):
142–9.
4 http://pediatrics.aappublications.org
/content/early/2014/03/11/peds.2013
-0652.full.pdf+html.

5 http://www.ncbi.nlm.nih.gov
/pubmed/21069673.
6 http://www.ncbi.nlm.nih.gov
/pubmed/19379128.
7 http://www.ncbi.nlm.nih.gov
/pubmed/25784748.
8 http://www.ncbi.nlm.nih.gov
/pubmed/19268266.
9 http://www.ncbi.nlm.nih.gov
/pubmed/26200040.

DIVERTICULITIS

1   http://www.ncbi.nlm.nih.gov
    /pubmed/26289102.
2   http://www.ncbi.nlm.nih.gov/pmc/articles
    /PMC3785555/.
3   http://www.ncbi.nlm.nih.gov
    /pubmed/26289102.
4   http://www.uptodate.com/contents/colonic
    -diverticulosis-and-diverticular-disease
    -epidemiology-risk-factors-and
    -pathogenesis/abstract/51.
5   http://www.ncbi.nlm.nih.gov
    /pubmed/26251177.

DRY EYES

1   http://www.ncbi.nlm.nih.gov
    /pubmed/24240351.
2   http://www.ncbi.nlm.nih.gov
    /pubmed/22336631.
3   http://www.ncbi.nlm.nih.gov/pmc/articles
    /PMC3874521/.
4   http://www.ncbi.nlm.nih.gov
    /pubmed/25697893.
5   http://www.ncbi.nlm.nih.gov
    /pubmed/25719253.
6   http://www.ncbi.nlm.nih.gov
    /pubmed/26269110.
7   https://ods.od.nih.gov/factsheets/VitaminA
    -HealthProfessional/.

DRY MOUTH

1   http://www.ada.org/~/media/ADA
    /Science%20and%20Research/Files/CSA
    _Managing_Xerostomia.ashx.
2   http://www.researchgate.net
    /publication/225062011_Established_and
    _Novel_Approaches_for_the_Management
    _of_Hyposalivation_and_Xerostomia
    ?enrichId=rgreq-63be0377-8bc4-4a32-81d5
    -4cf349821805&enrichSource=Y292ZXJQY
    WdlOzIyNTA2MjAxMTtBUzoxMDMwMz
    k3ODg2NTA1MDVAMTQwMTU3ODAw
    ODU2Mg%3D%3D&el=1_x_2.
3   http://www.ncbi.nlm.nih.gov
    /pubmed/25617026.

DRY SKIN

1   http://www.ncbi.nlm.nih.gov
    /pubmed/12376390; http://www.ncbi.nlm
    .nih.gov/pubmed/20620753.
2   http://www.ncbi.nlm.nih.gov
    /pubmed/26058417.
3   http://www.ncbi.nlm.nih.gov
    /pubmed/23685373.
4   http://www.ncbi.nlm.nih.gov
    /pubmed/26428734.
5   http://www.ncbi.nlm.nih.gov
    /pubmed/23682371.
6   http://www.ncbi.nlm.nih.gov
    /pubmed/22955355.
7   http://www.ncbi.nlm.nih.gov
    /pubmed/21084879.
8   http://lpi.oregonstate.edu
    /mic/micronutrients-health/skin
    -health/nutrient-index/essential
    -fatty-acids.
9   http://www.ncbi.nlm.nih.gov
    /pubmed/18761778.
10 http://lpi.oregonstate.edu/mic
    /micronutrients-health/skin-health
    /nutrient-index/vitamin-E.
11 http://www.ncbi.nlm.nih.gov/pubmed
    /?term=coconut+oil+epidermal
    +hydration.
12 http://www.ncbi.nlm.nih.gov
    /pubmed/26161938.

EARACHE

1   http://www.ncbi.nlm.nih.gov/pmc/articles
    /PMC3725497/.
2   http://www.ars.usda.gov/News/docs
    .htm?docid=6231
3   http://www.ncbi.nlm.nih.gov
    /pubmed/19460262.
4   http://www.ncbi.nlm.nih.gov/pmc/articles
    /PMC4391953/.
5   http://www.ncbi.nlm.nih.gov
    /pubmed/15871121.
6   https://www.nlm.nih.gov/medlineplus/ency
    /article/000619.htm.
7   http://www.ncbi.nlm.nih.gov
    /pubmed/26322459.
8   http://www.ncbi.nlm.nih.gov/pmc/articles
    /PMC2952292/.
9   http://www.ncbi.nlm.nih.gov/pmc/articles
    /PMC3259400/.

ECZEMA

1   http://www.ncbi.nlm.nih.gov /pubmed/25622761.
2   http://www.ncbi.nlm.nih.gov /pubmed/26198702.
3   http://www.ncbi.nlm.nih.gov /pubmed/23682371.
4   http://www.ncbi.nlm.nih.gov/pmc /articles/PMC4471811/.
5   http://www.ncbi.nlm.nih.gov /pubmed/22955355.
6   http://www.ncbi.nlm.nih.gov/pmc/articles /PMC4516989/.
7   http://www.ncbi.nlm.nih.gov /pubmed/26224067.
8   http://www.ncbi.nlm.nih.gov /pubmed/25869743.
9   http://www.ncbi.nlm.nih.gov/pmc/articles /PMC4470215/.
10 http://www.ncbi.nlm.nih.gov /pubmed/25967637.
11 http://www.ncbi.nlm.nih.gov /pubmed/26466117.
12 http://www.ncbi.nlm.nih.gov/pmc/articles /PMC3535097/.
13 http://www.ncbi.nlm.nih.gov/pmc/articles /PMC3529416/.
14 http://www.ncbi.nlm.nih.gov/pmc/articles /PMC3314669/.
15 N. S. Al-Waili, "Therapeutic and Prophylactic Effects of Crude Honey on Chronic Seborrheic Dermatitis and Dandruff," *European Journal of Medical Research* 6 (2001): 306–8.
16 http://www.ncbi.nlm.nih.gov /pubmed/21084879.
17 http://lpi.oregonstate.edu/mic /micronutrients-health/skin-health /nutrient-index/essential-fatty-acids.
18 http://www.ncbi.nlm.nih.gov /pubmed/18761778.
19 http://lpi.oregonstate.edu/mic /micronutrients-health/skin-health /nutrient-index/vitamin-E.

ERECTION PROBLEMS, ERECTILE DYSFUNCTION

1   http://www.ncbi.nlm.nih.gov /pubmed/16564129.
2   http://nutritiondata.self.com/foods -00008900000000000000000.html.
3   http://www.ncbi.nlm.nih.gov /pubmed/24362474.
4   http://www.ncbi.nlm.nih.gov/pmc/articles /PMC4460349/.
5   http://www.ncbi.nlm.nih.gov /pubmed/25764393.
6   http://www.ncbi.nlm.nih.gov/pmc/articles /PMC3575935/.
7   http://www.ncbi.nlm.nih.gov /pubmed/17568759.
8   http://www.ncbi.nlm.nih.gov/pmc/articles /PMC3622365/.
9   http://www.ncbi.nlm.nih.gov/pmc/articles /PMC3720104/.
10 http://synapse.koreamed.org/search .php?where=aview&id=10.4111 /kju.2009.50.2.159&code=0020KJU& vmode=FULL.
11 http://www.ncbi.nlm.nih.gov/pmc/articles /PMC4236337/.
12 https://ods.od.nih.gov/factsheets/Folate -HealthProfessional/.

FATIGUE

1   http://www.cdc.gov/nutritionreport /pdf/4Page_%202nd%20Nutrition %20Report_508_032912.pdf.
2   http://lpi.oregonstate.edu/mic/vitamins /vitamin-B6.
3   http://lpi.oregonstate.edu/mic/minerals /iron.
4   http://nutritiondata.self.com /foods-0001020000000000000000 .html.
5   http://www.ncbi.nlm.nih.gov /pubmed/23983338.
6   http://www.ncbi.nlm.nih.gov /pubmed/21315814.
7   http://nutritiondata.self.com/foods -009101000000000000000-1w.html.
8   http://lpi.oregonstate.edu/mic/vitamins /vitamin-C.
9   http://www.ncbi.nlm.nih.gov /pubmed/17955479.
10 http://www.ncbi.nlm.nih.gov /pubmed/23603951.
11 http://jop.sagepub.com/content/29 /5/642.
12 http://www.ncbi.nlm.nih.gov /pubmed/26244378.
13 http://www.ncbi.nlm.nih.gov /pubmed/17955479.

FIBROCYSTIC BREASTS

1   http://www.ncbi.nlm.nih.gov
    /pubmed/25922691.
2   http://www.ncbi.nlm.nih.gov
    /pubmed/24887724.
3   http://www.ncbi.nlm.nih.gov/pmc/articles
    /PMC2884331/.
4   http://www.ncbi.nlm.nih.gov/pmc/articles
    /PMC2884330/.

5   http://www.ncbi.nlm.nih.gov
    /pubmed/22492774.
6   http://www.ncbi.nlm.nih.gov
    /pubmed/24709924.
7   http://www.ncbi.nlm.nih.gov
    /pubmed/22622809.
8   http://www.ncbi.nlm.nih.gov/pmc/articles
    /PMC3782413/.

FIBROMYALGIA

1   http://www.sciencedirect.com/science
    /article/pii/S2255502115000899.
2   http://www.ncbi.nlm.nih.gov
    /pubmed/24373370.
3   http://www.ncbi.nlm.nih.gov
    /pubmed/25786053.
4   http://www.painphysicianjournal.com
    /linkout?issn=1533-3159&vol=18&page
    =E877; http://www.ncbi.nlm.nih
    .gov/pubmed/20498201.
5   http://www.ncbi.nlm.nih.gov
    /pubmed/24730754.
6   http://www.ncbi.nlm.nih.gov
    /pubmed/24315268.
7   http://www.ncbi.nlm.nih.gov
    /pubmed/24438771.

8   http://link.springer.com
    /article/10.1007%2Fs10067-006-0348-5.
9   http://nutritiondata.self.com/foods
    -000102000000000000000.html.
10 http://www.ncbi.nlm.nih.gov
    /pubmed/11408989.
11 http://www.ncbi.nlm.nih.gov
    /pubmed/22766026.
12 http://www.ncbi.nlm.nih.gov
    /pubmed/23765203.
13 http://www.ncbi.nlm.nih.gov/pmc/articles
    /PMC4209093/.
14 http://www.ncbi.nlm.nih.gov
    /pubmed/25119831.
15 http://www.ncbi.nlm.nih.gov
    /pubmed/25956352.

FLATULENCE

1   http://www.ncbi.nlm.nih.gov
    /pubmed/26393648.
2   http://www.ncbi
    .nlm.nih.gov/pubmed
    /24548289.

3   A full list can be found at http://www.ibsdiets
    .org/fodmap-diet/fodmap-food-list/ and
    http://www.researchgate.net/publication
    /272515985_Role_of_FODMAPs_in_Patients
    _With_Irritable_Bowel_Syndrome.

FOOD ALLERGIES

1   http://www.ncbi.nlm.nih.gov
    /pubmed/25481434.
2   http://www.ncbi.nlm.nih.gov
    /pubmed/26456449.
3   http://www.karger.com
    /Article/FullText/369340;
    http://www.ncbi.nlm
    .nih.gov/pubmed/26044855.
4   http://www.nejm.org/doi/full/10.1056
    /NEJMoa1414850#t=articleResults.

5   http://pediatrics.aappublications.org
    /content/136/3/600.long.
6   http://pediatrics.aappublications.org
    /content/early/2013/11/12/peds.2012
    -3692.full.pdf+html.
7   http://www.ncbi.nlm.nih.gov
    /pubmed/23594506.

FUNGAL INFECTIONS (GENERAL, YEAST INFECTIONS, CANDIDIASIS)

1   http://eds.a.ebscohost.com/eds/detail
    /detail?sid=c1596096-74e8-454b-919d
    -0be2995bcd0a%40sessio
    nmgr4003&vid=0&hid=4102&bdata
    =JnNpdGU9ZWRzLWxpdmU
    %3d#AN=89767667&db=f6h

2   Ibid.
3   Ibid.
4   http://www.ncbi.nlm.nih.gov
    /pubmed/25219289.
5   http://www.ncbi.nlm.nih.gov
    /pubmed/24057219.

6 http://femspd.oxfordjournals.org /content/70/3/432.long.

7 http://eds.a.ebscohost.com/eds/detail /detail?sid=104be252-4da3-4ef2-b9cd -99b32d2da64f%40session- mgr4004&vid=0&hid=4102&bdata =JnNpdGU9ZWRzLWxpdmU%3d #db=a9h&AN=99956496

8 http://www.ncbi.nlm.nih.gov /pubmed/23210319.

9 http://eds.a.ebscohost.com/eds/detail /detail?sid=ec3b8ce8-1472-4760-a7c3 -82a450736094%40session- mgr4001&vid=0&hid=4102&bdata =JnNpdGU9ZWRzLWxpdmU%3d#AN=89588573&db=a9h

10 http://www.ncbi.nlm.nih.gov/pmc/articles /PMC3903393/.

11 http://www.ncbi.nlm.nih.gov /pubmed/25362524.

12 http://www.ncbi.nlm.nih.gov /pubmed/17251510.

13 http://www.ncbi.nlm.nih.gov/pmc/articles /PMC4103721/; http://www.ncbi.nlm.nih .gov/pubmed/12174037/.

14 http://www.ncbi.nlm.nih.gov/pmc/articles /PMC1360273/.

15 http://www.ncbi.nlm.nih.gov /pubmed/17651080.

16 http://www.ncbi.nlm.nih.gov/pmc/articles /PMC3101062/.

17 http://www.ncbi.nlm.nih.gov /pubmed/25605775.

18 http://www.ncbi.nlm.nih.gov /pubmed/23721186.

FUNGAL INFECTIONS (NAILS)

1 http://www.ncbi.nlm.nih.gov /pubmed/26481920.

2 Ibid.

3 http://www.ncbi.nlm.nih.gov /pubmed/21209346.

4 http://www.ncbi.nlm.nih.gov /pubmed/26481920.

5 http://www.ncbi.nlm.nih.gov /pubmed/26427766.

6 http://www.ncbi.nlm.nih.gov/pmc /articles/PMC3770062/.

7 http://www.ncbi.nlm.nih.gov/pmc/articles /PMC3874089/#B21.

8 Ibid.

9 http://www.ncbi.nlm.nih.gov/pmc/articles /PMC4353666/

10 http://www.ncbi.nlm.nih.gov/pmc/articles /PMC4345801/.

11 http://www.ncbi.nlm.nih.gov /pubmed/25953414.

GALLSTONES

1 http://www.ncbi.nlm.nih.gov/pmc/articles /PMC4438647/.

2 http://www.ncbi.nlm.nih.gov /pubmed/26198295.

3 http://www.ncbi.nlm.nih.gov /pubmed/25020181.

4 http://www.cghjournal.org/article/S1542 -3565(13)01837-5/fulltext.

5 http://www.ncbi.nlm.nih.gov /pubmed/24045793.

6 http://www.ncbi.nlm.nih.gov /pubmed/12587687.

7 http://www.ncbi.nlm.nih.gov /pubmed/23495001.

8 http://www.ncbi.nlm.nih.gov/pmc/articles /PMC4310066/.

GASTRITIS

1 http://www.ncbi.nlm.nih.gov /pubmed/25901896

2 http://www.ncbi.nlm.nih.gov/pmc/articles /PMC3770045/; http://www.academia.edu /3468803/Herbs_Used_In_Peptic_Ulcer_A _Review; http://www.ncbi.nlm.nih.gov /pubmed/19399927; http://www.ncbi.nlm.nih .gov/pubmed/24647097; http://www.academia .edu/3468803/Herbs_Used_In_Peptic_Ulcer _A_Review; http://www.ncbi.nlm.nih.gov /pmc/articles/PMC3535097/; http://www.ncbi.nlm.nih.gov /pubmed/25799054; http://www.ncbi .nlm.nih.gov/pubmed/16621751.

3 http://www.wjgnet.com/1007-9327 /full/v20/i30/10368.htm #__sec4.

4 http://www.ncbi.nlm.nih.gov/pmc/articles /PMC4080703/.

5 http://www.ncbi.nlm.nih.gov/books /NBK92775/.

6 http://www.ncbi.nlm.nih.gov/pmc/articles /PMC4137549/.

7 http://www.ncbi.nlm.nih.gov/pmc /articles/PMC3123991/#B17; M. N. Asl and H. Hosseinzadeh, "Review of Pharmacological Effects of *Glycyrrhiza* sp. and Its Bioactive Compounds,"

HAIR LOSS

1. https://www.aad.org/public/skin-hair-nails /hair-care/female-pattern-hair-loss
2. http://www.ncbi.nlm.nih.gov /pubmed/26278532.
3. http://ndb.nal.usda.gov/ndb /nutrients/report/nutrientsfrm ?max=25&offset=0&totCount =0&nutrient1=203&nutrient2=& nutrient3=&subset=0&fg=&sort =c&measureby=m.
4. http://ndb.nal.usda.gov/ndb/nutrients /report/nutrientsfrm?max=25 &offset=0&totCount=0&nutrient1 =203&nutrient2=&nutrient3 =&subset=0&fg=&sort=c& measureby=m.
5. http://www.ncbi.nlm.nih.gov/pmc/articles /PMC3509882/.
6. http://www.ncbi.nlm.nih.gov/pmc/articles /PMC4389977/#B12.
7. http://onlinelibrary.wiley.com/doi/10.1111 /jocd.12127/epdf.
8. http://www.ncbi.nlm.nih.gov /pubmed/23772161.
9. http://www.ncbi.nlm.nih.gov /pubmed/23428658.
10. http://www.ncbi.nlm.nih.gov/pmc/articles /PMC4418416/.
11. http://www.ncbi.nlm.nih.gov /pubmed/26147750.
12. http://www.ncbi.nlm.nih.gov /pubmed/24371385.
13. http://www.ncbi.nlm.nih.gov /pubmed/24887725.
14. http://www.ncbi.nlm.nih.gov /pubmed/12715094.
15. http://www.ncbi.nlm.nih.gov /pubmed/25842469.

HALITOSIS

1. http://www.eurekalert.org/pub _releases/2003-05/uoia-tfb051403 .php; http://www.ncbi.nlm.nih.gov /pmc/articles/PMC4415245/; http://www.ncbi.nlm.nih.gov /pubmed/22226360.
2. http://consumer.healthday.com /dental-and-oral-information-9 /bad-breath-54/yogurt-may-chase -away-bad-breath-524456.html.
3. http://www.nature.com/ijos/journal/v4/n2 /full/ijos201239a.html#bib109.
4. S. Asokan et al., "Effect of Oil Pulling on Halitosis and Microorganisms Causing Halitosis: A Randomized Controlled Pilot Trial," *Journal of the Indian Society of Pedodontics and Preventive Dentistry* 29 (2011): 90–4.
5. http://www.ncbi.nlm.nih.gov /pubmed/18408265.
6. http://www.ncbi.nlm.nih.gov /pubmed/19336860?dopt=Abstract.
7. http://www.ncbi.nlm.nih.gov/pmc/articles /PMC2948765/.

HEADACHES/MIGRAINES

1. http://www.ncbi.nlm.nih.gov/pmc/articles /PMC4227630/.
2. http://headache.wwwss14.a2hosted.com /wp-contentuploads/2015/01/237149311 -Low-Tyramine-Headache-Diet-from-the -National-Headache-Foundation.pdf.
3. http://www.ncbi.nlm.nih.gov /pubmed/26252585.
4. http://www.ncbi.nlm.nih.gov /pubmed/26252588.
5. http://www.ncbi.nlm.nih.gov /pubmed/26120333.
6. http://www.ncbi.nlm.nih.gov /pubmed/25790451.
7. http://www.nlm.nih.gov/medlineplus /druginfo/natural/957.html.
8. http://www.ncbi.nlm.nih.gov/pmc/articles /PMC4359851/.
9. http://www.ncbi.nlm.nih.gov /pubmed/26056551.
10. http://lpi.oregonstate.edu/mic/vitamins /vitamin-B6.
11. http://www.ncbi.nlm.nih.gov/pmc/articles /PMC4586582/; http://www.ncbi.nlm.nih .gov/pubmed/22426836.
12. http://www.ncbi.nlm.nih.gov/pmc/articles /PMC4586582/.
13. http://www.ncbi.nlm.nih.gov/pubmed /20490742; http://www.ncbi.nlm.nih .gov/pubmed/22644176.

HEART DISEASE (CARDIOVASCULAR DISEASE)

1. https://www.heart.org/idc/groups /ahamah-public/@wcm/@sop/@smd /documents/downloadable/ucm _470704.pdf.
2. http://www.ncbi.nlm.nih.gov /pubmed/25894796.
3. http://www.ncbi.nlm.nih.gov /pubmed/26429084.

Phytotherapy Research 22 (2008): 709–24.

8   Ibid.

GINGIVITIS

1   http://www.ncbi.nlm.nih.gov /pubmed/26487430.
2   http://www.ncbi.nlm.nih.gov /pubmed/23507683.
3   http://www.ncbi.nlm.nih.gov /pubmed/25359326.
4   http://www.hsph.harvard.edu /nutritionsource/calcium-sources/.
5   http://europepmc.org/abstract /MED/16878680/reload=0;jsessionid =eXZz55eCzn35pKmXiwG8.24.
6   S. Slawik et al., "Probiotics Affect the Clinical Inflammatory Parameters of Experimental Gingivitis in Humans," *European Journal of Clinical Nutrition* 65 (2011): 857–63, doi: 10.1038/ejcn.2011.45.
7   http://onlinelibrary.wiley.com/doi/10.1111 /idh.12071/full.
8   http://www.njms.in/article.asp ?issn=0975-5950;year=2015;volume=6;issue =1;spage=67;epage=71;aulast=Singh.

9   http://www.ncbi.nlm.nih.gov/pmc/articles /PMC2995283/.

9   http://www.ncbi.nlm.nih.gov/pmc/articles /PMC3633300/.
10   http://www.ncbi.nlm.nih.gov /pubmed/25610918.
11   http://www.ncbi.nlm.nih.gov /pubmed/26321324.
12   http://www.ncbi.nlm.nih.gov /pubmed/22226360.
13   http://www.ncbi.nlm.nih.gov/pmc/articles /PMC3303561/
14   http://www.ncbi.nlm.nih.gov /pubmed/22030309
15   http://www.ncbi.nlm.nih.gov /pubmed/18408265
16   http://www.ncbi.nlm.nih.gov /pubmed/19336860?dopt=Abstract
17   http://www.ncbi.nlm.nih.gov /pubmed/25838632

GLAUCOMA

1   http://www.ncbi.nlm.nih.gov /pubmed/26340868.
2   http://www.ncbi.nlm.nih.gov/pmc/articles /PMC3703386/.
3   http://www.ncbi.nlm.nih.gov /pubmed/24912005.
4   http://www.ncbi.nlm.nih.gov/pmc/articles /PMC4149344/.
5   http://www.ncbi.nlm.nih.gov/pmc/articles /PMC2727664/.

6   http://www.ncbi.nlm.nih.gov/pmc/articles /PMC2734559/
7   http://www.ncbi.nlm.nih.gov/pmc/articles /PMC3448787/.
8   http://www.ncbi.nlm.nih.gov/pmc/articles /PMC3374099/.
9   http://www.ncbi.nlm.nih.gov /pubmed/24290344.
10   http://onlinelibrary.wiley.com/doi/10.1111 /j.1755-3768.2011.02356.x/epdf.

GOUT

1   http://www.ncbi.nlm.nih.gov /pubmed/23089274.
2   http://www.ncbi.nlm.nih.gov/pmc/articles /PMC4119792/.
3   http://www.ncbi.nlm.nih.gov /pubmed/25971955.
4   http://www.ncbi.nlm.nih.gov /pubmed/24527421.
5   http://www.ncbi.nlm.nih.gov /pubmed/15838248; http://www.ncbi .nlm.nih.gov/pubmed/21859653.
6   http://www.ncbi.nlm.nih.gov /pubmed/20035225.
7   http://www.ncbi.nlm.nih.gov /pubmed/23681955.
8   http://www.ncbi.nlm.nih.gov /pubmed/25287939.

9   http://www.ncbi.nlm.nih.gov /pubmed/21671418.
10   http://www.ncbi.nlm.nih.gov/pmc/articles /PMC4119792/; http://www.ncbi.nlm.nih .gov/pubmed/26082349.
11   R. Terkeltaub, "Are Cherries Now Ripe for Use as a Complementary Therapeutic in Gout? Appraisal of the State of Evidence," *Evidence Based Medicine* 18, no. 6 (December 2013): 230–31.
12   http://www.ncbi.nlm.nih.gov /pubmed/23023818.
13   http://www.ncbi.nlm.nih.gov /pubmed/26082349.

4   http://www.ncbi.nlm.nih.gov
    /pubmed/26279608.
5   http://www.ncbi.nlm.nih.gov/pmc/articles
    /PMC4332633/.
6   http://www.ncbi.nlm.nih.gov
    /pubmed/22875558.
7   http://www.ncbi.nlm.nih.gov
    /pubmed/25510863.
8   http://www.ncbi.nlm.nih.gov/pmc
    /articles/PMC4586551/.
9   http://www.ncbi.nlm.nih.gov
    /pubmed/25449821.
10 http://www.heart.org/HEARTORG
    /GettingHealthy/Nutrition
    Center/HealthyEating/Alcohol
    -and-Heart-Health_UCM
    _305173_Article.jsp#.Vh6wl3hNxxo.
11 http://www.ncbi.nlm.nih.gov
    /pubmed/25207479.
12 http://www.ncbi.nlm.nih.gov
    /pubmed/26363438.
13 http://www.nejm.org/doi/full
    /10.1056/NEJMoa1200303#t
    =articleDiscussion.
14 http://ajcn.nutrition.org/content/102/1/172
    .full.pdf+html.
15 http://advances.nutrition.org/content/3/1/39
    .full; http://www.ncbi.nlm.nih.gov/pmc
    /articles/PMC3262612/.
16 http://www.ncbi.nlm.nih.gov
    /pubmed/25915608.
17 Ibid.
18 http://nutritionreviews.oxford
    journals.org/content/73/suppl_2
    /120.long.

19 http://hyper.ahajournals.org
    /content/61/1/42.
20 http://www.ncbi.nlm.nih.gov
    /pubmed/26148914.
21 Ibid.
22 http://www.sciencedirect.com/science
    /article/pii/S0026049513003879.
23 http://www.europeanreview.org/wp
    /wp-content/uploads/441-445.pdf.
24 Ibid.
25 Ibid.
26 https://www.jstage.jst.go.jp/article
    /ihj/56/3/56_14-243/_pdf.
27 http://www.ncbi.nlm.nih.gov
    /pubmed/12442909.
28 http://www.ncbi.nlm.nih.gov
    /pubmed/26429077.
29 http://www.ncbi.nlm.nih.gov/pmc/articles
    /PMC4548168/.
30 http://www.ncbi.nlm.nih.gov/pmc/articles
    /PMC4477151/.
31 http://www.ncbi.nlm.nih.gov
    /pubmed/24941669.
32 http://www.ncbi.nlm.nih.gov
    /pubmed/25749238.
33 http://www.ncbi.nlm.nih.gov
    /pubmed/22944717.
34 http://www.ncbi.nlm.nih.gov
    /pubmed/25749238.
35 http://www.ncbi.nlm.nih.gov/pmc/articles
    /PMC4387232/.
36 http://www.ncbi.nlm.nih.gov
    /pubmed/24274771.
37 http://www.ncbi.nlm.nih.gov/pmc/articles
    /PMC4594054/.

HEARTBURN

1   http://www.ncbi.nlm.nih.gov
    /pubmed/25956834.
2   http://www.fda.gov/Food
    /FoodborneIllnessContaminants
    /CausesOfIllnessBadBugBook/ucm
    122561.htm.
3   http://foodscience.caes.uga.edu/extension
    /documents/FDAapproximatep
    Hoffoodslacf-phs.pdf.
4   http://www.ncbi.nlm.nih.gov/books
    /NBK92775/.
5   http://www.ncbi.nlm.nih.gov/pmc/articles
    /PMC4137549/.

6   http://www.ncbi.nlm.nih.gov/pmc/articles
    /PMC3123991/#B17; M. N. Asl and
    H. Hosseinzadeh, "Review of
    Pharmacological Effects of *Glycyrrhiza*sp.
    and Its Bioactive Compounds," *Phytotherapy
    Research* 22 (2008): 709–24.
7   http://umm.edu/health/medical/altmed
    /herb/licorice.
8   Ibid.
9   http://www.ncbi.nlm.nih.gov/pmc/articles
    /PMC2995283/.
10 http://www.ncbi.nlm.nih.gov/pmc/articles
    /PMC4080703/.

HEMORRHOIDS

1   http://www.ncbi.nlm.nih.gov
    /pubmed/16405552/.
2   http://www.ncbi.nlm.nih.gov
    /pubmed/24305429.
3   N. S. Al-Waili et al., "The Safety and
    Efficacy of a Mixture of Honey, Olive
    Oil, and Beeswax for the Management
    of Hemorrhoids and Anal Fissure:

A Pilot Study," *TSW Holistic Health &
Medicine* 1 (2006): 26–33, doi:10.1100
/tswhhm.2006.5.
4   http://www.ncbi.nlm.nih.gov
    /pubmed/26061489.

HIGH BLOOD PRESSURE (HYPERTENSION)

1 http://www.nhlbi.nih.gov/news/press -releases/2015/landmark-nih-study-shows -intensive-blood-pressure-management-may -save-lives.

2 http://content.onlinejacc.org/article .aspx?articleid=2445324.

3 http://www.ncbi.nlm.nih.gov /pubmed/22895979.

4 http://www.ncbi.nlm.nih.gov/pmc/articles /PMC4460349/.

5 http://www.ncbi.nlm.nih.gov /pubmed/25441094.

6 http://www.ncbi.nlm.nih.gov /pubmed/26016594.

7 http://www.ncbi.nlm.nih.gov /pubmed/25137341.

8 http://www.ncbi.nlm.nih.gov /pubmed/26141200.

9 http://www.ncbi.nlm.nih.gov/pmc/articles /PMC4123567/.

10 http://www.ncbi.nlm.nih.gov /pubmed/25557383.

11 http://www.ncbi.nlm.nih.gov /pubmed/25578927.

12 http://naturalmedicinejournal.com/journal /2013-04/pilot-study-evaluate-antihyper tensive-effect-celery-extract-mild-moderate.

13 http://www.ncbi.nlm.nih.gov/pubmed /23735001; http://www.ncbi.nlm.nih.gov /pubmed/25352064.

14 http://www.ncbi.nlm.nih.gov /pubmed/26101753.

15 http://www.ncbi.nlm.nih.gov/pmc/articles /PMC4116579/.

16 http://www.ncbi.nlm.nih.gov /pubmed/25809855.

17 http://www.ncbi.nlm.nih.gov/pmc/articles /PMC4484644/.

18 http://www.ncbi.nlm.nih.gov /pubmed/25740909.

19 http://www.ncbi.nlm.nih.gov /pubmed/26071633.

20 http://www.ncbi.nlm.nih.gov /pubmed/25403867.

21 http://www.ncbi.nlm.nih.gov/pmc/articles /PMC4525132/.

22 http://www.ncbi.nlm.nih.gov /pubmed/25683748.

23 http://www.ncbi.nlm.nih.gov/pmc/articles /PMC4245587/.

24 http://www.ncbi.nlm.nih.gov/pmc/articles /PMC4317480/.

25 http://www.ncbi.nlm.nih.gov /pubmed/26129945.

26 http://www.ncbi.nlm.nih.gov /pubmed/23558164.

27 http://www.ncbi.nlm.nih.gov /pubmed/25149893.

HIGH CHOLESTEROL

1 http://health.gov/dietaryguidelines/2015 -BINDER/meeting7/docs/DGAC-Meeting -7-SC-1.pdf.

2 http://www.ncbi.nlm.nih.gov/pmc/articles /PMC4330060/.

3 http://www.ncbi.nlm.nih.gov /pubmed/24394704.

4 http://www.ncbi.nlm.nih.gov/pmc/articles /PMC4415962/.

5 http://link.springer.com/article /10.1007%2Fs13197-014-1396-5.

6 http://www.ncbi.nlm.nih.gov /pubmed/25499941.

7 http://www.nmcd-journal.com/article /S0939-4753(09)00211-7/abstract.

8 http://www.ncbi.nlm.nih.gov /pubmed/26405440.

9 http://www.ncbi.nlm.nih.gov/pmc/articles /PMC4330049/.

10 http://www.ncbi.nlm.nih.gov /pubmed/26269239.

11 http://www.ncbi.nlm.nih.gov /pubmed/24360749.

12 http://www.ncbi.nlm.nih.gov /pubmed/25837212.

13 http://www.ncbi.nlm.nih.gov /pubmed/25267241.

14 http://www.ncbi.nlm.nih.gov /pubmed/26269373.

15 http://www.ncbi.nlm.nih.gov /pubmed/21631511.

16 http://www.ncbi.nlm.nih.gov /pubmed/24851570.

17 http://www.ncbi.nlm.nih.gov /pubmed/25489404.

18 http://www.ncbi.nlm.nih.gov /pubmed/23590705.

19 http://www.ncbi.nlm.nih.gov /pubmed/24976429.

20 http://www.ncbi.nlm.nih.gov/pmc/articles /PMC4521177/.

21 http://www.ncbi.nlm.nih.gov/pmc/articles /PMC4606102/.

22 http://www.ncbi.nlm.nih.gov/pmc/articles /PMC3875260/.

23 http://www.ncbi.nlm.nih.gov /pubmed/26224298.

24 http://ajcn.nutrition.org/content/94/2 /601?ijkey=82a401c05646aee007732e3 cef84ba38b2318185&keytype2=tf_ipsecsha.

25 http://www.ncbi.nlm.nih.gov /pubmed/26093535.

26 http://www.ncbi.nlm.nih.gov /pubmed/25266246; http://www.ncbi

.nlm.nih.gov/pmc/articles
/PMC4169558/.

27 http://www.ncbi.nlm.nih.gov
/pubmed/24972454.

28 R. R. He et al., "Beneficial Effects of Oolong
Tea Consumption on Diet-Induced Overweight
and Obese Subjects," *Chinese Journal of Integrated Medicine* 15 (2009): 34.

HIVES

1 http://www.ncbi.nlm.nih.gov
/pubmed/21905094.

2 https://www.nlm.nih.gov/medlineplus
/bvitamins.html; http://www.hsph.harvard
.edu/nutritionsource/vitamin-b/#bottom
-line; http://www.ijdvl.com/article.asp
?issn=0378-6323;year=2012;volume=78
;issue=2;spage=142;epage=145;aulast
=Pazyar.

3 http://www.ncbi.nlm.nih.gov
/pubmed/23333628.

4 http://www.ncbi.nlm.nih.gov/books
/NBK299046/; http://www.ncbi.nlm.nih.gov
/pubmed/15668926.

5 http://www.ijdvl.com/article.asp?issn
=0378-6323;year=2012;volume
=78;issue=2;spage=142;epage=145
;aulast=Pazyar#ft7.

6 http://www.ncbi.nlm.nih.gov
/pubmed/21144345; http://www.ncbi
.nlm.nih.gov/pubmed/24250539.

HYPERHIDROSIS (EXCESSIVE SWEATING)

1 http://www.ncbi.nlm.nih.gov
/pubmed/8402963.

2 http://www.ncbi.nlm.nih.gov
/pubmed/?term=sage+tea+throat.

3 http://www.drweil.com/drw/u/QAA400958
/Sage-for-Excess-Sweating.html#_ga=1.6695
6206.1428823967.1435580517.

4 http://www.ncbi.nlm.nih.gov/pmc/articles
/PMC4345801/.

5 https://www.aad.org/dermatology-a-to
-z/diseases-and-treatments/e---h
/hyperhidrosis/hyperhidrosis-tips-for
-managing.

HYPOGLYCEMIA

1 http://www.ncbi.nlm.nih.gov
/pubmed/26468155.

2 http://www.racgp.org.au/afp/2015/may
/diet-and-diabetes/.

3 Ibid.

INDIGESTION

1 http://www.ncbi.nlm.nih.gov
/pubmed/25628849.

2 http://www.ncbi.nlm.nih.gov/books
/NBK92775/.

3 http://www.ncbi.nlm.nih.gov
/pubmed/14653829.

4 http://www.ncbi.nlm.nih.gov
/pubmed/25954317.

5 http://www.ncbi.nlm.nih.gov/pmc/articles
/PMC4137549/.

6 http://www.ncbi.nlm.nih.gov/pmc/articles
/PMC4080703/.

7 http://www.ncbi.nlm.nih.gov/pmc/articles
/PMC4387228/#ref26.

8 http://www.ncbi.nlm.nih.gov
/pubmed/21488913.

9 http://www.ncbi.nlm.nih.gov/pmc/articles
/PMC3513878/.

10 http://www.ncbi.nlm.nih.gov/pmc/articles/PM
C3123991/#B17; M. N. Asl and H. Hosseinzadeh,
"Review of Pharmacological Effects of
Glycyrrhiza sp. and Its Bioactive Compounds,"
Phytotherapy Research 22 (2008): 709–24.

11 http://umm.edu/health/medical/altmed
/herb/licorice.

12 Ibid.

13 http://www.ncbi.nlm.nih.gov/pmc/articles
/PMC2995283/.

INFERTILITY

1 https://www.asrm.org/Not_Just_Obesity
_but_High_Fat_Diets_May_be_Enough_to
_Impact_Fertility/.

2 http://www.ncbi.nlm.nih.gov
/pubmed/25764357.

3 http://www.ncbi.nlm.nih.gov
/pmc/articles/PMC3717046
/#B24.

4 http://www.ncbi.nlm.nih.gov
/pubmed/26351959.

5   http://www.ncbi.nlm.nih.gov/pmc/articles
    /PMC3717046/#B24.
6   http://www.ncbi.nlm.nih.gov
    /pubmed/26351959; http://humupd
    .oxfordjournals.org/content/10/3
    /267.full.
7   http://www.ncbi.nlm.nih.gov/pmc/articles
    /PMC3066040/.
8   http://www.ncbi.nlm.nih.gov/pmc/articles
    /PMC3717046/#B23
9   http://www.fda.gov/Food/ResourcesForYou
    /Consumers/ucm079609.htm.
10 http://www.ncbi.nlm.nih.gov
    /pubmed/26298524.
11 http://www.ncbi.nlm.nih.gov
    /pubmed/24717915.
12 https://ods.od.nih.gov/factsheets/Vitamin
    D-HealthProfessional/.

13 http://www.ncbi.nlm.nih.gov
    /pubmed/26026343.
14 http://www.ncbi.nlm.nih.gov/pmc/articles
    /PMC3717046/#B24.
15 Ibid.
16 https://ods.od.nih.gov/factsheets/Folate
    -HealthProfessional/.
17 http://www.ncbi.nlm.nih.gov
    /pubmed/21546386/.
18 http://www.ncbi.nlm.nih.gov/pmc/articles
    /PMC3717046/#B24.
19 http://www.ncbi.nlm.nih.gov/pmc/articles
    /PMC4377061/.
20 http://humupd.oxfordjournals.org
    /content/10/3/267.full.

INFLUENZA

1   http://www.ncbi.nlm.nih.gov/pmc/articles
    /PMC3725497/.
2   http://www.ars.usda.gov/SP2UserFiles
    /Place/80400525/Data/Flav/Flav_R03-1.pdf.
3   http://nutritiondata.self.com/foods
    -00010200000000000000.html.
4   http://www.ncbi.nlm.nih.gov
    /pubmed/?term=l+reuteri+influenza;

    http://www.ncbi.nlm.nih.gov
    /pubmed/25604727; http://www.ncbi
    .nlm.nih.gov/pubmed
    /25294223.
5   http://www.ncbi.nlm.nih.gov
    /pubmed/24880005.
6   http://www.ncbi.nlm.nih.gov
    /pubmed/25847473.

INSECT/SPIDER BITES AND STINGS

1   http://www.ijdvl.com/article.asp?issn=0378
    -6323;year=2012;volume=78;issue=2;spage
    =142;epage=145;aulast=Pazyar#ft7.
2   http://www.ncbi.nlm.nih.gov/
    pubmed/24250539; http://www.ncbi.nlm.nih
    .gov/pubmed/21144345.

3   http://www.hindawi.com/journals
    /ecam/2013/681304/.
4   http://www.ncbi.nlm.nih.gov
    /pubmed/26061489.

INSOMNIA

1   http://www.ncbi.nlm.nih.gov/pubmed
    /25266053; http://www.journalsleep.org
    /ViewAbstract.aspx?pid=30153; http://
    www.escardio.org/The-ESC/Press-Office
    /Press-releases/Last-5-years/Poor
    -sleep-associated-with-increased
    -risk-of-heart-attack-and-stroke;
    http://www.ncbi.nlm.nih.gov/pubmed
    /26355726; http://hyper.ahajournals
    .org/content/65/3/644.long; http://
    www.ncbi.nlm.nih.gov/pubmed/26444730.
2   http://www.ncbi.nlm.nih.gov/pmc/articles
    /PMC4440346/.
3   http://www.ncbi.nlm.nih.gov
    /pubmed/22038497/.
4   Ibid.
5   http://www.ncbi.nlm.nih.gov/pmc/articles
    /PMC4440346

6   H. H. Lin et al., "Effect of Kiwifruit
    Consumption on Sleep Quality in Adults with
    Sleep Problems," *Asia Pacific Journal of
    Clinical Nutrition* 20, no. 2 (2011): 169–74.
7   https://sleepfoundation.org/sleep-topics
    /food-and-sleep.
8   http://www.researchgate.net
    /publication/225087663_Diet_promotes
    _sleep_duration_and_quality.
9   Ibid.
10 http://www.ncbi.nlm.nih.gov
    /pubmed/26354605.
11 http://www.ncbi.nlm.nih.gov
    /pubmed/17284739.
12 http://www.ncbi.nlm.nih.gov/pmc/articles
    /PMC4134283/.
13 http://www.ncbi.nlm.nih.gov/pmc/articles
    /PMC3703747/.

IRRITABLE BOWEL SYNDROME

1 http://www.ncbi.nlm.nih.gov/pmc/articles/PMC4202343/.
2 http://www.ncbi.nlm.nih.gov/pubmed/25982757.
3 A full list can be found at http://www.ibsdiets.org/fodmap-diet/fodmap-food-list/.
4 Ibid.; http://www.researchgate.net/publication/272515985_Role_of_FODMAPs_in_Patients_With_Irritable_Bowel_Syndrome.

KIDNEY STONES

1 http://www.ncbi.nlm.nih.gov/pubmed/26150027.
2 http://www.ncbi.nlm.nih.gov/pmc/articles/PMC4265710/.
3 http://urology.jhu.edu/kidney and click on the Prevention tab
4 http://lpi.oregonstate.edu/mic/minerals/potassium
5 https://www.kidney.org/atoz/content/kidneystones_prevent.
6 http://www.ncbi.nlm.nih.gov/pmc/articles/PMC4265710/.

LIGHTHEADEDNESS

1 http://www.ncbi.nlm.nih.gov/pubmed/26206997.
2 http://www.ncbi.nlm.nih.gov/pubmed/26077805; http://www

LUPUS

1 http://ncp.sagepub.com/content/25/1/61.short.
2 http://www.lupus.org/answers/entry/lupus-diet-and-nutrition.
3 http://www.scielo.br/scielo.php?script=sci_arttext&pid=S0482-50042012000300009&lng=en&nrm=iso&tlng=en.
4 http://www.sciencedirect.com/science/article/pii/S2255502114001515.
5 http://www.nutritionj.com/content/14/1/82.
6 http://www.ncbi.nlm.nih.gov/pmc/articles/PMC3898893/.
7 http://www.housemajority.org/wp-content/uploads/2014/03/10-Effect_of_Vitamin_D_supplementation_on_Inflammatory_and_Hemostatic_markers_and_Disease_activity_inpatients_with_systemic_lupus.pdf.

MACULAR DEGENERATION

1 http://archopht.jamanetwork.com/article.aspx?articleid=268224.
2 http://www.ncbi.nlm.nih.gov/pubmed/23644932.

5 http://www.ncbi.nlm.nih.gov/pmc/articles/PMC4223251/.
6 http://www.ncbi.nlm.nih.gov/pmc/articles/PMC4356930/.
7 http://www.ncbi.nlm.nih.gov/pmc/articles/PMC2886445/.
8 http://www.ncbi.nlm.nih.gov/pmc/articles/PMC2583392/?tool=pubmed.
9 http://www.ncbi.nlm.nih.gov/pubmed/26319955.

7 http://www.ncbi.nlm.nih.gov/pmc/articles/PMC4525130/.
8 http://www.niddk.nih.gov/health-information/health-topics/urologic-disease/diet-for-kidney-stone-prevention/Pages/facts.aspx.
9 https://ods.od.nih.gov/factsheets/Calcium-HealthProfessional/.
10 http://www.ncbi.nlm.nih.gov/pubmed/26382905.
11 http://www.ncbi.nlm.nih.gov/pubmed/25091135.

.ncbi.nlm.nih.gov/pubmed/26380428; http://www.ncbi.nlm.nih.gov/pubmed/22653692.

8 http://www.ncbi.nlm.nih.gov/pubmed/26227163.
9 http://www.ncbi.nlm.nih.gov/pmc/articles/PMC4198387/.
10 http://www.scielo.br/scielo.php?script=sci_arttext&pid=S0482-50042012000300009&lng=en&nrm=iso&tlng=en.
11 Ibid.
12 Ibid.
13 http://www.ncbi.nlm.nih.gov/pubmed/21742514.
14 http://www.ncbi.nlm.nih.gov/pubmed/17569223/.
15 http://www.ncbi.nlm.nih.gov/pubmed/20146265.

3 http://www.ncbi.nlm.nih.gov/pubmed/26447482.
4 http://www.ncbi.nlm.nih.gov/pubmed/26310706.

5 http://www.ncbi.nlm.nih.gov
   /pubmed/25225109.

6 http://nutritiondata.self.com/foods
   -0001260000000000000000.html.

MEMORY LOSS (SHORT TERM)

1 http://jn.nutrition.org/content/142/1/76.
2 http://www.ncbi.nlm.nih.gov/pubmed
   /?term=annals+of+neurology+devore.
3 http://www.ncbi.nlm.nih.gov
   /pubmed/26461383.
4 http://www.ncbi.nlm.nih.gov
   /pubmed/26280945.
5 http://www.ncbi.nlm.nih.gov
   /pubmed/25733635.
6 http://www.ncbi.nlm.nih.gov
   /pubmed/22468945.
7 http://www.ncbi.nlm.nih.gov
   /pubmed/26212523.
8 http://www.ncbi.nlm.nih.gov
   /pubmed/20838622.
9 http://www.ncbi.nlm.nih.gov
   /pubmed/25877495.

10 http://www.ncbi.nlm.nih.gov/pmc/articles
   /PMC4555146
11 http://onlinelibrary.wiley.com/doi/10.1002
   /hup.2259/abstract.
12 http://www.ncbi.nlm.nih.gov
   /pubmed/25352453; http://www.ncbi.nlm
   .nih.gov/pubmed/25114079.
13 http://www.ncbi.nlm.nih.gov/pmc/articles
   /PMC4555146/.
14 http://onlinelibrary.wiley.com/doi/10.1111
   /jcpp.12209/abstract.
15 P. Lehert et al., "Individually Modifiable
   Risk Factors to Ameliorate Cognitive
   Aging: A Systematic Review and Meta-
   Analysis," *Climacteric* 18, no. 5 (2015):
   678–89.

MENOPAUSE

1 http://www.ncbi.nlm.nih.gov
   /pubmed/25482487.
2 http://www.endocrinology.org/press
   /pressreleases/2015-11-02_SoybeanFoods
   MayProtecMenopausalWomenAgainst
   Osteoporosis.pdf.
3 http://ajcn.nutrition.org/content/100
   /Supplement_1/423S.long.
4 http://www.ncbi.nlm.nih.gov
   /pubmed/25660429.
5 http://ajcn.nutrition.org/content/97/5/1092.
6 http://www.ncbi.nlm.nih.gov/pmc/articles
   /PMC4161099/.
7 https://ods.od.nih.gov/factsheets/Folate
   -HealthProfessional/.

8 http://www.ncbi.nlm.nih.gov
   /pubmed/14644697.
9 http://www.ncbi.nlm.nih.gov
   /pubmed/22781782.
10 http://www.ncbi.nlm.nih.gov
   /pubmed/26428734.
11 http://www.ncbi.nlm.nih.gov
   /pubmed/?term=coconut+oil
   +epidermal+hydration.
12 http://www.ncbi.nlm.nih.gov
   /pubmed/26161938.
13 http://www.hindawi.com/journals
   /ogi/2011/949302/.

MENSTRUAL CRAMPS (DYSMENORRHEA)

1 http://www.ncbi.nlm.nih.gov/pmc/articles
   /PMC1459624/.
2 http://www.ncbi.nlm.nih.gov
   /pubmed/25389482.
3 http://www.ncbi.nlm.nih.gov
   /pubmed/25097605.
4 http://www.ncbi.nlm.nih.gov
   /pubmed/25399316.
5 http://www.ncbi.nlm.nih.gov
   /pubmed/22781186.
6 http://www.ncbi.nlm.nih.gov
   /pubmed/25389490.
7 http://www.ncbi.nlm.nih.gov
   /pubmed/24695380.
8 http://www.ncbi.nlm.nih.gov
   /pubmed/26023601.

9 http://www.ncbi.nlm.nih.gov
   /pubmed/26023350.
10 http://www.ncbi.nlm.nih.gov
   /pubmed/25363189.
11 https://ods.od.nih.gov/factsheets
   /Thiamin-HealthProfessional/.
12 http://lpi.oregonstate.edu/mic/vitamins
   /thiamin.
13 http://www.ncbi.nlm.nih.gov
   /pubmed/22261128.

MOTION SICKNESS

1 http://www.ncbi.nlm.nih.gov
   /pubmed/3277342.
2 http://www.ncbi.nlm.nih.gov
   /pubmed/2062873.
3 http://www.ncbi.nlm.nih.gov
   /pubmed/26452639.
4 http://www.ncbi.nlm.nih.gov
   /pubmed/12576305.

5 http://www.ncbi.nlm.nih.gov
   /pubmed/25502048.
6 http://www.ncbi.nlm.nih.gov
   /pubmed/22784340.
7 http://www.ncbi.nlm.nih.gov
   /pubmed/25095772.

MUSCLE CRAMPS

1 http://www.ncbi.nlm.nih.gov
   /pubmed/26446763.
2 https://www.nlm.nih.gov/medlineplus/ency
   /article/002066.htm.
3 http://www.hsph.harvard.edu
   /nutritionsource/calcium-sources/.
4 http://health.gov/dietaryguidelines/dga2005
   /document/pdf/Appendix_B.pdf.

5 http://www.ncbi.nlm.nih.gov
   /pubmed/19829096.
6 http://www.ncbi.nlm.nih.gov
   /pubmed/19997012.
7 http://www.ncbi.nlm.nih.gov
   /pubmed/25562454; http://www.ncbi.nlm
   .nih.gov/pubmed/23952039.

NAUSEA

1 http://www.ncbi.nlm.nih.gov
   /pubmed/25414888; http://www.ncbi.nlm
   .nih.gov/pubmed/24535321.
2 http://www.ncbi.nlm.nih.gov
   /pubmed/24693389; http://www.ncbi.nlm
   .nih.gov/pubmed/24218997; http://www
   .ncbi.nlm.nih.gov/pmc/articles/PMC3984021/.

3 http://www.ncbi.nlm.nih.gov
   /pubmed/26414587.
4 http://www.ncbi.nlm.nih.gov
   /pubmed/21818642.
5 http://www.ncbi.nlm.nih.gov
   /pubmed/22784340.

OSTEOPOROSIS

1 http://www.iofbonehealth.org/what-is
   -osteoporosis.
2 http://www.niams.nih.gov/Health_Info
   /Bone/Osteoporosis/osteoporosis
   _hoh.asp.
3 http://connection.ebscohost.com/c
   /articles/89040744/early-adult-osteoporosis
   -can-be-prevented-by-adequate-dietary
   -calcium-intake-during-childhood.
4 http://www.niams.nih.gov/Health_Info
   /Bone/Osteoporosis/bone_mass.asp.
5 http://www.ncbi.nlm.nih.gov
   /pubmed/22946650.
6 http://www.ncbi.nlm.nih.gov/pmc/articles
   /PMC3552690/.
7 http://www.ncbi.nlm.nih.gov/pmc/articles
   /PMC4425157/.

8 http://www.ncbi.nlm.nih.gov
   /pubmed/25412684.
9 http://www.ncbi.nlm.nih.gov/pmc/articles
   /PMC3894263/#SD1.
10 http://www.ncbi.nlm.nih.gov
   /pubmed/24975408.
11 http://www.ncbi.nlm.nih.gov/pmc/articles
   /PMC3836362/.
12 http://www.ncbi.nlm.nih.gov/pmc/articles
   /PMC3693746/.
13 http://www.ncbi.nlm.nih.gov
   /pubmed/24729336.
14 http://www.ncbi.nlm.nih.gov
   /pubmed/24989680.
15 http://www.ncbi.nlm.nih.gov/pmc/articles
   /PMC3831545/.

OVERWEIGHT AND OBESITY

1 http://www.hsph.harvard.edu/obesity
   -prevention-source/obesity-definition/.
2 http://healthintelligence.drupalgardens
   .com/content/trends-overweight-and
   -obesity-country-level.

3 http://apps.who.int/iris/bitstream
   /10665/148114/1/9789241564854
   _eng.pdf?ua=1.
4 http://onlinelibrary.wiley.com/doi/10.1111
   /pme.12158/abstract.

5   http://www.nature.com/mp/journal/vaop
    /ncurrent/full/mp2015129a.html.
6   http://health.clevelandclinic.org/2013/10
    /obesity-a-risk-factor-for-alzheimers/.
7   http://www.ncbi.nlm.nih.gov/pmc/articles
    /PMC4493396/.
8   http://www.ncbi.nlm.nih.gov/pmc/articles
    /PMC4234734/.
9   http://ajcn.nutrition.org/content/99/1
    /35.long.
10 http://aje.oxfordjournals.org
    /content/182/6/503.abstract.
11 http://www.ncbi.nlm.nih.gov/pmc/articles
    /PMC4166206/.
12 http://journals.cambridge.org/action
    /displayAbstract?fromPage
    =online&aid=9236077&-
    fileId=S0007114514000063.
13 http://journals.plos.org/plosone
    /article?id=10.1371/journal.pone.0139817.
14 http://www.thelancet.com/journals/landia
    /article/PIIS2213
    -8587%2815%2900367-8/abstract.
15 http://www.ncbi.nlm.nih.gov/pmc/articles
    /PMC4578962/.
16 http://www.ncbi.nlm.nih.gov/pmc/article
    s/PMC3464869/.
17 http://www.ncbi.nlm.nih.gov
    /pubmed/25079040.
18 http://www.ncbi.nlm.nih.gov
    /pubmed/24246368.
19 https://www.ikhebeenvraag.be
    /mediastorage/FSDocument/240
    /molecules-16-08919.pdf.

20 http://www.ncbi.nlm.nih.gov
    /pubmed/25456022.
21 http://www.jcimjournal.com/jim/FullText2
    .aspx?articleID=S2095-4964(15)60176-5.
22 http://www.ncbi.nlm.nih.gov
    /pubmed/24809437.
23 http://www.ncbi.nlm.nih.gov
    /pubmed/23357955.
24 http://www.ncbi.nlm.nih.gov/pmc/articles
    /PMC4222592/.
25 http://heb.sagepub.com/content/early/2015
    /10/15/1090198115610571.full.
26 http://jn.nutrition.org/content/145/9/2052
    .long.
27 http://www.ncbi.nlm.nih.gov/pmc/articles
    /PMC4239493/.
28 http://www.ncbi.nlm.nih.gov
    /pubmed/20216555.
29 http://www.ncbi.nlm.nih.gov
    /pubmed/23614897.
30 http://www.ncbi.nlm.nih.gov
    /pubmed/24558988.
31 http://www.ncbi.nlm.nih.gov/pmc/articles
    /PMC4322420/.
32 http://www.ncbi.nlm.nih.gov
    /pubmed/26093535.
33 R. R. He et al., "Beneficial Effects of Oolong
    Tea Consumption on Diet-Induced
    Overweight and Obese Subjects," *Chinese
    Journal of Integrated Medicine* 15 (2009): 34.
34 http://www.ncbi.nlm.nih.gov/pmc/articles
    /PMC4344557/.
35 http://www.ncbi.nlm.nih.gov/pmc/articles
    /PMC4502735/.

PMS (PREMENSTRUAL SYNDROME)

1   http://www.ncbi.nlm.nih.gov/pmc/articles
    /PMC3972521/.
2   http://www.ncbi.nlm.nih.gov/pmc/articles
    /PMC4177637/.
3   http://www.ncbi.nlm.nih.gov/pmc/articles
    /PMC4437117/.
4   http://www.ncbi.nlm.nih.gov/pmc/articles
    /PMC4177637/.
5   http://ccsenet.org/journal/index.php/gjhs
    /article/view/36220.
6   http://www.ncbi.nlm.nih.gov
    /pubmed/25363189.
7   https://ods.od.nih.gov/factsheets/Thiamin
    -HealthProfessional/.
8   http://lpi.oregonstate.edu/mic/vitamins
    /thiamin.

9   http://www.ncbi.nlm.nih.gov/pmc/articles
    /PMC3076657/.
10 http://lpi.oregonstate.edu/mic/vitamins
    /riboflavin.
11 http://www.ncbi.nlm.nih.gov/pmc/articles
    /PMC4277629/.
12 http://www.nutricionhospitalaria.com
    /pdf/6648.pdf.
13 http://www.hsph.harvard.edu
    /nutritionsource/calcium-sources/.
14 https://ods.od.nih.gov/factsheets
    /Magnesium-HealthProfessional/.
15 https://ods.od.nih.gov/factsheets
    /Iron-HealthProfessional/.
16 https://ods.od.nih.gov/factsheets
    /Iron-HealthProfessional/

PNEUMONIA

1   http://ajcn.nutrition.org/content/83/5/991
    .full.
2   http://ajcn.nutrition.org/content/86/4/1167
    .abstract.

3   http://nutritiondata.self.com/foods
    -000102000000000000000.html.
4   http://www.ncbi.nlm.nih.gov
    /pubmed/25920295.

5 http://www.ncbi.nlm.nih.gov
   /pubmed/25666113.
6 http://www.ncbi.nlm.nih.gov
   /pubmed/25516315.

PSORIASIS

1 https://www.psoriasis.org/advance
   /researchers-study-how-diets-affect
   -psoriatic-disease; http://www.ncbi.nlm.nih
   .gov/pmc/articles/PMC4104239
2 http://www.ncbi.nlm.nih.gov/pmc/articles
   /PMC4104239/.
3 http://www.ncbi.nlm.nih.gov
   /pubmed/21654830.
4 http://www.ncbi.nlm.nih.gov
   /pubmed/25662711.
5 http://www.ncbi.nlm.nih.gov
   /pubmed/10651693.

SHINGLES

1 http://www.cdc.gov/shingles/about
   /overview.html.
2 http://www.ncbi.nlm.nih.gov/pubmed
   /26478818; http://www.ncbi.nlm.nih.gov
   /pmc/articles/PMC4140624/.
3 http://www.ncbi.nlm.nih.gov
   /pubmed/23088666.
4 http://nutritiondata.self.com/foods
   -00010200000000000000.html.
5 http://www.ncbi.nlm.nih.gov/pmc
   /articles/PMC3725497/.

SINUSITIS

1 http://www.ars.usda.gov/SP2UserFiles
   /Place/80400525/Data/Flav/Flav_R03-1.pdf.
2 pdf Turmeric, the golden spice https://www
   .ncbi.nlm.nih.gov/pubmed/22887802
3 http://www.ncbi.nlm.nih.gov/
   pubmed/26228533.
4 http://www.ncbi.nlm.nih.gov/pmc/articles
   /PMC3529416/.

SORE THROAT

1 http://www.ncbi.nlm.nih.gov
   /pubmed/?term=sage+tea+throat.
2 http://www.ncbi.nlm.nih.gov
   /pubmed/26045910.
3 http://umm.edu/health/medical/altmed
   /herb/marshmallow.
4 http://www.ncbi.nlm.nih.gov
   /pubmed/15998989.

STRESS

1 http://joannabriggslibrary.org/jbilibrary
   /index.php/jbisrir/article/view/2298/2550.

7 http://www.ncbi.nlm.nih.gov
   /pubmed/24797941.

6 http://www.ncbi.nlm.nih.gov
   /pubmed/26422425.
7 http://www.ncbi.nlm.nih.gov
   /pubmed/23752669.
8 http://www.ncbi.nlm.nih.gov
   /pubmed/21492252.
9 http://www.ncbi.nlm.nih.gov/pmc/articles
   /PMC4134971/.
10 https://www.psoriasis.org/treating
   -psoriasis/complementary-and
   -alternative/diet-and-nutrition
   /anti-inflammatory-diet.

6 http://www.ars.usda.gov/SP2UserFiles
   /Place/80400525/Data/Flav/Flav
   _R03-1.pdf.
7 http://www.ncbi.nlm.nih.gov
   /pubmed/22735054.
8 http://www.ncbi.nlm.nih.gov/pmc/articles
   /PMC4500781/.
9 http://www.ncbi.nlm.nih.gov
   /pubmed/?term=turmeric+herpes.

5 http://www.ncbi.nlm.nih.gov
   /pubmed/26045910.
6 http://www.ncbi.nlm.nih.gov/pmc/articles
   /PMC4264806/
7 http://www.entnet.org/content/sinusitis.
8 http://www.ncbi.nlm.nih.gov/pmc/articles
   /PMC3904042/.

5 http://www.ncbi.nlm.nih.gov/pmc/articles
   /PMC4264806
6 http://www.ncbi.nlm.nih.gov
   /pubmed/23286823.
7 http://www.sciencedirect.com
   /science/article/pii
   /S0167779903000854.

2 http://www.ncbi.nlm.nih.gov
   /pubmed/25373096.

3 http://www.ncbi.nlm.nih.gov
/pubmed/26468409.

4 http://www.ncbi.nlm.nih.gov
/pubmed/22473079/.

5 http://www.ncbi.nlm.nih.gov
/pubmed/26238744.

6 http://www.ncbi.nlm.nih.gov
/pubmed/24811775.

7 http://www.ncbi.nlm.nih.gov
/pubmed/26404481.

8 http://www.ncbi.nlm.nih.gov
/pubmed/23347122.

9 http://www.ncbi.nlm.nih.gov
/pubmed/25780358.

10 http://link.springer.com/article/10.1007
%2Fs12671-014-0360-9.

11 http://www.tandfonline.com/doi
/abs/10.4161/gmic.2.4.16108.

12 http://www.ncbi.nlm.nih.gov
/pubmed/25470391.

13 http://www.maneyonline.com/doi/abs/10.117
9/1476830515Y.0000000023?url_ver=Z39.88
-2003&rfr_id=ori:rid:crossref.org&rfr
_dat=cr_pub%3dpubmed.

14 http://www.ncbi.nlm.nih.gov/pubmed
/?term=fermented+foods+neuroticism.

15 http://www.ncbi.nlm.nih.gov
/pubmed/19253862.

16 http://www.ncbi.nlm.nih.gov
/pubmed/26425385.

17 http://www.ncbi.nlm.nih.gov/pmc/articles
/PMC4290459

18 http://www.ncbi.nlm.nih.gov
/pubmed/21905094.

19 http://www.ncbi.nlm.nih.gov/pmc/articles
/PMC2748268/.

20 http://www.lib.okayama-u.ac.jp/www/acta
/pdf/67_2_99.pdf.

21 http://www.prevention.com/health/health
-concerns/carpal-tunnel-symptoms
-and-and-treatments.

22 U.S. Department of Agriculture, Agricultural
Research Service. 2013. USDA National
Nutrient Database for Standard Reference,
Release 26. Nutrient Data Laboratory Home
Page, http://www.ars.usda.gov/ba/bhnrc/ndl

23 http://lpi.oregonstate.edu/mic/vitamins
/vitamin-B12.

24 https://ods.od.nih.gov/factsheets
/Iron-HealthProfessional/.

25 http://www.ncbi.nlm.nih.gov
/pubmed/26353411.

26 http://www.joannabriggslibrary.org/index
.php/jbisrir/article/view/2298.

27 https://umm.edu/health/medical/altmed
/supplement/magnesium.

28 http://www.joannabriggslibrary.org/index
.php/jbisrir/article/view/2298.

29 http://www.ncbi.nlm.nih.gov/pmc/articles
/PMC2868080/.

STROKE

1 http://www.cdc.gov/stroke/.
2 http://www.cdc.gov/stroke/facts.htm.
3 Ibid.
4 http://stroke.ahajournals.org
/content/45/12/3754.long.

5 http://www.ncbi.nlm.nih.gov
/pubmed/26363438.

6 http://www.ncbi.nlm.nih.gov
/pubmed/22363060.

7 http://www.ncbi.nlm.nih.gov
/pubmed/23169473.

8 http://stroke.ahajournals.org
/content/45/12/3754.long.

9 https://www.nhlbi.nih.gov/health/health
-topics/topics/dash.

10 http://www.ncbi.nlm.nih.gov
/pubmed/24342529/.

11 http://www.ncbi.nlm.nih.gov
/pubmed/23073261.

12 http://www.ncbi.nlm.nih.gov/pmc/articles
/PMC4330060/; http://www.ncbi.nlm.nih
.gov/pubmed/25489404; http://www.ncbi
.nlm.nih.gov/pubmed/23590705; http://
www.ncbi.nlm.nih.gov/pubmed/25499941;
http://www.ncbi.nlm.nih.gov/pmc/articles
/PMC4330049/; http://www.ncbi.nlm.nih
.gov/pubmed/26269239; http://www.ncbi
.nlm.nih.gov/pubmed/25837212; http://
www.ncbi.nlm.nih.gov/pubmed/24360749;
http://www.ncbi.nlm.nih.gov
/pubmed/25267241; http://www.ncbi.nlm
.nih.gov/pubmed/21631511; http://www
.ncbi.nlm.nih.gov/pmc/articles
/PMC4521177/; http://www.ncbi.nlm.nih
.gov/pmc/articles/PMC4606102/; http://
ajcn.nutrition.org/content/94/2/601
?ijkey=82a401c05646aee007732e3cef
84ba38b2318185&keytype2=tf_ipsecsha.

13 http://www.ncbi.nlm.nih.gov/pmc/articles
/PMC3678213

14 http://www.ncbi.nlm.nih.gov
/pubmed/25190445.

15 http://stroke.ahajournals.org
/content/42/10/2746.abstract
?ijkey=84c117795293561643a6f0
ec5a65890e4e7fd696&keytype2
=tf_ipsecsha.

16 http://health.gov/dietaryguidelines/dga2005
/document/pdf/Appendix_B.pdf.

17 http://www.stroke.org/we-can-help
/survivors/stroke-recovery/first-steps
-recovery/preventing-another-stroke.

18 http://www.ncbi.nlm.nih.gov
/pubmed/26468409.

SUNBURN

1 http://www.skincancer.org/media-and
   -press/Press-Release-2008/stopping-skin
   -cancer-epidemic-starts-with-children.
2 http://www.ncbi.nlm.nih.gov
   /pubmed/21953695.
3 http://www.ncbi.nlm.nih.gov/pmc/articles
   /PMC3257702/.

4 http://www.ncbi.nlm.nih.gov
   /pubmed/21953695.
5 http://www.ncbi.nlm.nih.gov
   /pubmed/12871030.
6 http://onlinelibrary.wiley.com/doi/10.1111
   /j.1600-0625.2011.01294.x/full.

THYROID DISEASE

1 https://ods.od.nih.gov/factsheets/Iodine
   -HealthProfessional/.
2 http://www.environmentalnutrition
   .com/issues/37_6/youshouldknow
   /keep-your-thyroid-health-through
   -diet_152620-1.html.
3 Ibid.
4 http://nutritiondata.self.com/foods
   -00008700000000000000000.html.

5 http://www.jmnn.org/article
   .asp?issn=2278-1870;year=2014;volume=3
   ;issue=2;spage=60;epage=65;aulast=Sharma.
6 http://www.ncbi.nlm.nih.gov
   /pubmed/25932388.
7 http://www.ncbi.nlm.nih.gov
   /pubmed/25263477.
8 http://www.ncbi.nlm.nih.gov/pmc/articles
   /PMC3847753/.

TINNITUS

1 http://www.ncbi.nlm.nih.gov
   /pubmed/24408248.
2 http://www.ncbi.nlm.nih.gov
   /pubmed/23461976.
3 https://www.ata.org/managing-your
   -tinnitus/treatment-options/general
   -wellness.
4 http://www.ncbi.nlm.nih.gov
   /pubmed/20053154/.
5 http://www.ncbi.nlm.nih.gov
   /pubmed/24608016.
6 http://www.ncbi.nlm.nih.gov
   /pubmed/23313584.

7 http://www.ncbi.nlm.nih.gov
   /pubmed/24973579.
8 http://www.ncbi.nlm.nih.gov
   /pubmed/?term=tinnitus+aspartame.
9 http://www.ncbi.nlm.nih.gov
   /pubmed/26467416.
10 http://www.ncbi.nlm.nih.gov
   /pubmed/23543524.
11 http://www.ncbi.nlm.nih.gov
   /pubmed/26413574.

TOOTH DECAY

1 http://www.ncbi.nlm.nih.gov/pmc/articles
   /PMC4251936/.
2 http://www.ncbi.nlm.nih.gov
   /pubmed/25040739.
3 http://www.ncbi.nlm.nih.gov/pmc/articles
   /PMC3906556/.
4 http://www.researchgate.net/profile
   /Atsushi_Ishikado/publication/263318551
   _A_High-Fiber_Low-Fat_Diet_Improves_
   Periodontal_Disease_Markers_in_High
   -risk_Subjects_A_Pilot_Study/links
   /5508e58e0cf27e990e0d30fe.pdf.
5 http://www.researchgate.net
   /publication/260023945_Association_of
   _oral_hygiene_habits_and_food_intake
   _with_the_risk_of_dental_caries_among
   _undergraduate_university_women_in
   _Saudi_Arabia.
6 http://www.ncbi.nlm.nih.gov
   /pubmed/26371954.

7 http://www.researchgate.net/profile/Avron
   _Spiro/publication/281143397_The_Dietary
   _Approaches_to_Stop_Hypertension_Diet
   _and_New_and_Recurrent_Root_Caries
   _Events_in_Men/links/55df9acf08aede
   0b572b90e3.pdf.
8 http://www.e-jds.com/article/S1991
   -7902(12)00168-7/abstract.
9 http://www.nutritionandmetabolism.com
   /content/9/1/61#B59.
10 http://www.ncbi.nlm.nih.gov
   /pubmed/24993270.
11 Ibid.
12 http://www.ncbi.nlm.nih.gov
   /pubmed/18408265.
13 http://www.ncbi.nlm.nih.gov
   /pubmed/19336860?dopt=Abstract.

ULCERS (PEPTIC)

1 http://www.academia.edu/3468803/Herbs
_Used_In_Peptic_Ulcer_A_Review.
2 Ibid.
3 http://www.scielo.br/scielo.php?pid
=S0102-67202014000400298&script=sci
_arttext.
4 http://www.ncbi.nlm.nih.gov/pmc/articles
/PMC3770045/.
5 Ibid.
6 http://www.ncbi.nlm.nih.gov
/pubmed/25799054.
7 Ibid.
8 http://www.ncbi.nlm.nih.gov/pmc/articles
/PMC3770045/
9 Ibid.
10 Ibid.
11 http://www.niddk.nih.gov/health
-information/health-topics/digestive
-diseases/smoking/Pages/facts.aspx#peptic.
12 Ibid.
13 Ibid.
14 http://www.academia.edu/3468803/Herbs
_Used_In_Peptic_Ulcer_A_Review.
15 http://www.ncbi.nlm.nih.gov/
pubmed/19399927; http://www.ncbi.nlm.nih
.gov/pubmed/24647097.
16 http://www.ncbi.nlm.nih.gov/pmc/articles
/PMC3535097/.
17 http://www.ncbi.nlm.nih.gov
/pubmed/16621751.
18 http://www.scielo.br/scielo.php?pid=S0102
-67202014000400298&script=sci_arttext.

VAGINITIS

1 http://www.ncbi.nlm.nih.gov
/pubmed/24473986.
2 http://www.ncbi.nlm.nih.gov/pmc/articles
/PMC3529416/.
3 http://www.altmedrev.com
/publications/14/2/141.pdf.
4 http://www.ncbi.nlm.nih.gov
/pubmed/16117603.
5 http://www.ncbi.nlm.nih.gov/pmc
/articles/PMC3249897/; http://www
.ncbi.nlm.nih.gov/pubmed
/23583806.
6 http://www.ncbi.nlm.nih.gov
/pubmed/17595415.

VARICOSE VEINS

1 http://stmjournals.com/index.php
?journal=JoNSP&page=article
&op=view&path%5B%5D=4043.
2 http://www.ncbi.nlm.nih.gov/pmc/articles
/PMC3116297/.
3 http://www.ncbi.nlm.nih.gov/pmc/articles
/PMC4277013/#B76-nutrients-06-06020.
4 http://www.ncbi.nlm.nih.gov
/pubmed/26270637.
5 http://www.nutraceuticalsworld.com
/issues/2014-11/view_supplier-research
/pycnogenol-found-to-improve-varicose
-spider-veins-following-pregnancy/.
6 http://www.ncbi.nlm.nih.gov/pmc/articles
/PMC3933503/.
7 http://www.ncbi.nlm.nih.gov
/pubmed/23775628.

VERTIGO

1 http://www.ncbi.nlm.nih.gov/pmc/articles
/PMC4593901/.
2 http://www.ncbi.nlm.nih.gov/pmc/articles
/PMC4593901/.
3 http://www.ncbi.nlm.nih.gov
/pubmed/26503384.

WARTS (COMMON)

1 http://www.ncbi.nlm.nih.gov
/pubmed/24910383.
2 http://www.clinmedres.org/content/4/4/273
.long.
3 https://umm.edu/health/medical/altmed
/condition/warts.
4 Ibid.; http://www.ncbi.nlm.nih.gov
/pubmed/7301999.
5 http://www.hindawi.com/journals
/drp/2014/709152/.
6 http://www.ncbi.nlm.nih.gov
/pubmed/24915350.

WOUNDS

1. http://journals.lww.com/aswcjournal /Fulltext/2012/02000/The_Role_of _Nutrition_in_Wound_Care.5.aspx.
2. http://www.ncbi.nlm.nih.gov /pubmed/17595415.
3. http://www.annalsoflongtermcare.com /article/rationale-zinc-supplementation -older-adults-wounds.
4. http://www.ncbi.nlm.nih.gov /pubmed/21084879.
5. http://www.ncbi.nlm.nih.gov /pubmed/25373096.
6. http://www.ncbi.nlm.nih.gov /pubmed/23036226/.
7. http://www.ncbi.nlm.nih.gov/pmc/articles /PMC4217020/.
8. http://www.ncbi.nlm.nih.gov /pubmed/26081867.
9. http://www.ncbi.nlm.nih.gov/pmc/articles /PMC4217020/.
10. http://nutritiondata.self.com/foods -00008900000000000000-2.html?.
11. http://www.ncbi.nlm.nih.gov/pmc/articles /PMC4217039/.
12. http://umm.edu/health/medical/altmed /supplement/glutamine.
13. http://www.ncbi.nlm.nih.gov /pubmed/25876636; http://www.ncbi.nlm .nih.gov/pubmed/24165637.
14. http://www.ncbi.nlm.nih.gov /pubmed/25559730.
15. http://journals.lww.com/aswcjournal /Fulltext/2012/02000/The_Role_of _Nutrition_in_Wound_Care.5.aspx.
16. http://lpi.oregonstate.edu/mic /micronutrients-health/skin-health /nutrient-index/vitamin-C.
17. http://www.ncbi.nlm.nih.gov /pubmed/21084879.
18. http://lpi.oregonstate.edu/mic/vitamins /vitamin-A.
19. http://www.ncbi.nlm.nih.gov /pubmed/14653765.
20. http://ncp.sagepub.com/content/25/1 /61.short.
21. http://www.ncbi.nlm.nih.gov/pmc/articles /PMC3523510/.
22. http://www.ncbi.nlm.nih.gov /pubmed/22296524.
23. http://www.ncbi.nlm.nih.gov /pubmed/24305429.
24. http://www.ncbi.nlm.nih.gov /pubmed/25449450.
25. http://www.karger.com/Article /FullText/357477
26. http://www.ncbi.nlm.nih.gov /pubmed/26113180; http://www.ncbi .nlm.nih.gov/pubmed/22887802.
27. http://www.ncbi.nlm.nih.gov /pubmed/24793420; S. Prasad et al., "Curcumin, a Component of Golden Spice: From Bedside to Bench and Back," *Biotechnology Advances* 32, no. 6 (2014): 1053–64.
28. http://www.ncbi.nlm.nih.gov/pmc/articles /PMC4506744/.
29. http://www.ncbi.nlm.nih.gov /pubmed/21084879.

WRINKLES

1. http://www.ncbi.nlm.nih.gov/pmc/articles /PMC4106357/.
2. http://www.ncbi.nlm.nih.gov/pmc/articles /PMC3583891/.
3. http://www.ncbi.nlm.nih.gov/pmc/articles /PMC4492544
4. http://www.ncbi.nlm.nih.gov/pmc/articles /PMC4562654/.
5. http://www.ncbi.nlm.nih.gov/pmc/articles /PMC3136561/.
6. http://www.ncbi.nlm.nih.gov/pmc/articles /PMC4492544
7. http://www.ncbi.nlm.nih.gov/pmc/articles /PMC4265247/.
8. http://lpi.oregonstate.edu/mic /micronutrients-health/skin-health /nutrient-index/essential-fatty-acids.
9. http://www.ncbi.nlm.nih.gov /pubmed/22382828.
10. http://www.ncbi.nlm.nih.gov /pubmed/26454905.
11. http://www.ncbi.nlm.nih.gov /pubmed/25758427.
12. http://lpi.oregonstate.edu/mic/dietary -factors/phytochemicals/soy-isoflavones.
13. http://www.ncbi.nlm.nih.gov/pmc/articles /PMC3664913/.
14. http://www.ncbi.nlm.nih.gov/pmc/articles /PMC4321565/.
15. http://www.ncbi.nlm.nih.gov /pubmed/26428734.
16. http://www.ncbi.nlm.nih.gov /pubmed/26287529.
17. http://jn.nutrition.org/content/141/6/1202.long.
18. http://www.ncbi.nlm.nih.gov /pubmed/26114360.
19. http://www.ncbi.nlm.nih.gov/pmc/articles /PMC4390761/.

Index

Underscored page references indicate boxed text.

A

Abdominal fat, 22, 27, 77, 336, 398, 402, 403
Acid damage to teeth, 437, 438
Acid reflux, 148–50, 149, 322, 323, 438
Acne, 36, 151–52, 256, 262, 404, 406, 461
ADHD, 87, 176–79
Adrenal exhaustion/adrenal fatigue, 153–55
Age-related macular degeneration (AMD). See Macular degeneration
Alcohol. See also Wine
  anxiety and, 167
  fibrocystic breasts and, 271
  gout risk from, 300, 301
  limiting
    for cancer prevention, 206
    for heart health, 318, 319
    with peptic ulcers, 439
  lupus and, 371
  moderate consumption of, 18
Allergic rhinitis, 156–59, 175, 280
Allergies, food. See Food allergies
Almond oil, for treating
  dry skin, 256
  fungal nail infections, 286
Almonds
  paired with kefir, 72
  properties of, 72–73
  for treating
    high blood pressure, 331
    high cholesterol, 336

Alpha-linolenic acid
  food sources of, 77, 93, 94, 204, 208, 259
  for preventing
    cancer, 77, 208
    cardiovascular disease, 81
Aluminum, Alzheimer's disease and, 163
Alzheimer's disease, 160–64. See also Dementia
  foods preventing
    fish, 88, 89, 91
    fruits, 25, 31
    herbs and spices, 59, 61–62
    mushrooms, 124
    olive oil, 80
    tea, 15
  obesity and, 396–97
AMD. See Macular degeneration
Amino acids, for heart health, 320
Antibiotics, for treating urinary tract infections, 183, 185
Antioxidants
  food sources of, 264, 272–73, 305, 351, 376, 409, 414, 415, 443, 449
  for preventing
    allergic rhinitis, 157
    bruises, 188
    eczema, 261
    hair loss, 305
    macular degeneration, 374–75, 376
    shingles, 414
    vaginitis, 443
    wrinkles, 454–55

for treating
  acne, 152
  bronchitis, 186–87
  burns, 190–91
  bursitis, 192–94
  fibromyalgia, 272–73
  pneumonia symptoms, 409
  sinusitis, 415
  warts, 449
  wounds, 450
Anxiety, 165–70, 342, 420–21, 422
  dehydration and, 16, 17
  foods preventing, 24, 52, 59, 102, 131
Apple cider vinegar
  in salad dressings, 79
  for treating
    ear infections, 258
    fungal nail infections, 285
    insect bites and stings, 356
    psoriasis, 412
    yeast infections, 282
Applegate, Liz, 64
Apples
  for preventing
    cancer, 198
    fibrocystic breasts, 271
    peptic ulcers, 441
  properties of, 25–27
Apricot oil, for treating
  dandruff, 222
  fungal nail infections, 286
Argan oil, for preventing wrinkles, 456
Arginine, for wound healing, 451

Aronia berries
  for preventing urinary tract
    infections, 184
  properties of, 27–28
Arthritis, 171–73
  foods preventing or treating
    chile peppers, 128
    fruits, 30, 32, 43
    herbs and spices, 60, 69, 70
    seeds, 93, 95–96
    tea, 14
    tuna, 91
Artichoke leaf extract, for
    treating indigestion, 346
Artichokes
  cooking, 103
  properties of, 103–5
Artificial food dyes, ADHD and,
    178
Arugula, for preventing peptic
    ulcers, 441
Ask the Expert
  Applegate, Liz, 64
  Campanile, Giovanni,
    40–41
  Kadey, Matthew, 82–83
  Mohr, Christopher, 10–11
  Nisevich Bede, Pamela,
    106–7
Asparagus
  cooking, 105
  properties of, 105, 108
Asparagus root extract, for
    treating dandruff, 222
Aspartame
  avoiding, with fibromyalgia,
    274
  tinnitus and, 433, 434
Asthma, 156, 158–59, 174–75
  foods preventing or treating
    fruits, 25, 26–27, 43
    herbs and spices, 53, 69
    vegetables, 112, 126
Athletic performance, kefir
    improving, 12
Atopic dermatitis, 255, 256, 259,
    262
Attention deficit hyperactivity
    disorder (ADHD), 87,
    176–79
Avocado oil, for treating dry
    skin, 256

Avocados
  in desserts, 28
  pitting, 29
  for preventing wrinkles, 456
  properties of, 28–30, 219
  ripening, 29
  for treating high cholesterol,
    335
  for weight loss, 401

B

Back pain, 128, 180–82
Bad breath. See Halitosis
Banana pulp or peel, for
    treating
  warts, 448
  wounds, 453
Barberry, for treating peptic
    ulcers, 439–40
Barley
  cooking, 139
  properties of, 139–40
Basil
  handling and storing, 52
  for heart health, 321
  properties of, 51–52
  for treating insect bites and
    stings, 356
Basil oil, for treating earache,
    257
Bay leaves, for treating
    diabetes, 244
Beans
  black, properties of, 2
  for cancer prevention, 198–99
  canned, 5
  fiber in, 5, 64, 219
  gas from, 5, 276
  mung, properties of, 4
  red, properties of, 4–6
  for supercharged meals, 7
  white, properties of, 6–7
Beetroot juice, properties of,
    108–10
Beets
  properties of, 108, 110
  raw vs. cooked, 109
  for treating erection
    problems, 264
  uses for, 109

Bell peppers, properties of, 127
Bergamot oil, for treating
  excessive sweating, 341
  fungal nail infections, 286
Berries. See also specific berries
  buying and storing, 31
  for preventing
    cancer, 199–200
    memory loss, 377–78
    varicose veins, 445
  properties of, 27–28, 30–32,
    36–38, 46–48
Beta-carotene
  food sources of, 230, 298–99
  macular degeneration and,
    374, 375
  for preventing
    dementia, 230, 231
    fibrocystic breasts, 271
    osteoporosis, 395
    sunburn, 427
Bites and stings, insect/spider,
    354–56
Black bean extract, for cancer
    prevention, 198
Black beans, properties of, 2
Black cherry, for treating
    bronchitis, 187
Black chokeberries, for
    preventing urinary tract
    infections, 184
Black cumin
  for heart health, 321
  for treating indigestion,
    346
Black pepper
  curcumin and, 169–70, 173,
    181, 195, 205, 262
  properties of, 52–53
Black radish, for preventing
    gallstones, 289
Bladder infections, 16, 37,
    183–85, 381
Blood oranges, 36
Blood sugar dip, preventing, 15
Blueberries
  paired with spinach, 30
  for preventing dementia, 229,
    231
  properties of, 30–32, 219
  for treating high blood
    pressure, 329, 331

Body mass index (BMI)
    breast cancer risk and, 270
    effect on memory, 380
    recommended, for cancer
        prevention, 206
Boje, Andrea, 462
Bone health
    foods for, 12, 22, 35, 78, 381,
        392–93
    loss of (see Osteoporosis)
Borage oil, for treating dry skin,
    255, 262
Brazil nuts, properties of, 73
Breastfeeding, for preventing
    food allergies, 280
Broccoli
    paired with eggs, 110
    preparing, 111
    properties of, 110–12
    for treating peptic ulcers,
        440
Bromelain
    caution about, 194
    in pineapple, 43, 191, 194
    for treating
        bursitis, 194
        eczema, 262
        sinusitis, 416
        vaginitis, 443
Bronchitis, 186–87, 220, 221,
    308
Bruises, 188
Brussels sprouts
    preparing, 113
    properties of, 112–13
Buckwheat
    cooking, 141
    properties of, 140–42
Burns, 189–91
Bursitis, 192–95
Butterbur, for preventing
    migraines, 310–11
B vitamins. See also specific B
        vitamins
    deficiency of, insomnia from,
        358
    food sources of, 379
    for preventing memory loss,
        378
    for stress reduction, 339,
        421–22

C

Cabbage
    properties of, 113–15
    reducing cooking odor of, 114
Caffeine
    anxiety and, 166–67
    avoiding
        with fatigue, 268
        with peptic ulcers, 439
    fibrocystic breasts and, 270
    health benefits of, 201, 202
    pregnancy loss and, 350
    tinnitus and, 433
    for treating dry eyes, 250
Calcium
    food sources of, 180, 261, 294,
        366, 373, 388, 406, 435
    for lupus sufferers, 373
    paired with vitamin D, 106
    for preventing
        kidney stones, 365, 366
        muscle cramps, 388
        osteoporosis, 392, 394
        tooth decay, 435
    for treating PMS, 406
Calcium deficiency
    with ADHD, 179
    with gingivitis, 294
Campanile, Giovanni, 40–41
Cancer, 196–211
    foods causing, 18, 21
    foods preventing or treating,
        197–98, 206
        beans, 2, 4, 5, 198–99
        beverages, 8, 9, 12, 13, 14,
            16, 19, 200–202, 211
        dairy products, 20, 22
        fruits, 25–26, 27, 29–30, 31,
            33–34, 36, 37, 38, 39, 43,
            45, 46, 48, 49, 50, 198,
            199–200, 204–5, 209, 211
        herbs and spices, 51, 53, 54,
            56, 58, 60, 63, 65, 67, 68,
            69, 204, 205
        honey, 102, 205–7
        nuts, 72, 74, 76, 77, 207
        oils, 78–79, 84–85, 204, 207
        omega-3 sources, 208
        seafood, 87
        seeds, 93, 94, 96

        vegetables, 41, 104, 105,
            106, 111, 112, 114, 115–16,
            116–17, 119, 121, 123, 124,
            125, 127, 128, 130, 131,
            132, 133, 134, 135, 136,
            200, 202–3, 203–4, 207,
            208–10
        whole grains, 141, 143, 145,
            146, 211
    healthy habits preventing,
        206
    risk factors for, 196–97
Candidiasis, 55, 56, 281–83. See
        also Fungal infections
Capers, properties of, 53–54
Capsaicin, 128–30
    for heart health, 320–21
    for preventing obesity, 321
    for treating
        arthritis, 173
        peptic ulcers, 441
        shingles, 414
    for weight loss, 400
Carbohydrates, refined,
        diabetes risk from, 239
Cardiovascular disease (CVD).
        See also Heart disease
    causes of, 268, 357, 396, 419,
        436
    conditions associated with,
        160, 224, 407, 411
    foods preventing
        apples, 25
        beverages, 9, 14, 18, 19
        cocoa, 98, 99
        dairy products, 22
        fish, 88, 91
        legumes, 6
        nuts, 72, 74
        oils, 79, 81, 84
        seeds, 93
        turmeric, 69
        vegetables, 110, 111, 124,
            132, 133
        whole grains, 146
    healthy diet preventing, 263,
        399
Carnosine, for stress reduction,
    421
Carotenoids
    food sources of, 157, 298, 427

for preventing
  allergic rhinitis, 157
  cancer, 197
  osteoporosis, _395_
  sunburn, 427
for vision health, 298, 375
Carrots
  for cancer prevention, 200
  properties of, 115–16
  roasting, _115_
Catechins, for preventing heart
  disease, 315, 316
Cauliflower
  buying and using, _117_
  in cheese sauce, _116_
  properties of, 116–17
Cayenne pepper, paired with
  sweet potatoes, _136_
CDC's top 20 powerhouse fruits
  and vegetables, _122_
Celery, for treating high blood
  pressure, 331
Celiac disease, psoriasis and,
  410–11
Centella asiatica, for preventing
  varicose veins, 445
CFS (chronic fatigue syndrome),
  269
Chamomile, for treating
  acid reflux, 150
  anxiety, 167
  gastritis, 292
  heartburn, 324
  indigestion, 347
  menstrual cramps, 385
  PMS, 404–5
Charred meats, cancer risk
  from, _67,_ 197
Cheddar cheese, sardines
  paired with, _22_
Cherries
  buying and storing, _33_
  juicing, _33_
  for preventing or treating
    gout, 32, 302–3
  properties of, 32–34
Cherry juice, for treating
  arthritis, 173
  back pain, 181
Chewing gum, for gum health,
  294

Chia flour, for reducing blood
  pressure, 332
Chia seeds
  properties of, 92–93, 219
  uses for, _92_
Chile peppers. _See_ Peppers,
  chile (hot peppers)
Chocolate
  for heart health, 321
  properties of, 98–100
  for treating
    decreased libido, 224–25,
      264
    diabetes, 239–40
    high blood pressure, 328
Chokeberries
  for cancer prevention, 199
  properties of, 27–28
Chokecherries, fiber in, 219
Cholesterol, high. _See_ High
  cholesterol
Chronic fatigue syndrome (CFS),
  269
Cilantro, properties of, 54–55
Cineole, for treating
  bronchitis, 187
  coughs, 221
Cinnamon, for treating
  diabetes, 241
  menstrual cramps, 385
  PMS, 404
Cistanche tubulosa, for hair
  growth, _306_
Citrus fruits
  for preventing
    cancer, 200
    osteoporosis, _394_
  properties of, 34–36
Clay, for treating diarrhea,
  246–47
Clove oil, for treating fungal
  nail infections, 284
Cocoa
  for heart health, 321
  for preventing
    Alzheimer's disease, 164
    flu, 353
  for treating
    diabetes, 239–40
    high blood pressure,
      328

Coconut oil
  for preventing hair loss,
    306
  properties of, 84–85
  for treating
    dandruff, 222
    dry skin, 256
    yeast infections, 283
Coffee
  caution about, 202
  high blood pressure and,
    329
  pregnancy loss and, 350
  for preventing
    cancer, 200–202
    depression, 237
    diabetes, 240
    gallstones, 288, 289
    gout, 300
  properties of, 8–9
  storing, _9_
Colds, 214–17
Cold sores, 212–13
Colloidal oatmeal, for treating
  dry skin, 256
  hemorrhoids, 325
  hives, 340
  insect bites and stings, 354
  vaginitis, 442
Constipation, 218–19
  causes of, 104, 246, 248, 282,
    325, 360, 361, 404, 406,
    429
  preventing or treating, with
    fiber, 2, 325
    foods, 38, 50, 81, 118, 139,
      145
    probiotics, 346, 363
    water, 16
Copper, for preventing tooth
  decay, 435–36
Coriander, properties of, 54–55
Corticosteroids, for lupus, 371
Coughs, 220–21
  causes of, 156, 174, 186, 214,
    352, 407, 415, 429
  foods treating, 102, 142, 157,
    187, 408, 409, 417
Cramps, menstrual, 55, 384–85,
  405
Cramps, muscle, 388–89

Cranberries
  buying and preparing, <u>37</u>
  for preventing urinary tract
      infections, 183–84
  properties of, 36–38
Cranberry extract, for treating
    oral thrush, 282
Cranberry juice, for treating
    oral thrush, 282
    peptic ulcers, 440
Cruciferous vegetables
  for preventing
      arthritis pain, <u>173</u>
      cancer, 202–3
      diverticulitis, 248
      varicose veins, 444
  thyroid disease and, 430
Cucumbers, properties of, 38
Cumin, for weight loss, <u>400</u>
Curcumin. *See also* Turmeric
  black pepper and, 169–70, 173,
      181, 195, 205, 262
  gallbladder emptying from,
      289
  for preventing
      cancer, 205
      eczema, 262
      peptic ulcers, 441
  for treating
      allergic rhinitis, 157
      anxiety, 169–70
      back pain, 181
      bursitis, 194–95
      fatigue, 268
      gastritis, 291
      gingivitis, 294–95
CVD. *See* Cardiovascular
    disease
Cystitis. *See* Bladder infections

D

Dairy-free diet, 155, <u>461</u>, <u>462</u>
Dairy products. *See also* Eggs;
    Milk, dairy; Yogurt
  fermented, for acne, 152
  gas from, 276
  for preventing
      diabetes, 240–41
      eczema, 260

heart disease, 316
  osteoporosis, <u>394</u>
Dandruff, 102, 108, 222–23
Dark, leafy greens. *See* Greens,
    dark, leafy
DASH diet
  for brain health, 161–62, 228
  for preventing tooth decay,
      437
  for treating lupus, 371
Decreased libido, 153, 224–25,
    263, 264, 381, 383
Dehydration
  causes of, 245, 390–91
  effects of, 364, 368
Dementia, 226–31. *See also*
    Alzheimer's disease
  contributors to, 89, 312, 327,
      396, <u>436</u>
  foods preventing or treating,
      15, 68, 70, 380
Depression, 232–37
  foods preventing or treating
      beverages, 9, 14, 17, 18
      fermented foods, 167, 169
      in healthy diet, 166
      herbs and spices, 69, 167,
          405, 421
      olive oil, 78
      omega-3 fatty acids, 422
      probiotic, 24, 420–21
      seeds, 93, 94
      tomatoes, 48
      wheat germ extract, 406
  health conditions associated
      with, 153, 357, 396, 404,
      405, 406, 419, 429
Dermatitis
  atopic, 255, 256, 259, 262
  eczema as, 259–62
Diabetes, gestational, 238
Diabetes, type 1, 238
Diabetes, type 2
  dietary guidelines for, 238–44
  facts and statistics on, 238
  foods preventing or
      controlling
      beans and legumes, 3–4, 7
      beverages, 8, 14, 19
      chocolate, 98–99
      dairy products, 21, 24

fruits, 25, 27, 34, 35–36, 42,
    46, 47–48
  herbs and spices, 54, 55, 56,
      59, 60, 62, 65, 68, 69, 70
  honey, 102
  nuts, 75–76
  olive oil, 78
  seeds, 95
  vegetables, 110, 112, 123,
      128, 132, 133
  whole grains, 141, 145–46
  high blood pressure and, 327
  reversal of, <u>460–61</u>
  tinnitus with, 433
Diarrhea, 245–47
  causes of, 165, 248, 278, 282,
      325, 360, 361, 404, 407
  preventing or treating, with
      foods, 69, 104, 118, 131, <u>362</u>
  probiotics, 216, 219, 346,
      408
Dill, for treating menstrual
    cramps, 384
Diosmectite, for treating
    diarrhea, 246–47
Dishwashing, for stress relief,
    <u>420</u>
Diverticulitis, 248–49
Dry eyes, 16, 39, 250–51, 252,
    370
Dry mouth, 16, 252–53, 272
Dry skin, 254–56
  causes of, 262, 381, 382–83,
      410, 429
  dandruff from, 222
  treating, 96, 222, 262, 383,
      457
Dysmenorrhea, 55, 384–85, 405

E

Earache, 257–58
Eczema, 222, 259–62
  dry skin from, 254, 255
  food allergies and, 278, 279,
      280
  foods treating, 143, 152
EGCG
  in green tea, 14
  for preventing

heart disease, 316
sunburn, 427
for treating yeast infections,
283
for weight loss, 402
Eggs
broccoli paired with, 110
properties of, 20–21
as salad topper, 20
Erection problems and erectile
dysfunction, 50, 224,
263–65
Essential fatty acids, 169, 222,
255, 262, 304. *See also*
Omega-3 fatty acids;
Omega-6 fatty acids;
Omega-9 fatty acids
Essential oils, for treating
fungal nail infections,
284–86
Eucalyptus, for treating
coughs, 221
pneumonia symptoms, 408,
409
Eucalyptus oil, for treating
fungal nail infections,
285
EVOO. *See* Extra-virgin olive
oil
Excitotoxin elimination diet,
for fibromyalgia, 274
Excitotoxins, tinnitus and,
433–34
Exercise
for immune system support,
107
for preventing
Alzheimer's disease,
160–61, 163
cancer, 206
diabetes, 242
glaucoma, 298
for stress reduction, 314
Extraordinary people,
extraordinary healing
Aaron and Jen, 461
Boje, Andrea, 462
Gordon, Maria, 460–61
Huber, Lia, 459–60
Rosenberg, Lisa Rae, 460
Yeager, Samantha, 461

Extra-virgin olive oil (EVOO).
See also Olive oil
for preventing
Alzheimer's disease, 162
cancer, 207
properties of, 78–81

F

Fat, abdominal, 22, 27, 77, 336,
398, 402, 403
Fat, dietary. *See also* specific
oils and omega fatty
acids
gallbladder emptying and,
288–89
paired with vegetables,
78, 82
Fatigue, 266–69
adrenal, 153–55
treating, with
coconut oil, 85
herbs and spices, 55, 60, 62
hydration, 16, 17, 237
Feingold diet, for ADHD, 178
Fennel
properties of, 118–19
for treating
acid reflux, 149
gastritis, 291
heartburn, 323
indigestion, 346
PMS, 404
Fenugreek
properties of, 55–56
for treating
diabetes, 241
menstrual cramps, 385
Fermented foods
for preventing diabetes,
240–41
for treating
acne, 152
anxiety, 167, 169
Fever blisters, 212–13
Fiber
deficient in diet, 40
food sources of, 5, 40, 218,
219, 288, 325, 425, 444,
447

for gastrointestinal health, 2
for preventing
cancer, 198, 199, 206
diverticulitis, 248
stroke, 425
varicose veins, 444
for treating
constipation, 218–19, 325
diverticulitis, 248
high cholesterol, 64, 335
for weight loss, 2, 64
Fibroadenomas, 270–71
Fibrocystic breasts, 270–71
Fibromyalgia, 69, 272–75,
460
Fish, 86–91. *See also* Seafood
buying, 89
garlic paired with, 90
lacking in diet, 82
wine paired with, 40
Flatulence, 2, 276–77
reducing, 5, 69, 118, 346,
363
Flavonoids
food sources of, 257, 414,
424–25
for preventing
dementia, 229, 231
diabetes, 239, 243
ear infections, 257
flu, 352–53
glaucoma, 297
heart disease, 315–16
memory loss, 377–78
shingles, 414
stroke, 424–25
for treating
asthma, 174
high blood pressure,
328–29, 331
Flaxseed oil, 93
for preventing cancer, 204
properties of, 81
for treating dry skin, 255,
256, 262
Flaxseeds, 93
for preventing cancer, 204
properties of, 93–94
for treating high blood
pressure, 331–32
Flu. *See* Influenza

FODMAPs. *See also* Low-
    FODMAP diet
  diarrhea and, 246
  gas and, 276–77
Folate, food sources of, 225, 265,
    350–51, 382
Folic acid, for treating
  erection problems, 265
  hot flashes, 382
  menopausal symptoms, 225
Food allergies, 278–80
  conditions related to, 156,
    159, 245, 259, 290, 339,
    345
Food combinations for overall
    health, 10, 40, 64, 82, 106
Food dyes, ADHD and, 178
Food triggers. *See* Trigger
    foods, for specific
    conditions
Free radicals, aging and, 454
Fruit juices. *See also specific*
    juices
  for preventing
    kidney stones, 364
    memory loss, 378
  during wound healing, 453
Fruits. *See also specific fruits*
  CDC-recommended, 122
  cleaning, 26
  for weight loss, 399
Fungal infections, general, 108,
    222, 281–83
  preventing or treating, 43, 55,
    65, 408
Fungal infections, nail, 284–86

G

Gac fruit, properties of, 38–39,
    456
Gallstones, 287–89, 345
Garlic
  fish paired with, 90
  onions paired with, 56
  for preventing
    cancer, 204
    colds, 11, 41, 215–16
    vaginitis, 443
  properties of, 56–58
  roasting, 57

  for treating
    bronchitis, 186
    ear infections, 258
    fatigue, 269
    high blood pressure, 329
    high cholesterol, 337–38
    warts, 448
    yeast infections, 283
Garlic oil, for treating fungal
    nail infections, 285
Gas. *See* Flatulence
Gastritis, 290–92, 345
Gastroesophageal reflux
    disease (GERD), 148, 220,
    308, 322, 438
GI. *See* Glycemic index of foods
Ginger
  buying, 59
  for fertility, 351
  in marinades, 59
  for preventing
    colds, 41, 215
    vaginitis, 443
  properties of, 58–60
  for treating
    acid reflux, 148–49
    arthritis, 172
    asthma, 175
    bronchitis, 186–87
    bursitis, 195
    coughs, 221
    decreased libido, 225
    diabetes, 243–44
    gastritis, 291
    heartburn, 323
    indigestion, 346
    menstrual cramps, 384
    motion sickness, 386–87
    nausea, 64, 390
    pneumonia symptoms,
      408–9
    sinusitis, 416
Gingivitis, 293–96, 435, 436
Ginkgo biloba
  for memory improvement,
    380
  tinnitus and, 434
Ginseng
  properties of, 60–62
  for treating
    bronchitis, 187
    erection problems, 264–65

Glaucoma, 297–99
Glutamine, for wound healing,
    451
Gluten-free diet, 275, 410–11,
    461, 462
Gluten-free grains, 154
Glycemic index (GI) of foods
  acne and, 151
  diabetes and, 242
  sleep quality and, 358–59
  white beans reducing, 7
Glycine, for treating hot flashes,
    382
Goitrogenic foods, effect
    on thyroid function,
    430–31
Gordon, Maria, 460–61
Gout, 32, 300–303
Grapefruit juice
  for arterial health, 34
  scopolamine and, 386
Grape juice, for cancer
    prevention, 204–5
Grapes
  paired with raspberries, 46
  for preventing
    cancer, 204–5
    wrinkles, 455–56
  properties of, 39, 42
Grape seed extract, for treating
  peptic ulcers, 440
  wounds, 453
Grape seed oil, for dry skin,
    256
Greens
  cooking, 120
  dark, leafy
    for cancer prevention,
      203–4
    for heart disease
      prevention, 314, 315
    for osteoporosis prevention,
      394–95
  in smoothies, 119, 121
  in soup, 119
  paired with olive oil, 78
  properties of, 119–21, 123
Green tea. *See* Tea
Green tea extract, for wound
    healing, 453
Grilled meat, rosemary paired
    with, 67

H

Hair loss, 95, 153, 222, 223, 262, 304–6, 370, 429
Halitosis, 307–8
  causes of, 252, 293, 415, 435
  preventing, 16, <u>126</u>, 295, 308
Hay fever, 156–59, 175, 280
Headaches, 309–12. *See also* Migraines
  causes of, 153, 156, 165, 272, 282, 343, 352, 369, 370, 404, 413, 423, 446
  preventing or treating, 16, 55, 242, 385, 406
Healing Foods
  for ADHD, <u>177</u>
  for arthritis pain, <u>173</u>
  for common cold, <u>215</u>
  for eczema, <u>261</u>
  for gout, <u>301</u>
  for insect/spider bites and stings, <u>356</u>
Healthy Insights
  dishwashing for stress relief, <u>420</u>
  exercise for glaucoma prevention, <u>298</u>
  kudzu for fatigue, <u>267</u>
  rosemary for memory, <u>227</u>
  sake yeast for sleep quality, <u>358</u>
  smoking and ulcers, <u>440</u>
  tooth loss and health risks, <u>436</u>
Heartburn, 63, 148, 150, 292, 322–24, 345, 347, 439
Heart disease, 313–21. *See also* Cardiovascular disease (CVD)
  foods preventing, 313–21
    cocoa, 321
    dairy products, 22
    fish, 88
    legumes, 2, 3
    nuts, 72, 75, 207, 336
    olive oil, 79
    soy isoflavones, 382
    tea, 14
    vegetables, 123, 130, 134
    whole grains, 320
  lupus and, 373
  risk factors for, 293, 300, 313–14, 320, 334, 337, 381, 419
  stroke risk from, 423
  tinnitus and, 433
  types of, 313
Heavy metals
  detoxifying from, <u>375</u>
  macular degeneration from, 375–76
Helicobacter pylori
  bad breath and, 308
  gastritis and, 290, 291
  peptic ulcers from, 439
Hemorrhoids, 325–26, 445
Herbs. *See also specific herbs*
  drying and storing, <u>61</u>
  for preventing
    cancer, 205
    osteoporosis, 393, <u>395</u>
High blood pressure, 327–33
  benefits of lowering, 327
  foods lowering, 328–32
    beans and legumes, 2, 6
    beverages, 13, 14
    chocolate, 98, 99, 100
    fruits, 27, 28, 31, 36, 45, 50
    herbs and spices, 53, 56, 58
    nuts, 75, 76, 77
    oils, 80, 84
    seeds, 92–93, 94, 96, 97
    vegetables, 108, 123, 125
    whole grains, 141
    yogurt, 24
  minerals affecting, 332–33
  recommended range of, 327–28
  sodium and, 432–33
  as stroke risk factor, 423
High cholesterol, 334–38
  foods lowering, 425
    beverages, 12, 14, 19, 316, 402
    cocoa, 239, 321
    fruits, 25, 28, 29, 34, 36, 38, 46, 47, 48, 49
    herbs and spices, 56, 58, 68, 69, <u>90</u>, 241, 243, 244, 321, <u>400</u>
    honey, 102
    legumes, 2, 4, 6, <u>64</u>
    nuts, 72, 73, 74, 75, 76, 77, 317, 331
    oils, 80, 81, 84
    omega-3 fatty acids, 317, 320
    seeds, 96, 97
    soy, 13, 381–82
    vegetables, 104, 111, 114, 125, 126, 128, 133, 134, 331
    whole grains, <u>64</u>, 139, 140, 141, 142, 145
    yogurt, 24
  gout and, 300, 302
  as heart disease risk factor, 313
  with hypothyroidism, 429
  as stroke risk factor, 423, 425
  from trans fats, 350
  vegan diet lowering, 310, <u>460</u>
  vertigo and, 447
  yoga lowering, <u>314</u>
High-fat diet, infertility and, 348–49, 350
High-fructose corn syrup, gout risk from, 300, <u>301</u>
Himalayan salt, for preventing eczema, 260
Hives, 278, 339–40
Holy basil
  properties of, 51–52
  for treating
    diabetes, 241–43
    stress, 421
Honey
  for preventing
    cancer, 205–7
    colds, 216
    tooth decay, 437
  properties of, 100–102
  as sugar swap, <u>101</u>
  for treating
    allergic rhinitis, 156–57
    bronchitis, 187
    burns, 189–90
    cold sores, 213
    coughs, 157, 187, 220–21
    dandruff, 222–23
    eczema, 262
    flu, 353
    hemorrhoids, 325–26
    insect bites and stings, 355

Honey (*cont.*)
    for treating (*cont.*)
        pneumonia symptoms,
            408–9
        sinusitis, 416
        wounds, 452–53
Hot flashes, 102, 225, 381, 382
Hot peppers. *See* Peppers, chile
HRSV, 214–15
Huber, Lia, 459–60
Human respiratory syncytial
    virus (HRSV), 214–15
Hydration. *See also* Water;
    specific beverages
    during diarrhea, 245–46
    during flu, 353
    for preventing
        dry eyes, 250
        gout, 300
        kidney stones, 364
        muscle cramps, 388
    for treating
        dry mouth, 252
        dry skin, 254
        lightheadedness, 368
        pneumonia, 408
        vertigo, 446
    after vomiting, 390–91
    during wound healing, 453
Hyperhidrosis, 341–42
Hypertension. *See* High blood
    pressure
Hyperthyroidism, 429, 430, 431
Hypoglycemia, 343–44
    health effects of, 312, 342,
        368, 369, 446
Hypothyroidism, 429, 430, 431

I

IBS. *See* Irritable bowel
    syndrome
Immune system support
    exercise for, 107
    for preventing shingles,
        413–14
Indian gooseberries, for
    treating peptic ulcers,
    440
Indigestion, 54, 69, 104, 118,
    150, 292, 324, 345–47

Indulgent foods, expert-
    recommended, 11, 41, 83,
    107
Infertility, 348–51, 396
Influenza, 112, 217, 352–53, 407
Insect/spider bites and stings,
    354–56
Insomnia, 357–59
    causes of, 165, 170, 381, 419,
        422
    effects of, 266, 309, 454
    treating, 32, 100, 236
Insulin resistance, 164, 229,
    302, 331, 397. *See also*
    Diabetes, type 2
Iodine, for thyroid function,
    430
Iron
    food sources of, 261, 267, 273,
        306, 406, 422
    for preventing
        fatigue, 267
        PMS, 406
    for treating
        ADHD, 178–79
        anxiety, 168, 170
        fibromyalgia, 273
        stress, 422
Iron absorption
    from lentils and lemons, 3
    vitamin C for, 64, 106
Iron deficiency
    with ADHD, 178
    hair loss from, 305–6
Irritable bowel syndrome (IBS),
    91, 104, 246, 272, 274, 345,
    360–63
Ivy leaf extract, for bronchitis,
    187

J

Joint pain, 171–73. *See also*
    Arthritis

K

Kadey, Matthew, 82–83
Kaffir limes, properties of, 36
Kale, in soups, 119

Kale juice, for reducing blood
    pressure, 332
Kefir
    paired with almonds, 72
    properties of, 9, 12
    for treating constipation, 219
Kidney stones, 16, 17, 364–67,
    396
Korean red ginseng, for treating
    tinnitus, 434
Kudzu, for fatigue, 267

L

Lactose intolerance, 12, 21, 23,
    245, 276, 394
Laminaria japonica, for hair
    growth, 306
L-arginine, for increased sex
    drive, 224, 264
Lavender, for treating anxiety,
    169
Lavender oil, for treating
    fungal nail infections, 285
    insect bites and stings,
        354–55
Legumes. *See also* Beans;
    Lentils; Split peas
    for treating high cholesterol,
        336
Lemongrass oil, for treating
    dandruff, 222
Lemons or lemon juice
    for iron absorption, 3
    for treating
        high blood pressure, 36
        insect bites and stings, 356
        nausea, 390
Lemon zest, 35
Lentils
    lemons and, for iron
        absorption, 3
    properties of, 3–4, 219
Libido, decreased. *See*
    Decreased libido
Lichen planus, 461
Licorice
    cautions about, 158, 291–92,
        323–24, 347, 369, 409, 414,
        417
    for preventing colds, 214–15

properties of, 62–63
for treating
  acid reflux, 149–50
  allergic rhinitis, 158
  coughs, 221
  gastritis, 291–92
  heartburn, 323–24
  indigestion, 346–47
  lightheadedness, 369
  pneumonia symptoms, 408,
    409
  shingles, 414
  sinusitis, 416
  sore throat, 417
Lightheadedness, 16, 165,
  368–69, 446
Lignans, for weight loss, 398–99
Lime juice, for treating insect
  bites and stings, 356
Limes, Kaffir, properties of, 36
Low-carb diet, for weight loss,
  399
Low-flatulogenic diet, for
  reducing gas, 276
Low-FODMAP diet
  for preventing diarrhea, 246
  for treating IBS, 360–61
Low Tyramine Headache Diet,
  310
Lupus, 250, 370–73, 459, 460
Lutein, for vision health, 375,
  376
Lycopene
  for improving fertility, 350
  for preventing wrinkles, 456

M

Maca
  for improving fertility, 351
  for increased sex drive, 225
Macular degeneration, 87, 88,
  115, 374–76
Magnesium
  food sources of, 2, 312, 358,
    388, 406, 422
  glaucoma risk and, 298,
    299
  for preventing
    headaches, 312
    muscle cramps, 388

for treating
  anxiety, 168, 170
  insomnia, 358
  PMS, 406
  stress, 422
Malassezia fungus, dandruff
  from, 222, 223
Mammy apples, fiber in, 219
Manganese, for preventing
  macular degeneration,
  376
Marshmallow root, for treating
  dry mouth, 253
  sore throat, 417
Mayonnaise substitute, 23
Meal timing, for weight loss,
  400–401
Meats
  charred, cancer risk from,
    67, 197
  gout risk from, 300–301
  processed, cancer risk from,
    197
  red, limiting, 206
Mediterranean diet
  foods in, 3, 17, 19, 26, 38, 63,
    77, 78, 80
  for preventing
    Alzheimer's disease,
      161–62
    cancer, 198, 207
    dementia, 228
    depression, 233–34
    fatigue, 266
    heart disease, 79, 313–14
    memory loss, 80, 380
    osteoporosis, 393
    stroke, 424
  for treating
    asthma, 175
    decreased libido, 224
    erection problems, 263
    high blood pressure,
      79–80
    high cholesterol, 338
    hot flashes, 382
    lupus, 370–71
    tinnitus, 433, 434
  for weight loss, 40, 398
  wine in, 19
Memory, rosemary improving,
  227

Memory loss. *See also*
  Alzheimer's disease;
  Dementia
  short-term, 377–80
  from vitamin B$_{12}$ deficiency,
    236
Ménière's disease, 432
Menopause, 225, 270, 381–83,
  392
Menstrual cramps, 55, 384–85,
  405
Metabolic syndrome
  foods preventing or treating
    beans, 2
    coffee, 240
    dairy products, 21, 22
    fruits, 28, 29, 36, 46
    mushrooms, 125
    nuts, 75, 77, 316
    olive oil, 79
    probiotic, 402
    turmeric, 69–70
  health effects of, 224, 263
  lupus and, 370
MEWS diet, for food allergies,
  280
Migraines, 128, 309–12,
  343, 446, 461. *See also*
  Headaches
Milk, dairy
  for preventing gout, 303
  properties of, 21–22
  for treating insect bites and
    stings, 356
Milk, plant-based, properties
  of, 12–13
Milk allergy, 12, 21
Milk thistle
  for preventing gallstones,
    289
  for treating diabetic
    complications, 244
MIND diet, for preventing
  Alzheimer's disease, 161–62
  dementia, 228–29
Mint, for treating
  bad breath, 307
  nausea, 390
Mohr, Christopher, 10–11
Monosodium glutamate. *See*
  MSG avoidance
Mood-boosting foods, 234–35

Moringa stenopetala plant, for bronchitis, <u>187</u>
Motion sickness, 386–87, 390, 446
MSG avoidance
with fibromyalgia, 274
with tinnitus, 434
Mulberry leaves, for treating peptic ulcers, 440
Mullein oil, for treating ear infections, 258
Multivitamins, <u>107</u>, <u>163</u>
Mung bean extract, for cancer prevention, 198–99
Mung beans, properties of, 4
Muscle cramps, 388–89
Mushrooms
for preventing cancer, 207
properties of, 123–25
for treating
bronchitis, 187
colds, 214
fatigue, 268–69
Myrrh oil, for treating fungal nail infections, 285

N

Nail infections, fungal, 284–86
Nasal irrigation, for treating
allergic rhinitis, <u>158</u>
sinusitis, 416
Nausea, 390–91
causes of, 148, 165, 202, 218, 248, 278, 281, 287, 290, 343, 345, 364, 386, 406, 407, 413, 439, 446
foods treating
cinnamon, 385
fennel, 119, 149, 291, 323, 346
fenugreek, 55, 385
ginger, 58–59, 148, 323, 346, 386, 387, 390
licorice, 63
New Nordic diet, for weight loss, 398
Niacin
food sources of, 255, <u>261</u>, 358
for treating insomnia, 358
Nisevich Bede, Pamela, <u>106–7</u>

Nitrates
for blood pressure reduction, 332
for erection problems, 264
Nitric oxide (NO)
for erection problems, 263–64
for increased sex drive, 224
Nordic diet
for treating lupus, 371
for weight loss, 398
Nuts. *See also specific nuts*
for preventing
cancer, 207
heart disease, 316–17
as snack, <u>11</u>
for treating
high blood pressure, 331
high cholesterol, 336–37

O

OAG (open-angle glaucoma), 298
OAS (oral allergy syndrome), 159
Oats. *See also* Colloidal oatmeal
cooking, <u>143</u>
properties of, 142–44
for treating
high cholesterol, <u>64</u>, 337
insect bites and stings, 354
psoriasis, 412
Obesity. *See* Overweight and obesity
Oil pulling, for oral health, 295–96, 308, 437–38
Oils, 78–85. *See also specific oils*
Olive oil. *See also* Extra-virgin olive oil (EVOO)
for burn healing, 191
grades of, <u>80</u>
paired with leafy greens, <u>78</u>
for preventing osteoporosis, 393, <u>395</u>
for treating
dandruff, 222
dry skin, 256
fungal nail infections, 286
high cholesterol, 338
yeast infections, 282

Omega-3 fatty acids
deficiency of, <u>10</u>
food sources of, 162, 251, <u>379</u>, 385, 412, 416, 422, 428, 451
for preventing
Alzheimer's disease, 162–64
cancer, 208
depression, 235–36
effects of stress, 422
glaucoma, 299
hair loss, 305
heart disease, 317, 320
migraines, 311
sunburn, 428
wrinkles, 455
for treating
acne, 152
ADHD, 176, 178
anxiety, <u>168</u>, 169
arthritis, 171
asthma, 175
back pain, 181
bursitis, 192
dry eyes, 250–51
high cholesterol, 338
high triglycerides, <u>10</u>
hives, 340
lightheadedness, 369
lupus, 371–72
menstrual cramps, 385
psoriasis, 411–12
sinusitis, 416
wounds, 450–51
Omega-6 fatty acids
anxiety and, 169
asthma and, 175
cancer prevention and, 208
delaying wound healing, 451
glaucoma and, 299
hair loss and, 305
lupus and, 371
Omega-9 fatty acids, <u>168</u>, 169, 335
Onions
for cancer prevention, 208–9
paired with garlic, <u>56</u>
preventing bad breath from, <u>126</u>
properties of, 125–26
Open-angle glaucoma (OAG), 298
Oral allergy syndrome (OAS), 159

Oral hydration therapy, 245–46, 368
Orange juice, for bone health, 35
Oranges, 34, 36
Oregano
    for heart health, 321
    properties of, 63, 65
Oregano oil, for treating fungal nail infections, 285
Osteoporosis
    causes of, 180, 373, 381, 392–95, 396
    preventing, with
        calcium and vitamin D, 110, 180, 381
        foods, 12, 22, 34, 80, 118, 134
Otitis media, 257–58
Overweight and obesity, 396–403
    abdominal fat with, 22, 27, 77, 336, 398, 402, 403
    health conditions from
        Alzheimer's disease, 160, 227
        back pain, 180
        cardiovascular disease, 232, 313
        cognitive decline, 380
        decreased libido, 224
        diverticulitis, 248, 249
        gallstones, 288
        infertility, 348, 349
        muscle cramps, 388
        psoriasis, 411
        stroke, 423
    from insomnia, 357
    preventing, with
        capsaicin, 321
        diet, 7
        foods, 14, 69, 76, 98, 174, 240, 331
        milk thistle, 244, 289
    tooth loss and, 436
Oxalates, kidney stones and, 364–66
Oysters, properties of, 86–87

P

Panic attacks, 165, 170
Papayas
    properties of, 42–43
    for wound healing, 452

Parsley
    for fresh breath, 126
    for heart health, 321
    properties of, 65–66
Passion fruit, fiber in, 219
PCOS, 350
Peanut allergy, 279
Peanuts
    for preventing fibrocystic breasts, 271
    properties of, 73–74
Peas, split, properties of, 6, 219
Pecans, properties of, 74–75
Pepper, black, properties of, 52–53
Pepper, cayenne, paired with sweet potatoes, 136
Peppermint oil, for treating
    fungal nail infections, 286
    hives, 340
    IBS, 363
    insect bites and stings, 354
Peppers, bell, properties of, 127
Peppers, chile (hot peppers)
    cooking, 129
    properties of, 128–30
    for weight loss, 400
Peptic ulcers. See Ulcers, peptic
Persian shallot, for treating yeast infections, 282
Pesto, pistachios in, 76
Pickle juice, for treating muscle cramps, 389
Pineapples
    bromelain in, 43, 191, 194
    buying and preparing, 44
    properties of, 43–44, 171, 262
    for treating
        bursitis, 194
        sinusitis, 416
Pistachios
    in pesto, 76
    properties of, 75–76
    for treating
        high blood pressure, 331
        high cholesterol, 336–37
Plant-based milk, properties of, 12–13
Plant sterols, for lowering cholesterol, 335–36
PMS. See Premenstrual syndrome

Pneumonia, 407–9
Polycystic ovary syndrome (PCOS), 350
Polyunsaturated fatty acids. See PUFAs
Pomegranate extract, for treating
    fungal nail infections, 286
    peptic ulcers, 440–41
Pomegranate juice, for treating erection problems, 264
Pomegranates
    in anti-inflammatory diet, 171
    for cancer prevention, 209
    properties of, 44–46
Potassium
    food sources of, 107, 261, 333, 388, 425–26
    for lowering blood pressure, 333
    for preventing
        muscle cramps, 388
        stroke, 425–26
Potassium citrate, for preventing kidney stones, 364
Power Pairs
    almonds and kefir, 72
    broccoli and eggs, 110
    eggs and salad, 20
    garlic and fish, 90
    garlic and onions, 56
    green tea and toast, 15
    leafy greens and olive oil, 78
    lentils and lemons, 3
    raspberries and grapes, 46
    rosemary and grilled meats, 67
    salmon and tomatoes, 88
    sardines and Cheddar cheese, 22
    spinach and blueberries, 30
    sweet potatoes and cayenne pepper, 136
Prebiotics
    for preventing food allergies, 280
    for weight loss, 399–400, 401–2
    for wound healing, 451–52

Premenstrual syndrome (PMS),
     110, 119, 272, 404–6
Probiotics
     deficiency of, 64
     food sources of, 9, 383, 408,
          418, 443
     for preventing
          bad breath, 307–8
          colds, 216
          diarrhea, 246
          eczema, 259, 261
          flu, 353
          food allergies, 280
          pneumonia, 408
          sore throat, 418
          urinary tract infections,
               184–85
          wrinkles, 457
     for treating
          allergic rhinitis, 157–58
          anxiety, 167, 168, 420–21
          constipation, 219
          depression, 420–21
          diarrhea, 246
          dry skin, 255, 382–83
          gingivitis, 294
          IBS, 361, 363
          indigestion, 346
          peptic ulcers, 440
          sore throat, 418
          vaginitis, 442–43
          yeast infections, 282–83
     for weight loss, 399–400, 402
     for wound healing, 451–52
Processed meats, cancer risk
     from, 197, 206
Protein
     animal, kidney stones from,
          366–67
     for heart health, 320
     for preventing hair loss,
          304–5
     for treating
          adrenal exhaustion, 154
          anxiety, 168
          lightheadedness, 369
Psoriasis, 69, 128, 143, 222, 254,
     262, 410–12
PUFAs, for preventing
     depression, 235–36
     heart disease, 317, 320
     memory loss, 378, 380

Pumpkin
     canned, uses for, 95
     for preventing peptic ulcers,
          441
Pumpkin seeds
     for preventing peptic ulcers,
          441
     properties of, 94–95
Pycnogenol, for treating
          varicose veins, 445

Q

Quercetin
     food sources of, 261, 315
     for preventing heart disease,
          315–16
     for treating
          allergic rhinitis, 157
          asthma, 174
          bursitis, 194
          cold sores, 213
          eczema, 262
          high blood pressure, 329
          hives, 339–40
Quince juice, for treating peptic
     ulcers, 440
Quinoa
     cooking, 144
     in desserts, 142
     properties of, 144–45

R

Raspberries
     paired with grapes, 46
     properties of, 46–47
Red beans, properties of, 4–6
Red clover extract
     for increased sex drive, 225
     for menopausal symptoms,
          383
Red ginseng, for preventing
          wrinkles, 457
Red palm oil, properties of, 81,
     84
Red wine
     as anti-inflammatory, 173,
          181
     for heart health, 318, 424

Restaurant foods, expert-
     recommended, 11, 41, 107
Resveratrol
     for heart health, 318, 424
     for preventing
          cancer, 204
          fatigue, 268
          memory loss, 378
          wrinkles, 456
     for treating
          arthritis, 173
          back pain, 181
          cold sores, 213
          hot flashes, 382
          peptic ulcers, 440
     for vision health, 207
Riboflavin
     for preventing migraines, 310,
          311
     for treating PMS, 405
Rosemary
     for memory improvement, 227
     paired with grilled meat, 67
     properties of, 66–67
Rosemary oil, for hair growth,
     306
Rosenberg, Lisa Rae, 460

S

Safflower oil, for treating yeast
     infections, 282
Saffron, for weight loss, 400
Sage
     for heart health, 321
     properties of, 67–68
     for treating
          excessive sweating, 341
          sore throat, 417
Sage leaf extract, for treating
     diabetes, 244
Sage oil, for treating fungal nail
     infections, 285
Sake yeast, for sleep quality,
     358
Salad dressing, apple cider
     vinegar in, 79
Salads
     eggs topping, 20
     with fat source, 40
     olive oil on, 78

Salicylate-free diet, for ADHD, <u>177</u>, 178
Salmon
    paired with tomatoes, <u>88</u>
    properties of, 87–89
Salt. *See* Sodium
Sardines
    paired with Cheddar cheese, <u>22</u>
    properties of, 89–90
Sauerkraut, properties of, 130–31
Scarborough Fair Diet, for preventing osteoporosis, 393
Scopolamine, for motion sickness, <u>386</u>
Sea cucumbers, 209–10
Seafood, <u>86</u>, 86–87. *See also* Fish
    oysters, 86–87
    for preventing hair loss, 304–5
Sea vegetables and seaweed
    for cancer prevention, 209–10
    introducing, in diet, <u>132</u>
    iodine in, 430
    properties of, 131–33
Seborrhea. *See* Dandruff
Seizures, <u>106</u>
Selenium
    deficiency of, depression from, 236
    food sources of, <u>234</u>
    for thyroid function, 430
    for treating asthma, 174–75
Sesame oil, for treating yeast infections, 282
Sesame seeds, properties of, 95–96
Sex drive, decreased. *See* Decreased libido
Shallot oil, for treating fungal nail infections, 286
Shellfish. *See* Seafood
Shingles, 413–14
Silymarin
    for preventing gallstones, 289
    for treating diabetic complications, 244
Sinusitis, 44, 156, 308, 415–16
Skin irritation, cleanse for treating, <u>461</u>

Smoking, ulcer risk from, <u>440</u>
Smoking cessation, for cancer prevention, <u>206</u>
Smoothies, <u>7</u>, <u>30</u>, <u>82</u>, <u>92</u>, <u>119</u>, <u>121</u>
Snacks, grab-and-go, <u>11</u>, <u>83</u>, <u>107</u>
Sodium
    increasing blood pressure, 332, 432
    kidney stones from, 366
    reducing intake of, <u>365</u>, 444–45
    stroke risk from, 424
    tinnitus and, 432–33
Sore throat, 186, 214, 415, 417–18
Sorghum, properties of, 145–46
Soy isoflavones
    for improved memory, 380
    for preventing wrinkles, 456
    in soy milk, 13
    for treating menopausal symptoms, 381–82
Soy milk, 13
Soy products
    for preventing fibrocystic breasts, 270
    properties of, 133–35
    for supercharging diet, <u>134</u>
Spices. *See specific spices*
Spicy foods, for treating sinusitis, 416
Spinach
    paired with blueberries, <u>30</u>
    for reducing blood pressure, 332
Split peas, properties of, 6, 219
Strawberries
    for preventing dementia, 229, 231
    properties of, 47–48
Stress, 419–22
    foods treating, 24, 52, 98, 118, 166–67, 169, <u>362</u>
    health effects of
        acne, 151
        adrenal exhaustion, 153
        back pain, 180
        cold sores, 212
        decreased libido, 224
        diarrhea, 245
        excessive sweating, 342
        fatigue, 266

        free radical damage, 170
        gastritis, 290
        headaches, 309
        heartburn, 322
        heart disease, 313, <u>314</u>
        hives, 339
        IBS, 360, 363
        indigestion, 345
        insomnia, 357
        lightheadedness, 368
        menstrual cramps, 384
        peptic ulcers, 439
        shingles, 413
        stroke, 423, 426
        tinnitus, 434
        vertigo, 447
        wrinkles, 454
        yeast infections, 281
Stroke, 423–26
    foods preventing
        beverages, 14, 15, 18
        chocolate, 99
        citrus fruits, 35
        dairy, 22
        vegetables, 123
        whole grains, 146
Sugar
    ADHD and, 178
    avoiding
        with fatigue, 268
        for weight loss, 399
    cancer risk from, <u>206</u>
    honey as substitute for, <u>101</u>
    tooth decay from, 268, 437
Suicide risk, foods preventing, coffee, 8–9
Sunburn, 189, 217, 260, 427–28
Sunflower seed oil, for treating dandruff, 222
Sunflower seeds, properties of, 96–97
Supercharge Your Meals, with
    apple cider vinegar, <u>79</u>
    avocados in desserts, <u>28</u>
    beans, <u>7</u>
    beets, <u>109</u>
    canned pumpkin, <u>95</u>
    cauliflower in cheese sauce, <u>116</u>
    chia seeds, <u>92</u>
    Greek yogurt as mayo substitute, <u>23</u>

Supercharge Your Meals, with
(*cont.*)
kale in soups, <u>119</u>
pistachios in pesto, <u>76</u>
quinoa, <u>142</u>
seaweed, <u>132</u>
smoothie additives, <u>121</u>
tofu, <u>134</u>
vegetables as cream
substitute in soup, <u>118</u>
Sweating, excessive, 341–42
Sweet potatoes
paired with cayenne pepper,
<u>136</u>
properties of, 136, 138
storing and preparing, <u>137</u>

T

Tai chi, for stress reduction,
<u>314</u>
Tea
for oral health, 295
paired with toast, <u>15</u>
for preventing
Alzheimer's disease, 162
bad breath, 307
cancer, 211
colds, 217
depression, 237
diabetes, 240
heart disease, 316
osteoporosis, 395, <u>395</u>
stroke, 425
sunburn, 427
warts, 449
wrinkles, 457
properties of, 13–16
for treating
anxiety, 166–67, <u>168</u>
arthritis, 171–72
high blood pressure,
328–29
high cholesterol, 338
insect bites and stings,
<u>356</u>
sinusitis, 416
sore throat, 417–18
yeast infections, 283
for weight loss, 402–3
during wound healing, 453

Tea tree oil, for treating
fungal nail infections, 284
psoriasis, 412
yeast infections, 283
Testosterone levels, sex drive
and, 225
Thiamin. *See* Vitamin B$_1$
Thrush, 281, 282
Thyme, properties of, 68–69
Thyme and ivy leaf extract, for
treating bronchitis, 187
Thyme and primrose, for
treating bronchitis, 187
Thyme oil, for treating fungal
nail infections, 284–85
Thyroid disease, 211, 429–31
TIA, 423, 426
Tinnitus, 432–34
Tofu, <u>134</u>, <u>135</u>
Tomatoes
for cancer prevention, 211
homemade sun-dried, <u>49</u>
paired with salmon, <u>88</u>
properties of, 48–49, 456
Tooth decay, 252, 268, 295, 308,
435–38
Tooth loss, health risks and,
<u>436</u>
Top foods to avoid, <u>40</u>, <u>82</u>, <u>106</u>
Top recommended foods, <u>10</u>,
<u>40–41</u>, <u>82</u>, <u>83</u>, <u>106–7</u>
Trans fats
cancer risk from, <u>206</u>
eliminating, for heart health,
<u>318</u>
infertility and, 348, 350
Transient ischemic attack (TIA),
423, 426
Trigger foods, for specific
conditions
acid reflux, <u>149</u>
bladder infection pain, 185
cold sores, 212
eczema, 260
excessive sweating, 342
headaches, 309–10
heartburn, 322
hives, 339
indigestion, 345
vertigo, 446–47
Triglycerides, omega-3 fats
lowering, <u>10</u>

Tryptophan, for treating
hot flashes, 382
insomnia, 358
Tulsi. *See* Holy basil
Tuna, properties of, 90–91
Turmeric. *See also* Curcumin
properties of, 69–71
for treating
arthritis, 172–73
bronchitis, 187
diabetes, 241
heartburn, 324
indigestion, 346
lupus, 373
shingles, 414
sinusitis, 416
wounds, 453
Turmeric oil, for treating fungal
nail infections, 285
Tyramine, as headache trigger,
310
Tyrosine, for thyroid function,
430

U

Ulcers, peptic, 290, 345,
439–41
foods treating, 12, 43, 51, 63,
125, 130, 149, 150, 291,
292, 323, 324, 347
Uric acid, gout from, 300–303
Urinary tract infections (UTIs),
16, 37, 183–85, 381

V

Vaginal yeast infections, 281,
282–83
Vaginitis, 442–43
Varicose veins, 53, 188, 444–45
VCO. *See* Virgin coconut oil
Vegan diet, 310, 431, <u>460</u>
Vegetables. *See also specific
vegetables*
CDC-recommended, <u>122</u>
cleaning, <u>26</u>
as cream substitute in soup,
<u>118</u>
fat paired with, <u>78</u>, <u>82</u>

green, for preventing heart disease, 315
for weight loss, 399
Vegetarian diet, 165, 166, 233, 236, 336, 369, 431
Vertigo, 368, 386, 432, 446–47
Vinegar. *See also* Apple cider vinegar
for treating ear infections, 258
Virgin coconut oil (VCO). *See also* Coconut oil
properties of, 84–85
for treating yeast infections, 283
Vitamin A
corticosteroids and, 371
food sources of, 257–58, <u>261</u>, 299, 371, 452
for preventing
ear infections, 257–58
eczema, <u>261</u>
glaucoma, 298–99
for treating dry skin, 255, 262
for vision health, 251
for wound healing, 452
Vitamin B$_1$
for preventing glaucoma, 298, 299
for treating
menstrual cramps, 385
PMS, 405
Vitamin B$_2$. *See* Riboflavin
Vitamin B$_6$
food sources of, 267, 311, 366, 422
headaches and, 311
for preventing
fatigue, 267
kidney stones, 366
for treating
anxiety, <u>168</u>, 170
stress, 421–22
Vitamin B$_9$. *See* Folic acid
Vitamin B$_{12}$
deficiency of, 236, 421
food sources of, <u>234</u>, 422
for preventing
Alzheimer's disease, <u>163</u>
depression, 236–37
for treating
anxiety, <u>168</u>, 170
back pain, 182

Vitamin C
food sources of, <u>215</u>, <u>230</u>, 249, 267–68, 273, 293, <u>301</u>, 306, 340, 373, <u>394</u>, 422, 455
for iron absorption, <u>64</u>, <u>106</u>
kidney stones and, 365–66
for preventing
bruises, 188
colds, 214, <u>215</u>
dementia, <u>230</u>, 231
fatigue, 267–68
gout, <u>301</u>, 302
wrinkles, 455
for treating
anxiety, <u>168</u>, 170
cold sores, 212
diverticulitis, 249
fibromyalgia, 273
gingivitis, 293
hives, 340
lupus, 373
stress, 422
for wound healing, 452
Vitamin D
calcium paired with, <u>106</u>
for preventing
back pain, 180–81
cancer, 249
colds, <u>215</u>, 216–17
eczema, 260
fatigue, 267
fibrocystic breasts, 271
flu, 352
osteoporosis, 392, 394–95
tooth decay, 435
sources of, <u>215</u>, <u>230</u>, <u>234</u>, <u>261</u>, 267, 274, 306, 350, 352, 372–73, 408–9, 413–14, 415, 435
for treating
dry eyes, 251
fibromyalgia, 273–74
gingivitis, 293–94
infertility, 350
lupus, 372–73
sinusitis, 415
Vitamin D deficiency, <u>64</u>, <u>82</u>
with ADHD, 179
effects of
back pain, 180
dementia, 231
depression, 236

hair loss, 306
osteoporosis, 394–95
with fibromyalgia, 273
with lupus, 372–73
Vitamin E
food sources of, <u>230</u>, 256, <u>261</u>, 389, 455
for preventing
Alzheimer's disease, <u>163</u>
dementia, <u>230</u>, 231
eczema, 260
muscle cramps, 388–89
wrinkles, 455
for treating
dry skin, 255–56, 262
hot flashes, 382
Vitamin K, for preventing bruises, 188

W

Walnuts
properties of, 76–77
for treating high cholesterol, 336
Warts (common), 448–49
Water, 16–17. *See also* Hydration
for preventing
depression, 237
kidney stones, 364
for treating
acid reflux, 150
adrenal exhaustion, 154
burns, 191
dry skin, 254
heartburn, 324
Watermelon, properties of, 49–50
Weight gain, menopausal, 382
Weight loss
diet for, <u>40</u>, 180
experts' recommendations for, <u>10</u>, <u>40</u>, <u>64</u>, <u>82</u>, <u>106</u>
rapid, gallstones from, 288
stories about, <u>460</u>, <u>461</u>, <u>462</u>
for treating
coughs, <u>220</u>
infertility, 349, 350
psoriasis, 411
Wheat germ, for treating
menstrual cramps, 385
PMS, 405–6